MW00835498

BSAVA Manual of Ornamental Fish
Second edition

Editor:

William H. Wildgoose
BVMS CertFHP MRCVS

Midland Veterinary Surgery
655 High Road, Leyton
London E10 6RA, United Kingdom

Published by:

British Small Animal Veterinary Association
Woodrow House, 1 Telford Way, Waterwells
Business Park, Quedgeley, Gloucester GL2 4AB

A Company Limited by Guarantee in England.
Registered Company No. 2837793.
Registered as a Charity.

First edition published 1992.
Reprinted 1996.

A catalogue record for this book is available from the British Library.

ISBN 0 905214 57 9

Typeset by: Fusion Design, Fordingbridge, Hampshire, UK

Printed by: Grafos, Barcelona, Spain

Other titles in the BSAVA Manuals series:

Manual of Advanced Veterinary Nursing
Manual of Canine and Feline Emergency and Critical Care
Manual of Canine and Feline Gastroenterology
Manual of Canine & Feline Haematology and Transfusion Medicine
Manual of Canine and Feline Nephrology and Urology
Manual of Companion Animal Nutrition and Feeding
Manual of Canine Behaviour
Manual of Exotic Pets
Manual of Feline Behaviour
Manual of Canine and Feline Infectious Diseases
Manual of Psittacine Birds
Manual of Rabbit Medicine and Surgery
Manual of Raptors, Pigeons and Waterfowl
Manual of Reptiles
Manual of Small Animal Anaesthesia and Analgesia
Manual of Small Animal Arthrology
Manual of Small Animal Clinical Pathology
Manual of Small Animal Dentistry
Manual of Small Animal Dermatology
Manual of Small Animal Diagnostic Imaging
Manual of Small Animal Endocrinology
Manual of Small Animal Fracture Repair and Management
Manual of Small Animal Neurology
Manual of Small Animal Oncology
Manual of Small Animal Ophthalmology
Manual of Small Animal Reproduction and Neonatology
Manual of Veterinary Care
Manual of Veterinary Nursing

For information on these and all BSAVA publications please visit our website: www.bsava.com

Contents

List of contributors   v

Foreword   vii

Preface   viii

Part I: General background and management

1	**The aquatic environment** *Jane Lloyd*	1
2	**Ornamental fish trade** *Keith Davenport*	9
3	**Ornamental fish farming** *Chris Walster*	13
4	**Aquatic traders** *Bernice Brewster*	19
5	**Pond fish keeping** *Frank Prince Iles*	25
6	**Freshwater aquaria** *David Pool*	37
7	**Marine aquaria** *Dick Mills*	45
8	**Public aquaria** *Ian D.F. Walker and Brent R. Whitaker*	53

Part II: Clinical investigation

9	**General approach** *Ray L. Butcher*	63
10	**Examining the environment** *Todd R. Cecil*	69
11	**Restraint, anaesthesia and euthanasia** *Lindsay G. Ross*	75
12	**Clinical examination** *Gregory A. Lewbart*	85
13	**Laboratory techniques** *Peter J. Southgate*	91
14	**Diagnostic imaging and endoscopy** *Mark D. Stetter*	103

Part III: Diseases – by system

15	**Skin disease** *William H. Wildgoose*	109
16	**Internal disorders** *William H. Wildgoose*	123
17	**Respiratory disease** *Sara Childs and Brent R. Whitaker*	135
18	**Ocular disorders** *Brent R. Whitaker*	147
19	**Behavioural changes** *Ruth Francis-Floyd and William H. Wildgoose*	155
20	**Sudden death** *William H. Wildgoose*	163

Part IV: Diseases – by cause

21   **Parasitic diseases**   167
Matt Longshaw and Stephen W. Feist

22   **Bacterial diseases**   185
Gavin Barker

23   **Fungal diseases and harmful algae**   195
Andrew Holliman

24   **Viral diseases**   201
David Bucke

25   **Environmental disorders**   205
Todd R. Cecil

26   **Toxins**   213
Peter J. Southgate and Edward J. Branson

27   **Neoplasia and developmental anomalies**   219
John C. Harshbarger

28   **Nutritional disorders**   225
Roy P.E. Yanong

29   **Reproductive and genetic disorders**   231
Roy P.E. Yanong

Part V: Treatment and prophylaxis

30   **Therapeutics**   237
William H. Wildgoose and Gregory A. Lewbart

31   **Surgery**   259
Craig A. Harms and William H. Wildgoose

Part VI: Miscellaneous

32   **Aquatic invertebrates**   267
Colin Grist

33   **Legislation**

    a   **UK legislation**   275
Peter W. Scott

    b   **US legislation**   281
Roy P.E. Yanong

34   **Health and safety**   285
Colin Grist

Appendices

    1   **Conversion factors**   291

    2   **Scientific names of fish and aquatic invertebrates mentioned in the text**   292

    3   **Fish health societies and related organizations**   294

Index   295

Contributors

Gavin Barker PhD
formerly at CEFAS Weymouth Laboratory, Barrack Road, The Nothe,
Weymouth, Dorset DT4 8UB, UK

Edward J. Branson BVetMed BSc MSc MRCVS
Red House Farm, Llanvihangel, Monmouth, Gwent NP25 5HL, UK

Bernice Brewster BSc MIBiol CBiol MIFM
Aquatic Consultancy, 9 Charlton Lane, West Farleigh, Maidstone, Kent ME15 0NX, UK

David Bucke MPhil CBiol MIBiol MIFM
D.B. Aquatic Pathology Services, Chaser's Folly, 3b Roundhayes Close,
Weymouth, Dorset DT4 0RN, UK

Ray L. Butcher MA VetMB MRCVS
The Wylie Veterinary Centre, 196 Hall Lane, Upminster, Essex RM14 1TD, UK

Todd R. Cecil DVM
Western Aquatic Animal Veterinary Service, PO Box 900584, San Diego, CA 92190-04584, USA

Sara Childs DVM
Department of Animal and Avian Sciences, University of Maryland, College Park, MD 20742, USA

Keith Davenport BSc MIBiol CBiol
Ornamental Aquatic Trade Association (OATA), Unit 5, Narrow Wine Street,
Trowbridge, Wiltshire BA14 8YY, UK

Stephen W. Feist PhD
CEFAS Weymouth Laboratory, Barrack Road, The Nothe, Weymouth, Dorset DT4 8UB, UK

Ruth Francis-Floyd DVM MS DipACZM
Professor, Department of Large Animal Clinical Sciences,
Department of Fisheries and Aquatic Sciences, University of Florida,
7922 NW 71 Street, Gainesville, FL 32653, USA

Colin Grist
New England Aquarium, Central Wharf, Boston, MA 02110, USA

Craig A. Harms DVM PhD DipACZM
North Carolina State University, College of Veterinary Medicine, Department of Clinical Sciences,
Center for Marine Sciences and Technology, 303 College Circle, Morehead City, NC 28557, USA

John C. Harshbarger PhD
Professor of Pathology, Registry of Tumors in Lower Animals, Department of Pathology,
George Washington University Medical Centre, 2300 I Street N.W., Washington, DC 20037, USA

Andrew Holliman BVSc BA MSc MRCVS
Veterinary Laboratories Agency, Merrythought, Calthwaite, Penrith, Cumbria CA11 9RR, UK

Gregory A. Lewbart MS VMD DipACZM
Department of Clinical Sciences, North Carolina State University, College of Veterinary Medicine,
4700 Hillsborough Street, Raleigh, North Carolina 27606, USA

Jane Lloyd BSc CertEd
Aquatic Training & Consultancy, 26 Greenway, Child Oakeford, Dorset DT11 8DZ, UK

Matt Longshaw BSc MSc
CEFAS Weymouth Laboratory, Barrack Road, The Nothe, Weymouth, Dorset DT4 8UB, UK

Dick Mills
10 Rosken Grove, Farnham Royal, Slough, Berkshire SL2 3DZ, UK

David Pool BSc PhD
Tetra, Lambert Court, Chestnut Avenue, Eastleigh, Hampshire SO53 3ZQ, UK

Frank Prince Iles
3 Sunnydale Avenue, Brighton, East Sussex BN1 8NR, UK

Lindsay G. Ross BSc PhD
Professor, Institute of Aquaculture, University of Stirling, Stirling FK9 4LA, UK

Peter W. Scott BVSc MSc FRCVS
Zoo & Aquatic Veterinary Group, Keanter, Stoke Charity Road, Kings Worthy,
Winchester, Hampshire SO23 7LS, UK

Peter J. Southgate BVetMed MSc MRCVS
Fish Vet Group, Rowandale, By Dunscore, Dumfries, Dumfries & Galloway DG2 0UE, UK

Mark D. Stetter DVM DipACZM
Veterinary Services Director, Disney's Animal Programs, Post Office Box 10000,
Lake Buena Vista, FL 32830-1000, USA

Ian D.F. Walker BVM&S MRCVS
Associate Veterinarian, National Aquarium in Baltimore, Pier 3, 501 East Pratt Street,
Baltimore, MD 21202-3194, USA

Chris Walster BVMS MRCVS
Island Veterinary Clinic, 132 Lichfield Road, Stafford ST17 4LE, UK

Brent R. Whitaker MS DVM
Director of Animal Health, National Aquarium in Baltimore, Pier 3, 501 East Pratt Street,
Baltimore, MD 21202-3194, USA

William H. Wildgoose BVMS CertFHP MRCVS
Midland Veterinary Surgery, 655 High Road, Leyton, London E10 6RA, UK

Roy P.E. Yanong VMD
Assistant Professor, Tropical Aquaculture Laboratory,
Department of Fisheries and Aquatic Sciences, Institute of Food and Agricultural Sciences,
University of Florida, 1408 24th Street SE, Ruskin, FL 33570-5434, USA

Foreword

For most of us in first opinion veterinary practice, a fish is an unusual patient. Not so for the team of 29 international authors of this entirely new 2nd edition of the *BSAVA Manual of Ornamental Fish* who, under the editorial guidance of William Wildgoose, have shared with us their wealth of experience.

The opening section on general background includes information on the fish trade and farming. Clinical investigation is followed by a section on disorders by system. Parts 4 and 5 list specific causes of disease and their treatment. The final section covers legislation in the UK and the USA. Veterinary surgeons, nurses, students and enthusiastic hobbyists will find this text an invaluable guide and it will have an essential place in the practice library.

It is the experience of practice that the more unusual species are presented at a late stage of disease when failure of individual treatment is common. In part this may relate to a lack of client faith in the expertise available. The better our education in aquaculture, the better equipped we are to advise confidently and the more likely we are to see the patient at a time when diagnosis and treatment have more chance of success. The practical nature of this well illustrated text will provide the basis for better care, offers more specialist reference where appropriate, and also highlights the availability of expert referral if necessary.

BSAVA is justifiably proud of the Manual series and this volume adds to the worldwide reputation enjoyed by the Publications department who are to be congratulated once again.

Julian Wells BVSc MRCVS
BSAVA President 2001–2002

Preface

Ornamental fish medicine has progressed enormously since 1992 when Ray Butcher edited the first edition of the *BSAVA Manual of Ornamental Fish*. In this fully revised edition we again guide the reader through the now vast subject of ornamental fish from a veterinary perspective.

The book is aimed at anyone involved in ornamental fish health in a recreational or professional capacity. It should prove useful to veterinary surgeons, researchers and fish pathologists, as well as hobbyists and those in the aquatic trade and public aquaria. Twenty-nine authors from the UK and US have written this book for an international readership.

Following on from the principles of the aquatic environment, we present a broad overview of the whole ornamental fish industry, including production, trade and methods of fish keeping. These important background issues provide a greater understanding of the management and complex environmental aspects of fish health. They highlight areas where professional involvement is eagerly required, such as in the growth of public aquaria, which are subject to zoo licensing regulations and require regular veterinary inspections.

The second section discusses the clinical investigations involved in tackling fish health problems and covers methods of restraint, clinical and pathological examination and diagnostic imaging procedures. Because cases are usually presented according to clinical signs rather than by aetiology, a problem-oriented approach has been used. Chapter plans have been provided to enable a quick review of differential diagnoses and help direct the reader to the relevant area. In section four, the causative agents are presented in more detail and provide information relevant to each disorder. A greater understanding of these facts should then enable the reader to select the most appropriate action with regard to medical or surgical treatment as outlined in the fifth section.

Despite its size, my main aim was to produce a book that was concise and practical. It is not perfect but we have done our best. Every day we learn more about fish health and I am painfully aware that some areas of this book will rapidly become out of date. This is inevitable but I hope that our efforts will be regarded as a starting point. New medical disorders, investigations, treatments and surgical procedures will continue to emerge but a line had to be drawn somewhere. It will never be complete and it could easily have been three times longer but there is a limit to the practical nature of such a publication.

I am grateful to many people – too many to name individually – for their help and enthusiasm during the production of this book. I am grateful to BSAVA for giving me the opportunity to pursue this important project and publish many of my photos, thus allowing me to justify to myself the vast expense on film and camera equipment. Special thanks go to Marion Jowett (BSAVA Publishing Manager), Val Porter (copy editor), Sam Elmhurst (illustrator) and Graeme and Matthew at Fusion (design and typesetting) for their efforts and for keeping this a light-hearted experience – we were only producing a book. Thanks also go to all the authors who wrote such inspiring chapters that helped me to remain motivated and without whom this book would never exist. I am grateful to my clients who have allowed me to do my best for their pets, regardless of cost and also to my work colleagues for allowing me to develop my skills and experience in fish health. To my fellow fish professionals who have helped me over the years, I am pleased to say that your advice was never wasted and I am indebted to you for your time and efforts. I am also grateful to several dealers and public aquaria for allowing me to turn up unannounced and take photos of their facilities and sharing their knowledge. And, finally, I am immensely grateful to my wife and family for their love and support during a long and challenging experience and for tolerating my unhealthy passion and interest in sick fish.

It goes without saying that I am grateful to you, the reader, for buying this book and confirming that there is a great need for this publication. As words of advice, I would add that we all have much to learn about ornamental fish medicine and that you will often discover new fish health problems. I would urge you to investigate these cases thoroughly and write them up for the benefit of everyone, not least the fish. In order to develop your skills further, it is essential to follow up all cases: you will be surprised how rewarding it can be. Fish medicine is a truly fascinating subject and despite the technical frustrations, it has immense potential for further veterinary involvement.

William H. Wildgoose
September 2001

The aquatic environment

Jane Lloyd

The importance of understanding the relationship between water quality, stress and disease cannot be overemphasized. The aquatic environment is very different from the terrestrial one but most husbandry problems may be avoided by routine monitoring of water quality: poor water quality is generally a precursor to disease in fish. Usually it is only when fish present with clinical signs of disease that a water quality problem is identified and action taken.

Healthy fish are in equilibrium with their environment and with any pathogen within it. Changes in environmental conditions may upset this balance and influence the development of disease in a number of ways:

- Direct toxic effect of the environmental parameter
- Indirect effect by altering the toxicity of another parameter
- Indirect effect causing stress which subsequently reduces the fish's resistance to disease from another source.

Acclimation is the physiological adaptation of a fish to a new environment or change in its existing environment. When a fish is unable to adapt and the change is extreme, the fish will experience the same physiological changes that are associated with stress in mammals.

This chapter discusses the most important physical and chemical properties of the aquatic environment that influence the health of ornamental fish. A comprehensive account of these water parameters is outside the scope of this book and only relevant background detail can be provided here. Methods of measurement, the ideal environmental requirements of the fish and underlying factors that may result in changes to the environment are also discussed. The consequences of poor water conditions are discussed in Chapter 25.

Physical properties

Temperature and stratification

Water has a high specific heat capacity, causing it to warm up and cool down more slowly than the surrounding air or soil. Larger bodies of water are more stable, with temperatures changing slowly with the season rather than on a daily basis. Water stratifies in static and large open bodies such as ponds. The differences in temperature cause a layering effect, which is most pronounced in summer and winter. These layers are:

- Epilimnion or top layer
- Thermocline or transitional layer
- Hypolimnion or bottom layer.

Fish are ectothermic (poikilothermic), since their body temperature varies with that of their surrounding environment (to within $\pm 0.5°C$). The body temperature affects enzyme activity and the metabolic rate of the fish. For example, a rise of $10°C$ effectively doubles the metabolic rate. Feeding rates and therefore growth rates also depend on water temperature.

Breeding patterns are often linked to seasonal temperature changes and generally coincide with increased availability of natural food sources. Artificially imitating this may stimulate spawning.

Requirements

Fish are found in a wide range of temperatures; extreme examples are the Antarctic icefish at $-2°C$ and the desert pupfish at up to $51°C$. All fish have an optimum range in which they survive best and some may tolerate a wide range of temperatures (e.g. goldfish can withstand temperatures from 2 to $40°C$). In this context, fish are grouped as:

- Eurythermic (adaptable over a wide range of temperatures)
- Stenothermic (only tolerating a narrow range).

Abnormality

Rapid temperature changes – particularly sudden and extreme increases – are often harmful to fish, causing stress and reducing their resistance to disease. Most fish will cope with temperature changes of several degrees Celsius, if they are gradual.

Coldwater fish exported from warm climates are often chilled before transportation, in order to reduce their metabolic rate and hence excretion of metabolic wastes. Lower water temperatures reduce the toxicity of ammonia and have a calming effect on some species. Ice packs may be used inside the transport container to maintain the low temperature during the journey. When unpacking the fish, care must be taken to allow the water temperature of both the container and the facility to equalize during the acclimation period.

Conductivity, specific gravity and water density are temperature-dependent. In addition, as the temperature increases, dissolved oxygen decreases, and ammonia becomes more toxic due to the conversion of ionized ammonia (NH_4^+) to un-ionized (or free) ammonia (NH_3).

Density

Water density is greatest at 4°C. At higher temperatures it becomes less dense and lighter, so that warmer water floats on top of colder water. Below 4°C, cold water floats at the top and turns to ice, which is less dense than water. It is therefore recommended that outdoor ponds are at least 1 m deep to enable fish to survive in the warmer water beneath the ice.

Surface tension

Water has a high surface tension and cohesion, allowing some animals (e.g. pond skaters) to live on the surface.

Sound

Sound travels more than four times faster in water than in air and can carry for long distances. This allows some species to communicate with one another and enables some carnivorous species to find their food.

Light

Light is very important for photosynthesis in plants, algae and symbiotic algae that live in many invertebrates, such as corals and anemones. Turbidity is caused by suspended materials, often fine solids, and can greatly affect light penetration.

pH

The pH is a measure of the relative amounts of positively charged hydrogen ions (H^+) and negatively charged hydroxyl ions (OH^-):

$$H_2O \rightleftharpoons H^+ + OH^-$$

The pH is neutral when there are equal numbers of H^+ and OH^- ions in the same solution, such as in pure water. Because it is such a good solvent, water is rarely pure and it expresses the pH of the salts it dissolves. A pH value of 7 is neutral; values less than 7 are acidic and those greater than 7 are alkaline. The scale is logarithmic; for example, pH 3 is 10 times more acidic than pH 4 and 100 times more acidic than pH 5. Therefore, only a small change in pH means a dramatic change in acidity. A change of less than one unit may have fatal effects on some fish. A change of not more than 0.3 pH units per day is recommended during any acclimation period.

Measurement

- Indicator test strips (litmus paper)
- Chemical test kits
- Electronic meter.

Requirements

As a rule, fish survive best within a pH range of 6–8. Some species may survive in extreme conditions, but these fish are not generally kept by hobbyists. Each species has its own optimum pH at which it functions normally. For example, Malawi cichlids are alkalophiles and prefer a high pH (7.8–8), whereas acidophiles, such as discus, prefer acidic water of pH 6 and marine fish must be kept at pH 8.2–8.4. Fish may survive outside these ranges but they will be stressed and their growth retarded.

Many freshwater fish are now bred in captivity and may not tolerate the extreme conditions of their native habitat. The neon tetra is now intensively bred in the Far East and rarely experiences the water conditions found in its native Peru.

It is strongly recommended that the pH be monitored regularly, since a change in pH often indicates an underlying water quality problem.

Abnormality

Several underlying causes may result in a consistently low or high pH or produce dramatic fluctuations.

Low pH

- When the water is changed, the pH of the tap water may differ from that in the pond or aquarium
- Chlorine in tap water produces a mildly acidic solution of hydrochloric acid and the use of a commercial dechlorinating agent or sodium thiosulphate is recommended
- Carbon dioxide builds up in the sealed bags during transport and forms carbonic acid
- Carbon dioxide is occasionally added to water to promote plant growth and therefore the pH should be carefully monitored
- Medicinal products, such as anaesthetic agents, alter the pH and must be buffered before use
- Ageing or maturation of a system lowers the pH, due to the effect of nitrification; the breakdown of ammonia to nitrates lowers the pH, due to the release of hydrogen ions
- Runoff from peaty soil during heavy rain or due to poor drainage design may contaminate pond water.

High pH

- Ammonia is alkaline, therefore the pH will rise if the filtration system is not operating efficiently or if excessive decomposing waste matter is present
- Runoff from limed soil and concrete may contaminate pond water.

Fluctuating pH

- Diurnal rhythm in a well planted pond or aquarium can produce very dramatic pH swings if the water is not properly buffered. These fluctuations are due to the effects of photosynthesis on the balance of carbonate and hydrogen ions in the water. The pH will rise during the day and fall during the night: it should be measured at the same time each day so that the results are not affected by this diurnal change. Equally, measurements can be taken at different times of the day (e.g. early morning and late afternoon) to see this effect
- The buffering capacity of water limits pH change, but the pH will fluctuate rapidly when this is exhausted. This is particularly important in marine systems, since fish and invertebrates will not survive a sudden drop in pH.

Hardness

Water contains a range of dissolved substances. The type and amount of those found in freshwater depend upon the water source and the rocks and soils through which the water passes. Hardness is a measure of the divalent metal ions present in the water, notably calcium and magnesium and, to a lesser extent, aluminium, barium, copper, iron, strontium and zinc. These are mainly present as hydroxide, carbonate and bicarbonate salts.

- Temporary (carbonate) hardness (KH) is derived from calcium carbonate ($CaCO_3$) and calcium bicarbonate ($CaHCO_3$) and is readily removed by boiling
- Permanent hardness consists of non-carbonate metal (e.g. magnesium) salts, namely sulphates, nitrates, chlorides and silicates, which are not removed from solution by boiling
- Total (or general) hardness (GH) is the sum of temporary hardness and permanent hardness.

Measurement

- Chemical test kits (colorimetric and titrametric)
- Colorimetric photometer.

Hardness is often expressed in mg/l as $CaCO_3$ but there are several other scales (Figure 1.1). The German (deutsch) scale of degrees hardness (°dH) is commonly used by hobbyists.

Water with a hardness value of less than 50 mg/l (3°dH) is termed 'soft', whereas a value over 300 mg/l (18°dH) is termed 'hard' (Figure 1.2).

Scale	Country of origin	Conversion (mg/l as $CaCO_3$)
°hardness	USA	1
°Clark	UK	14.3
°dH	Germany	17.9
°fH	France	20
mEq/l		50
µS/cm		2

Figure 1.1 Comparison of different scales of water hardness and approximate conversion factors.

Hardness	(mg/l as $CaCO_3$)	°dH
Soft	0–50	3
Moderately soft	50–100	3–6
Slightly hard	100–200	6–12
Moderately hard	200–300	18–18
Hard	300–450	18–25
Very hard	> 450	> 25

Figure 1.2 Ranges of water hardness.

Requirement

The preferred hardness for fish is usually within the range 50–400 mg/l as $CaCO_3$ (3–22°dH). To maintain a stable pH and good buffering capacity in the captive environment, it is beneficial to keep the fish at over 100 mg/l (5.5°dH).

Abnormality

Hardness affects the fish's ability to osmoregulate and control its fluid balance. If a freshwater fish is placed in softer water, then it must remove the extra water that enters the tissues by osmosis. Extremely hard water may cause renal calculi or nephrocalcinosis, due to inability to control the balance of calcium salts in the body. Hardness also has an effect on the hardening of incubating egg capsules.

Health problems related to hardness are usually linked to changes in pH. Soft water tends to be acidic, because it readily absorbs carbon dioxide. Hard water is more alkaline, due to the buffering effect of the bicarbonates. Heavy metal toxicity is increased and some medications (benzalkonium chloride, chloramine-T, copper sulphate and formalin) are more toxic in soft water.

Alkalinity

Total alkalinity is the total concentration of bases (carbonates and bicarbonates) in water. It is related to hardness and is expressed in mg/l as $CaCO_3$. Temporary hardness values are often similar to those for alkalinity, due to measurement of similar salts. Alkalinity may be considered as a measure of the resistance or buffer to pH change. In a marine aquarium, it is also called the 'marine reserve' or 'marine buffering'.

Measurement

- Chemical test kits (titrametric).

Buffering capacity

If an acid or alkali is added to pure water, then there is an immediate change in its pH. If a buffer agent (for example, calcium carbonate and calcium bicarbonate) is present in the water, then no such immediate change will occur. Thus, when acid is added to hard water, little or no change in pH occurs until a large amount has been added, because the acid is neutralized by the carbonate (CO_3^{2-}) and bicarbonate (HCO_3^-) present (Figure 1.3). The carbonate and bicarbonate have buffered the water sample against the acid. When all the calcium carbonate has attached to the free hydrogen ions, the buffering capacity is said to be depleted or 'used up' and the pH of the sample then changes.

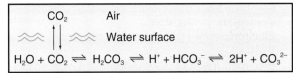

$$CO_2 \quad Air$$
$$\text{Water surface}$$
$$H_2O + CO_2 \rightleftharpoons H_2CO_3 \rightleftharpoons H^+ + HCO_3^- \rightleftharpoons 2H^+ + CO_3^{2-}$$

Figure 1.3 Buffering effects.

Hard water has a large buffering capacity and small additions of acid do not change its pH. If similar amounts of acid were added to a soft water supply, then there would be a large shift in pH. In heavily planted aquaria and ponds with soft water, the diurnal rhythm of photosynthesis will cause dramatic pH changes; therefore, to maintain a stable pH, the temporary hardness should be kept above 100 mg/l as $CaCO_3$ (5.5°dH).

Marine water is also buffered by the presence of carbonates and bicarbonates, in particular. A pH below 7.8 will kill many marine fish and invertebrates. If these buffering carbonates become depleted, then the pH will fall and a partial water change or the addition of a commercial buffer will become necessary.

Dissolved gases

Under any given set of conditions, there is an equilibrium between gases entering and leaving the water. Less gas can be dissolved at higher temperatures or in water with increasing levels of dissolved solids. The solubility of different gases in water varies considerably: carbon dioxide is 70 times more soluble than nitrogen but oxygen is only twice as soluble as nitrogen.

Oxygen

One-fifth of the atmosphere is composed of oxygen and terrestrial animals have an abundant supply of this vital gas in the air. Water holds only 5% of the oxygen contained in the same volume of air and therefore aquatic animals must be more efficient at extracting oxygen from their environment. With such a low concentration of dissolved oxygen in water, it is easy for this to decrease to fatal hypoxic levels. Hypoxia is one of the main problems faced by pond keepers and fish farmers during hot summer months. Environmental hypoxia may arise if ponds are overstocked, if fish are overfed or if there is a lot of rotting organic matter being actively degraded by bacteria.

In most bodies of water, photosynthesis by submerged plants is the main source of dissolved oxygen. Oxygenating plants are very useful in a pond or aquarium but they also require oxygen to respire. In heavily planted systems, this may cause huge oxygen reductions at night, the lowest levels being found early in the morning. Measuring dissolved oxygen levels later in the day may not reveal environmental hypoxia, as plant photosynthesis will have altered the levels of dissolved oxygen. Because of this and the low solubility of oxygen in warm water, mechanical aeration should be provided through the night in hot summer weather.

Measurement

- Chemical test kits (colorimetric and titrametric)
- Ion-specific photometer
- Electronic meter with polarographic probe.

Electronic meters used to determine dissolved oxygen levels usually express the results in milligrams per litre (mg/l) or parts per million (ppm). Occasionally, the percentage saturation is given and this represents the percentage of oxygen dissolved in one litre of water.

Dissolved oxygen levels should be monitored throughout the day (particularly early in the morning), using an oxygen meter. Ideally, the water should be maintained at 100% saturation but the actual level will often vary depending on the temperature and dissolved solids.

Requirement

Dissolved oxygen is one of the most important water quality parameters and the requirement varies with the species, size, age and health of the fish. Feeding and stress increase the oxygen requirements of fish. Whilst some species may tolerate levels of dissolved oxygen as low as 4 mg/l, most fish require at least 6 mg/l. Below these levels, most fish become physiologically stressed or die. The total oxygen requirement is called the biological oxygen demand (BOD) and includes that required by all the aquatic animals, plants and micro-organisms within a system.

Bacteria are often the largest consumer of oxygen in a system and may survive at the lowest levels of dissolved oxygen. At very low oxygen levels, anaerobic bacteria produce toxic gases such as hydrogen sulphide.

Abnormality

Gases dissolve into water through its surface by diffusion. Aeration and water movement increase the surface area of water, thereby increasing the rate of diffusion. If the surface is covered with a film of oils or dust from some foods, then the oxygen diffusion may be significantly reduced. Excessive growth of surface plants may also significantly reduce the available water surface area. The vigorous aeration in protein skimmers creates bubbles that will remove these materials in the waste foam.

The total amount of oxygen that can be dissolved in water depends mainly upon the following.

- Water temperature: this is the most important factor determining the amount of oxygen that may be dissolved in water. As the temperature increases, the BOD increases but the solubility of oxygen decreases
- Salinity: full strength sea water holds significantly less oxygen than freshwater
- Atmospheric pressure: this is only significant during unusual weather conditions, or at altitude during air transportation. A sudden decrease in atmospheric pressure during hot summer nights before a storm may cause oxygen levels to fall even lower. Sudden mass mortalities in overstocked ponds are not uncommon.

Supersaturation

In heavily planted systems or ponds with heavy algal growth, excessive light from sunlight or continuous artificial lighting may result in supersaturation with oxygen. In most cases, this rarely causes a health problem but occasionally it may result in gas bubble disease in some fish.

Nitrogen

Most dissolved nitrogen in water originates from diffusion from the atmosphere but a small amount may be produced by denitrification by anaerobic bacteria.

Measurement

- Electronic meter (total gases).

Supersaturation

Excessive levels of dissolved nitrogen occur when air is forced into the water under high pressure, at a rate faster than it can diffuse out. This may occur due to air being drawn into leaking pipework by pumps, by an over-efficient venturi or by using fresh borehole water in outdoor systems. The nitrogen levels may reach over 102% saturation and cause gas emboli in the fish, often referred to as 'gas bubble disease' and similar to 'bends' in divers. The water should be aerated vigorously to help the excess gas to escape.

Carbon dioxide

Carbon dioxide is very soluble in water and often exceeds atmospheric concentrations. It is produced by respiration by fish and bacteria, and also by plants during the night. Consequently, dissolved levels are highest just before dawn.

Measurement

- Chemical test kits (titrametric).

Abnormality

Levels above 10 mg/l are considered harmful. High levels of dissolved carbon dioxide also develop over lengthy periods inside the sealed bags used to transport fish. Hypercarbia reduces the uptake of oxygen by haemoglobin and may cause hypoxia. Chronic high levels of dissolved carbon dioxide have been associated with nephrocalcinosis in some species.

Salinity

Water is an ideal solvent for other compounds. Because of its readiness to take up other chemicals, it is rarely found in a pure form. It may dissolve more substances and in greater quantities than other solvents, because it consists of a positive and a negative charge that form weak bonds with other polar substances (e.g. salts).

Elements dissolve in water, allowing the ions to become free-moving and thus able to conduct electricity. Pure water is not a good conductor of electricity, but hard water and sea water are excellent. Many fish use electricity to communicate and to locate food.

Sea water has a specific composition of several salts: sodium chloride, magnesium chloride, magnesium sulphate, calcium sulphate, potassium sulphate, calcium carbonate, potassium bromide and sodium bromide. These are called conservative elements and are always present in the same proportions, regardless of the salinity. 'Trace elements' vary in concentration and include zinc, copper, iodine, pigments and proteins.

Salinity is a measure of the total quantity of dissolved material in a water sample. It is expressed in parts per thousand (ppt or $^o/_{oo}$) and occasionally in g/l water (1 ppt = 1 g/l).

Freshwater has a low salinity (less than 0.5 ppt), whereas natural sea water has a high salinity (about 35 ppt). Between these two extremes are various concentrations of brackish (estuarine) water. The salinities are classified as:

- Freshwater: < 0.5 ppt
- Oligohaline: 0.5–5 ppt
- Mesohaline: 5–15 ppt
- Polyhaline: 18–30 ppt
- Euryhaline: 30–40 ppt
- Hyperhaline: > 40 ppt.

Measurement

Salinity is difficult to measure directly and several indirect methods are used, including the following.

Specific gravity: Specific gravity (SG) is the comparison of the weight of a water sample with the weight of an equal volume of distilled water at 4°C. It is expressed as a ratio, where the weight of pure water is 1.000. Sea water has a specific gravity of between 1.023 and 1.027 (Figure 1.4). Specific gravity is temperature-dependent, since water density varies with temperature. For example, sea water with a salinity of 35 ppt has a specific gravity of 1.026 at 15°C and 1.024 at 24°C.

Specific gravity	Salinity (g/l)
1.015	20.6
1.016	22.0
1.017	23.3
1.018	24.6
1.019	25.9
1.020	27.2
1.021	28.5
1.022	29.8
1.023	31.1
1.024	32.4
1.025	33.7
1.026	35.0
1.027	36.3
1.028	37.6
1.029	38.9
1.030	40.2

Figure 1.4 Comparison between specific gravity and salinity at 15°C.

Specific gravity is measured using a hydrometer, which is a float with a calibrated scale. Most hydrometers are calibrated to be accurate only at a specific temperature, normally 24°C. They are useful to show any changes in salinity.

Refractive index: A hand-held refractometer (salinometer) may be used to measure the refractive index of a solution. These small but expensive instruments are accurate and require only a small sample volume. They are calibrated to give readings in ppt and for use at a specific temperature but some new models incorporate automatic temperature compensation.

Electric conductivity: Electric conductivity is defined as the ability of a substance to conduct an electric current and is the reciprocal of electrical resistivity. The unit of measurement commonly used is Siemens per centimetre, as milliSiemens/cm (mS/cm) or microSiemens/cm (μS/cm). In aqueous solutions conductivity is directly proportional to the

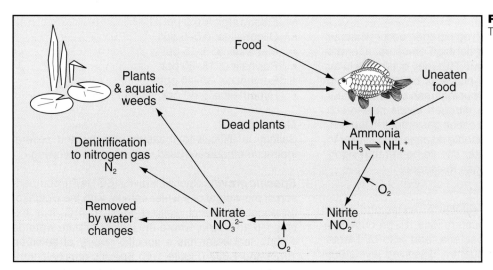

Figure 1.5
The nitrogen cycle.

concentration of dissolved solids. For example, the conductivity of distilled water is 0.5 μS/cm, domestic tap water is 500–800 μS/cm and full-strength sea water is 45–55 mS/cm.

Sodium ion-selective meter: An ion-selective meter uses a sodium-sensitive electrode that measures salinity and expresses the result in g/l. Since sodium chloride is the main sodium salt in sea water, there is a direct relationship between sodium content and salinity.

Chlorinity: Chlorinity is a measure of the total amount of halides in a given sample. There is a constant relationship between chlorinity and salinity and it may thus be used to calculate salinity. It is also expressed in ppt and is determined by titration.

Requirement
Most marine fish are stenohaline: they only tolerate a relatively narrow range of salinity (because it is relatively constant in oceanic waters). Salinities outside this range or rapid fluctuations in salinity result in changes in the osmotic pressure in the fish, producing stress and a lower resistance to disease. Brackish-water fish (e.g. scats, blue acaras) are euryhaline: they are more tolerant of salinity change than marine fish but cannot tolerate rapid changes. Consequently, most estuarine fish move with the tide to stay in a stable and desirable salinity.

Salinity in the small volume of a marine aquarium may progressively increase due to evaporation of water. To maintain the same salinity, it is important to add water regularly or use an automatic top-up system.

As the water in a tank ages, the trace elements change. Dissolved metabolic wastes increase and iodine is readily removed by plants and by protein skimming. Trace elements are maintained by water changes or the addition of commercial preparations.

Medicinal use
Salt is used as a treatment for freshwater fish and many exporters add about 1 g salt/l to the water to reduce osmotic stress during the journey. Tonic salts are commonly used instead of sea salt.

Nitrogenous compounds

In a confined body of water, the excretion of metabolic wastes (and the consequences of their accumulation in the environment) is one of the most important aspects of aquatic life. Ammonia is produced as the main waste product of protein metabolism and excreted by the gills and, to a lesser extent, by the kidneys.

Autotrophic bacteria (e.g. *Nitrosomonas*) in the water and on the surface of filter media (where oxygenated water is constantly flowing) metabolize ammonia as an energy source. This is oxidized to nitrite (NO_2), which is very toxic to fish. Other nitrifying bacteria (e.g. *Nitrobacter*) oxidize nitrite into nitrate (NO_3), which accumulates in the water and is tolerated by most fish or is taken up by plants. Fish often eat plant matter and hence complete the nitrogen cycle (Figure 1.5).

New tanks and ponds take several weeks for this bacterial flora to establish and for the filter system to function efficiently (Figure 1.6). Initially, ammonia levels will increase due to waste production by the fish. As the bacterial populations multiply in response to this 'nutrient', the ammonia level will fall but the resulting nitrite levels will rise. Other bacteria will then multiply over the following few weeks to utilize these nitrites. The final product of this nitrification is nitrate, which gradually increases unless it is removed from the system.

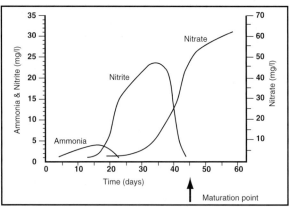

Figure 1.6 Typical ammonia, nitrite and nitrate concentrations during the first 60 days after adding fish to new tank or pond (from Bower, 1983).

Disease problems that develop during this maturation period are often referred to as 'new tank/pond syndrome' and are directly related to poor water quality and opportunist pathogens. As a result, new facilities must not be overstocked and fish numbers should be built up gradually. Some medications may destroy the bacterial population and cause the same effect.

Ammonia

Ammonia dissolves in water and rapidly dissociates to produce ammonium ions (NH_4^+) and un-ionized (or free) ammonia (NH_3). The total ammonia nitrogen is the sum of both the ionized and un-ionized ammonia. The equilibrium shifts towards un-ionized ammonia when:

- pH is higher (i.e. alkaline)
- Temperature is higher
- Salinity is lower (i.e. in freshwater).

$$NH_3 + H_2O \rightleftharpoons NH_4^+ + OH^-$$

Measurement

- Chemical test kits (colorimetric)
- Ion-specific photometer.

Toxicity

Un-ionized ammonia is much more toxic to fish than ammonium. Most test kits and electronic meters measure the total ammonia nitrogen. In order to assess toxicity, it is necessary to calculate or measure the un-ionized ammonia levels. Figure 1.7 enables the percentage of un-ionized ammonia to be calculated from the total ammonia nitrogen at different temperatures and pH.

Different species vary in their susceptibility to ammonia poisoning. Fish eggs and fry are very sensitive to even low levels. The lethal limit of un-ionized ammonia for many freshwater aquarium fish is 0.2–0.5 mg/l. Below these levels, fish may survive but they are stressed and more vulnerable to secondary disease. Therefore, the only safe level in which to keep fish is 0 mg/l.

Causes of ammonia toxicity: The accumulation of ammonia may arise for several reasons, including:

- Immature filter (when there are insufficient numbers of bacteria present in a filtration system to cope with the amount of ammonia being produced)
- Overstocked system (too many fish present or introduced too quickly, producing too much ammonia for an inadequate biological filter)
- Decomposition (rotting dead fish or plants, or excess food not eaten immediately by fish)
- Irregular over-feeding (causes irregular patterns of ammonia production)
- Damaged biological filter (caused by the use of some antibacterial medications, pump failure or other interruption of water supply to the filter leading to hypoxia/anoxia; poor filter maintenance and over-zealous cleaning).

Nitrite

Ammonia is oxidized to nitrite (NO_2^-) by *Nitrosomonas* bacteria and other microorganisms. New tanks are most commonly afflicted by high nitrite levels, due to the slow multiplication and insufficient numbers of *Nitrobacter* and the other microorganisms that convert nitrite into nitrate. High levels of ammonia also inhibit the growth of *Nitrobacter*.

pH Value	Temperature (°C)														
	4	6	8	10	12	14	16	18	20	22	24	26	28	30	32
7.0	0.11	0.13	0.16	0.18	0.22	0.25	0.29	0.34	0.39	0.46	0.52	0.60	0.69	0.80	0.91
7.2	0.18	0.21	0.25	0.29	0.34	0.40	0.46	0.54	0.62	0.72	0.83	0.96	1.10	1.26	1.44
7.4	0.29	0.34	0.40	0.46	0.54	0.63	0.73	0.85	0.98	1.14	1.31	1.50	1.73	1.98	2.26
7.6	0.45	0.53	0.63	0.73	0.86	1.00	1.16	1.34	1.55	1.79	2.06	2.36	2.71	3.10	3.53
7.8	0.72	0.84	0.99	1.16	1.35	1.57	1.82	2.11	2.44	2.81	3.22	3.70	4.23	4.82	5.48
8.0	1.13	1.33	1.56	1.82	2.12	2.47	2.86	3.30	3.81	4.38	5.02	5.74	6.54	7.43	8.42
8.2	1.79	2.10	2.45	2.86	3.32	3.85	4.45	5.14	5.90	6.76	7.72	8.80	9.98	11.29	12.72
8.4	2.80	3.28	3.83	4.45	5.17	5.97	6.88	7.90	9.04	10.31	11.71	13.26	14.95	16.78	18.77
8.6	4.37	5.10	5.93	6.88	7.95	9.14	10.48	11.97	13.61	15.41	17.37	19.50	21.78	24.22	26.80
8.8	6.75	7.85	9.09	10.48	12.04	13.76	15.66	17.73	19.98	22.41	25.00	27.74	30.62	33.62	36.72
9.0	10.30	11.90	13.68	15.67	17.82	20.18	22.73	25.46	28.36	31.40	34.56	37.83	41.16	44.53	47.91
9.2	15.39	17.63	20.08	22.73	25.58	28.61	31.80	35.12	38.55	42.04	45.57	49.09	52.58	55.99	59.31
9.4	22.38	25.33	28.67	31.80	35.26	38.84	42.49	46.18	49.85	53.48	57.02	60.45	63.73	66.85	69.79
9.6	31.36	34.96	38.68	42.49	46.33	50.16	53.94	57.62	61.17	64.56	67.77	70.78	73.58	76.17	78.55
9.8	42.00	46.00	50.00	53.94	57.78	61.47	64.99	68.31	71.40	74.28	76.92	79.33	81.53	83.51	85.30
10.0	53.44	57.45	61.31	64.98	68.44	71.66	74.63	77.35	79.83	82.07	84.08	85.88	87.49	88.92	90.19
10.2	64.53	68.15	71.52	74.63	77.46	80.03	82.34	84.41	86.25	87.88	89.33	90.60	91.73	92.71	93.38

Figure 1.7 Percentage of total ammonia nitrogen that is un-ionized ammonia in freshwater at different temperatures and pH values (after Emerson *et al.*, 1975).

Measurement

- Chemical test kits (colorimetric)
- Ion-specific photometer.

Toxicity

Nitrite is less toxic than ammonia and is considered lethal at levels between 10 and 20 mg/l. Nitrite is actively absorbed by the gills, though this may be inhibited by chloride ions and is therefore less toxic in salt water and hard water. It oxidizes haemoglobin to methaemoglobin, which cannot transport oxygen so efficiently. Nitrite levels should be maintained below 0.1 mg/l but the optimum level is 0 mg/l.

Nitrate

Nitrite is oxidized to nitrate (NO_3) by *Nitrobacter* bacteria and other microorganisms. In the absence of regular partial water changes, nitrates may accumulate in fish tanks and ponds. They may also originate from domestic tap water or from fertilizers washed into ponds from the surrounding soil by rainwater.

Measurement

- Chemical test kits (colorimetric)
- Ion-specific photometer.

Toxicity

Nitrate is less toxic than ammonia or nitrite but levels of 50–300 mg/l may be lethal to some species. Nitrate is more toxic in salt water and at low pH. High levels may encourage algal blooms.

Other solutes

Chlorine

Chlorine is used in domestic tap water supplies as a disinfectant against bacteria and algae. It is forced into the water under high pressure, driving off other gases. In the UK, it is dosed to produce a residual level of 0.2–0.5 mg/l at the end-user's tap. In solution, free chlorine and water associate to form hypochlorous acid (HOCl) and chlorine ions (Cl⁻). The acid is the disinfecting agent and is toxic to fish. Chlorine may also originate from equipment that has been inadequately rinsed following cleaning with chlorine-based disinfectants.

$$Cl_2 + H_2O \rightleftharpoons HOCl + H^+ + Cl^-$$

Toxicity depends upon the pH, temperature, residual chlorine, toxic chemicals, dissolved oxygen and the species of fish or invertebrate. Lethal levels are considered to be 0.2–0.3 mg/l but it is recommended not to exceed 0.003 mg/l for most species.

Chlorine is unstable in water, particularly at high temperatures or in the presence of organic matter. It may be removed by vigorous aeration, by being left to stand for 24 hours in an open-topped vessel or by the addition of a commercial water dechlorinating agent or sodium thiosulphate.

Chloramine

This compound is produced by combining chlorine with a nitrogenous compound, namely ammonia. It is more stable than chlorine and releases hypochlorous acid at a steady rate. Chloramine may be removed by using sodium thiosulphate to neutralize the chlorine component, leaving ammonia, which may then be filtered through zeolite or carbon or metabolized by the bacterial filter.

Metals

Copper, iron and lead may be found in water supplies, having leached out of the metal pipework, particularly in soft and seawater conditions. Some metals may also leach from poor-grade plastics.

Copper is very soluble in soft water, where it exists in the toxic 'free copper' form. The lethal level in fish is species-dependent and is approximately 0.015 mg/l. Invertebrates and plants are not tolerant, even of these levels. In hard water, copper forms copper carbonate, which precipitates and is less toxic. Copper is added to water as a treatment against ectoparasites and is commonly used for marine fish.

Iron and lead are toxic to fish, particularly in soft water at low pH. The lethal level for both is about 0.03 mg/l.

Heavy metals may produce various clinical signs, with damage to the gills and internal organs, or sudden death. Running the tap for 5 minutes before taking water to add to a tank or pond will reduce the metal content by flushing the pipes.

Pesticides

Domestic water supplies occasionally contain insecticides such as pyrethrins and permethrin used to kill water lice (*Asellus*) in the pipework. The water companies usually dose in the spring and autumn at 5–10 µg/l over several days. Do not use water for a further 14 days, because residual levels may kill fish and invertebrates in particular. Contact the water supply companies to enquire when they will be using these pesticides.

Domestic hazards

Fish are very sensitive to a variety of household substances that may pollute the water, including aerosol sprays and tobacco smoke. Particular care should be taken if a venturi or air pump is used on the system because this forces the air into the water, concentrating the pollutant. Equally, traces of chemicals such as aftershave, hairspray or hair gel on the hands of the operator may enter the water during routine aquarium maintenance.

Further reading

Adey WH and Loveland K (1991) *Dynamic Aquaria: Building Living Ecosystems.* Academic Press, London

Andrews C, Exell A and Carrington N (1988) *The Interpet Manual of Fish Health.* Salamander Books, London

Bower CE (1983) *The Basic Marine Aquarium.* Charles C Thomas, Springfield, Illinois

Emerson K, Russo RC, Lund RE and Thurston RV (1975) Aqueous ammonia equilibration calculations: effect of pH and temperature. *Journal of the Fish Research Board of Canada* **32**, 2379–2383

Kelly LA (1998) Water quality and rainbow trout farming. *Fish Veterinary Journal* **2**, 31–47

Moe MA (1992) *The Marine Aquarium Reference: Systems and Invertebrates.* Green Turtle Publications, Plantation, Florida

Moe MA (1992) *The Marine Aquarium Handbook: Beginner to Breeder.* Green Turtle Publications, Plantation, Florida

Spotte S (1979) *Seawater Aquariums: the Captive Environment.* John Wiley, New York

Stoskopf MK (1993) *Fish Medicine.* WB Saunders, Philadelphia

Ornamental fish trade

Keith Davenport

Ornamental fish can be broadly defined as fish that are not kept as a source of food. However, in different parts of the world, one man's pet may be another man's food item. With the growth of ornamental fish keeping, there is now awareness in the less developed countries that some species of fish are more valuable as an export item than as a source of food. Consequently, there has been a significant growth in trade to meet the demand from hobbyists and this now forms an important part of some local economies.

Before discussing specific aspects of fish health and disease in this book, it is important to have an appreciation of the global ornamental fish industry. The trade can be divided into three sections: coldwater, tropical freshwater and tropical marine (Figure 2.1).

The bulk of the trade (99%) in the UK is in freshwater fish with about half of this as coldwater species for outdoor ponds and the rest as tropical species for indoor aquaria. The keeping of marine fish requires more elaborate filtration and facilities: this sector of the hobby represents about 1% of fish sold. Of the marine fish kept, most are tropical species and only a few are temperate species, which are more commonly kept in public aquaria rather than by hobbyists. The keeping of aquatic invertebrates is a growing area and requires a greater degree of experience and care, particularly in mixed reef systems. Equally, maintaining healthy aquatic plants in some fish tanks and ponds is an important part of the hobby but it is often overlooked.

Many freshwater species are now produced by commercial fish farms in tropical areas but many of the tropical marine species are still caught from the wild, due to the difficulty of breeding them. Small barrier nets and hand nets are almost universally used for collecting these species. The use of poisons to collect fish is roundly condemned by all responsible businesses in the industry. The often repeated assertion that dynamite is used to collect fish for the industry is entirely incorrect.

The collection and trade of some species (hard corals and arowana) are monitored and controlled by the Convention on the International Trade in Endangered Species (CITES).

The global industry

Over the last 10 years, records from the Food and Agriculture Organization (FAO) of the United Nations show that 146 countries exported and 133 countries imported ornamental fish.

Although there can be slight variation in recorded figures due to differences in the stocking density used to pack the fish, freight weight most accurately reflects the numbers of fish that pass through the trade. However, very few countries other than the UK report this accurately and the USA has not reported any freight weights to the FAO for at least 10 years.

Comparing volumes based on financial values is problematic. The cost of fish and freight vary and so do the exchange rates. In 1998, global exports amounted to US$174 million and global imports were US$257 million. The values of ornamental fish exported by the largest producers in 1998 are shown in Figure 2.2.

The countries that import most fish are shown in Figure 2.3. Because of domestic production, US consumption of ornamental fish is far larger than its imports (production occurs mainly in Florida and was estimated to be worth US$56.2 million in 1998). If the figures for the European Union (EU) are aggregated, then the combined buying power of its members makes the EU the largest market for ornamental fish in the world.

Category	Main sources	Species	Wild/farmed
Coldwater	Japan, Israel, USA, China	20 species principally koi and goldfish	100% farmed
Tropical freshwater	Singapore, Brazil, Czech Republic	1000+ species	95% farmed
Tropical marine	Indonesia, Philippines and Pacific Islands	1000+ species	99% wild-caught

Figure 2.1 Categorization and origin of ornamental fish.

Country	Value (US$ million)
Singapore	43.0
USA	10.7
Czech Republic	10.6
China – Hong Kong	10.3
Malaysia	8.6
Sri Lanka	8.2
Japan	7.5
Israel	6.4
Philippines	4.5

Figure 2.2 Global exports of ornamental fish by value (1998).

Country	Value (US$ million)
USA	67.3
Japan	39.3
Germany	24.7
France	21.1
UK	20.1
Netherlands	11.7
Belgium	10.1
Italy	9.9
Singapore	9.0
Spain	6.0

Figure 2.3 Global imports of ornamental fish by value (1998).

IATA regulations

International Air Transport Association (IATA) regulations stipulate criteria for the correct transportation of fish and other animals. These include details on package design, construction and labelling, the preparations before dispatch and general care and loading.

Fish are packed in strong polyethylene bags that are filled one-third with water, then fully inflated with oxygen and sealed. The bags are often sealed inside a second bag and placed inside a rigid leak-proof outer container.

Small fish should be packed to survive for up to 48 hours from the time of acceptance by the airline. Larger fish (over 40 cm) should be packed to be able to survive for at least 18 hours. To minimize severe temperature changes, adequate insulation material should be used, particularly for tropical species. Sealed packets of crushed ice packed around the transport bags can be used to keep coldwater species cool in warm weather.

Sharks, and other species that must swim constantly, require the use of specially designed transport containers with a submersible pump and a constant oxygen supply. These fish must be accompanied by an experienced attendant.

UK aquatic industry

The UK imports in excess of 30 million ornamental fish annually, of which 300,000 are marine species. During 1999, ornamental fish were imported from 42 countries, not including imports from other EU member states. The value of this trade amounted to approximately £12 million and was represented by almost 1800 tonnes of freight (including water and packaging).

Within the EU, the UK was the largest importer (by value) of ornamental fish in 1999. Trade between EU member states amounted to some £9.2 million in 1999 (though this is probably an underestimate, because of the recording system used). To prevent the introduction of diseases that might affect native stocks, the UK imports coldwater fish from approved disease-free farms in the EU. Tropical ornamental species do not represent a disease risk and are imported from elsewhere in the EU without such stringent controls applied.

From a trade point of view, choosing the source of ornamental fish depends on a large number of factors, including:

- Health status
- Species availability
- Price of fish
- Price of freight
- Import/export restrictions
- Currency fluctuation
- Availability of flights (historically, the best flight routes are from ex-colonies).

During 1999, imported fish entered the UK via Heathrow (64%), Manchester (30%) and Gatwick (5%) airports. There is a seasonal variation, with a large upsurge in imports of coldwater fish in the spring. There was a marked downturn in trade during the early 1990s but the industry is now growing, due to improvement in the general economic climate and an increase in disposable income.

Supply chain in the UK

Figure 2.4 illustrates the various stages in the supply chain in the UK. Similar chains operate in many countries, but the balance between the sectors may vary.

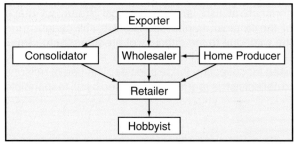

Figure 2.4 The chain of supply of ornamental fish in the UK.

Wholesalers import stock, unpack the fish and hold them until orders arrive from retailers. The fish are then repacked and dispatched.

Consolidators buy on behalf of a number of clients (retailers and wholesalers), thus gaining an advantage by buying both fish and freight in bulk. The consolidator then delivers the boxes of fish (unopened) to the client, at which point the boxes are opened and the fish unpacked. Due to the cost of putting together a consignment, only very large retailers import on their own behalf.

There are approximately 100 businesses licensed to import ornamental fish into the UK. These in turn supply some 2000 retailers, 600 of which are entirely aquatic outlets. There are several hundred manufacturers of dry goods such as aquaria, pumps, pond liners, accessories and food. It is estimated that the industry turnover is in excess of £250 million per year, including sales of dry goods.

The scale of breeding and production of ornamental fish in the UK has not yet been measured but is estimated to be 4 million fish per year. Most production involves coldwater species, but tropical freshwater and marine species are also produced commercially in the UK.

Pet shops

The majority of ornamental fish in the UK are sold through pet shops and aquatic outlets. These are required by the Pet Animals Act 1951 to be licensed annually. Licences are issued following an inspection by environmental health officers of the local council and, on occasion, by a veterinarian. Guidelines for these inspections have been published in the *Model Standards for Pet Shop Licence Conditions*, which were produced by a working group of the Local Government Association, the British Veterinary Association, the Chartered Institute of Environmental Health, the Pet Care Trust and the Ornamental Aquatic Trade Association.

The recommendations cover: retailers selling pet livestock; wholesalers stocking pet livestock; dealers in pet livestock; livestock importers and exporters; and pet auctions and one-day auctions. Any businesses offering domestic pets for gain should be subject to licensing conditions.

Water quality standards

It is virtually impossible to determine the quantity of fish to be kept in any facility based purely on a ratio of weight per volume or numbers of fish per volume. The variation in system design, types of fish involved and husbandry techniques would render any such method too simple to be useful or too complicated to be practical. Therefore, the essential maintenance of water quality standards is a simple but effective way to determine stocking densities. Basic water quality criteria have been established and are recommended as minimum standards to be maintained (Figure 2.5).

Water quality testing should be carried out at least once per week in facilities with a centralized filter system and in 10% of tanks with individual filtration systems. Unsatisfactory test results must be recorded in a register, together with the corrective action taken. Further tests must be carried out as required following visual inspection of the tanks.

In pet shops and commercial facilities, the stocks of fish held vary rapidly and dramatically; thus, small amounts of ammonia and nitrite might be present before the filter matures. In contrast, domestic aquaria and ponds with stable stocking levels should have no ammonia or nitrite, and sea water should be maintained at a pH value of 8.3.

UK aquatic hobby

In the UK, ornamental fish are the third most popular pets after dogs and cats. A recent survey revealed that there are approximately 5.3 million households with dogs, 5.0 million with cats and 3.0 million with ornamental fish. In the USA, over 10 million homes own ornamental fish.

In a survey of 4000 visitors to aquatic outlets in 1995, it was estimated that there was a pet fish population of over 100 million in the UK, compared with 7 million each of cats and dogs and 1.5 million each of pet rabbits, guinea pigs, hamsters and budgerigars.

UK legislative controls

As with the importation of any animal, there is always concern about the introduction of exotic diseases that may harm the native wild population or food-producing species. Consequently, there are several legislative controls on the importation of ornamental fish into the UK (Figure 2.6). These will be covered in more detail in Chapter 33. In the vast majority of instances, ornamental fish enter closed water systems such as ponds and aquaria and should pose no threat to other fish.

Parameter	Coldwater	Tropical	
		Freshwater	Marine
Dissolved oxygen (min., mg/l)	6	6	5.5
Un-ionized ammonia (max., mg/l)	0.02	0.02	0.01
Nitrite (max., mg/l)	0.2	0.2	0.125
Nitrate (max. above ambient tap water, mg/l)	50	50	40 [a]
pH (min.)			8.3

Figure 2.5 Water quality criteria.
[a] Absolute figure – does not relate to ambient tap water.

Laws	Effects
Animal Transport Regulations (91/628)	Apply IATA Regulations to all animals (including ornamental fish) imported into the EU All transport in EU is regulated and subject to inspection
Veterinary Checks Directive (91/496) (imports from third countries)	All consignments of animals entering the EU are subject to checks by the state veterinary service All consignments must enter via identified border inspection posts Two working days pre-notification of import is required
Veterinary Checks Directive (91/428)	Requires health certificates to accompany coldwater fish consignments All animal consignments subject to 24 hours prior notification to state veterinary service
Fish Health Regulations 1997 (SI 1997 No. 1881)	Implement Council Directive 91/67. Control movement of fish into UK from elsewhere in the EU
Fish Diseases Act 1937, as amended	Controls import of fish from non-EU member states Requires health declarations or certificates to accompany all shipments. Meets the requirements contained in Council Directive 91/67 that are to be applied in all member states
Wildlife and Countryside Act 1981	Prohibits the release of non-native species to the wild
Import of Live Fish (England and Wales) Act 1980	Requires that certain species are held or kept only under licence
Pet Animal Act 1951	Requires pet shops to be licensed annually by district authority

Figure 2.6 A brief overview of the legislative controls on the ornamental fish industry in the UK.

Further reading

International Air Transport Association (2000) *Live Animal Regulations.* Container requirements 51 and 52 for ornamental fish and 56 for corals

Lewbart GA (1992) Familiarizing yourself with the ornamental fish industry. *Journal of Small Exotic Animal Medicine* **2**, 29—34

Local Government Association (1998) *The Pet Animals Act 1951: Model Standards for Pet Shop Licence Conditions.* Local Government Association, London

Further information on the industry may be found at the websites of the Ornamental Aquatic Trade Association at www.ornamentalfish.org and www.aquaticsworldwide.org

3

Ornamental fish farming

Chris Walster

Ornamental fish farming has been practised for over a thousand years and began with the breeding of gold-fish in China. Today the variety of commercial enter-prises producing ornamental fish is as wide as the species produced. The degree of intensification and species farmed depends on the following:

- *Water availability.* Production can be limited by the cost and availability of water resources
- *International and local transportation.* The ability to move fish to a place of export and then distribute to foreign markets
- *Climate.* Cold climates make it too expensive to heat water to produce tropical fish. Warm climates may allow year-round spawning and growth
- *Local socio-economics.* In many Asian and South American countries, the farms are small family concerns with an additional need to produce food fish.

Many facilities originally began as farms for the production of food fish (Figure 3.1) and much of the technology and management systems used is identi-cal. Like any industry today, the most successful farms are those that are larger and employ more intensive systems (Figure 3.2). As well as economics, this is because of the ability to comply with regulations relating to the importation of fish in major markets such as Europe.

Intensive farms rely heavily on filtration and recirculation technology, with stocking densities as high as $300 \, kg/m^3$ (depending on the species involved). Regardless of the scale of the farm, broodstock selec-tion and grading of fish are still done by hand. This is labour-intensive and requires experienced personnel.

Health controls

These can be divided into three parts:

- *On-farm.* These relate to the scale of the facility and are often carried out by farm staff or veterinary surgeons. They are based on the principles of 'herd health' and follow management policies used in terrestrial farming. They include broodstock isolation, implementing an 'all in, all out' policy and strategic use of immunostimulants and chemotherapeutics
- *Holding facilities.* These are commonly found in areas where farms are small individual units, as in Asia. Prior to export, fish are moved from the farms to a central holding facility, where they are examined and treated as necessary before shipping
- *Regulatory.* All imports into the European Union (EU) are licensed and should be accompanied by a health declaration signed by the local competent authority in the exporting country. Certain countries, such as Singapore, require that the exporting farm be a member of an accredited farm scheme.

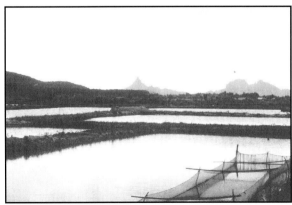

Figure 3.1 Koi-rearing ponds in the Far East. In Japan, most koi are reared in large earth ponds on an extensive basis. (Courtesy of R. Hale.)

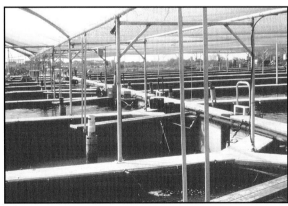

Figure 3.2 These large purpose-built holding ponds are typical of intensive farming systems used in Israel. (Courtesy of Mag Noy.)

The above, together with legislation preventing the shipment of fish in ill health, and customer concerns, generally mean that fish health on farms is good.

Problems

Three general problems are faced by all facilities:

- *Quality.* Consistent quality is important for the farm and gives buyers confidence in the product. This can be achieved by concentrating on an individual species or type of fish, or, in the case of large facilities, by extra production and grading of fish
- *Health.* Few countries outside Europe and the United States have adequate resources for checking fish health. Several Asian countries have only one fish health laboratory, which is often inaccessible to individual farmers. In these cases, sampling can be done at the central holding facility or by sending live fish to outside laboratories, such as CEFAS in Weymouth in the UK. The costs of this service are high but compliance with regulatory conditions is essential to enable the export of fish
- *Size.* Ornamental fish are sold according to their size. The breeding of tropical fish can be manipulated so that there is a short cycle of production and farms are compact. However, with coldwater species the supply of small fish can be a problem, since the area and volume of water required and the costs for each annual production cycle are too high to make it economical. Fish between 5 and 15 cm in size are the most popular. To ensure an adequate supply of these fish, growth must often be limited by means of restricted nutrition and stocking density, and this may inadvertently promote disease.

Production

Each production cycle must be carefully planned to ensure that the appropriate facilities are available at the correct time. In addition, it is necessary to anticipate market trends so that there is neither surplus nor deficiency of the correct size, nor are fish ready at the wrong time of year. The following is based on koi production but much is applicable to other species.

Selection for breeding

Broodstock are selected according to body conformation, colour and pattern. Conditioning of broodstock is important, since this increases fecundity. The health status of the stock should be assessed and it is good practice to keep broodstock in isolation. Records should be kept of fertility, fecundity, rate of survival to fry, cross-mating, and the nature and percentage of deformities. These records can be inspected subsequently in assessing the breeding potential of any fish.

Manipulation of breeding

Koi are induced to spawn by increasing daylight length and water temperature. Under hatchery conditions, this involves a photoperiod cycle of up to 16 hours light and 8 hours dark, and a water temperature of 22–25°C. It is essential that the temperature be maintained within this range, otherwise there may be spasmodic release of eggs by the female. Under more natural conditions in a pond, spawning will start at water temperatures of 15°C. To synchronize male and female, carp pituitary extract is injected. Male koi are injected only once. Females receive a second injection 12 hours later. After a further 12 hours, the eggs can be stripped from the females (Figure 3.3) and milt collected from the males (Figure 3.4).

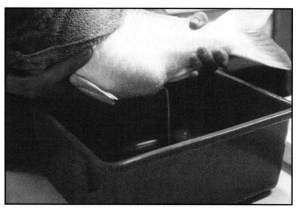

Figure 3.3 Manual stripping of female koi. The fish is sedated and gentle manual pressure applied to the abdomen to massage the eggs through the vent. (Courtesy of Mag Noy.)

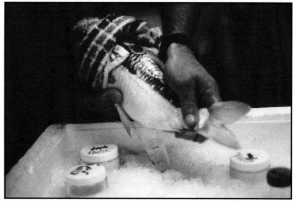

Figure 3.4 Milt (sperm) is collected from male koi and placed in containers immersed in ice. (Courtesy of Mag Noy.)

Eggs and milt are thoroughly mixed (Figures 3.5 and 3.6) and a solution of salt, urea and water is added to prevent the eggs from sticking and clumping. Mixing continues for a few further minutes. Fertilized eggs absorb the fluid and swell up to 10 times their original size. This process can take up to 90 minutes and sufficient fluid should be added until the eggs have stopped swelling. At this point, the eggs are given a final rinse in a weak solution of tannic acid to remove any residual stickiness before being placed in Zuger jars (Figure 3.7).

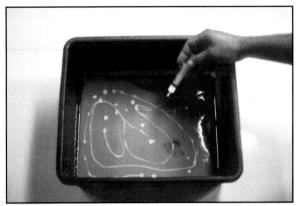

Figure 3.5 Adding milt to freshly stripped eggs from koi. (Courtesy of Mag Noy.)

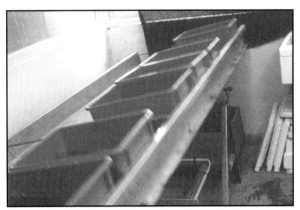

Figure 3.6 Gentle and thorough mixing of milt and eggs is achieved on a mechanical rocking table. (Courtesy of Mag Noy.)

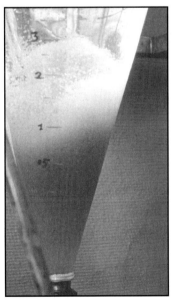

Figure 3.7 Fertilized eggs are incubated in Zuger jars. These open-topped glass funnels have an upflow of fresh water which keeps the eggs in constant motion. (Courtesy of Mag Noy.)

Egg incubation

Development starts immediately after fertilization and embryogenesis takes 3–4 days. During the first few hours, the egg is sensitive to physical damage so care should be taken to prevent any mechanical shock. At this point, oxygen demand is minimal and water flow rates through the jars are low. As the eggs develop,

the flow rate is gradually increased. Due to the development of the embryo, the colour of the egg changes to orange and this will give an indication of the fertilization rate.

Unfertilized eggs will die and become infected with fungi such as *Saprolegnia*, which can quickly spread through the whole egg mass. To prevent this, malachite green is added to the jars. After a couple of days, unfertilized eggs start to disintegrate. Dead eggs turn white, rise to the top (due to their light weight) and can be siphoned off.

Once the eggs start to hatch there are two options:

1. Hatching can be left to proceed naturally. It takes 3–4 days for the swim-bladder to develop; larvae then swim out of the jar and can be collected into vats
2. The water flow rate can be reduced for 5–10 minutes and then increased slightly. This induces hatching and the whole mass can be siphoned into a large flat-bottomed bowl. All the eggs will hatch after a few minutes.

Larval husbandry

Larvae are sensitive to rapid changes in the environment and are easily damaged. The digestive tract develops at the same time as the swim-bladder and the larvae will actively seek out food when they are ready to accept it. In the hatchery, they can be fed on brine shrimp (e.g. *Artemia*) or hard-boiled egg yolk mixed in water.

Where possible, they should be moved into fry-rearing ponds within a day or two of starting to eat. These ponds should be small, have excellent water quality and provide plenty of natural food. They should be built within a polyethylene tunnel (Figure 3.8) in order to maintain water temperature and protect the larvae from predation.

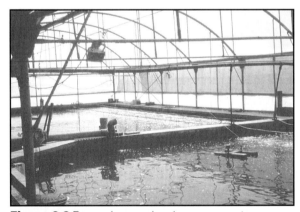

Figure 3.8 Fry-rearing ponds, where warm water temperatures are maintained inside polyethylene tunnels.

The ponds should be prepared for stocking about 2 weeks in advance. The pond bottom is cleaned and quicklime applied to eliminate pathogens. After flooding, organic and inorganic fertilizers are applied to promote the growth of algae and lower crustaceans.

Rotifers are the preferred food of first-feed fry and the pond is managed to increase the prevalence of these microscopic animals by using chemicals that selectively kill zooplankton that feed on rotifers. After a few days, larger plankton are required. Where chemical treatments have been used, plankton must be inoculated into the pond. The final food used in this stage of production is *Daphnia* (water fleas), which should be abundant in the pond from about 3 weeks following introduction of the fry.

The type and abundance of natural food should be checked between initial flooding and the stocking of the pond. The presence of cyclops (the larval stages of some copepods) in the pond will cause fry mortality and should be closely monitored.

Where outside ponds are not available, there are several commercial indoor systems for the culture of algae and these can provide a more controlled feeding programme. From the first day, fry should be offered a 'flours' diet. The fry will not initially take this very fine artificial feed but it encourages them to take artificial diets and provides additional nutrition for plankton.

Fry will stay in these ponds for 3–6 weeks. During this time, a white plate placed under the water surface helps to monitor their development: the dark fry can be easily seen against the white background.

Growing-on

At about 6 weeks of age, the fry can be graded and placed in growing-on ponds (Figures 3.9 and 3.10). Here they remain until ready for sale. The ponds can be

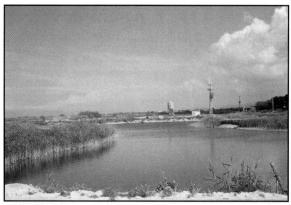

Figure 3.9 Massive outdoor ponds where koi are grown on to a size suitable for sale.

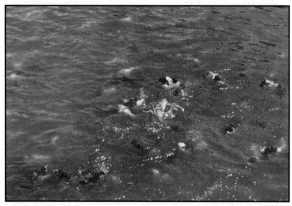

Figure 3.10 Koi in natural earth ponds. The water clarity is often very different from that in hobbyist ponds. (Courtesy of R. Hale.)

up to several thousand square metres in size, depending on the final stocking density. (The larger ponds may also act as water reservoirs for irrigation.) Subsequent procedures include:

- Daily visual inspection for signs of illness and to ensure that they are feeding well (healthy fish normally gather around the feeding units)
- As the fish grow, the diet is changed according to their nutritional requirements. Depending on water temperature and rate of growth required, they are fed between 2% and 10% bodyweight per day
- Fish should be sampled weekly, examined for parasites and their general health status monitored (both internal and external examination). Frequency of inspection decreases as the fish grow
- Treatment should be given when required. Before using any medication the cost, potential harmful effect of chemicals, discharge consents and exact need for treatment must be considered. With a well managed pond, the use of medication will be infrequent
- When netting ponds, the least stressful method should be used (Figure 3.11). This may include netting only part of the pond and restricting the catch to 20 minutes
- Predators will be attracted to ponds where large numbers of fish are held. Measures should be taken to control predator numbers.

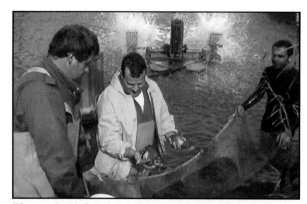

Figure 3.11 Goldfish being netted in the rearing ponds prior to transfer to holding tanks and sale. A paddle-wheel aerator is operating in the background. (Courtesy of Mag Noy.)

As they grow, the fish will be graded according to size. In general, this will be when they reach about 5 cm, 15 cm and 30 cm in length. Koi are also graded according to quality of coloration and conformation. About 90% of fish from an average spawning will have been culled or lost by the time of second grading, when only those fish that show good potential will be allowed to continue to grow.

Pond management

Each year all ponds should be drained and allowed to dry (Figure 3.12). This allows examination and repair of

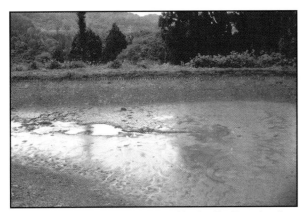

Figure 3.12 A natural earth pond in the Far East that has been drained as part of an annual pond management programme. (Courtesy of B. Brewster.)

banks and dams. It also allows the pond bottom to regenerate and decreases the incidence of disease. Ponds that are continuously under water become significantly less productive.

Slaked lime (calcium hydroxide) is applied to the bottom of the drained pond at 750–1000 kg/ha. Only half this dose is used if there is a thin layer of mud. Lime has the following benefits:

- Raises pH and increases buffering capacity of the water
- Increases decomposition and mineralization of organic material
- Precipitates any organic matter in suspension
- Has mild disinfectant properties
- Provides calcium for the shells and exoskeletons of invertebrates.

Prior to refilling with water, the pond should be fertilized to help to generate a natural food supply. In a large mud pond the vegetation and aquatic life act as a natural filter. The stocking level must be adjusted according to the feeding rate and growth of fish.

Routine health checks and water quality monitoring

Health checks should be carried out as described earlier. Both healthy and diseased fish should be examined. Where on-farm expertise is limited, a private veterinarian should be contracted to visit monthly. Government agencies may also be involved in routine health monitoring, often on a 3-monthly basis.

Water quality should be tested daily in fry-rearing ponds and weekly in growing-on ponds. Where possible the test samples should be collected at the same time of day. Standard parameters should be measured and recorded. Other factors may need to be monitored periodically, depending on the management system and source of water. In warmer climates, particular attention should be paid to dissolved oxygen levels and algal blooms. Changes in water quality should always be investigated promptly. On smaller facilities or in the hatchery it can be economic to install electronic monitoring and alarm systems.

Distribution

This is the most stressful stage for the fish, due to the amount of handling involved.

Dealer selection and sales

Koi are sold according to their grade. The fish are checked in the holding ponds before being brought to the packinghouse (Figure 3.13), where they are treated if necessary and rested prior to dispatch. The dealers visit the producers and personally select fish of the highest quality. This involves a lot of handling and fish that are not picked should be returned to the growing-on pond for a period of recuperation. Once fish are selected for dispatch, packing starts immediately.

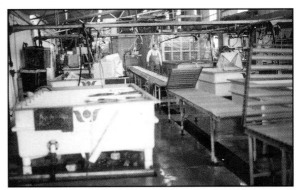

Figure 3.13 Packing facility in Israel, where fish are prepared for export.

Packing and transportation

To ensure maximum survival of fish during lengthy flights, various management tools are employed:

- The fish are starved for 24–48 hours to empty the digestive tract. This reduces ammonia production and faecal excretion during transportation
- The water temperature is reduced to 10°C, which slows down their metabolism, reducing oxygen consumption and ammonia production
- Fish are packaged following IATA regulations, which state that the fish must be able to survive for up to 48 hours in the container
- Fish are packed using a double-bag system where one polyethylene bag is placed inside another. The inner bag is filled with one-third water at 10°C and two-thirds pure oxygen. Both bags are sealed separately with rubber bands and then placed inside either insulated cardboard (Figure 3.14) or polystyrene boxes
- Ice or dry ice (solidified carbon dioxide) may be packed around the outside of the transport bag containing the fish to help to maintain the low water temperature, particularly in warm weather
- Zeolite (clinoptilolite) can be used to absorb the ammonia produced by fish during transportation. Water pH often drops to 6 or less, due to carbon dioxide produced by respiration. Ammonia is not toxic below pH 6.5; therefore the addition of zeolite is not necessary. Other proprietary products may be added to the transport water to help to prevent physical damage to scales

- Transport to the airport should be in temperature-controlled vehicles. At the airport, the boxes should be kept out of direct sunlight to prevent temperature increases
- Strict regulations dictate how the boxes should be handled and placed in the cargo hold. In general, direct flights are preferred since substantial delays can occur when the cargo changes planes
- Appropriate documents must accompany the consignment. In the UK, the Fisheries Inspectorate should be given at least 24 hours notice of arrival of the shipment so that they may perform their statutory inspections
- On arrival in the EU, the boxes must pass through a border inspection post. In the UK, Heathrow and Manchester are the main airports used to receive live fish
- The dealers collect the boxes of fish only after release by the authorities.

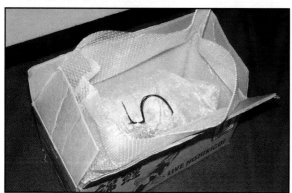

Figure 3.14 Typical container for exporting koi. Using a double-bag system, the inner bag is filled to one third of its volume with water, inflated with oxygen and placed inside an insulated cardboard box. (© W.H. Wildgoose.)

Distribution within the UK

Due to the large financial value of each shipment, most imports are distributed by consolidation. Here, the consolidator makes up an order from several retailers and the boxes of fish are distributed directly upon their arrival. Alternatively, the fish are taken to the wholesaler's facility for collection by the retailer.

From a health perspective, consolidation is not ideal but it allows the retailer to pay a better or lower price. Retailers often overstock or have insufficient space to rest fish prior to sale. With a wholesaler, fish can be rested in a quiet environment and it is often more practical to administer any medications necessary at this time.

Fish should be rested for a minimum of 48 hours before being sold on to customers. Fish under treatment should only be moved if absolutely necessary. The practice of routinely dipping fish in baths of medications on arrival is not condoned and may contribute to further stress. In practice, it can be a minimum of a week before any harmful effects from transportation may be noted.

Costs involved

The major costs in farming ornamental fish vary, depending on the facility and species reared. The main expenses are for food and labour. Transportation costs are generally borne by the importer and are incorporated in the cost of the fish or as a separate charge.

Further reading

Horvath L, Tamas G and Seagrave C (1992) *Carp and Pond Fish Culture.* Fishing News Books, Oxford

Pillay TVR (1999) *Aquaculture Principles and Practices.* Fishing News Books, Oxford

Plumb JA (1999) *Health Maintenance and Principal Microbial Diseases of Cultured Fishes.* Iowa State University, Ames, Iowa

Stoskopf MK (1993) Carp, koi and goldfish reproduction. In: *Fish Medicine*, ed. MK Stoskopf, pp. 470–472. WB Saunders, Philadelphia

Acknowledgements

The author is grateful to Modi Bracha of Mag Noy, Israel, Richard Hale of Berry Ring Herpetological & Aquatic Supplies Ltd and Bernice Brewster for the use of their photographs.

4

Aquatic traders

Bernice Brewster

Fish have been kept in captivity for thousands of years, originally to maintain a reliable and regular food resource. In the UK, the opening of the public aquarium at the Zoological Society in London in 1852 initiated the keeping of fish as a hobby and owning an aquarium rapidly became a status symbol. Indigenous species of fish and invertebrates were kept in parlour aquaria during the Victorian and Edwardian periods.

It is uncertain when large numbers of exotic species of tropical fish first appeared in the UK but after the First World War transportation of fish in metal canisters by sea routes became possible. Fish keeping as a hobby entered a new phase after the Second World War, with more efficient air transportation and the availability of plastic bags inside insulated boxes for moving delicate species. This in turn led to the increased availability of a wider range of exotic species. Consequently, improvements in the technology associated with keeping fish as pets promoted the growth of the retail aquatics industry as a whole.

In recent years, there has been renewed interest in coldwater species of fish, notably fancy varieties of goldfish for indoor aquaria and koi for purpose-built ponds. The retail value of the fish stocks depends on the rarity of some species and the quality of fin attributes, coloration and pattern in many fancy varieties of coldwater fish.

The commercial businesses involved in the trade of ornamental fish include importers, breeders, wholesalers and retailers. Importers may sell fish to retailers or direct to the public and may not be involved in the sale of 'dry goods' such as fish food and equipment. Retailers, on the other hand, sell a substantial amount of dry goods in addition to livestock (Figures 4.1 and 4.2).

Filtration systems

Aquaria

Large volumes of water are chemically more stable. Therefore, for most species, it is preferable to link a number of aquaria to a single filtration system (Figure 4.3). In an ideal situation, there should be two or three separate filtration systems, allowing related species to be held together in different systems and to reduce the potential spread of infectious diseases.

In many instances, aquaria and filtration systems can be purchased and installed as functional units from specialist manufacturers (Figure 4.4). These units often

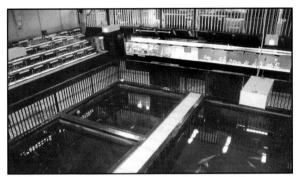

Figure 4.1 A large specialist centre with separate coldwater ponds for large koi, and banks of aquaria for freshwater tropical fish and marine fish. (Courtesy of Maidenhead Aquatics. © W.H. Wildgoose.)

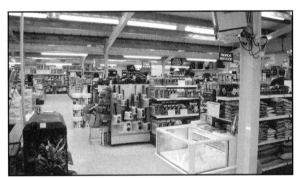

Figure 4.2 Although selling fish is important, the sale of dry goods (food, equipment and accessories) often forms a major part of the business. (Courtesy of Swallow Aquatics. © W.H. Wildgoose.)

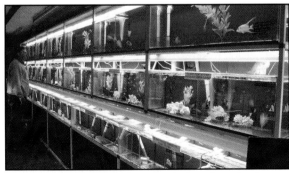

Figure 4.3 A large number of tanks housing mixed species of tropical marine fish sharing a central filtration system. The tanks are linked so that the water supplies and drains from each tank in parallel. (Courtesy of Home Marine. © W.H. Wildgoose.)

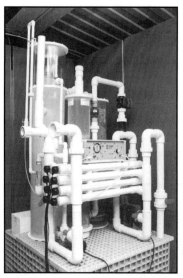

Figure 4.4 A large-capacity commercial filtration system available from a specialist manufacturer. This unit houses several ultraviolet tubes, a protein skimmer, fluidized sand-bed filter and a trickle tower biological filter. An ozone generator and heating and cooling elements are optional extras. (Courtesy of Tropical Marine Centre.)

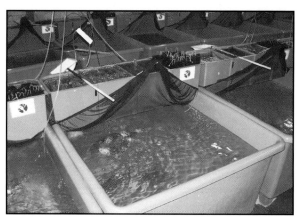

Figure 4.5 Self-contained fibreglass tanks for coldwater fish at an importer's premises. These units are made by a specialist manufacturer and have their own individual filtration system mounted above and at the rear of the tanks. (Courtesy of Koi Company.)

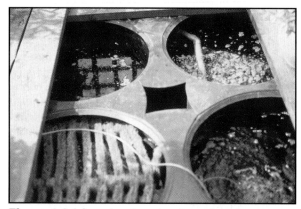

Figure 4.6 A four-chambered vortex unit partly concealed under some wooden decking. These are commonly used in many coldwater retail outlets and hobbyists' ponds. Some chambers contain Japanese filter matting and gravel while others are empty and allow centrifugal force to remove any suspended solids.

incorporate disinfection systems that use ultraviolet light or ozone. Some use fluidized-bed filtration systems (see Chapter 5), since these are generally more efficient than conventional biological filtration units. Disposable paper cartridges and bag filters are also used in some systems and these can remove suspended solids and some free-swimming parasites as small as 5 μm.

Some retail outlets have systems that are designed and built in-house but many have been sited to maximize retail space, making maintenance difficult, if not impossible.

Ultraviolet lights are commonly used as a means of disinfection but the unsuitable positioning of these units close to the pump often reduces their efficiency by shortening exposure time, due to the high flow rate of water. A few retail outlets use undergravel filtration systems in each aquarium and maintain these as separate entities. Routine maintenance and monitoring of water quality for many of these aquaria are very labour intensive, whether because of poor design or the large number maintained.

Pond systems

Pond fish such as fancy goldfish, carp, orfe, tench and rudd tend to be held in large tanks or ponds linked to a single filtration system. The filter units are either one of many manufactured systems or purpose-built.

For koi, each pond may be separately filtered (Figure 4.5) or linked to one central system that treats all the water. One problem with central filtration systems in a retail outlet is that the whole system must be treated to achieve an effective dose of medication. Currently, vortex systems (Figure 4.6) that use centrifugal force to remove suspended solids are commonly used for koi ponds. However, the flow rate from the pond to the vortex unit is often too slow, causing organic detritus to settle in the intermediate pipework and resulting in various environmental problems. In recent years, fluidized-bed filtration systems have been adapted for use in pond systems and these are now available as an additional component for filtration systems.

Water quality management

For all freshwater and marine systems, regardless of the method of filtration employed, standard water quality parameters must be monitored regularly. The frequency of monitoring and the scope of tests performed will vary depending on the efficiency of the filtration system, the stocking density and stock turnover. As a recommended minimum, the levels of ammonia, nitrite, nitrate, temperature, pH and dissolved oxygen should be measured and recorded. In many cases, these parameters are checked using standard commercial test kits, but, due to the labour and time involved, this may be performed less frequently than is desirable. Electronic equipment, using ion-specific probes and other analytical methods, is used where it is considered economical. In a few large facilities, 24-hour monitoring is performed by specialist electronic equipment (Figure 4.7) but at present the range of parameters monitored is limited and standard methods also need to be employed.

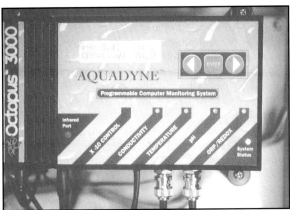

Figure 4.7 Electronic equipment for continuous monitoring of water quality. Various parameters can be measured and some units will activate other equipment (e.g. heaters, ozone generator) and adjust the water quality accordingly. This unit can monitor conductivity, temperature, pH and oxygen-reduction potential.

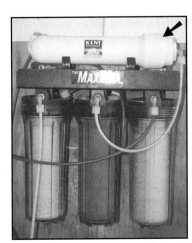

Figure 4.8 A reverse osmosis unit (arrowed) that produces purified water by allowing domestic tap water to pass through a semi-permeable (thin film composite) membrane using mains water pressure. Water first passes through the lower canisters, which are prefilters: these remove particles as small as 5 μm and 1 μm; then activated carbon removes chlorine that may damage the membrane. (Courtesy of Home Marine. © W.H. Wildgoose.)

Many wholesalers and retailers of ornamental fish belong to the Ornamental Aquatic Trade Association (OATA), which sets out recommended guidelines on water quality criteria for its members (see Chapter 2).

Coldwater

In general, water quality in coldwater systems remains relatively stable, often due to the larger volume of water involved. Outdoor ponds are vulnerable to seasonal temperature changes and occasional algal blooms.

Tropical freshwater

The tropical environment is generally very stable but many tropical species are sensitive to slight changes or fluctuations in temperature or pH.

Marine

The heat from lighting and equipment used for tropical marine systems results in water evaporation. To maintain a constant salinity, it is essential to monitor the specific gravity of the tank water and top up with freshwater.

As part of the management of all these systems, routine water changes are required in order to replenish many of the trace elements that become depleted. The water used for tropical marine systems and sensitive tropical freshwater species is generally obtained using reverse osmosis (Figure 4.8), a filtration system for removal of selective ions from tap water. The treated water can then be used for mixing with synthetic sea salts or specific minerals suitable for the required freshwater ecosystem.

Water quality and effect of transportation

Many species of fish are imported into the UK from around the world. Fish are transported in sealed plastic bags, about one-third of which contains water and the remainder is inflated with pure oxygen. The bags are placed inside insulated boxes. The water conditions in the shipping bag deteriorate considerably during transportation and, on arrival of freshwater fish, bag water has a low pH due to dissolved carbon dioxide levels produced during respiration. Although dissolved oxygen levels usually remain high, carbon dioxide levels are often greatly elevated. The ammonia concentration in the water is often excessive but, in theory (due to the low pH of the water), the less toxic ionized form predominates. However, ionized ammonia also accumulates in the blood and tissues. When the bags are opened, dissolved carbon dioxide will escape as gas, causing the pH of the water to rise. As the water becomes more alkaline, the ionized ammonia is converted into the un-ionized form, becoming more toxic to the fish.

The consequence of transport is that fish are in a stressed condition on arrival at the wholesale or retail premises and require a considerable time to recuperate. This interval between shipping and sale depends on the length of the original journey but, as a guide, it is recommended that fish that have been in transit for 24–36 hours should be rested for at least 2 weeks. The reality is that fish stocks tend to be moved quickly from the wholesaler to either a retailer or the public before the fish have fully recovered, rendering them more susceptible to infectious disease.

It appears that marine fish are less susceptible to these changes in pH, due to the buffering capacity of sea water, but there are few data on marine water quality following transportation.

Stocking levels

In many cases, there is little planning with regard to the numbers of fish that any particular system should or can hold. The criteria commonly applied are that the water should be free of ammonia and nitrite, indicating that the filtration system is able to cope with a particular stocking level.

Tropical freshwater

The stocking density of tropical freshwater aquaria is often related to the sales of individual species and these may be topped up on a regular basis, usually with new fish arriving weekly. New stocks tend to be added to the depleted tanks of existing fish.

Marine

More care is given to the stocking of marine aquaria, often because these fish are more expensive and aggression between fish of the same or different species can be a problem. Most wholesalers and retailers of marine stocks tend to adhere to recommended stocking levels (which are also applicable to the hobbyist):

- Fish (total length, including the tail): 1 cm per 3.5 litres in a system with a mature filter
- Invertebrates per 100 litres: five colonial animals, 15 anemones (3–5 cm disc), one pair of boxing shrimps and five small cleaner shrimps.

These levels are very low compared with most tropical freshwater systems.

Coldwater

A guideline for stocking pond fish, as recommended by OATA, is 8 kg bodyweight per 1000 litres of water.

Traditionally, the Easter holiday heralds the start of the UK 'pond season', which ends in September or October, depending on the ambient temperature. Therefore, the duration of this retail market is very short. In the winter, sales of pond fish virtually cease and this in turn affects stocking policies. Through the winter months, systems may be closed down completely or run with minimal numbers of fish.

As Easter approaches, the systems are often suddenly stocked with large numbers of fish in anticipation of the forthcoming season, resulting in poor water conditions with high concentrations of ammonia and nitrites. These problems are ameliorated by adding common salt (sodium chloride) and by frequent partial water changes. This sudden change in water quality can be minimized by seeding the filter with nitrifying bacteria, commercially available in suspensions of nutrient medium or as dry cultures. Despite this, serious deterioration of water quality with accompanying disease and mortality of fish stocks can still occur.

An alternative to seeding the filtration system is to 'feed' it with a source of inorganic ammonia, such as ammonium sulphate or ammonium chloride. To do this requires estimating the total bodyweight of fish held in that system and the total feed requirement. The latter is calculated at 2% bodyweight per day for adult fish and 5% bodyweight per day for juveniles. On average, 1 gram of food produces 40 mg of ammonia (Bryant *et al.,* 1980). Therefore, from the total amount of feed required by the fish, it is possible to estimate the amount of ammonium salt required to maintain the filtration system.

Stock management

In the majority of retail outlets, all fish stocks on display are intended for sale and usually operate an 'all in, all out' policy. A limited number of retailers may hold one or more large specimen fish such as koi, sturgeon or occasionally sharks that are not for sale but to encourage members of the public to visit the outlet (Figure 4.9). Some shops also operate quarantine tanks that are used to house their own sick or injured fish and occasionally offered as a service to customers. A few retailers use these facilities to accommodate recently arrived fish and allow them to recover from the stress of shipping before going on display. Maintaining strong, healthy fish for retail sale requires considerable care and management of both stocks and systems.

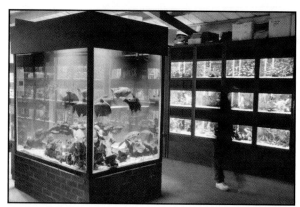

Figure 4.9 A large show tank at a retail outlet. This centrepiece exhibit is designed to attract potential customers. The large specimen fish are often long-lived staff pets or rare species. (Courtesy of Swallow Aquatics. © W.H. Wildgoose.)

Fish management in many retail outlets involves the removal of dead or sick specimens from public view on a daily basis. Occasionally, records of mortalities are maintained and where a tank or holding system seems to be affected by some disease, these stocks are usually withdrawn from sale. Few retailers will knowingly sell sick fish, for fear of loss of reputation and litigation.

Many wholesalers and importers are less fastidious with regard to hygiene, as the fish are not on public display and it is quite possible to find sick or dead fish amongst stock that are available for sale. Stocks are moved on as quickly as possible, with a few exceptions, and imported fish are often available for sale on the same day that shipment has arrived. After the fish have been despatched to the retailer, any mortalities must be notified within 24 hours and replacements are given for these with the next consignment. Rarely is any responsibility accepted outside of this period by the wholesaler, importer or even breeder. Many breeders routinely treat fish prior to shipment but it is not uncommon to find that sick fish have been included in the consignment.

On arrival, many wholesalers open the transport boxes and immediately dip or bathe the fish in a strong solution of a proprietary medication. The view is that this will kill any ectoparasites and that if the fish die in the process then they were weak and would not have survived anyway. The effect of such dips on stressed fish immediately following shipment is rarely taken into consideration. In many cases, dip treatment immediately following shipment is unnecessary, because outbreaks of common ectoparasites such as *Ichthyobodo*, *Chilodonella*, *Trichodina* and flukes tend to occur several days later, probably because of stress-induced immunosuppression.

Some wholesalers and retailers possess their own microscopes, which are used for identifying ectoparasites prior to the administration of an appropriate medication, but some medications are given on a prophylactic basis to new arrivals in the hope of controlling infectious diseases. Chemicals are occasionally administered to these fish, regardless of the presence or absence of a pathogen.

Common health problems

Many of the problems commonly encountered in retail outlets are related to stress, the effect of which is cumulative and begins with the netting and transport of fish. Although most freshwater tropical fish are farmed, a limited number of retail outlets will purchase wild-caught exotic species for the experienced and specialist hobbyist. In recent years, increasing numbers of marine fish are being successfully bred in captivity, such as several species of goby, clownfish, sea-horses and shrimps. Although there is increasing awareness of the importance of rearing marine fish and invertebrates for the aquarium market, many species are still wild-caught. Techniques for capturing wild fish (such as netting and use of toxic chemicals), accompanied by transportation, are extremely stressful to these animals.

Stress

The consequences of stress result in outbreaks of common ectoparasite infections such as white spot in freshwater and marine fish. In addition, stressed fish become more susceptible to common bacterial infections resulting in fin rot and skin ulceration. In most instances, the fish are treated with a proprietary brand of medication, which controls the disease. Some species of tropical freshwater fish, notably the mollies, are intolerant of slight temperature fluctuation, which often results in outbreaks of white spot. Correct temperature control, by heating each aquarium separately, minimizes this problem.

Physical injury

Injuries resulting from poor handling and netting procedures are not uncommon. Fish with spiny dorsal fins become ensnared in nets and the delicate tissue of the fin becomes torn, exposing the bony ray. Secondary bacterial infection of the torn tissue is common, often leading to erosion of the fin. Damage to the lateral body surfaces commonly produces raised scales and localized oedema where the fish has been struck during netting. Often these areas of tissue damage heal without intervention but occasionally they lead to necrosis of the epidermis, with loss of scales. Various injuries to the eye can occur during netting and may result in corneal ulceration, cataract or extensive intraocular damage.

Disease control

Prophylaxis

Prophylactic treatment of ornamental fish is common practice and may vary from regular dips or long-term baths in chemicals to the routine use of antibiotic and antimicrobial drugs. The use of chemicals and drugs in this way is carried out irrespective of any contraindications or the effects of repeated long-term exposure. In many cases, prophylactic treatment is used as a substitute for good fish husbandry and stock management, though there is an entrenched belief held by some that prophylaxis is a sound practice and beneficial to the fish's welfare.

Medication

The level of treatment given to fish stocks is varied and often proportional to their retail value. Inexpensive fish are generally given proprietary brands of medication but no further action is taken if these fail to be effective, because the cost of treatment may exceed the total stock value. Valuable stock tends to receive more care, though in some instances the medication given may be inappropriate, and occasionally professional help from veterinarians or independent fish health consultants may be requested. Regrettably, many retailers fear the impact of adverse publicity about a disease problem and prefer to cull affected fish than seek professional assistance.

Disinfection

The standards of routine disinfection of equipment and nets vary considerably. This important aspect of fish husbandry and hygiene is complex and often poorly understood. In many cases, unsuitable chemicals are used, often at ineffective concentrations for an insufficient exposure time, giving a false sense of security. Occasionally, disinfection of the whole premises may be required following an outbreak of a notifiable disease such as spring viraemia of carp.

Although many effective disinfectants are available, only a few are suitable and safe to use in the aquatic environment, since some residues may be lethal to fish. Advice on the use of suitable chemical disinfectants can be obtained from the relevant fish disease authority.

In addition to the cost of the chemical agent, disinfecting a commercial facility is very labour intensive and re-establishing biological filters is a slow process. As a result, total disinfection is only performed when it is economically viable.

Veterinary approach

In general, the veterinary profession and independent fish health consultants are viewed with some scepticism by the retail industry and only a small number of outlets employ veterinary services. This mistrust is partly historical, because prior to the 1990s only a few veterinarians were interested in treating pet fish – simply due to lack of demand from retailers and hobbyists. From the late 1970s, the popularity and price of koi meant that retailers and fish keepers increasingly turned to the veterinary profession for access to prescription drugs for treating sick fish.

Many retailers are very knowledgeable on the ethology of many species of fish and there seems to be a general opinion among them that they know more than the average veterinarian about fish husbandry and disease management. Yet in many instances there is little understanding of basic fish anatomy and physiology, the influence of good husbandry practices, epidemiology and the correct use of proprietary medicines and prescription drugs.

There is an increased awareness of the value of further education, and qualified members of staff are now employed by larger retail outlets. Various continuing education programmes are available for staff as full-time courses or distance learning. Many of these emphasize the importance of good husbandry and the value of veterinary consultation.

In the UK, veterinarians are also required to inspect retail outlets regularly on behalf of local government authorities as part of the licensing procedure for pet shops.

For veterinary involvement in the pet fish trade to progress, it is important that veterinarians should demonstrate a sound knowledge of basic filtration systems and fish keeping, and be able to generate more confidence within the industry. Although any approach needs to be conducted with sensitivity, there is certainly a need for the veterinary profession to develop relationships within the industry in order to improve the welfare of pet fish.

Further reading

Banister KE (1979) *Aquarial Fish.* Frederick Muller, London

Bassleer G (1996) *Diseases in Marine Aquarium Fish: Causes, Development, Symptoms, Treatment.* Bassleer Biofish n.v., Westmeerbeek

Bryant P, Jauncey K and Atack T (1980) *Backyard Fish Farming.* Prism Press, Dorchester

Debelius H and Baensch, HA (1994) *Marine Atlas: the Joint Aquarium Care of Invertebrates and Tropical Marine Fishes.* Mergus, Melle

Francis-Floyd R (2000) Approaches to aquarium stores and wholesalers. In: *Proceedings of the North American Veterinary Conference.* NAVC, Orlando, Florida

Lundegaard G (1990) *Keeping Marine Fish: an Aquarium Guide.* Blandford, London

Spotte S (1993) *Marine Aquarium Keeping*, 2nd edn. John Wiley & Sons, New York

Acknowledgements

The author gratefully acknowledges the assistance given by Peter Gostling and the staff at Badshot Lea Garden Centre, and their permission to photograph the Aquatic Centre. Thanks are also due to Tony Lewis and Dave Skilleter for their constructive appraisal of draft copies of the manuscript.

5

Pond fish keeping

Frank Prince-Iles

Over the last decade, there have been substantial changes in pond fish keeping, mainly due to the increased popularity of koi. This has led to changes in sizes and types of ponds, filtration methods and ancillary equipment used by hobbyists. However, despite improvements in fish-keeping equipment and filtration, the major cause of fish health problems is due to poor environmental conditions, irrespective of the system used.

Pond construction

Position

Garden ponds should be situated in open areas where they will receive the sun for most of the day. A pond should have some shade from the midday sun and shelter from winter winds, which can usually be achieved by careful use of plants adjacent to the pond. Plants that cover the water surface, such as lilies, will give fish additional shade. Ideally, ponds should be sited away from trees and overhanging bushes, as leaf litter in the autumn can cause considerable pollution.

Ponds should be on level ground to prevent the risk of water 'run-off' from surrounding garden areas carrying fertilizers or pesticides into the pond.

For the normal garden pond, access to water for topping up and electricity to run pumps and other equipment will also be necessary. For koi ponds, it may be necessary to consider access to drains for water discharges.

Construction

The initial choice for the pond keeper is between a preformed plastic pond and constructing their own pond. While the easiest method is to use the preformed type (Figure 5.1), these are generally small and suitable for only a few small fish. For larger ponds (Figure 5.2) there are various methods of construction.

The simplest and cheapest method is to use a flexible butyl rubber liner, which is put into a lined excavation. Butyl rubber liners suffer from the disadvantages of creases and folds and a susceptibility to damage from sharp objects.

Concrete is still sometimes used but, while it provides a strong durable finish, it can often crack. An alternative is to use concrete blocks, which are rendered (often using reinforcing fibres) and lined with a variety of finishes, including pond paints,

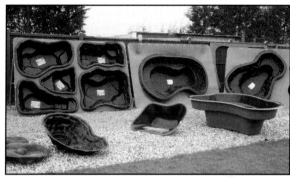

Figure 5.1 Preformed garden ponds are available in heavy duty plastic and fibreglass. Due to their limited size, these ponds are only suitable for goldfish and small koi. (Courtesy of Shotgate Koi. © W.H. Wildgoose.)

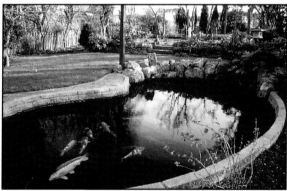

Figure 5.2 A large formal koi pond. (© W.H. Wildgoose.)

specialist sealants or fibreglass. The fourth (but little used) option is a natural pond lined with clay.

Shelves and ledges are often incorporated to allow for marginal plants but these are rare in koi ponds, because of the tendency of koi to uproot the plants.

Size

Pond size is an important consideration and can have a direct effect on many aspects of fish health. Very small ponds suffer from fluctuations in water quality and temperature but it may be easier to see and treat the fish in a small pond. Larger ponds usually offer more stable conditions but catching and treating the fish can be a problem.

Although ponds can be of any size, there are a few basic considerations. A minimum depth of 0.5 m is needed to provide protection for fish during the winter months but a depth of 1 m should be considered as the minimum if koi are being kept. Overall, a size of 2 m × 1.5 m with a depth of 0.5 m should be considered as the minimum size for any garden pond. However, this size would only be suitable for smaller species, such as goldfish and possibly tench.

Fish such as koi and orfe need a larger area, which is dependent on the intended stocking density. A size of 3 m × 2.5 m with a depth of 1 m should be considered as the minimum for a koi pond. It is essential to know the exact volume of the pond in order to calculate the correct stocking density, filtration requirements and quantities of medication. Initially, the pond should be filled using a water meter to check the exact volume of water; otherwise, it will be necessary to calculate the volume from various measurements.

A purpose-built koi pond can represent a considerable investment in both time and money, with costs of about £2–4 per 10 litres volume, including filtration.

Filtration

Fish are continually polluting the water in which they live, excreting substantial amounts of metabolic ammonia (50–100 mg/kg bodyweight per 24 hours). This is in addition to urine and faeces. In an established well planted pond with moderate stocking densities, these waste products are rapidly utilized by nitrifying bacteria and plants. However, as stocking densities increase, additional biological filtration is often needed to deal with the increase in organic and nitrogenous pollution.

All biological filtration systems work by passing polluted water over a medium that has a relatively large surface area for microbial colonization. In addition to providing biological nitrification, most filters will act as a mechanical filter by trapping solid wastes.

Types of filter

There are essentially three different methods of pond filtration:

- Pump-fed external filters
- Gravity-fed filters
- Undergravel filters.

Pump-fed external filters

These use a submersible pump in the pond to pump water into the filter. Water passes through the filter medium and returns to the pond (Figure 5.3). The advantage of this type of filter is the simplicity of installation and low cost, but there are several disadvantages. Because the pump is in the pond, it will often clog and will need regular (perhaps daily) cleaning. Solids drawn into the pump tend to be liquidized. The typical box-type filter tends to become clogged rapidly with solids and requires regular maintenance to keep it clean. Because of the relatively small size, this type of filter is generally only suitable for smaller ponds.

Gravity-fed filters

These are an alternative to pump-fed filtration systems. They are connected by pipework to the pond, often by bottom drains, and are at the same level as the pond (Figures 5.4 and 5.5).

Clean, treated water is pumped out of the last stage of the filter and back into the pond, thus drawing polluted water and solids into the first stage. The filter medium is usually supported off the bottom of the chamber to create a void. Water from the final chambers is often pumped back into the pond through an ultraviolet lamp and a venturi (a simple aeration device). Each chamber usually has a bottom drain leading to a standpipe chamber. When the standpipes are removed, solid wastes at the bottom of each chamber are flushed out and usually discharged to mains drainage or a soakaway.

The first stage is usually a large empty settlement chamber or, alternatively, a 'vortex' that gently spins the water so that solids settle out by centrifugal force and are discharged to waste. The water then passes through

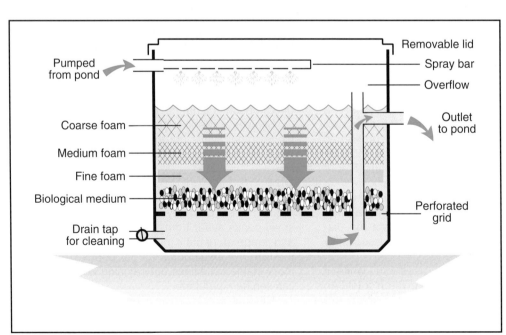

Figure 5.3
Pump-fed external filter. Water is pumped from the pond and distributed over the medium through a spray bar. It flows through the medium and returns to the pond, often via a waterfall. (© W.H. Wildgoose.)

Pumped from pond

Removable lid
Spray bar
Overflow

Coarse foam

Outlet to pond

Medium foam

Fine foam

Biological medium

Drain tap for cleaning

Perforated grid

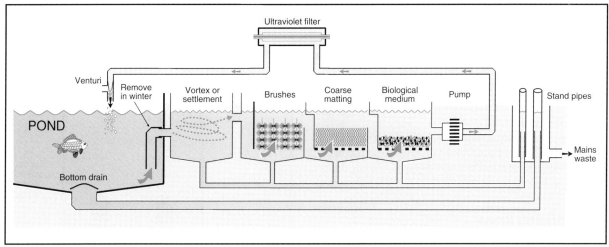

Figure 5.4 Diagram of a gravity-fed filter. Water from the pond enters the settlement chamber or vortex, where heavy solids settle out. The water passes through a transfer port into the next chamber, where filter brushes trap finer suspended solids. It then passes through a series of chambers containing various types of medium before being pumped back into the pond. (© W.H. Wildgoose.)

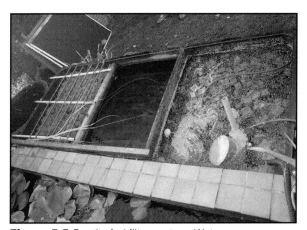

Figure 5.5 Gravity-fed filter system. Water passes through the circular vortex chamber on the far left then through a chamber of brushes, plastic matting and finally plastic medium before being pumped back into the pond. (© W.H. Wildgoose.)

one or more chambers of different media, where additional mechanical straining and biological filtration take place, before being pumped back into the pond.

Generally, this type of system is used for koi ponds. The disadvantages are that these filters are more expensive and difficult to instal. Even this type of system can become clogged with solids and regular maintenance is necessary to keep all chambers clean. Poorly maintained filters, leading to high levels of organic pollution, are a common underlying cause of many fish health problems.

Undergravel filters

This system, though less popular now, is still used in many ponds. It consists of a network of perforated pipes under a layer of gravel. Water is drawn down through the gravel and pumped back into the pond (Figure 5.6). The gravel acts as a mechanical and biological filter. The system is usually situated within the pond.

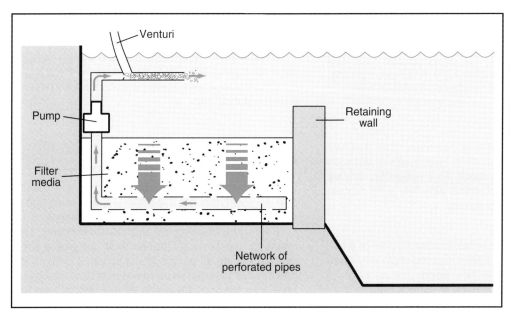

Figure 5.6
Internal undergravel filter. Water is drawn down through the medium (usually gravel) into a pipework matrix and then pumped back into the pond, often through a venturi.

Although undergravel filters are often built on the pond bottom, the best option is to have a raised, walled section where it is possible to isolate the filter for maintenance by lowering the pond water level. While cheap and easy to instal, these filters are almost impossible to clean and are liable to be affected by pond medications.

Vegetable filters

This is an optional extension of biological and mechanical filtration. Treated water is passed through a bed of fast-growing plants, often watercress (*Nasturtium officinale*), to help to remove nitrates and thus discourage algal blooms.

New filtration ideas

Some new approaches to pond filtration look promising. These should result in easier maintenance and more effective filtration.

Trickle tower filters

Water, either directly from the pond or after it has passed through a settlement chamber, is pumped up to the top of the filter where it is sprayed, usually via a rotating head, over the medium. It then trickles through the medium and returns to the pond (Figure 5.7).

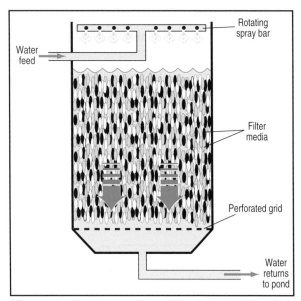

Figure 5.7 Trickle tower filter. Water is pumped from the pond or settlement chamber, usually passing through a UV lamp. A rotating spray bar distributes the water over the medium.

These filters are taller and contain more medium than external pump-fed filters. High levels of aeration together with thin-film water flow make this a very effective filter system. There is very little solid deposition, so maintenance is simple.

Fluidized filters

Pre-cleaned water is pumped into the bottom of a tall, narrow chamber partly filled with sand or plastic beads (Figure 5.8). The water flow keeps the particles in suspension, providing a massive surface area for bacterial colonization.

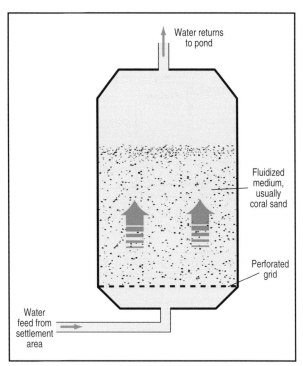

Figure 5.8 Fluidized-bed filter. Water pressure keeps the medium in constant suspension. Flow rates are critical to keep the medium suspended and prevent it rising too high in the column.

Bubble-bead filters

These use an innovative approach. Water is pumped directly from the pond into the bottom of the filter vessel that contains plastic beads. There are two basic designs. The most common is packed with beads that act as both biological and mechanical media. In one design, the plastic beads float on top of the water, acting as a mechanical strainer and trapping the solids as the water passes through (Figure 5.9).

In the other design, two types of bead are used: one heavier than water and the other lighter. The lighter beads float on the top of the water, while the heavier ones are kept in motion by the water flow and act as a fluidized-bed filter.

Maintenance of both types is simple, using a multiport valve to reverse the water flow, flushing the trapped solids to waste. These filters are expensive and require a heavy-duty pump.

Filtration media

Filtration media can be broadly divided into mechanical or biological types but it is important to realize that all media carry out both functions to some degree.

Foam and brushes are the most commonly used media for mechanical filtration; both are highly effective at trapping all but the finest solids. It is important that they are cleaned (in pond water) on a regular basis, otherwise the trapped solids simply decompose and pollute the water.

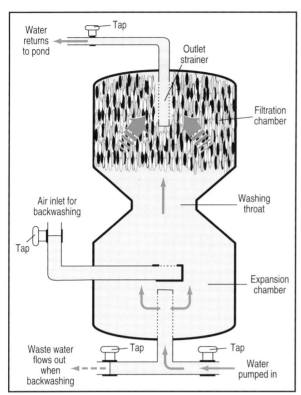

Figure 5.9 Bubble-bead filter. Water is pumped under pressure into the chamber. The lightweight beads float to the top, providing a large surface area for bacterial colonization and acting as a mechanical filter by trapping solids. Another design includes heavier beads that are kept in suspension by the water flow and provide additional surface area for biological filtration.

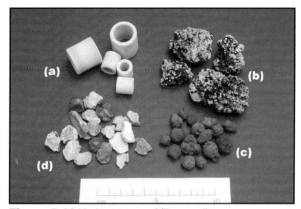

Figure 5.10 Various types of filter medium: (a) Siporax; (b) Alfagrog; (c) Lytag; (d) Canterbury spar. (© W.H. Wildgoose.)

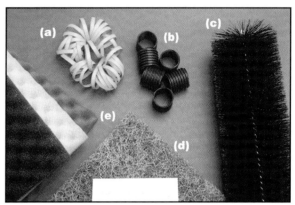

Figure 5.11 Various types of plastic filter medium: (a) Springflo; (b) Flocor; (c) filter brush; (d) Japanese filter matting; (e) foam sheet. (© W.H. Wildgoose.)

There is a range of media to encourage biological filtration or nitrification (Figures 5.10 and 5.11). Essentially all these media provide a large surface area for microbial colonization (Figure 5.12). They include:

- Natural stone (e.g. Canterbury Spar)
- Baked clay granules (e.g. Lytag®)
- Porous sintered ceramic media (e.g. Alfagrog)
- Sintered glass (e.g. Siporax®)
- Plastic media (e.g. Flocor® – corrugated tubes; Springflo® – dimpled plastic tape; Japanese filter matting – sheets of bonded plastic fibres).

Medium	Specific surface area (m^2 surface area per m^3 medium)
Gravel/stone	100–200
Flocor®	230
Springflo®	300
Filter matting	300–350
Foam	400–500
Siporax®	1800*

Figure 5.12 Surface area of commonly used filter media.
* Includes internal vaults

In sufficient quantity, any of these media will provide ample surface area for nitrification. With most ponds producing less than 10 g of ammonia daily, the required 'active' surface area is modest (1 m^2 of biologically active medium can process 1 g of ammonia every 24 hours). The most significant factors affecting the choice of medium are cost and the ease of cleaning. Stone and gravel are the cheapest but are the most difficult to clean, while lightweight media such as matting and plastics are far easier to clean but considerably more expensive.

Flow rates

Flow rates through the filter are dependent on stocking levels but, as a general rule of thumb, the flow rate should be approximately one-third to half the volume of the pond per hour. The aim is to pass the volume of the pond through the filter every 2–3 hours. It is necessary to measure actual pump flow rates, as these are often significantly different than the quoted pump output because of frictional losses caused by pipework and the backpressure from the head of water.

Retention time

Water retention times within the filter are important. If the filter is too small, there will be very little settlement of solids or time for any significant biological activity. The flow rate through the filter should be such that water passes through relatively slowly and is retained for a few minutes – ideally 5 minutes or more. Longer retention times generally result in better water quality. Filter media density and water displacement will have a significant effect on retention times. Lightweight media displace less water and thus increase retention time for a given filter volume. Obviously, as flow rates increase, the filter size has to be increased to allow for the retention time.

Pond equipment

There are many additional pieces of equipment available for the pond keeper.

Nets

There is a wide range of nets for catching and handling fish. This is particularly important with koi, where a large pan-type net with a robust handle is needed if fish are to be caught safely and quickly. Another useful net is the 'sock net', which is like a long sock but open at each end. With the fish safely inside and both ends held, the fish can be handled without any fear of dropping or damaging it.

Pumps

Pumps vary in size and can be used to provide fountains or waterfalls, which help with water movement and aeration. A pump is essential if any form of filtration is used and will need to be left running continuously to prevent the death of aerobic microorganisms in the filter.

Air pumps

When connected to porous air-stones or porous pipes these can be used to provide additional aeration in the pond or filter. This is especially useful in warm weather and when oxygen-depleting pond treatments such as formalin are used.

Venturis

These simple devices are fitted to the end of the water return pipe. A constriction inside the unit results in a change in pressure, which in turn pulls air into the venturi. This gives a high-pressure return full of bubbles and thus improves aeration of the pond.

Ultraviolet (UV) lamps

Water is pumped through these very useful and effective devices to kill single-cell algae and other microorganisms that pass through. The lamps have little effect on the bacterial levels within the pond, but effectively control suspended single-cell algae. The bulbs have a limited effective life and need to be changed every 6 months.

Pond vacuums

These enable detritus and 'mulm' (solid wastes) to be removed from the bottom without the need to empty the pond. They are very useful for larger ponds and almost essential for large koi ponds without bottom drains.

Pond heaters

These range from small 100 W heaters that keep a small surface area free of ice during the winter, to gas or electrical systems that maintain warm water throughout all or part of the winter months.

Water purifiers

Based on activated carbon and ion exchange resins, these units remove impurities such as chlorine and heavy metals from the domestic water supply. They are supplied as a series of two or three pods, with each pod carrying out a different function. The cartridges need regular changing, depending on the water throughput and its ionic content.

Water test kits

Regular water testing is essential to ensure optimum conditions. There is a range of cheap, simple, reliable kits. Typical kits use either liquid or tablet reagents to perform either titration or colour comparative tests.

Sand pressure filters

These act as mechanical filters, removing fine particulate solids. Water is passed, under pressure, through a layer of sand inside the filter. This method is less popular now because the filters need to be operated by a swimming-pool pump and need regular backflushing to prevent blockage. In use, they often fail to maintain 'crystal clear' water but they do return very clean water to the pond.

Foam fractionators

These work on the same principle as aquarium 'protein skimmers', removing surface-active molecules such as proteins and other organics. Water is passed through a large-diameter pipe in which a porous air-stone or a venturi produces a continuous stream of bubbles, usually counter-current to the water flow. This creates, at the top of the column, an organic-rich foam that is either removed or drained off.

Stocking ponds

Many varieties of fish are kept, but the most popular are goldfish, orfe, tench and koi (Figures 5.13, 5.14, 5.15 and 5.16).

Stocking levels

Stocking densities are arguably the single most important factor affecting water quality, fish health, system requirements and routine husbandry. As stocking densities increase, the safety margin between good and poor conditions is reduced and system management becomes more critical. Overstocking and poor maintenance are common problems.

Stocking densities are based on the mass of fish per volume of water, rather than numbers or length of fish. Increases in bodyweight are not proportional to increased body length (excluding caudal fin), which complicates the calculation of stocking levels when larger fish such as koi are kept (Figure 5.17).

While it is possible to give guidelines for the number of goldfish that can be kept safely in a given volume of water, it is less clear when koi are involved as the relative sizes of the fish must also be taken into account.

As a very general rule of thumb, a reasonable stocking density would be 2 kg of fish per 1000 litres, in an established pond. For example, a medium-sized

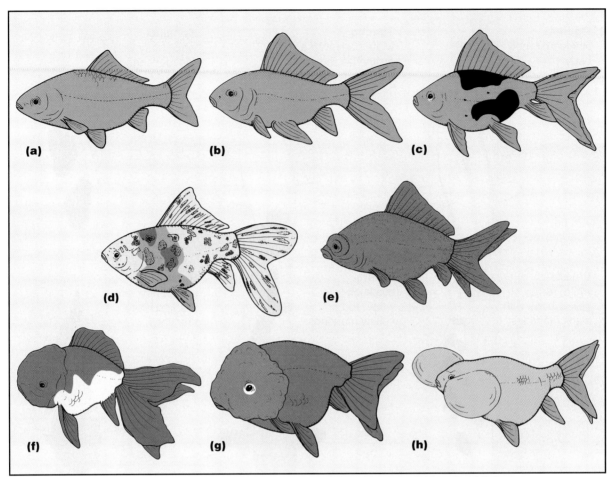

Figure 5.13 Common varieties of fancy goldfish: (a) common goldfish; (b) comet; (c) fantail goldfish; (d) shubunkin or calico goldfish; (e) black moor; (f) oranda; (g) lionhead goldfish; (h) bubble eye.

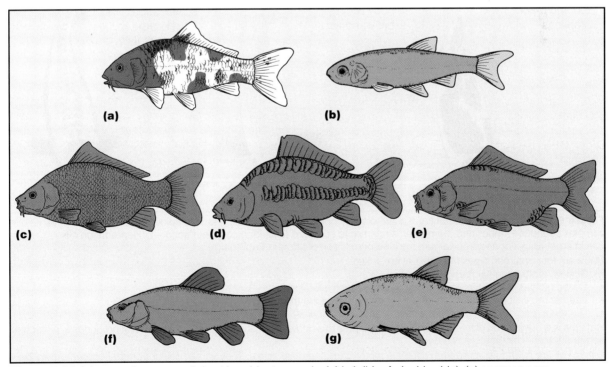

Figure 5.14 Other species commonly kept in coldwater ponds: (a) koi; (b) orfe (golden ide); (c) common carp; (d) mirror carp; (e) leather carp; (f) tench; (g) rudd.

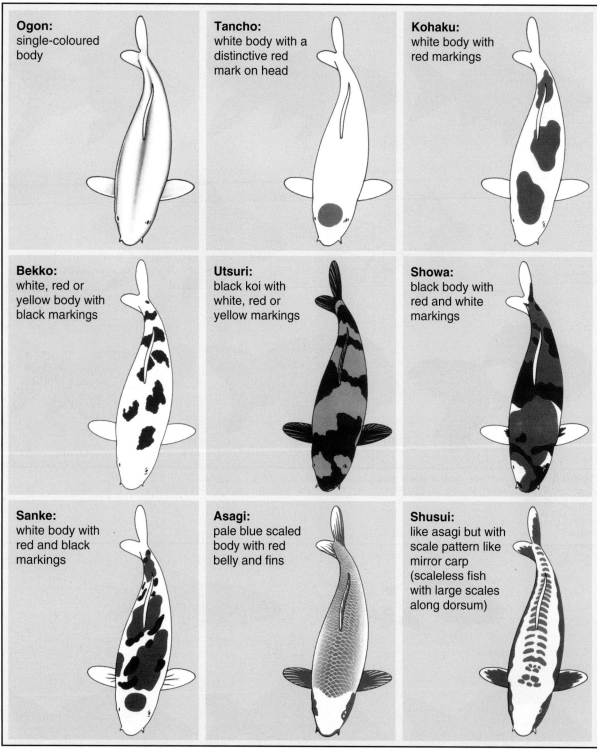

Ogon:
single-coloured
body

Tancho:
white body with a
distinctive red
mark on head

Kohaku:
white body with
red markings

Bekko:
white, red or
yellow body with
black markings

Utsuri:
black koi with
white, red or
yellow markings

Showa:
black body with
red and white
markings

Sanke:
white body with
red and black
markings

Asagi:
pale blue scaled
body with red
belly and fins

Shusui:
like asagi but with
scale pattern like
mirror carp
(scaleless fish
with large scales
along dorsum)

Figure 5.15 Common varieties of koi. Koi are classified into groups according to their colour patterns. These have complex Japanese names and the reader is referred to standard texts for a complete account. (Reproduced from The Interpet Encyclopaedia of Koi with the kind permission of Interpet Publishing.)

There are four common types of scale pattern in koi:
- Scaled (typical regular carp scale formation)
- Doitsu (scales along dorsum and occasionally along lateral line)
- Leather (no visible scales except for very small ones along the dorsum)
- Gin rin (a gold or silver mirror-like effect on individual scales).

Matsuba is a description of the scale pattern and relates to a darkening in the centre of the scales that produces a 'pine-cone' appearance on a single-coloured body.

'Ghost koi' are hybrid fish bred from a female mirror carp and male sanke. They vary in colour from dark green-brown like a common carp to a light silver colour, particularly around the head.

Grass carp are a different species with olive green or dark green body and small scales.

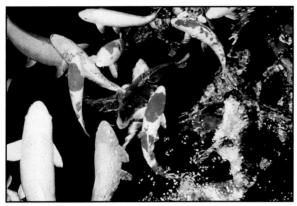

Figure 5.16 Mixed varieties of koi. (© W.H. Wildgoose.)

Fish length (excludes tail) (cm)	Fish weight (approx) (g)
10–15	100–300
15–20	300–400
25–30	800–1000
30	1000
38	2000
46	3000

Figure 5.17 Approximate weights of different-sized fish (goldfish and koi).

garden pond of 2500 litres with a small box filter could support 12 to 15 medium-sized goldfish or five 30 cm koi. These modest densities would allow a reasonable margin of safety. Initial stocking densities would have to be slightly lower to take account of pond/filter maturation time and fish growth. These densities could be exceeded by experienced pond keepers, especially when more sophisticated filtration is used.

Disease prevention

There is a very real risk that new fish will introduce infectious diseases or parasites into a pond and therefore all new fish should be quarantined, examined and, if necessary, treated prior to being put in the main pond. Such facilities need to be reasonably spacious, with well filtered water. Good water quality is paramount during quarantine.

The reality is that very few fish keepers will have adequate quarantine facilities to hold fish for several weeks and few hobbyists will have the skill or equipment to carry out a basic examination of fish. In the absence of such facilities, a minimum precaution would be a short-term bath against parasites, though this would not be effective against *Ichthyophthirius* (the organism that causes 'white spot'). All fish should be floated in their plastic bag for 15–20 minutes to let water temperatures equalize prior to release.

Lifespan

There is limited information about the natural lifespan of coldwater ornamental fish. In general, healthy fish of most species will live in excess of 15 years, with koi and goldfish occasionally exceeding 25 years.

Invertebrates and amphibians

Many pond keepers add invertebrates such as snails, mussels and crayfish to ponds in the belief that they will purify and clean the pond. These claims are dubious.

Amphibians such as frogs, toads and newts can coexist with fish. Generally, amphibians do not pose a threat to fish, the exception being at mating time when the amorous male may grab and attach itself to a passing fish and often needs to be removed manually. Frog spawn and to a lesser degree toad spawn can pose a problem with some filtration systems, either by blocking them or by being drawn into the discharge area. In such circumstances, the spawn is best removed to a separate pond.

Pond planting

Plants generally have a beneficial effect. Apart from being visually appealing, plants provide shelter and shade for fish and areas for spawning, as well as assisting water quality by removing excess nutrients such as nitrates and phosphates from the water. However, large fish such as koi will often knock over baskets or uproot plants, which is why koi ponds tend to be devoid of plants.

Aquatic plants are usually planted in sterilized soil in lined purpose-made baskets, with a topping of small stones or gravel to prevent the fish disturbing the soil. If plants are used in koi ponds, a different method has to be used, such as suspending the basket on brackets so that it is just below the water surface, where the koi cannot disturb it.

There are several types of suitable pond plants, including marginal and floating plants, lilies and submerged plants. Water lilies (*Nymphaea*) are particularly useful, providing large areas of shade for the fish as well as reducing algal blooms caused by direct sunlight.

There is often confusion about the role of 'oxygenating' plants such as *Elodea* (Canadian pondweed). These only release oxygen during daytime photosynthesis. At night they remove oxygen when photosynthesis ceases but normal respiration continues, which in heavily planted ponds can affect dissolved oxygen levels. If pondweed growth is excessive, it can make normal pond maintenance difficult, as well as reducing water circulation.

All plants should be disinfected with a potassium permanganate solution (5 mg/l for 5 minutes) to kill any attached parasites and snails before putting them in the pond.

Nutrition

The nutritional needs of fish are similar to those of most animals. They require carbohydrates, proteins, lipids, vitamins and minerals. One significant difference is that protein is a major energy source and fish require 30–36% in their diet. Deficiency in essential amino acids can cause retarded growth.

Pathological conditions can be caused by diets high in saturated fats, deficient in essential fatty acids, or containing oxidized lipids. Fish food should be used within 60 days of opening, because of the risk of lipid oxidation and vitamin loss.

In a well planted pond, fish will be able to find substantial amounts of natural food of both plant and animal origin and it is unlikely there would be any nutritional deficiencies.

In barren koi ponds and heavily stocked ponds, there is more reliance on fish food to supply a balanced diet. There are various types of commercially prepared fish food, including floating and sinking pellets, flakes and sticks. Ideally, the food should have a high mixed protein content and contain a range of vitamins and minerals. There are several health problems associated with vitamin deficiencies.

Standard fish foods can be supplemented with occasional treats of brown bread, sweetcorn, cockles, prawns, sliced oranges, lettuce and frozen and live foods. Koi foods often include dried *Spirulina* algae that contain carotenoids, a group of fat-soluble pigments used to enhance coloration in koi. Live foods such as water fleas (*Daphnia*) and tubificid worms should be used with caution, due to the risk of introducing pathogens.

Water temperatures influence fish appetite. During the summer months, fish should be fed two or three times daily and given only as much as they will eat within 2–3 minutes. Any uneaten food should be removed from the pond to avoid polluting the water. As seasonal temperatures decrease, feeding should be reduced to a light feed once daily and stopped entirely when water temperatures are below 8°C (the fish will virtually stop feeding anyway). Although fish can be fed small amounts on warmer winter days, there is a danger that the food could remain undigested in the gut if water temperatures should fall sharply.

Breeding

Mature fish mate during the spring and summer months. As fish prepare to mate, the male starts to chase the female, gently nudging her sides with his mouth. It can become rough when several males are involved in the chase, as they jostle for position and in shallow water the female may be lifted clear of the water. Physical injury during mating is not uncommon.

The results of such a mating, particularly with koi, are totally unpredictable. For selective breeding, it is normal to remove the female and place her in a breeding tank with two males of choice.

In the pond, the fertilized eggs will be deposited over plants and the pond walls. The fish will start to eat the eggs as soon as mating has finished and only well hidden eggs will survive and hatch.

In koi ponds, it is common to put spawning material (such as ropes, soft brushes or strips of foam) into the pond to encourage the female to deposit her eggs on these rather than on the hard pond wall. The spawning material can then be removed after mating and placed in a well aerated hatching tank.

Pond maintenance

Maintaining water quality is essential, as the majority of health problems are related to poor environmental conditions. The amount of regular maintenance required will depend on the type of pond and filter system.

Water testing

The water quality of all ponds should be regularly monitored, particularly during the summer months. The core water parameters to be tested are pH, ammonia, nitrite, nitrate and water hardness (carbonate and general hardness).

Required levels for koi, goldfish, tench and orfe are:

- pH 7–8.5
- ammonia and nitrites < 0.1 mg/l
- nitrates < 50 mg/l
- calcium carbonate 100–300 mg/l.

Cleaning

A moderately stocked, heavily planted 'natural' pond will need little in the way of maintenance beyond removing excess food and occasionally netting out any decaying leaves and other detritus on the pond bottom. One or two partial water changes of 10–15% during the summer months will help to restore mineral levels. Major cleaning will be required every few years to remove the build-up of decaying sediment on the bottom of the pond.

A mixed pond with a simple filter system will need more attention. In summer, the pump is placed near the bottom as far away from the water return as possible, to maximize water flow around the pond. The pond bottom needs to be kept reasonably clear of decaying matter. The filter (usually a pump-fed box type) should be kept reasonably clean, with sponges and other media being regularly rinsed in pond water to remove solid wastes. This practice is often neglected, leading to a substantial build-up of sludge and decomposing organic matter in the filter. This can affect filter function as well as producing high levels of dissolved organic carbon compounds, which can impact on fish health and water quality. Decaying organic material in the pond or filter can produce toxic hydrogen sulphide.

Purpose-built koi ponds with specialist filtration systems need regular attention because of the amount of waste produced. Settlement areas should be cleaned on a daily basis, while mechanical straining sections, such as foams and brushes, should be cleaned weekly during the summer months. The biological area needs to be kept clear of solid wastes by regular backflushing or other means of forcing settled solids out of the medium. This helps to prevent blockage of the medium, as well as reducing organic and inorganic pollution levels. Lack of routine filter maintenance is a common cause of pollution and koi health problems.

Winter maintenance

Routine maintenance is reduced during the winter months. If the pond does freeze over, a small area should be kept clear of ice by using a pond heater.

During extended cold periods of 4°C or less, the water pump may need to be turned off since excessive water movement can reduce the thermal inversion that occurs below 3.94°C. As water temperatures approach freezing, warmer water sinks to the bottom and cold water rises to the surface, providing an area at the bottom of the pond that is a degree or two warmer than the top. During the winter months, submerged pumps should be lifted clear of the bottom and placed near to the water return from the filter to minimize water movement. Filter maintenance is also reduced during winter months but some cleaning may still be required.

Seasonal aspects
Garden ponds are subject to seasonal variations in temperature and sunlight. These have a major effect on many aspects of fish health and pond maintenance. Most books and magazines cover these variations in detail, but some major considerations are highlighted below.

Plant growth
Plants will grow throughout the spring and summer months and then die back in the autumn. Dead and dying plant material should be removed from the pond. Additionally, autumn leaves from nearby trees should be removed from the pond on a regular basis to prevent water pollution, or alternatively a net may be put over the pond.

Algal blooms
Problems caused by either single-cell algal blooms that turn the water green, or attached filamentous algae, commonly called blanketweed, are not uncommon. Growth of both types can be particularly troublesome in spring. Small amounts of algal growth do little harm, and indeed may be beneficial, utilizing metabolic fish wastes as well as providing an alternative food source. However, in excess they pose a threat to fish as well as looking unsightly.

In common with all submerged green plants, algae will consume oxygen during the hours of darkness when photosynthesis ceases. This can affect the dissolved oxygen levels. A sudden algal die-back can lead to large amounts of algae rotting on the pond bottom, causing pollution and a reduction in dissolved oxygen levels. Very green water can make it difficult to see or catch fish and will interfere with many fish treatments.

Additionally, in poorly buffered water, algal blooms can create a diurnal pH shift. Plant photosynthesis removes carbon dioxide and increases pH, which peaks around sunset and falls during the night as carbon dioxide is released during respiration. This can lead to significant diurnal pH variations, with levels sometimes reaching pH 10.

Excessive algal growth is caused by many factors, including too much direct sunlight, inadequate shading, rainwater washing fertilizer into the pond from the surrounding garden, or poor routine maintenance of the pond or filter leading to increased organic and inorganic pollution. Elevated nitrate and phosphate levels in particular encourage algal growth.

There are several proprietary anti-algal treatments available, but they should be used with care due to the risk of massive algal die-back. Green water is most effectively controlled by the use of a UV lamp, which kills algal cells. The aerobic decomposition of barley straw has been shown to inhibit the growth of suspended algae and small quantities are available in convenient proprietary packs. There are many products such as magnetic or electrical devices that

claim to control filamentous algae, but results from these are variable. The long-term solution to algal blooms involves minimizing the major causes of algal growth (such as nutrient-rich water) and providing surface shading.

Common health problems
The majority of all common health problems are related directly or indirectly to poor environmental conditions. Common underlying causes include:

- Overcrowding
- Elevated ammonia or nitrite levels
- Inappropriate pH or high diurnal fluctuation
- Inappropriate water hardness leading to poor pH buffering or increased osmotic stress
- High levels of organic pollution resulting from inadequate system maintenance.

Pond fish are susceptible to a range of diseases and some of the most common health problems are shown in Figure 5.18.

Clinical sign	Cause
Fin rot	Bacterial infection by *Cytophaga–Flavobacterium–Flexibacter* group
Body ulcers	Bacterial infection by aeromonads and pseudomonads
'Flashing'/rubbing	Ectoparasites Poor water quality
Lacerations/fin damage	Trauma
Dyspnoea	Ectoparasites Bacterial gill disease Oxygen deficiency

Figure 5.18 Common diseases of pond fish. Most diseases are secondary infections resulting from poor environmental conditions.

New pond syndrome
This is a very common problem affecting almost all new ponds. In an established pond, ammonia excreted by the fish is converted step-wise by nitrifying bacteria into nitrate. In a new system it can take 6–8 weeks for these bacteria to become established in the pond and filter, during which time levels of ammonia and nitrite can rapidly rise to toxic levels. Zeolite can be used to reduce the ammonia and nitrite levels at this stage. Regular testing, gradual stocking and water changes are required throughout this difficult start-up period.

Water temperature effects
Because fish are ectotherms, environmental temperatures affect their metabolism and physiology. Their immune response is reduced at lower temperatures and is only fully effective at temperatures above 12°C. This can lead to health problems in early spring, or even during mild winters when water temperatures can hover between 8 and 12°C, which is warm enough to stimulate bacterial and parasite reproduction but not warm enough for the fish to mount an effective response.

Medication

Many pond medications are affected by water chemistry and conditions; for example, formalin, malachite green, chloramine-T and benzalkonium chloride are more toxic in acidic soft water. For most medications, the dosage and frequency of use should be reduced when water temperatures are below 12°C. High levels of particulate and dissolved organic material, including single-cell algae, will interfere with many treatments, such as potassium permanganate, formalin and malachite green.

The large size of many koi ponds often makes it impractical to perform substantial water changes quickly, particularly in emergencies. Their size also necessitates the use and careful handling of large quantities of harmful chemicals. Distributing these evenly around the pond is improved by good water circulation and airstones. If bath treatments are used, it is essential to use a tank or bowl of sufficient size, particularly if treating large koi. A smooth circular tank minimizes injury and netting the top will prevent fish from jumping out.

Some antibacterial treatments will affect the biological filter, and the filter system should be isolated for 24 hours following medication. However, it is important to treat both the filter and the pond to eliminate the environmental stages of some parasites. The UV units should be switched off and the water aerated during medication. It is important that water quality is monitored during and after any treatment.

Koi shows

Koi showing, in which the quality of the fish is assessed by a panel of experienced judges, is a significant factor in the popularity of koi keeping by hobbyists. These shows popularize the hobby but they also bring some threats to koi health.

Fish are normally starved for 3 days prior to a show to reduce the amount of faeces excreted while in the show vats. Fish are usually transported to the show 'double-bagged' in polythene bags containing enough water to cover a fish's head. Sometimes oxygen is added prior to the bags being tied. The bags are laid on their sides inside polystyrene containers. It is normal to transport them so that the fish are sideways to the direction of travel, to minimize the trauma of braking. Obviously handling and transport can be stressful.

The fish are kept for the period of the show (which may be one or two days) in large aerated vats. Zeolite is often added to the vats to reduce ammonia build-up. Despite this, water quality can still be a problem and each vat must be regularly monitored for ammonia, water temperature and pH. If water quality deteriorates, then partial water changes are usually required.

There are essentially two types of show. In 'Japanese style' shows, all fish of the same variety and size are exhibited in the same vat, irrespective of owner. Although this makes judging easier, it predisposes fish to the risk of cross-infection. In 'western style' shows, each owner has his own vat and judging is made more difficult, because direct comparisons are not possible.

Further reading

Andrews C, Excell A and Carrington C (1988) *The Manual of Fish Health*. Salamander Books, London
Dawes J (1998) *Pond Owners Handbook*. Ward Lock, London
McDowall A (1989) *The Interpet Encyclopaedia of Koi*. Salamander Books, London
Schimana W (1994) *Garden Ponds for Everyone*. TFH Publications, New York

6

Freshwater aquaria

David Pool

Keeping fish in an aquarium is a popular pastime around the world. This chapter examines the requirements in setting up and maintaining a freshwater aquarium. Freshwater aquaria may be divided on the basis of the temperature of the water they contain. Tropical aquaria are generally heated, and contain a selection of fish and plants from tropical areas of the world. Coldwater aquaria are unheated, and contain goldfish and other species from temperate regions.

Tanks

Provided that certain guidelines are followed, establishing and successfully maintaining a freshwater aquarium is relatively straightforward.

Selection

The wide variety of aquaria and other water containers that can be used to keep freshwater fish ranges from small goldfish bowls (Figure 6.1) and *Betta* containers (for keeping Siamese fighting fish, *Betta splendens*) to large showpiece aquaria (Figure 6.2). As a general rule, the larger the aquarium the better, since the greater the volume of water, the more stable the water quality will be. A 36 litre tank (30 × 30 × 45 cm) should be regarded as the minimum in which to keep even a small number of fish.

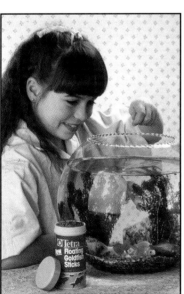

Figure 6.1 Goldfish bowls are only suitable for a few small fish. Severe fluctuations in water quality may result from the lack of filtration. The bowls should be only partially filled with water, so as to provide a greater surface area for gas exchange.

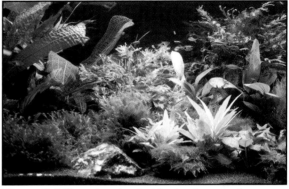

Figure 6.2 Showpiece tropical freshwater aquarium. These are often heavily stocked with a variety of fish species and plants to simulate a natural environment. Regular maintenance and efficient filtration systems are required to ensure good water quality. (© W.H. Wildgoose.)

The water surface area is important and permits good gas exchange. A tall thin tank has a smaller water surface area in comparison with a wide shallow tank of similar volume; consequently, fewer fish can be kept. Goldfish bowls are unsuitable for fish keeping but are still widely used, despite adverse publicity. If a bowl has a narrow neck, it is important to ensure that there is the maximum possible surface area by only partially filling the bowl.

A cover or condensation tray prevents evaporation, reduces heat loss and prevents fish from escaping.

Positioning

The aquarium must be sited away from draughts and room heaters, because these may produce temperature fluctuations. Direct sunlight should also be avoided: it can stimulate unsightly algal growth and can potentially cause overheating.

An aquarium filled with water is heavy: an aquarium of average size (60 × 30 × 30 cm) plus gravel will weigh approximately 115 kg and should be positioned on a secure stand.

The availability of an electricity supply for lighting, filtration and heating (if used) and easy accessibility to enable routine maintenance must also be considered.

Heating

With tropical fish, it is necessary to use an aquarium heater to maintain the water temperature above room temperature. In most cases the heater is supplied with a thermostat, often combined into one unit. The heater and thermostat should be positioned at the rear of the aquarium, in a good water flow. To avoid overheating, the heater and thermostat must be completely covered by water.

The volume of water and the presence of room heating determine the size of the heater. In a heated room, 1 watt per litre should be allowed; in an unheated room this should be doubled. Using a heater that is too small can result in the aquarium not reaching the desired temperature and the heater being 'on' all of the time, thereby reducing its lifespan.

Lighting

Aquarium hoods usually provide a space for the installation of artificial lighting. This is preferable to sunlight because the intensity and duration can be accurately controlled to enable the fish to be seen. Plant growth is encouraged but not the growth of unsightly algae.

Most freshwater aquarists use fluorescent tubes for aquarium illumination. As well as being economical, they provide light along the length of the tank and are available with light patterns developed specifically for aquarium use. The light output of fluorescent tubes tends to diminish after 6–12 months and they need to be replaced after 10–12 months to ensure that the plants still receive sufficient light. Failure to provide adequate illumination will result in the plants failing to grow or appearing thin and unhealthy.

The volume of water determines the lighting intensity for a particular aquarium. As a general rule 0.5 watts of fluorescent lighting per litre of aquarium water will encourage healthy plant growth. Therefore a 100 litre aquarium would require a lighting intensity of 50 watts, which should be left on for 10–12 hours per day in order to encourage healthy plant growth. A reflective surface above the light improves illumination within the aquarium.

Aeration

The filter usually provides aeration and good water circulation. This can be increased by adding a venturi fitting to the outflow of some canister filters, which will draw air into the water flow. In the majority of aquaria, the water movement created by the filter outflow will be sufficient to ensure that the water contains adequate oxygen. Additional aeration can be added to an aquarium by using an air pump and air-stone in order to power ornaments for decorative reasons or to supplement the existing supply.

Décor

As a rule, any item for tank décor that is purchased from an aquarium shop should be safe to use. Most metals, limestone, cement and chalk rocks should be avoided in most freshwater aquaria: they can cause the pH and water hardness to rise to an unacceptable level.

Green wood can rot and release undesirable substances into the water. Bogwood, a type of decorative wood used in freshwater aquaria, may add a brown coloration to the water; this will not adversely affect fish but can be minimized by soaking the wood before adding it to the aquarium.

Filtration

The many commercial designs for aquarium filtration systems all perform the same basic tasks of removing suspended debris from the water (mechanical filtration)

and encouraging bacteria and other microorganisms to remove the ammonia and nitrite (biological filtration). The filter should be operated continuously to ensure that the biological activity of the filter is maintained.

In many cases, small aquaria and goldfish bowls are not filtered and water quality is maintained by regular partial water changes. While this may ensure adequate water quality, it can lead to other problems due to the sudden changes in water chemistry (e.g. pH and hardness). Therefore, some form of filtration is advisable for most aquaria. The choice of filter is determined by tank size, fish species, available space and cost. The size of the filter is generally determined by the size of tank: the filter should circulate the total volume of water every 30–60 minutes.

Foam filter

An air pump and air-stone are used to draw water through a foam cartridge (Figure 6.3), which mechanically removes any particulate matter and provides a large surface area for bacterial growth.

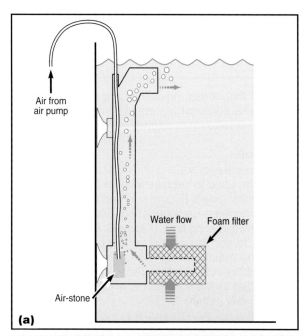

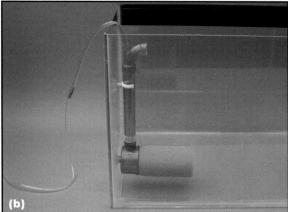

Figure 6.3 Foam filter. (a) These basic systems use a stream of fine air bubbles to draw water gently through the foam cartridge and through the uplift tube to the top of the aquarium. (b) A commercially produced foam filter is connected to an air pump by an airline. (© W.H. Wildgoose.)

Advantages

- Gentle water flow – ideal for tanks containing sick or young fish
- Inexpensive.

Disadvantages

- Inefficient in large tanks
- Unsightly.

Maintenance: Remove the foam every 2–3 weeks and clean in old aquarium water to remove excess debris.

Undergravel filter

Perforated plates are positioned beneath 5–8 cm of gravel (Figure 6.4). Water is drawn through the gravel and returned via an uplift tube by an air pump or power head (water pump). The gravel acts as a mechanical and biological filter, providing a very large surface area for colonization by nitrifying microorganisms.

Advantages

- Large surface area for biological activity
- Inexpensive.

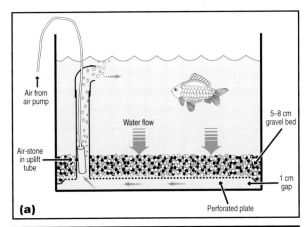

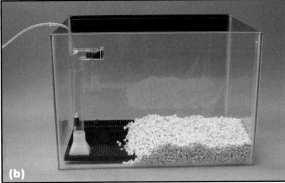

Figure 6.4 Undergravel filter. (a) Water is drawn through a gravel bed and into a void beneath the perforated plate by a current created from a stream of rising air bubbles in the uplift tube. (b) This commercially available unit has a small cartridge containing activated carbon at the top of the uplift tube. (© W.H. Wildgoose.)

Disadvantages

- Filter plates can be exposed by the digging activities of goldfish and cichlids
- Debris not removed from tank and can be disturbed by the digging activity of fish
- May adversely affect plant growth.

Maintenance: The debris collecting in the gravel should be removed using a gravel cleaner (Figure 6.5). It is advisable to remove debris from under the filter plates occasionally by siphoning through the uplift tube.

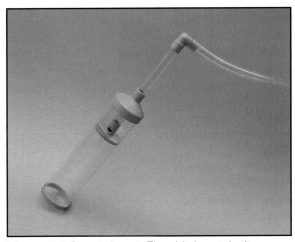

Figure 6.5 Gravel cleaner. The wide-bore tube is attached to a length of tubing and uses a siphon principle to remove light sediment and mulm from the bottom of the aquarium. This unit is self-priming and has a loose plastic flap that acts as a one-way valve. (© W.H. Wildgoose.)

Power filter

Water is drawn through a canister filled with a variety of filter media by means of an electrical pump (Figure 6.6). Depending on their design, canister filters may be located either in or outside the aquarium. The media should be positioned within the canister so that the water passes through the mechanical filter medium first, then the biological medium and finally any chemical medium (e.g. activated carbon or zeolite).

Advantages

- Powerful and efficient
- Easy to maintain
- Adjustable flow rate
- Ideal for large fish.

Disadvantages

- Unsightly inside aquaria
- Some models expensive to purchase.

Maintenance: Filter media should be rinsed in old aquarium water to remove the debris every 2–3 weeks. Activated carbon sachets, where used, must be changed every 2 months.

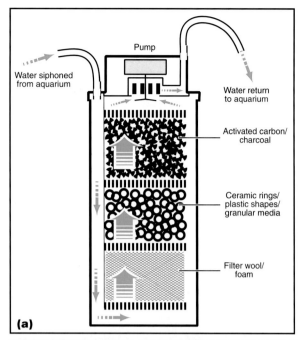

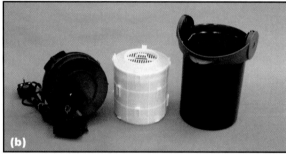

Figure 6.6 Power filter. (a) An electric pump draws water through the media. The inner compartments can be filled with one or more types of medium. (b) An external unit, disassembled to show the lid with integral pump, the three chambers for the filter media and the outer casing. (Courtesy of Wildwoods Ltd, © W.H. Wildgoose.)

Hang-on filters

The filter hangs on the outside of the aquarium (Figure 6.7), with water being pumped into the filter by an electric pump. These units are more popular and more widely available in the USA than in the UK.

Advantages

- Powerful and efficient
- Very easy to maintain
- Adjustable flow rate
- Ideal for large fish.

Disadvantages

- Unsightly
- Specially designed aquarium lid required.

Maintenance: Filter media should be rinsed in old aquarium water to remove the debris every 2–3 weeks. Some models use replacement filter media cartridges: to maintain adequate numbers of nitrifying microorganisms only one cartridge should be replaced at a time.

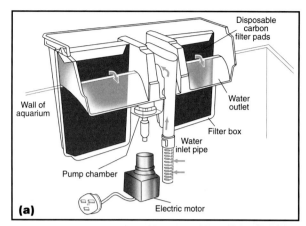

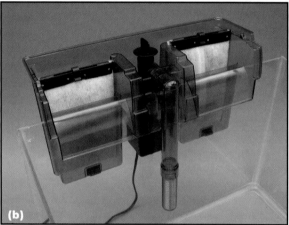

Figure 6.7 Hang-on filter. (a) The unit hooks on to the wall of the aquarium. Water is drawn up through the inlet pipe, into the pump chamber, then around the back into the filter box. Water permeates through the disposable carbon filter pads and returns to the tank over the outlet flap. (b) A double-chambered hang-on filter unit for home aquaria. (Courtesy of Tetra, © W.H. Wildgoose.)

Trickle (wet and dry) filters

The filter medium is not continually submerged (Figure 6.8), thereby improving the oxygen supply to the biological filter (see Chapter 7).

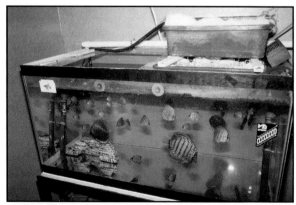

Figure 6.8 Trickle filter. Discus are often considered difficult fish and are frequently kept in sparsely furnished tanks. They require very specific and stable water conditions, namely soft acidic warm water. In this system, water is pumped into a homemade trickle filter that is situated above the main tank. (© W.H. Wildgoose.)

Advantages

- Very efficient
- Generally smaller than other filters for the same sized tank.

Disadvantage

- Some models expensive.

Maintenance: The foam or fibre matting at the inlet requires regular cleaning. Debris at the bottom of the unit may require occasional removal. Activated carbon sachets, where used, must be changed every 2 months.

Aquatic plants

The addition of plants to the aquarium greatly enhances its overall appearance, as well as performing a number of vital tasks. Healthy, growing plants will remove nutrients from the water, thus reducing or even eliminating algal problems. They also provide areas of retreat and shade for the fish.

The range of freshwater plants is very wide and not all are suitable for an aquarium. The plants originate from tropical areas of the world and, not surprisingly, require different water conditions (e.g. temperature, acidity or alkalinity and light intensity).

Before planting, it is advisable to trim back the root tips to encourage growth. The plants should not be allowed to dry out prior to planting and any decaying or torn leaves should be removed. Insufficient light or unsuitable conditions will result in poor plant growth.

A number of fish species (e.g. goldfish, tinfoil barbs, oscars) will consume or dig up the plants. The use of plastic plants is recommended with these species.

Captive species

The aquarium should be set up for 2–3 days before the first fish are added. About 500 varieties of tropical fish and 10 varieties of goldfish are commonly stocked by dealers (Figure 6.9).

Compatibility

Not all fish can be kept together and it is important to obtain information on their environmental requirements and tolerance of other species. Fish that have more or less the same requirements (Figure 6.10) should be kept together.

Goldfish

These fish are by far the most popular coldwater fish in aquaria across the world and are kept by both beginner and expert. The hardy varieties such as the comet, shubunkin and 'common' goldfish are ideal for anyone starting in the hobby, including children. More fancy varieties such as bubble-eye, ranchu and pearl-scale are more sensitive to poor conditions; they should be kept in larger aquaria, and not mixed with the more robust varieties.

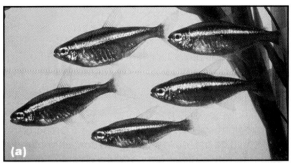
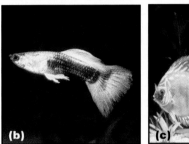
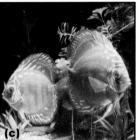
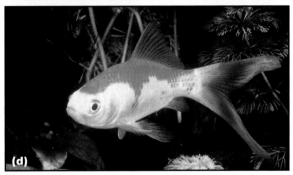

Figure 6.9 Common freshwater species suitable for home aquaria: (a) cardinal tetra; (b) guppy; (c) discus; (d) goldfish.

Group	Requirements		Species
	pH	General hardness (dH)	
Hardy fish with non-specific requirements	6.5–8.5	3–20	Rosy barb Tiger barb Siamese fighting fish *Corydoras* catfish Zebra danio Platy White cloud mountain minnow
Fish that prefer soft water conditions	6.0–7.5	0–5	Ram cichlid Pencilfish Cardinal tetra Neon tetra Suckermouth catfish Angelfish Dwarf gourami Discus Killifish
Fish that prefer hard water conditions	7.5–8.5	8–20	Guppy Black molly Swordtail Rainbow fish

Figure 6.10 Examples of fish that have similar requirements.

Selection and transport

When buying fish it is important to select only healthy specimens. Their appearance and behaviour in dealers' aquaria will provide clues to the health of the fish. Fish that show any lesions or abnormal behaviour should be avoided.

For transport, the fish should be packed into a sealed polyethylene bag containing one-third water and two-thirds air (or oxygen). During transport, the bag should be placed in a darkened container and not subject to any sudden temperature changes or jolts. On arrival, the bag should be floated in the aquarium for 20 minutes so that the water in the bag gradually adjusts to the temperature in the aquarium.

Stocking density

In a new aquarium, the first fish should be left for at least a week before any others are introduced. The stocking level can be increased to its maximum over the following 6–8 weeks.

The stocking density is largely influenced by the surface area of the water through which gas exchange can occur. The accepted rule for tropical fish is 2.5 cm of fish length (excluding tail fins) for every 72 cm^2 of water surface area. For goldfish, allow 144 cm^2 of water surface area for every 2.5 cm of fish length.

Overstocking or a rapid increase in the stocking level should be avoided since this can result in problems with poor water quality, commonly referred to as 'new tank syndrome' (Chapter 1).

Lifespan

The lifespan of aquarium fish varies considerably. For example, the typical lifespan of a killifish may be as little as 6–12 months; guppies, platies and other livebearing fish may live for 2–3 years; *Corydoras* catfish, angelfish and other cichlids may live for 4–6 years; whereas goldfish can live for up to 40 years.

The lifespan of aquarium fish is affected by the conditions in which they are kept and in particular by the water temperature: the higher the temperature, the shorter the lifespan.

Quarantine

New fish should be quarantined for 4 weeks in a separate aquarium before being added to the main tank. The quarantine tank need not be elaborate and can comprise a small aquarium (with a cover), fitted with a heater and foam filter. Keeping new fish in isolation enables observation and, if necessary, treatment with medications. Not all aquarists have a quarantine aquarium; in such cases, treatment with a general ectoparasite remedy should be added to the aquarium when the fish are introduced.

Nutrition

Removed from their natural environment and maintained under aquarium conditions, fish become dependent upon owners to provide them with a balanced diet. A good quality commercial food will provide a suitable balanced diet for most aquarium fish.

Quantity

Avoid overfeeding! The golden rule when feeding all aquarium fish is to feed 'little and often'. Fish should be fed two to four times per day with only as much food as is consumed within a few minutes. Any uneaten food should be removed, as it will decompose and may pollute the water.

The fish should rise eagerly to the surface at each feeding time. If not, they are probably being overfed or there are other problems within the aquarium. Small fish fry require more frequent feeds to ensure that they receive a constant supply of food for growth, but overfeeding must be avoided at all costs.

Variety

The overall benefits of feeding a nutritionally balanced diet will be seen in good health, vitality, coloration and resistance to disease. Coloration is worthy of special note, since fish cannot produce their own pigments but are dependent on colour enhancers contained in their diet.

The nutritional requirements of each species vary slightly. As community aquaria may contain 10–20 different species, it is advisable to use more than one food. For example, a staple food is an ideal basic diet for most tropical fish, but for herbivorous species this diet should be supplemented with a plant-based food.

The position where the fish feed in the water is also important. Surface-feeding fish should be given a flaked or floating stick food. Flaked foods will also slowly sink; they and slowly sinking granular foods are ideal for mid-water feeders. Bottom-dwelling fish need food that sinks, such as tablet foods.

The size of the food should be considered. Fry require a powdered diet whereas small and medium-sized fish need a flaked food. Larger individuals should be given a stick or pellet food.

Fresh foods

Live foods, although enjoyed by many fish, may introduce disease organisms into the aquarium. There are fewer risks associated with live foods of non-aquatic origin, such as earthworms and white worms (*Enchytraeus* spp.) or with cultured live foods. To eliminate any risk of disease, fish may occasionally be fed on frozen or freeze-dried foods.

Breeding

Most aquarium fish can be bred in captivity. Generally, this is on a small scale by specialist hobbyists, although a number of fish will breed in a normal 'community' aquarium. Live-bearing fish are relatively easy to breed and species such as guppies, swordtails, mollies and platies are very popular with new and young fish keepers because of the ease with which they will produce live young. Egg-laying species often require more specific conditions in which to breed. The young are often only 2–3 mm in length and are quickly eaten by other fish if breeding occurs in a community aquarium.

Breeding behaviour and the conditions necessary to encourage successful breeding of individual species are beyond the scope of this chapter (see Andrews, 1997).

Aquarium maintenance

Procedures

Once set up, an aquarium requires a minimum of care and attention to keep it looking attractive, and the fish and plants within it in the best of health. Without this basic maintenance, the aquarium can quickly degenerate into an unhealthy place for the fish to live and they will experience various health problems. The routine tasks involved are simple and are not time-consuming, but are essential for successful fish keeping.

Routine maintenance of an aquarium involves tasks that need to be undertaken either daily or every 2–3 weeks or only occasionally (Figure 6.11).

Daily	Every 2–3 weeks	Occasionally
Check fish numbers and behaviour	Measure water quality	Replace activated carbon
Feed fish	Remove algae from glass	Replace fluorescent tubes
Check water temperature	Perform partial water change	Check electrical equipment
Check filter and air pump	Clean out tank	Clean air pump valves
Turn lights off/on	Clean out filter	Clean condensation tray
	Trim plants	Remove dead plant leaves
		Thin out plants

Figure 6.11 Routine maintenance of freshwater aquaria.

Water quality

Regular measurement of water quality with a test kit will enable any problems within the aquarium to be detected and corrected before they adversely affect the fish or plants. When an aquarium is first established, hardness and pH values of both aquarium and tap water should be measured regularly in order to determine which species of fish can be kept. Thereafter the tap water should be tested before it is added to the aquarium, to ensure that it remains suitable. Ammonia, nitrite and nitrate should be tested at intervals of 2–3 weeks and preventive measures taken if the values exceed the safe limits. The maximum recommended levels for un-ionized ammonia and nitrite are 0.02 mg/l and 0.2 mg/l, respectively; nitrate levels should be no more than 50 mg/l above the level in tap water. The preferred levels of pH and hardness vary according to the species being kept.

Partial water changes

Once established, it is rarely necessary for an aquarium to be completely emptied and cleaned out. However, regular partial water changes and cleaning are important to ensure that the fish and plants remain healthy. Removing about 20–30% of the tank volume is sufficient. The fish can often be seen to be more active and show better coloration following the introduction of clean water. Adding fresh water to the aquarium dilutes any pollutants (e.g. nitrates, phosphates) that may be present. While the nitrate concentration within an

aquarium will rarely reach lethal levels, it can retard the growth and fin development of the fish and make them more lethargic even at relatively low levels (50 mg/l).

Removing water from the aquarium should be combined with a general clean up, particularly the removal of any debris or uneaten food. Using a gravel cleaner, any debris can be removed from the gravel without polluting the water. Regular use of a gravel cleaner prevents the gravel from becoming clogged with debris and allows the undergravel filter, if used, to function more efficiently. It is advisable occasionally to insert the siphon tube down the uplift tube of an undergravel filter and remove water from under the filter plates.

When replacing the water, it is important to ensure that it is at the same temperature and quality as the water in the aquarium. Large variations can stress the fish, making them more susceptible to infection and disease. The replacement water should always be treated with a proprietary water conditioner to remove any potentially harmful chlorine and metal ions.

Tap water contains some of the nutrients and trace elements found in natural waters but many are missing. To ensure that plants receive all of the nutrients they require to grow well, a good quality plant fertilizer can be added at each water change.

Cleaning

With the water level reduced during a partial water change, other routine maintenance tasks can be carried out. Algae can be removed from the aquarium glass using commercially available algae scrapers. Only the front glass of the aquarium needs cleaning. A small quantity of algal growth on the back and sides not only looks natural but also provides valuable food for herbivorous fish and removes large quantities of nitrates from the water. Where the algal growth is excessive, it can be controlled using an algicide. Heavy growth of algae should be partially removed using a scraper and siphoned out before any treatment is added. Following use of an algicide, any dead algae should be removed after 5–7 days. Recurrent algal growth in the aquarium suggests incorrect maintenance such as overfeeding, too much light or too few live plants.

Any debris in the filter unit should be removed. The filter medium in canister or foam filters should be removed and rinsed in old aquarium water. Tap water should not be used because the residual levels of chlorine present may kill many of the nitrifying microorganisms, thus reducing the effectiveness of the biological filter. When cleaning media, the aim is to remove the excess debris without removing the microorganisms; therefore a quick gentle wash is adequate.

Plant maintenance

Aquarium lights should be left on for 10–12 hours each day to encourage healthy plant growth. The plants grow at different rates and it will be necessary to prune the faster growing species. Removing the top 5–8 cm of plants with stems encourages lateral shoots and produces a more bushy growth. This can be done at any time but is easier when the water level is reduced during a partial water change. This also allows the removal of any dead leaves, which not only look unsightly but also decompose and adversely affect the water quality.

To ensure that the aquarium light reaches the plants, it is important to keep the condensation tray as clean as possible. Any dirt or algae on the tray may absorb certain wavelengths of light and reduce plant growth.

Holidays

Adult fish can be left for several days without any food. During such times they will consume algae and other material in the aquarium, as well as relying on their body fat reserves. This can be supplemented by 'holiday food sticks', which break down slowly, releasing food for the fish to consume. By using these 'holiday foods' or the automatic feeders that are available, an aquarium can safely be left for 10–14 days without supervision. During such periods the filter will continue to function by removing particulate matter and pollutants from the water. If plants are present, then the lighting should be operated by a time switch to keep them healthy.

Common health problems

Most health problems in tropical or coldwater fish are not new and in many cases are linked to a basic failure in maintenance, which can be easily corrected. Poor water quality accounts for the majority of problems, either directly (e.g. high levels of metabolic wastes caused by overstocking or by a rapid increase in stocking density) or indirectly (e.g. poor water quality causing stress and making fish more susceptible to disease). Figure 6.12 provides details of the most common problems encountered by coldwater or tropical fish keepers.

Clinical sign	Cause
White spots on skin	'White spot' (*Ichthyophthirius*) Nuptial tubercles
White cotton wool-like growth on skin	*Saprolegnia* (secondary to poor water quality)
Very small white spots on skin	'Freshwater velvet' (*Piscinoodinium*)
Colour change	Poor water quality Old age (goldfish) *Mycobacterium*
'Fin rot'	Bacterial disease (secondary to poor water quality)
Excess mucus	Ectoparasites Poor water quality
Skin ulceration	*Aeromonas* *Pseudomonas* *Mycobacteria*
Swollen abdomen	Polycystic kidneys (in goldfish) Gravid female Internal neoplasia
Buoyancy problems	Swim-bladder disorder Gastrointestinal tympany Internal neoplasia CNS lesion
Anorexia	Disease Poor water quality Inappropriate diet

Figure 6.12 Common disorders of freshwater aquarium fish.

Andrews C (1986) *A Fishkeeper's Guide to Fancy Goldfishes*. Salamander Books, London

Andrews C (1997) *A Fishkeeper's Guide to Fish Breeding*. Salamander Books, London

Andrews C and Baensch U (1991) *Tropical Aquarium Fish – Comprehensive Edition*. Tetra Press, Melle, Germany

Gratzek JB and Mathews JR (eds) (1992) *Aquariology – The Science of Fish Health Management*. Tetra Press, Melle, Germany

Mills D and Vevers G (1982) *The Practical Encyclopaedia of Freshwater Tropical Aquarium Fishes*. Salamander Books, London

Sandford G and Crow R (1993) *The Manual of Tank Busters*. Salamander Books, London

Further reading

Adey WH and Loveland K (1991) *Dynamic Aquaria: Building Living Ecosystems*. Academic Press, London

Acknowledgement

The author is very grateful to Tetra for assistance in the production of this chapter and the supply of illustrations.

7

Marine aquaria

Dick Mills

The marine aquarium hobby is the newest and therefore the smallest area of fish keeping. It is also one of the fastest growing and requires the highest technical skill from its participants.

Success is aided by the reliability of modern equipment, together with the increasing numbers of fish arriving in good health from distant collection points around the world. Although the majority of fish are still wild-caught, the number of species being raised in captivity is increasing, which ensures that natural stocks are put at less risk.

Tanks

Construction

One of the greatest obstacles to marine fish keeping in past years was the inability of aquaria to withstand the corrosive effects of salt water. The tanks were usually of metal-frame construction with glass panels held in place by putty. The metal frames were soon corroded and it was not until the introduction of 'all-glass' aquaria that this problem was solved. Today's aquarium can be all-glass or of extruded or moulded acrylic material; neither type is affected by salt water.

Due to the number of filtration components, it is common for the marine aquarium to be housed in a cabinet so that the water purification equipment can be kept out of sight and yet in close proximity to the tank (Figures 7.1 and 7.2). The wood finish should be resistant to salt spray, as many inexpensive veneers may become damaged. More sophisticated systems may be custom built by specialist companies (Figure 7.3).

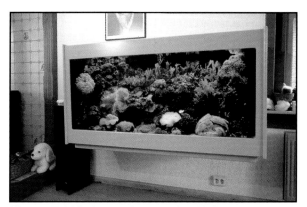

Figure 7.1 Modern marine aquaria with fish and invertebrates require efficient filtration systems to maintain good water quality. (© Bill Tomey.)

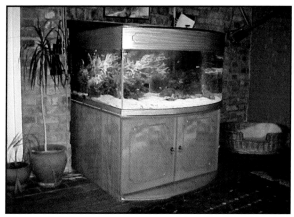

Figure 7.2 A modern marine aquarium housed in a wooden cabinet that conceals a compact filtration system below the tank. (Courtesy of Aquarium Rentals.)

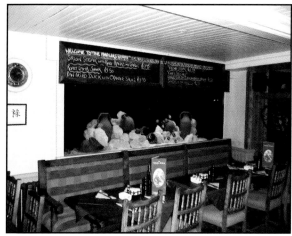

Figure 7.3 A large custom-built display tank in a restaurant. Impressive systems such as this are often designed and maintained by professional companies on a contract basis. (Courtesy of Aquarium Rentals.)

Heating

Most hobby marine fish come from tropical waters and the water in the aquarium must be maintained at around 25°C, using a heater and thermostat. An accurate thermometer should be used to warn of loss of heat through power failure, or overheating from a faulty thermostat or heater. Suitable and reliable equipment is readily available from aquatic suppliers. Fish from temperate climates, collected from the local seashore, may require the use of cooling equipment.

Lighting

Lighting depends on the type of aquarium. In 'fish-only' collections, with tank decoration consisting of dead skeletal corals and rocks, a simple system using one or two fluorescent tubes will suffice. For a mixed collection with fish, live invertebrates and live corals, more powerful lighting is required: often twice as many fluorescent tubes are needed to maintain beneficial live algae that grow within coral and the bodies of some invertebrates.

The colour spectrum of lamps is also important and the use of actinic lamps brings the necessary blue and ultraviolet wavelengths required for invertebrate growth. Where deep tanks are used, with water depths over 38 cm, fluorescent tubes may not be powerful enough and metal-halide or mercury discharge lamps are more useful.

The standard photoperiod should be between 12 and 14 hours per day. Shorter or longer photoperiods result in the growth of nuisance algae and may be stressful to some fish.

Water management

Unlike their freshwater counterparts, marine fish do not come from a variety of waters and the composition of their water is usually stable. This means that the marine fish is completely intolerant of changes in water quality and so the fish keeper must learn to maintain water conditions within very close tolerances at all times.

Salinity

Modern synthetic salt mixtures provide excellent water quality, are readily available and are easy to use. It is preferable to use a de-ionizer, a reverse osmosis unit or nitrate-removing resin to purify household tap water for preparing the sea water. Salinity is expressed in grams per litre (g/l) or parts per thousand (ppt). However, it is usually measured with an aquarium-calibrated hydrometer to ensure that the specific gravity (SG) of the resulting water is correct – generally between 1.020 and 1.025. Special calibrated refractometers and conductivity meters can also be used.

Water quality

The quality of the water will deteriorate after living organisms are placed in it. A good guide to evaluating this is by checking the pH regularly. Normally, sea water has a pH value of around 8.3 or higher. A steadily falling pH is a sign that a partial water change is due. This involves replacing 10–20% of the aquarium water with new, pre-mixed 'sea water'.

The main priority in maintaining water quality is the control of toxic substances in the water. These are nitrogenous metabolic waste products of the fish and invertebrates, and breakdown of uneaten food due to overfeeding. Ammonia and nitrites should ideally measure 0 mg/l. Nitrate levels should be less than 20 mg/l in a fish-only tank and less than 5 mg/l if invertebrates are present.

Filtration systems

Water filtration in marine aquaria uses four methods of water purification:

- Mechanical – removes suspended material with fine foam
- Chemical – adsorbs materials by using activated carbon
- Biological – converts ammonia to progressively less toxic nitrite and nitrate by bacterial action (in advanced systems, further anaerobic bacterial action may be used to convert nitrate back into free nitrogen)
- Foam fractionation – removes organic matter from the water by 'protein-skimming'.

Mechanical, chemical and foam fractionation all work instantly upon installation. Biological filtration performance depends on the prior establishment of bacteria and takes several weeks or months before it becomes fully active. It is sensitive to any overload, therefore livestock levels must be built up gradually so that the biological filter keeps in step with the workload.

During the establishment of the biological filter, nitrite levels rise and then fall after 2 or 3 weeks. Only when nitrite is at a consistently low level (hopefully zero) is it safe to introduce fish into the aquarium. This establishment period can be shortened by introducing one or two hardy, inexpensive, nitrite-tolerant fish (such as damselfish and clownfish) to produce the necessary metabolic wastes for the colonies of bacteria. Alternatively, the filter can be seeded with some substrate from an already established aquarium or by using a commercially produced bacterial culture. The rate of flow of water through a filter system should be approximately three times the total tank volume per hour.

Several different filtration systems, utilizing one or more of the above methods, are used in marine aquaria. The principles and design of some are explained in Chapters 5 and 6.

Undergravel filters

Undergravel filters work on the biological principle. Those driven by air pumps are not ideal for marine tanks, due to their low flow rates, but a submersible water pump (powerhead) fitted to the uplift pipe will improve the flow through the gravel and provide the strong water currents required by many fish and invertebrates.

A new technology is the use of 'live sand' or variations of the Jaubert system (Figure 7.4), especially in reef systems. A static anaerobic body of water is held beneath the substrate (the plenum) into which oxygen diffuses downwards through the substrate, sustaining nitrifying bacterial colonies. Some denitrification (from nitrate back to nitrogen) will occur in the plenum, thus completing the 'nitrogen cycle'.

Power filters

Self-contained external canister units are very efficient and available for all aquarium sizes. They can be filled with various media, including filter wool, ceramic shapes and activated carbon. They are being increasingly used in conjunction with protein skimming and live rock to form a complete filtration system.

Trickle filters

These modern filter units employ a 'wet and dry' system (Figure 7.5) and are up to 20 times more effective than undergravel filters.

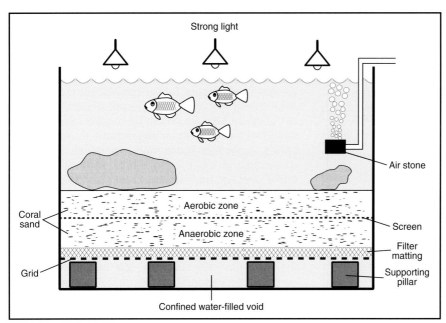

Figure 7.4 'Live sand' filtration system. A layer of calcareous sand 8–10 cm thick is supported 2 cm above a confined body of water by a grid covered in a thin layer of fibre matting. A screen below the surface of the sand prevents disturbance by fish and turbulence. Strong illumination and constant aeration are essential. (Redrawn after Jaubert, 1989.)

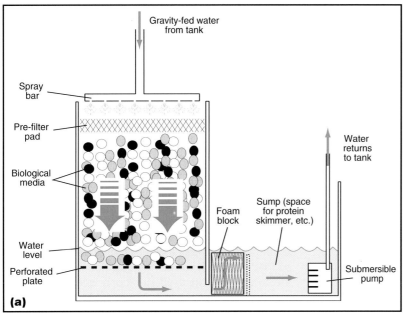

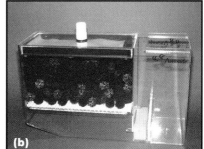

Figure 7.5 (a) A trickle filter system. This is positioned beneath the tank to allow water to gravitate through the spray bar and prefilter pad. Water trickles through the medium into the sump and is then pumped back into the aquarium. (b) A ready-made trickle filter for home aquaria. (Courtesy of Class 1 Koi. © W.H. Wildgoose.)

Sand filters

A more efficient method of biological filtration is provided by the external 'fluidized-bed' system in which the bacterial substrate (usually silica sand) is held in suspension within a column of upwardly flowing water, thus maximizing bacterial numbers.

Accessories

Ultraviolet (UV) units: These help to control algae and some waterborne pathogens by UV irradiation. To perform effectively, the UV tubes must be replaced regularly.

Protein skimmer: This mechanical device removes waste substances by 'air stripping' or foam fractionation. It produces a large water/air interface that attracts waste molecules, creating a scum or foam that rises to the surface (Figure 7.6).

Ozone: This gas-sterilizing agent is produced by an electric generator (Figure 7.7). Since ozone is highly toxic to fish and invertebrates, it must not enter the main tank and is usually linked to the protein skimmer. Ozone is also harmful to humans (see Chapter 34).

Redox: The redox (reduction–oxidation) value is defined as a measure of the ability of a system to eliminate waste, but in practical terms it is the ability of the aquarium water to conduct electricity and is measured in millivolts (mV). A healthy aquarium would typically show a reading of around 350 mV but this will vary according to the time of day and the effects of feeding, water changes and adding new fish.

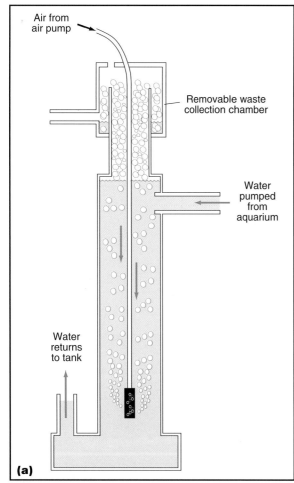

Air from air pump

Removable waste collection chamber

Water pumped from aquarium

Water returns to tank

(a)

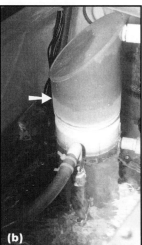

(b)

Figure 7.6 (a) A counter-current protein skimmer. Water is pumped into the unit against the flow of rising air bubbles. Organic matter binds to the surface of the bubbles to produce a foam that collects in the chamber at the top.
(b) A venturi-type protein skimmer in the sump of a trickle filter, showing the reservoir (arrowed) with proteinaceous waste. (Courtesy of Aquarium Rentals. © W.H. Wildgoose.)

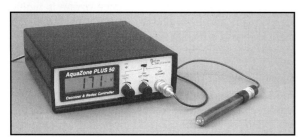

Figure 7.7 A modern ozone generator with oxygen reduction potential (ORP) controller. The platinum redox electrode requires periodic cleaning and calibration. (Courtesy of Interpet. © W.H. Wildgoose.)

Captive species

The domestic home aquarium contains specimens that are captured in shallow waters around the coral reefs in tropical seas. Certain precautions need to be exercised to ensure that a compatible collection is established. For example, different species exhibiting extremes of size would not be a good choice. Similarly, fish that prey upon invertebrate life (sedentary corals as well as more mobile animals) should be excluded from a collection, though separate 'species tanks' are not uncommon. Latest trends appear to favour the more modest-sized species, with particular emphasis on clownfish, damselfish, gobies and blennies (Figure 7.8).

One area of disappointment to many newcomers is that not all fish offered for sale are entirely suitable for the aquarium. For example, the butterflyfish group contains several members that are specialized feeders in the extreme, and whose dietary requirements cannot be provided in captivity, with the result that such fish starve to death. Other species, such as the sea-horse, may fail to acclimatize to aquarium conditions. The sea-horse is under threat from collectors in the curio and medical trades and there is a distinct possibility that some species may soon become endangered.

Compatibility

If the collection of fish is to remain stable then compatibility between species is vital. Unlike some freshwater species, it is uncommon to find shoals of marine fish being kept in the home aquarium. Many species are intolerant of their own kind, except when coming together to breed, and even of other species that are similar in shape and colour. Territorial disputes are likely to be frequent and violent if not enough hiding places are available within the aquarium. Such disputes inevitably occur when introducing new fish into an established collection and the remedy is to re-arrange the tank decor slightly before the introduction, so that every fish will be so busy 'house-hunting' that the newcomer is ignored. Another peace-keeping ploy is to feed the existing fish population at one end of the tank whilst introducing the new fish (perhaps with the tank lights subdued) at the other.

Lifespan

Lifespan is often proportional to size but knowledge about the natural lifespan of species commonly held in captivity is still very limited. Under ideal conditions, sea-horses may live for up to 3 years, puffers up to 8 years, surgeonfish to 10 years and clownfish to 12 years.

Stocking levels

The stocking density for marine fish is considerably lower than for freshwater fish. A common formula recommends 2.5 cm of fish length per 9 litres after the first year, when the system has matured. For example, in a tank measuring 90 cm × 38 cm × 30 cm and holding 90 litres of water, a total body length of approximately 25 cm is recommended, representing six 4 cm or four 6 cm fish.

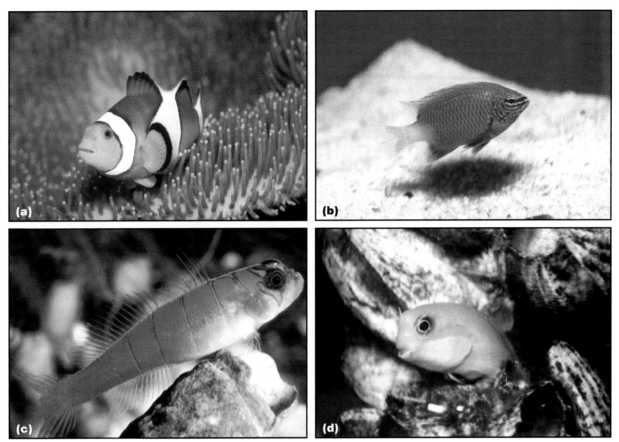

Figure 7.8 Various commonly kept species: (a) common clownfish; (b) yellow-tailed damselfish; (c) Catalina goby; (d) Midas blenny. (Courtesy of: Manor Aquatics; Home Marine; Tetra; Class 1 Koi.)

Due to the delicate balance that must be maintained in providing optimal water conditions at all times, the total fish-holding capacity of the tank can only be achieved over a relatively long period of time. The above example is the theoretical maximum; allowance must also be given for growth and only half this stocking density should be used for the first 6 months. In mixed tanks containing fish and invertebrates, only one-third of this density should be used.

Nutrition

Marine fish fall into the same three feeding categories as their freshwater counterparts: carnivores, herbivores and omnivores. Providing the required diets is not difficult: specialist foods are available as flakes, wafers or tablets. Previously, live foods such as shellfish, small fish and crustaceans were used but, to prevent the introduction of disease-carrying organisms, these are also readily available as gamma-irradiated frozen or freeze-dried foods.

It is important to know to which category each species belongs and also how it feeds. Many species, especially tangs and surgeonfish, are herbivorous grazers and their tank should contain ample growths of green algae; failing this, their diet must be supplemented with vegetable matter, including peas and scalded lettuce or spinach leaves (briefly dipped into boiling water to break down indigestible leaf cellulose).

Bottom-dwelling fish such as gobies and blennies should be fed with fast-sinking foods, since intercepting midwater-feeding fish will deny them their food. Consideration must also be given to nocturnal feeding species, with suitable food being given just after the aquarium lights have been turned off.

NEVER OVERFEED. Any uneaten food will pollute the aquarium. Only give as much food as will be readily consumed within a few minutes, twice daily. During holiday periods it is often preferable and safer to leave the fish unfed for up to 2 weeks than to ask an inexperienced neighbour to feed them.

Breeding

Due to the lack of space, many marine fish will not breed in captivity. In nature, their eggs are generally scattered and fertilized at the top of a spiralling chase through the water column. Fortunately, some species follow the example of some freshwater species, laying and subsequently guarding their eggs in selected locations. Since these fish are also of more modest proportions, they often form a popular core of interest for the marine fish keeper. These are the species whose young have been raised successfully in captivity and include the clownfish, damselfish, gobies and blennies. Other species may well breed in the aquarium but raising the fry to maturity has usually been unsuccessful, due to an inability to provide enough suitable first foods for the young.

Disease prevention

Attention to aquarium hygiene, modest stocking levels and quarantining of all new stock will do much to avoid stress and disease in the aquarium.

When buying fish, select only those that are brightly coloured and with well defined colour patterns. They should swim without effort and be able to maintain a steady position in the water. Check fins for splits. The skin and scales should be free of spots and wounds. Fish from a tank containing sick or dead fish must be avoided. The fish should be taking food readily. Most marine fish die in captivity because they are not provided with the correct diet.

A low-maintenance dose of a copper-based treatment can be used in fish-only systems. An accurate test kit should be used to monitor the copper levels and avoid toxic levels being reached. Activated carbon can be used to remove the chemical from the water at a later date.

The use of ozone and UV units may control some pathogenic organisms in the environment. True cleaner wrasse can be used to control ectoparasites on the gills and skin, although this diminishing diet may not be enough to make them a viable long-term addition in an aquarium of healthy fish.

Maintenance

Procedures

Constant monitoring and developing a routine maintenance schedule (Figure 7.9) are the keys to success with marine fish:

- The best time to do a head-count is at feeding time. Any missing fish should be located without delay, since a sick or dead fish may infect or pollute the aquarium
- Knowledge of each fish's normal behavioural characteristics is essential so that abnormalities can be identified immediately. Unlike freshwater species, some marine fish swim with their fins held close to the body: this is a normal characteristic, not an indication of disease
- Check the pH value and salinity of the water on a regular basis. Measure ammonia, nitrite and nitrate levels every 2 weeks in an established system, and every 2–3 days in new tanks. Ensure that the test kits are suitable for salt water
- Check the temperature regularly. If a heater fails, the tank will retain most of its heat for several hours while the repairs are made
- Remove algal growth from the front glass of the tank and keep cover-glasses scrupulously clean to make efficient use of all available light. Some algal growth should be left on the rear and side walls and aquarium decor for the benefit of herbivorous species
- Filter maintenance should be limited to periodic rinsing (in some aquarium water) of foam filter medium. This should be carried out on a rotational and partial basis when soiled: only half the medium should be washed at any one time, in order to preserve some of the bacterial colonies. Activated carbon should be renewed

	Daily	Weekly	Periodically (every 2–3 weeks)	Monthly	If fish are ill
General					
Check temperature	✓				✓
Count number of fish	✓				✓
Check air supply	✓				✓
Clean air pump valves and air filter			✓		✓
Remove algae from front glass			✓		
Check for signs of illness, bullying or overcrowding	✓				✓
Water quality					
Check ammonia, nitrite, nitrate, pH and specific gravity	✓ for first few weeks		✓		✓
Perform 20% water change			✓		✓
Filters					
External box: clean foam media		✓			
Replace foam medium on rotational basis to preserve bacteria				✓	
Undergravel filter: rake gravel gently to maintain water flow			✓		
Fluidized-bed filter: ensure water flow from outlet is well aerated before return to aquarium	✓				
Lighting					
Renew fluorescent tubes as necessary					
Clean cover glass				✓	

Figure 7.9 Routine maintenance schedule for marine aquaria.

every 2 months. Where biological filtration is provided by means of an undergravel bed, periodic raking of the substrate and use of a gravel-cleaner will ensure adequate water flow through the bed. External fluidized-bed filters will produce oxygen-deficient water at their outlet and so some form of aeration of this water should be provided before it returns to the main tank

- Empty the collecting cup on top of the protein skimmer regularly
- Partial water changes (20%) should be carried out every 2 weeks. This routine replaces trace elements and removes accumulated waste products. Replacement synthetic sea water should be made up in advance, so that it can be aerated and brought up to required temperature prior to use. To replace evaporation losses, only use fresh water (preferably distilled) since water alone will have evaporated; the salts remain in solution, therefore the specific gravity should always be monitored.

Common health problems

Fish health problems invariably occur and prevention rather than cure is desirable. The aquarium conditions and water quality parameters must always be checked when health problems are suspected. Diseases are often triggered by stress and abrupt changes in conditions, such as the introduction of new fish. Many diseases can be identified from external clinical signs and it is far better to treat early, before the disease becomes too advanced. Various common diseases in marine fish are listed in Figure 7.10.

Clinical sign	Cause
White spots on skin	Marine 'white spot' (*Cryptocaryon irritans*)
Very small spots on skin	Marine velvet (*Amyloodinium ocellatum*)
Respiratory distress	Low dissolved oxygen Parasitic disease
'Fin rot'	Bacterial infection
Excess mucus	Ectoparasitic disease Following trauma
Skin ulcerations	*Vibrio* *Mycobacteria* *Aeromonas*
Septicaemia	*Vibrio*
Head and lateral line erosion ('hole in the head')	Poor water quality? Nutritional deficiency? Viral infection
Wasting/emaciation	Mycobacteria
Exophthalmos ('pop-eye')	Bacterial disease? Poor handling injury
Small skin nodules	Lymphocystis

Figure 7.10 Common diseases of marine fish.

Medication

It may be best to remove sick fish to a separate treatment tank if medication is to be used, since some remedies are harmful to the nitrifying bacteria in biological filter systems. However, this may be stressful to sick fish and there may be a need to treat parasite stages found in the environment.

Activated carbon must be removed from the filtration system before dosing, since it adsorbs some therapeutic chemicals. Similarly, the UV and ozone units must be switched off during medication. When treating fish in a separate tank, water conditions in the treatment tank should be stabilized so that they are similar to those in the main tank before the fish are returned.

Correct dosing with medications is vitally important; underdosing will not effect a cure and overdosing might kill the fish. Many remedies are copper-based and fatal to invertebrates: they should not be used in mixed collections.

Some protozoan ectoparasites can be treated with a freshwater bath. Bathing an affected fish in fresh water for 3–10 minutes (less if the fish shows signs of distress) is usually sufficient.

Need for experience

At one time it was thought that marine fish keepers needed first to serve an 'apprenticeship' in the freshwater hobby for some years. Whilst any practical experience of fish keeping is bound to provide some beneficial advantage, it is only an appreciation of how the marine aquarium works that will guarantee success in the long term.

Modern marine aquaria are entirely reliable, provided that both the workings and the responsibilities involved are clearly understood. There are many books written for the marine hobbyist by knowledgeable authors; they should be mandatory reading before starting to keep these beautiful creatures. It is vital to know which species are unlikely to survive in captivity, and to avoid purchasing those captured by unscrupulous methods or those threatened with extinction.

Further reading

Bassleer G (1996) *Diseases in Marine Aquarium Fish*. Bassleer Biofish, Westmeerbeek

Dakin N (1992) *The Book of the Marine Aquarium*. Salamander Books, London

Fenner RM (1998) *The Conscientious Marine Aquarist*. Microcosm, Shelburne

Fosså SA and Nilsen AJ (1996) *The Modern Coral Reef Aquarium*, Vol. 1. Birgit Schmettkamp Verlag, Bornheim

Hall S (2001) *Understanding Marine Fish*. Interpet Publishing, Dorking

Jaubert J (1989) An integrated nitrifying–denitrifying biological system capable of purifying seawater in a closed circuit aquarium. *Bulletin of the Institute of Oceanography* **5**, 101–106

Mills D (2001) *Essential Guide to choosing your Marine Tropical Fish*. Interpet Publishing, Dorking

Mills D (2001) *Practical Guide to setting up your Marine Tropical Aquarium*. Interpet Publishing, Dorking

Moe MA Jr (1992) *The Marine Aquarium Reference: Systems and Invertebrates*. Green Turtle Publications, Plantation

Spotte S (1979) *Seawater Aquariums: the Captive Environment*. Wiley Interscience, New York

Tullock JH (1997) *Natural Reef Aquariums*. Microcosm, Shelburne.

8

Public aquaria

Ian D.F. Walker and Brent R. Whitaker

Modern public aquaria typically hold thousands of fish of many different species. This great diversity poses many challenges for veterinarians responsible for the health management of these collections. Apart from wide variations in the fishes' anatomy, physiology, environmental needs and disease processes, veterinarians are also faced with the complexities of aquatic life support systems and water chemistry. In addition, they must understand how medical treatments can affect exhibits and the husbandry staff that maintain them.

Life support systems

Aquatic animals have evolved a variety of physiological mechanisms that enable them to thrive in their specific environmental niches. Fish in captivity must be provided with artificial habitats in which critical environmental parameters are effectively reproduced and maintained. New fish introduced into a tank may die rapidly if conditions are inadequate. More often, suboptimal conditions cause stress, which may subsequently lead to increases in disease prevalence and mortality. Public aquaria attempt to reproduce many different habitats for their diverse collections, often on a huge scale, with some tanks containing several million litres of water and a multitude of species (Figure 8.1). Understanding the life support systems used to create and maintain these habitats is essential to the successful management and outcome of medical cases.

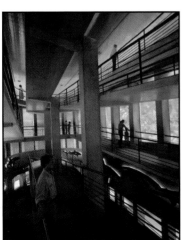

Figure 8.1 This Atlantic coral reef exhibit contains 1.2 million litres and incorporates a spiral ramp for visitors through its centre. Its inhabitants include Caribbean fish, invertebrates and stingrays. (© National Aquarium in Baltimore.)

Open systems

The water chemistry of oceans, lakes and rivers is often stable because of the vast volumes of water involved and the currents, tides and other factors that help to maintain their uniformity. Aquaria with open or 'flow-through' systems utilize this stability by drawing from large natural bodies of water and passing this water through the tanks before returning it to the original source. The advantages of open systems include:

* Natural water that continually has the correct ratio of chemical, biological and physical properties necessary for fish health
* Low or negligible concentrations of metabolic wastes
* Natural tank decoration by waterborne organisms (e.g. anemone and coral larvae)
* Relatively low maintenance costs.

Disadvantages include:

* Possible introduction of diseases and disease vectors, pollutants and unwanted organisms (e.g. algae)
* Restrictions on location (must be close to the water source to be cost effective)
* Possible limitations on chemical tank treatments because of pollution hazards when water is returned to the natural environment.

Closed systems

Closed systems (Figures 8.2 and 8.3) are more complex and often costly to operate and maintain. Marine water must either be imported from distant natural bodies or be synthesized using standard commercial or in-house methods. Once introduced into the exhibit tanks, the water is filtered and recirculated by filter systems that must be of the correct size and properly maintained. Frequent water quality monitoring and periodic water changes are essential for these systems to operate successfully.

Filtration methods

Both open and closed systems may use one or more of the following filtration methods.

Mechanical filtration

Suspended particles are physically removed from the water by a filter medium such as sand or floss. However, these filters may harbour infectious organisms. Complete disinfection of a system will require the filter medium to be replaced with new material.

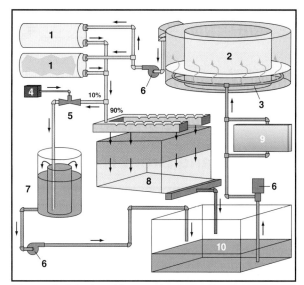

Figure 8.2 A closed-loop recirculating filtration system used by the National Aquarium in Baltimore: (1) sand filters, (2) exhibit tank, (3) undergravel filter, (4) ozone generating equipment, (5) venturi gas injector, (6) pumps, (7) ozone contact chamber, (8) bio-filtration, (9) heat exchanger and (10) sump. (Courtesy of Andy Aiken.)

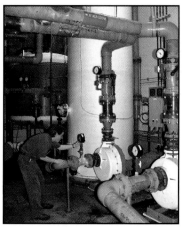

Figure 8.3 This picture illustrates the scale of the life support systems needed to support the exhibit in Figure 8.1. The large white tower in the background is an ozone contact chamber and the blue tower is a sand filter. (© Ian Walker.)

Biological filtration

Aquaria using recirculated water depend on active biological filters to maintain good water quality. Two types of biological filter are used in public aquaria: undergravel filters and trickle or wet-dry filter systems.

Biological filters can become disrupted in several ways, including sudden increases in stocking densities, decaying organic matter and exposure to certain antibacterial agents (e.g. tetracyclines, aminoglycosides, potentiated sulphonamides).

Chemical filtration

Chemical filtration refers to the removal of dissolved organic compounds from the water column. Public aquaria use several forms of chemical filtration successfully.

WARNING: All of the following must be disabled or removed before addition of any medications.

Ozone: Ozone is a powerful oxidizing agent. The safest method of administration is to inject it into ozone contact chambers or foam fractionators where it reduces nitrogenous waste, destroys potential pathogenic organisms and removes suspended organic materials from the water column. Contact time and dosage must be regulated carefully.

Residual ozone in the water can be dangerous to fish and plants and should be monitored with an oxidation-reduction potential (ORP) meter and alarm system. Excess residual ozone in the system can be detected when ORP levels approach 500 mV, or if there is a distinct ozone smell and crystal-clear water. Clinical signs of ozone exposure include respiratory distress, lethargy, incoordination and sudden death.

Prior to treating water with organic compounds, sufficient time should be allowed for venting after disabling ozone production.

Foam fractionation: Foam fractionation, or 'protein-skimming', is a method of chemically filtering dissolved organic compounds, proteins and fatty acids from the water by adsorption. Either air or ozone can be used; the latter greatly enhances the efficiency of the protein skimmer.

Activated carbon: Removal of undesirable organic compounds by activated carbon will improve water quality. The type and grade of carbon filter must be matched to the type and size of the system. Periodic changes of carbon are necessary for the filter to work effectively. After completion of treatments, fresh carbon can be added to facilitate the removal of medications from the water system.

Ultraviolet sterilization: Ultraviolet (UV) radiation is an effective method of water disinfection in aquaria. The high-intensity lights must be in close proximity to the water and have sufficient contact time.

Water quality

Excellent water quality and appropriate environmental parameters are critical to fish health (see Chapter 1) and should be routinely monitored. The range of acceptable values for these parameters varies, depending on the species and, in some cases, the age and health of individual fish.

Temperature

- Some species are more sensitive to temperature fluctuations
- The temperature of an aquarium system should be relatively constant and maintained within the appropriate range for the species.

pH

- In the wild, freshwater fish and invertebrates live within pH 5.0–9.0
- All marine fish and invertebrates must be maintained within pH 7.8–8.3
- Regular monitoring is essential
- pH may decrease over time in closed systems as natural buffers are utilized.

Salinity

- The salinity of an aquarium system should be maintained within the appropriate range for the species
- Salinity increases slowly in closed systems due to evaporation
- Marine fish with osmotic stress from gill or skin lesions may benefit from decreased salinity to 20–25 ppt
- Freshwater species with osmotic stress may benefit from increased salinity
- Any changes should be gradual, over a period of several hours.

Dissolved oxygen

- Should be maintained at levels close to saturation
- Water should be de-gassed before re-entering the tank, by spraying or using a gravity-return trickle filter
- Fish that die from hypoxia often have flared opercula
- Supersaturation can cause gas emboli.

Ammonia, nitrite and nitrate

- Fully functional and operational filtration systems should have no detectable trace of ammonia or nitrite
- Nitrate can accumulate in closed systems and interfere with osmoregulation. Regular water changes ensure no significant build-up over time.

Lighting and noise

Photoperiod, light spectrum and light intensity play major roles in the physiology of aquatic animals. Because public aquaria often conduct activities such as visitor events or construction during evening hours, disruption of photoperiod can occur. During such activities, displays containing sensitive fish should be shielded with light-tight materials.

Noise may have an impact on fish and should be kept to a minimum. Noise pollution can come from pumps, filtration equipment, other machinery and the general public.

Nutrition

Providing the correct diets, especially in exhibits of mixed species, can be challenging. Most of the nutritional research for aquatic animals has centred on commonly cultured commercial species (e.g. salmonids, shellfish); little is known, for example, about the nutritional requirements of tropical marine fish. Some general aspects of nutrition are covered in Chapter 28 but specific issues relating to larger species are discussed here.

Veterinarians must develop a nutritional plan based upon available nutritional data, personal experience, and the fishes' natural history, anatomy and physiology. Even the most nutritionally complete diet will be of little value if fish are unable or unwilling to consume it.

A variety of foods is generally provided in multiple species exhibits and diets typically include combinations of commercial pellets and flake foods, gelatin preparations, fish, grass shrimp, brine shrimp, clams, squid, algae, blackworms and vegetables.

Feeding regime

Foods must be of excellent quality. Proper storage and preparation are vital to the preservation of nutritional value.

- Frozen foods should be thawed slowly in a refrigerator and removed from it shortly before feeding, to prevent spoilage
- Gelatin foods are easy to prepare and can be stored frozen. Once thawed, they can be grated into different sizes and fed with minimal leaching of nutrients into the water. Oral medications can be added to the mixture
- Fresh green vegetables (e.g. broccoli, Romaine lettuce) are often fed to herbivorous fish (iceberg lettuce should be avoided – it has little nutritional value). Adequate refrigeration is needed to store these products for short periods. Since many herbivorous fish are bottom-grazers, vegetables must be weighted so that they sit on the bottom of the aquarium. Uneaten foods must be removed within 24 hours
- Live foods may be needed for recently captured fish, species that tend to refuse frozen or manufactured foods (e.g. trumpetfish and sea horses) and sick fish. Live prey can serve as disease vectors and should therefore be reared on-site or obtained only from trusted vendors. A quarantine period of 30 days for feeder fish is strongly advised; those that appear unhealthy must not be fed to carnivorous species. Live food can also be used as a route for providing medications to fish.

Energy requirements

The basal energy requirements of teleosts and elasmobranchs vary considerably. Most teleosts should be fed 1–3% of their bodyweight daily. Calorie-limiting diets are often used and fish should therefore be monitored for evidence of weight loss.

The most common causes of inadequate calorie intake are competition and aggression by tankmates. In larger tanks it may be difficult to feed uniformly. Particular species or individuals can be targeted by feeding by pole or by hand.

Sharks

On average, sharks should be fed 1.5–3.7% of their bodyweight two to three times per week. Feeding regimes for captive sharks are based on species and age. Adults and sedentary species (e.g. nurse sharks) require fewer calories than juveniles or more active species (e.g. lemon shark). Optimal feed rates can be developed for each fish by visually monitoring and weighing the fish on a regular basis. The use of whole or chopped fish, rather than fillets, reduces the risk of dietary deficiencies.

Anorexia following transport is common in sharks but generally should not persist more than 3–4 weeks. Failure to eat after 4 weeks may require veterinary intervention: a full physical examination should be performed to determine if there is a specific problem. Treatment may include fresh water and vitamin B complex delivered via stomach tube as an appetite stimulant.

Dietary deficiencies

Lipids
Many fish and elasmobranchs require omega-3 fatty acid, which is found in the oils of fish that consume marine and freshwater algae. Deficiency can lead to reduced growth rates, tissue oedema, fatty degeneration of the liver, decreased haemoglobin in red cells, fin erosions, and increased susceptibility to disease.

Polyunsaturated fatty acids are also subject to lipid autoxidation (peroxidation and rancidification). The resulting peroxides and aldehydes are toxic to fish and, presumably, other aquatic animals. Ingestion of these compounds can lead to emaciation, dark coloration, scale loss, fin necrosis, pale gills and increased mortalities. Proper handling and storage of frozen food should limit this problem. It is prudent to add the antioxidant vitamin E to the diets of any animals being fed frozen fish.

Vitamins
Clinical signs of vitamin deficiency are generally non-specific and therefore the diets of all species should be supplemented with multivitamins. Thiaminase, an enzyme found in the tissues of most feed fish, breaks down thiamine, which is essential in nervous tissue function. Thiamine supplements are important for preventing nervous system disorders. Many fish are unable to synthesize ascorbic acid, and supplementation with this vitamin is recommended for the promotion of wound repair, bone formation and disease resistance.

Minerals
Many ions (including calcium, zinc, iodine, selenium, sodium, chloride and potassium) are obtained by fish from their diets and from the water in which they live. In large closed systems where water changes are infrequent, serious imbalances or deficiencies of waterborne macroelements can occur as elements are utilized. Monthly monitoring of macroelements by laboratories with atomic absorption capabilities is advised. Corrections can be made by directly adding minerals to the water, supplementing the diet and frequent water changes. It is important to note that commercially available synthetic sea salt mixes often vary in chemical composition from one batch to another.

Thyroid hyperplasia: Thyroid hyperplasia or goitre is a common disorder in captive elasmobranchs and both freshwater and marine fish. It is recognized by a pathognomonic swelling of the thyroid gland that is visible under the gills in fish and as a ventral swelling in sharks. It can result from a lack of iodine in the diet or water, or the presence of goitrogenic substances.

Treatment of sharks with this condition can be achieved by supplementing the diet with calcium iodate or potassium iodide at 10 mg/kg once weekly in the food. Commercial multivitamin supplements are available for oral administration.

Quarantine

Quarantine, which typically lasts 30–90 days for fish, is designed to protect established exhibit populations from diseases that may be imported with newly acquired fish. Invertebrates (e.g. anemones, corals and live rock) and plants are also possible vectors for parasitic disease and should be quarantined separately from fish for long enough (30–60 days) to disrupt parasite life cycles. Guidelines in Whitaker *et al.* (1994) may be useful for the joint development of practical protocols by husbandry and veterinary personnel.

- Fish that have been recently transported are often stressed and are subsequently more susceptible to opportunistic pathogens. It is important that their acclimatization to the captive environment be as free of stress as possible
- Newly acquired specimens should be grouped by species while in quarantine so that the specific environmental and dietary needs of each species can be better met
- To prevent contamination of the established collection, quarantine systems should be housed in a different location and equipped with separate filtration. Any quarantine tanks sharing the same water and filtration systems must be considered as one group and quarantined together
- System design and décor must:
  - facilitate easy cleaning, removal and disinfection
  - provide adequate space and hiding places to reduce stress and aggression among tankmates
  - allow environmental parameters (including lighting and water quality) to be optimally maintained for each species
- All staff working with quarantined systems must follow strict hygienic practices. Where possible, personnel should perform all required duties for established healthy populations before working with quarantine tanks. Attention should be given to strict personal hygiene, the use of disinfectant, and separate equipment for each tank.

New arrivals
New fish should be visually inspected for signs of disease immediately on arrival and again 24 hours later. This includes an assessment of the colour, skin, fins, respiration rate, eyes and general behaviour.

Physical handling can be stressful to the fish and, unless absolutely necessary, should be delayed until they have acclimatized to captivity. Physical examinations include skin scrapes, fin and gill biopsies and (in larger fish) blood collection for culture and complete haematology and biochemistry analysis.

Physical examination of larger fish, such as sharks and rays, requires experienced staff to handle the fish safely. Sharks and rays often become quiescent – a state known as tonic immobility – when placed in dorsal recumbency. This state allows a full physical examination to be completed by veterinary staff with relatively little risk to handlers and fish alike.

Newly acquired fish – especially those collected recently – may be initially reluctant to feed. Feeding behaviours need to be encouraged by attempting to mimic natural conditions. It can be helpful to offer foods native to the natural environment of the species while slowly introducing the fish to a more practical captive diet, such as gelatin food.

Quarantine records

An individual quarantine record (see Figure 8.7) and a separate tank should be assigned to each group of fish. Good record keeping is essential and it is useful if records are easily accessible. For efficient interpretation, data should be laid out in a calendar-type format. This will allow clinicians to ascertain quickly the overall health status for each tank. Historical analysis of these records will show successful treatment regimes, problematic shipment sources, disease epidemiology and other invaluable data.

Prophylactic medication

The use of chemotherapeutics in quarantine programmes must be carefully balanced against their potential effects on the fish, biological filtration and water quality. At the National Aquarium in Baltimore, invertebrates, elasmobranchs and known sensitive fish are often given 90-day quarantine periods with physical examinations at the end in lieu of prophylactic medications.

The majority of freshwater and marine fish enter a minimum 30-day quarantine period with predetermined prophylactic treatment dates that are laid out on their quarantine records. These treatments are based on the likelihood that the fish are harbouring potential pathogens. The treatment regimen (Figure 8.4) is based on previous models of disease outbreaks: stress-related bacterial disease often occurs within 14 days of arrival whereas parasitic infestation usually occurs between days 14 and 21. The quarantine protocol can

be modified according to diagnosed diseases and clinical circumstances.

It is important to note that many of the treatments and their methods of administration are derived empirically, due to the lack of scientific therapeutic studies on these fish.

Disease treatments

Quarantine and exhibit tanks should be assessed regularly for evidence of disease. Early warning signs may be subtle and include changes in behaviour, decreased appetite, cloudy eyes, excessive mucus production, increased respiration, rubbing or 'flashing' on tank décor and increased mortalities in previously stable tanks. To prevent an epidemic, these clinical signs should be considered a medical emergency and investigated immediately.

In some cases, advanced warning can be achieved using sentinel fish that are particularly susceptible to certain infectious diseases. For example, fine-scaled slow-moving fish such as porcupinefish are more susceptible to external parasites and are easily caught from large aquaria for evaluation.

The onset of an epidemic is often associated with poor water quality or fluctuations in water temperature. For example, many large aquaria are faced with periodic outbreaks of external monogenetic trematodes in fish populations. These parasites are often present in low numbers, with fish exhibiting few clinical signs. When fish are exposed to a stressor, such as increased water temperature, an outbreak is likely to follow.

Treatment of a disease outbreak can be challenging and several special factors need to be considered when developing a treatment plan.

- Systems can contain several million litres of water, multiple species and, in some cases, aquatic vegetation
- Daily maintenance and feeding are usually accomplished using staff and volunteer divers
- These systems are prominent exhibits that attract large numbers of visitors.

Day	Marine fish	Freshwater fish
1–10	Furazone green® (proprietary product containing nitrofurazone, furazolidone and methylene blue) added once on day 1, removed on day 10	As for marine fish
11–12	Fenbendazole in gel food	As for marine fish
14–18	Copper therapy started and increased gradually to therapeutic levels[a]	Formalin and malachite green: 3 doses, 72-hour intervals with 50% water changes between doses
19–39	Therapeutic levels maintained at 0.18–0.20 mg/l	
17–21	Metronidazole in gel food	As for marine fish
26–27	Fenbendazole in gel food	As for marine fish
31–33	Praziquantel in gel food	As for marine fish

Figure 8.4 A medication protocol for quarantine in public aquaria.

[a]Copper is added to aquaria over 24-hour periods using intravenous giving sets. The amount added is adjusted according to daily monitored results. Substantial water changes (50%) are performed at the end of each course of in-water medication. Activated carbon is also used to remove the chemicals if necessary.

Bearing these factors in mind, the following steps should enable successful treatment:

- A rapid accurate diagnosis must be made through physical and postmortem examinations and a review of tank records
- A treatment's potential adverse effects on mixed species (e.g. copper toxicity in elasmobranchs and invertebrates) and vegetation must be taken into account. Certain species or plants may need to be removed and treated separately. Treatments that colour the water or stain the décor may not be practical in exhibit tanks
- The method of delivery (bath, in-feed or injectable), potential human health hazards and costs associated with the chosen medication must be evaluated
- Before treatment, life support engineers and husbandry personnel must be notified so that water filtration systems that would remove or affect medication (e.g. charcoal, protein skimmers, ozone, UV) can be disabled
- A plan to remove pharmaceuticals at the end of the treatment regime should be considered. Personnel must be informed when the treatment ends and given specific instructions on when to enable filtration systems. For large systems, significant amounts of fresh carbon may be required to adsorb dissolved medications
- Water quality laboratories must be warned to modify normal testing schedules. Increased monitoring is often necessary, to ensure that water quality is not deteriorating and becoming detrimental to the fish. It may also be necessary to monitor the water to ensure that drugs are maintained within therapeutic levels (e.g. copper levels must be maintained between 0.18 and 0.20 mg/l) and then completely removed at the end of treatment
- Divers must be notified before any treatments. All diving must be suspended when using medications known to be hazardous to human health
- Fish and other animals should be assessed regularly throughout the treatment period to ensure that the desired effect is being achieved.

Zoonoses

Certain fish diseases, poor water quality and some tank medications can have adverse effects on human health. The following procedures will minimize zoonotic disease transmission and other risks to human health:

- Development of a veterinary disease surveillance programme that includes identification and investigation of potential zoonotic pathogens (Figure 8.5) and notification of relevant personnel
- Implementation of health and safety protocols for staff, visitors and fish (Figure 8.6)
- Insistence on proper hygiene in all work areas
- Education of husbandry and veterinary staff to recognize and avoid potential pathogens.

Aeromonas hydrophila	*Mycobacterium marinum*
Campylobacter spp.	*Mycobacterium chelonia*
Edwardsiella tarda	*Pseudomonas* spp.
Escherichia coli (enteropathogenic)	*Salmonella* spp.
Escherichia coli (enterotoxic)	*Vibrio fluvialis*
Erysipelothrix spp.	*Vibrio parahaemolyticus*
Legionella pneumophila	*Vibrio vulnificus*
Mycobacterium fortuitum	*Yersinia enterocolitica*

Figure 8.5: Examples of pathogenic bacteria that may be contracted by people working in aquatic environments.

Animal care staff should:

- Cover all wounds
- Observe proper hygiene: wash well after handling fish or working in their environments
- Avoid exposure if immunosuppressed
- Avoid close contact with fish and their environment when ill
- Receive proper first aid immediately following injury
- Be informed of possible zoonotic disease and hazardous environments.

Laboratory staff should:

- Wear laboratory coats when working in the laboratory
- Cover all wounds
- Observe proper hygiene: wash well after handling specimens and samples
- Work with all microbes and other potential pathogens in a biological containment cabinet
- Avoid exposure to potential pathogens if immunosuppressed
- Not work with potential pathogenic pathogens when ill
- Not eat or drink in the laboratories
- Not store food in the same refrigerator as biological samples
- Receive proper first aid immediately following injury.

Divers should:

- Receive annual physical examinations
- Not dive with open wounds unless they can be completely covered
- Be informed of possible zoonotic diseases and hazardous environments
- Receive proper first aid immediately following injury.

Visitors should:

- Observe proper hygiene following any interaction with fish and their environments. Touch pools and other open exhibits should have hand-washing stations available for visitors. Open exhibits should be monitored vigilantly for signs of disease and be closed immediately to the public at the discretion of the veterinary departments.

Figure 8.6 Health and safety protocols for staff and visitors.

Record keeping

Record-keeping systems vary and include paper files, word-processing files, ISIS, ARKS, Medarks and a host of small individual databases. Whatever the method, good record keeping and fish identification are essential.

- Records should be maintained for quarantine, feeding, mortality, water quality, medical cases and general husbandry (Figure 8.7)
- All tanks should be individually and permanently labelled to ensure proper identification and allow cross-referencing of information

Record	Information	Comments
Feeding	Date, diet, amount fed, caloric value and appetite (e.g. good, moderate or poor)	Feeding trends easily evaluated
Quarantine	Arrival date, animal source, number of species and animals, pre-arrival medications, start and finish dates of treatments, water quality parameters, food intake, mortalities, quarantine release date and final destination	Helpful if presented in a calendar-type format; may allow more rapid historical analysis of treatment regimes, problematic shipment sources, disease epidemiology and other valuable data
Pathology log	Pathology number, date, location, genus and species, fish identification number	Unique pathology number allows tracking of cultures, gross pathology findings, histology, etc.
Case log	Case number, date initiated, genus and species, location, problem, animal ID if available and date closed	Allows cases to be followed
Clinical record	Case number, date(s), genus and species, location, history, assessment, clinical tests performed, medical plan and clinician's initials	Working clinical record for daily assessment and treatment
Medical record	Animal ID if available, date of acquisition/disposition, date of problem, assessment and treatment	In-depth animal record; typically includes clinical problem with a subjective evaluation, objective evaluation, assessment and plan for each entry
Water quality	Date, and system ID All systems: temperature, pH, dissolved oxygen, ammonia, nitrite, nitrate, macroelements (calcium, magnesium, phosphorus, sodium, chloride and others) *In addition:* Freshwater: hardness and alkalinity Marine: salinity	Allows water quality of systems to be monitored over time
Husbandry	Date and system ID; may incorporate feeding records, animal additions and mortalities, water changes and notes of special procedures	General log kept by aquarist to show daily activities

Figure 8.7 Record keeping in public aquaria.

- It is useful to have records readily available beside the tanks
- Additional data on species, fish numbers and optimum water quality for each tank will enable prompt identification of problems
- Tanks containing venomous fish must be clearly marked and should include medical contact and first aid information.

Dangerous species

The following sections outline the practices at the National Aquarium in Baltimore. All elasmobranchs undergo annual physical examinations that include assessment of the eyes, gills, oral cavity, skin, cloaca and blood. Abdominal palpation and ultrasonography are also performed. As many of these fish are large and can be dangerous to handle, the procedures must be well planned and utilize experienced staff members.

Sharks

- Gates and divers armed with barriers are used to isolate and steer sharks into an off-exhibit area (Figure 8.8a)
- A large stretcher is positioned in front of the shark and its head is guided into a hooded portion of the stretcher (Figure 8.8b)
- Once in place, the stretcher is closed and the poles are cinched together with 'rapid-release' dive belts

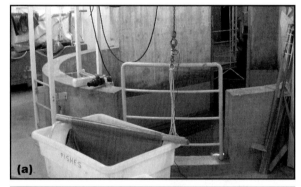
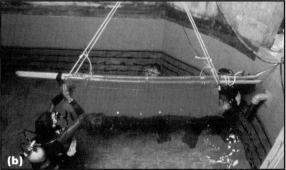

Figure 8.8 (a) The shark acclimation area is an important off-exhibit area used to acclimate, examine and treat large sharks. The area is directly off the main exhibit through a small access tunnel. It is large enough to allow even the largest sharks to swim freely for short periods and a tracked crane over the centre of the pool allows sharks to be handled easily. (© Ian Walker.) (b) View above the shark acclimation area. A large sand tiger shark has been placed into the hooded stretcher and hoisted above the water to obtain the fish's bodyweight. (© Ian Walker.)

- A large overhead mechanical crane is used to lift the shark from the water. The water is allowed to drain from the stretcher so that a reasonably accurate bodyweight can be obtained
- The fish is placed in a water-filled shark transport box, where a submerged pump pushes oxygenated water over the gills in a process known as ram ventilation (Figure 8.9)
- When rolled into dorsal recumbency and restrained, many sharks and rays enter a state of tonic immobility (Figure 8.10), which allows an examination (Figure 8.11) to be performed with relatively little risk.

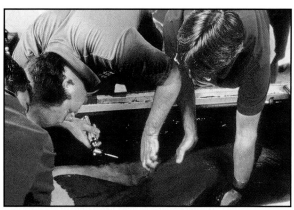

Figure 8.11 Annual physical examinations are performed on each elasmobranch in the National Aquarium in Baltimore's collection. This fish has not been sedated but is restrained by trained animal husbandry personnel. An auroscope is being used to inspect the gills through the gill slits. (© National Aquarium in Baltimore.)

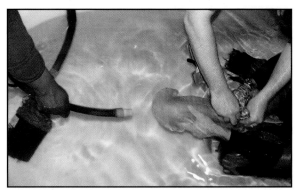

Figure 8.9 Ram ventilation being used to force water into the mouth and over the gills of a bonnet head shark to maintain adequate oxygenation during a medical procedure. (© Ian Walker.)

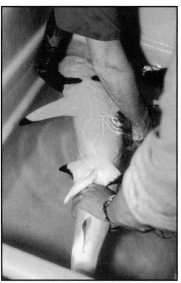

Figure 8.10 This black tip reef shark has been placed into tonic immobilization. Rolling some elasmobranchs into dorsal recumbency can elicit this unreactive state, which facilitates handling and medical examination. (© National Aquarium in Baltimore.)

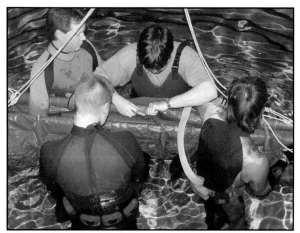

Figure 8.12 Blood being collected from the base of the dorsal fin of a sand tiger shark, with the fish restrained in a large hooded stretcher. (© Brent Whitaker.)

EDTA and sodium heparin have been used successfully as anticoagulants for fish blood. Elasmobranch blood differs significantly from that of other fish and relatively little published information on haematology is available.

Stingrays

For these fish (including southern and cownose rays), staff must take care to avoid the venomous spine at the base of the tail.

- The fish are collected in large nets and placed directly into square stretchers
- Bodyweights are obtained and the fish are transferred into a round tub containing 60 cm of water
- An experienced handler restrains the fish from the front to allow medical staff to remove the spine, using ordinary garden shears. Safety goggles should be worn. Once removed, the spine is placed into a sealed plastic container to prevent accidental envenomation

Blood sampling

In sharks, blood can be drawn from the ventral tail vein by inserting a 40 mm × 1.1 mm needle along the midline between the anal and tail fins. The needle is directed perpendicular to the body and advanced slowly until the ventral tail vein is reached. Larger fish may require a 90 mm × 1 mm spinal needle for successful phlebotomy.

Alternatively, blood can be collected from the base of the dorsal fin (Figure 8.12): a 40 mm × 1.1 mm needle is directed cranially along the midline at an angle of 10 degrees into either pocket at the caudal base of the dorsal fin.

- The fish can then be safely placed into tonic immobility for examination (Figure 8.13)
- Blood is collected from the ventral tail vein (Figure 8.14) using a 25 mm × 1.1 mm needle, which is directed cranially along the ventral midline at an angle of 45 degrees.

Venomous fish

Venomous fish, such as stonefish and lionfish, must be treated with care. Staff must always work in pairs and be aware of the potential risks of envenomation. Tanks should be labelled with information on the species, toxins and immediate first aid for envenomation.

Before any medical procedures are performed, venomous fish should be fully anaesthetized and restrained. The use of heavy rubber gloves (e.g. linesmen electrical gloves) and clear plastic 'nets' (to avoid spine entanglement) is recommended. Stonefish antivenin is available (CSL Stonefish Antivenin: Commonwealth Serum Laboratories, 45 Poplar Road, Parkville, Victoria 3052, Australia) and should be kept within reach whenever these fish are handled.

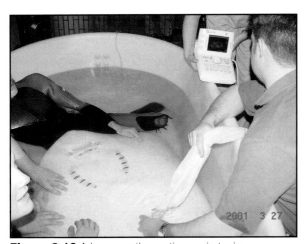

Figure 8.13 A large southern stingray in tonic immobilization (dorsal recumbency) for an ultrasound examination. (© Brent Whitaker.)

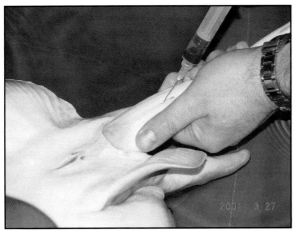

Figure 8.14 Blood being collected from the ventral tail vein of a southern stingray. Alcohol and povidone can cause skin irritation and ulceration in elasmobranchs; therefore the site area was cleansed by flushing with sterile saline. The venomous spine on the dorsal aspect of the tail has been removed to prevent injuries. (© Brent Whitaker.)

For any postmortem examination:

- Staff should wear protective goggles and heavy rubber gloves
- All spines should be removed and placed in a rigid container
- Following the examination, all tissues should be double bagged and packaged in well marked rigid cardboard boxes for safe disposal.

Fish removal

Sometimes fish need to be removed permanently from a collection. This can be accomplished through transfer to other institutions, release into the wild or, when other options are exhausted, euthanasia. The latter two solutions are controversial and require careful forethought and planning.

Release

Whether a fish is to be returned to the wild or transferred to another facility, a complete physical examination is essential. Both husbandry and veterinary staff should be confident that the fish is fit for the journey ahead.

The potential risks and benefits associated with releasing captive fish into wild populations must be thoroughly examined by veterinary and husbandry staff. Issues to consider include:

- Exposure to infectious diseases
- Exposure to medical treatments and the reasons for doing so
- Carrier state for resistant bacteria following antimicrobial medication
- Potential risk of introducing diseases into naïve populations as a result of being housed with fish from other habitats
- Ability to survive in the wild following habituation to captivity.

Euthanasia

Euthanasia of sharks and large fish can be accomplished by using an overdose of anaesthetic such as tricaine methane sulphonate (MS222), given by prolonged immersion. Alternatively, pentobarbitone can be given intravenously or by an intracardiac route. Free-swimming sharks can be sedated initially with xylazine (6 mg/kg) and ketamine (12 mg/kg) administered using a pole syringe and injected into the dorsal musculature between the gill slits and dorsal fin.

Further reading and references

Aiken A (1995) Use of ozone to improve water quality in aquatic exhibits. *International Zoo Yearbook* **34**, 106–114

Grguric G, Komas JA and Gainor LA (1999) Differences in major ions composition of artificial seawater from aquarium tanks at the New Jersey State Aquarium. *Aquarium Sciences and Conservation* **2**(3), 145–159

Nemetz TG and Shotts EB (1993) Zoonotic diseases. In: *Fish Medicine*, ed. MK Stoskopf, pp. 214–219. WB Saunders Company, Philadelphia

Sabalones J (1995) Considerations on the husbandry of sharks for display purposes. *International Zoo Yearbook* **34**, 77–87

Stoskopf MK (1993) Marine tropical fish nutrition. In: *Fish Medicine*, ed. MK Stoskopf, pp. 625–628. WB Saunders Company, Philadelphia

Stoskopf MK (1993) Shark pharmacology and toxicology. In: *Fish Medicine*, ed. MK Stoskopf, pp. 809–816. WB Saunders Company, Philadelphia

Whitaker BR (1999): Preventive medicine programs for fish. In: *Zoo and Wild Animal Medicine*, 4th edn, ed. ME Fowler, pp. 163–181. WB Saunders Company, Philadelphia

Whitaker BR, Hecker B and Andrews C (1994) Establishing a quarantine program for fishes. *American Zoo and Aquarium Association Conference Proceedings*, Atlanta, pp. 282–287

Acknowledgements

The authors would like to thank Mrs Susie Ridenour, who was invaluable in searching for and providing numerous articles for this paper. We would also like to thank Ms Valerie Lounsbury and the rest of the Review Committee at the NAIB for their constructive editing.

9

General approach

Ray L. Butcher

Veterinary surgeons are often reluctant to investigate disease problems in fish. However, the basic principles are the same as for any species: the appropriate treatment and advice can only be given once a diagnosis is made, and this in turn requires a standard logical approach.

Fish-keeping clients frequently complain, sadly with some justification, that veterinarians are not interested in their aquatic pets. There may therefore be a degree of prejudice with respect to a veterinarian's ability to diagnose and treat fish diseases, and the client may well have sought advice from other sources and used a whole range of medications for the existing problem. To achieve credibility, the veterinary surgeon must begin by asking the right questions, and this requires a basic understanding of the husbandry systems involved.

Importance of the environment

The establishment of a disease in fish often requires the interaction of a number of factors. The majority are a sequel to poor water quality or other husbandry factors. Even when specific pathogens or parasites are identified, environmental factors may well have predisposed the fish to infection or have influenced the response to treatments given. Thus, consideration of the environment and husbandry is of prime importance in the investigation of all disease outbreaks.

A further dilemma is that ornamental fish are kept in an intensive husbandry system and yet are often considered by their owners as individual companion animals. The diagnostic method involving slaughtering a percentage sample for autopsy is clearly not appropriate in these cases.

Stepwise approach

Given the above, the investigation should ideally address the following.

1. History – consideration of the underlying management system
2. History – the current problem
3. Evaluation of the water quality and environment
4. Observation of the fish in its environment and comparison with other in-contact fish
5. Clinical examination of individual fish within and out of the water, as appropriate (with or without the aid of sedation or anaesthesia)

6. Analysis of laboratory samples taken from live fish
7. Analysis of postmortem material
8. Further techniques – endoscopy, radiography, ultrasonography, etc.

The importance of a complete history cannot be overstressed. This was well emphasized by Wall (1993) in his consideration of the veterinary approach to salmon farming: '...the initial impression of the farm, and the stockman's history and opinion of the problems are very important. Keep your hands in your pockets and start by asking a lot of questions.'

The rest of this chapter will deal with the preliminary steps. The examination of the environment and the fish will be dealt with in subsequent chapters.

Home visits versus examination at the clinic – the economic realities

Much can be gained from a home visit, as this allows a direct assessment of the management system and observation of the fish in their environment. However, economic realities mean that this is not always possible and so an alternative strategy must be employed that makes as much of this information available as possible. This requires the meticulous recording of the history, not only of the current problem but also of the underlying management system. It must be accepted that this is second best to actual observation – the fact that a particular type or size of filter is present does not necessarily mean it has been installed correctly or is being used appropriately.

Taking the history

A full history is an essential element in the investigation of diseases in any species but this is especially important for fish, where the information from the physical examination may be relatively limited. History taking is an acquired skill, requiring careful questioning which may need to be modified to suit the knowledge and intelligence of the client. Veterinary surgeons in companion animal practice are well aware of the differences in dealing with pet-owning clients as opposed to breeders or even those involved with showing. Stoskopf (1988) classified fish clients as:

- Single-tank owners
- Multiple-tank owners
- Pond owners
- Commercial clients.

These tend to have different degrees of experience and knowledge (and sometimes tolerance to questioning) and need to be handled in different ways. It is essential to assess the client at an early stage.

Stoskopf (1988) was also sensitive to the economic pressures on the practitioner and stressed the need to limit phone time to a minimum. He suggested that the initial phone enquiry should address the following four steps:

1. Determine whether there really is a problem
2. Determine whether you can do anything about it
3. Determine whether the client wants anything done about it
4. Instruct the client on how to come in and what to bring.

Client expectations of what is possible are not always realistic and the cost implications should be made clear at this time, especially if home visits are considered appropriate. Once it has been agreed to proceed with the investigation, a full history should be taken. To avoid wasting time on the phone, this is best achieved using preprinted sheets, examples of which are given in Figures 9.1 and 9.2. These only represent a framework for questioning, and some of the basic questions may give leads that need to be explored in more depth.

The veterinary surgeon should then assess the urgency of the problem, and how best to deal with it given the practical and financial constraints. In many cases, the client will not have contacted the veterinarian until the situation had become a real emergency. In addition, it is important at this stage to assess whether the problem is likely to be infectious or non-infectious, as this may affect the approach to the case. Factors to consider are the percentage of fish affected, time scale and whether the problem has followed the introduction of new fish. A sudden-onset 100% mortality is much more likely to be a toxin or environmental catastrophe than an infectious agent.

When the case involves seeing the fish at the clinic rather than at a home visit, the history must include supplementary questions that attempt to give additional information on behaviour.

- Are the affected fish swimming with the others or remaining solitary?
- Are the fish 'flashing' or rubbing against objects in the pond or tank?
- Are the fish collecting at water inlets or at the surface of the water?
- Are there any other behavioural abnormalities?

Non-medicinal first aid

In emergencies, advice on first aid measures will often be of use until the fish can be dealt with properly. These measures may be life saving and at the very least the client will feel that they are doing something positive. The first aid measures that may be considered include:

- Isolating affected fish
- Withholding food
- Improving aeration/oxygenation of the water
- Checking filters
- Checking water quality parameters and repeating daily
- Performing regular partial water changes
- Reducing stocking density if possible.

The isolation of affected fish may be ideal but this does require that the fish be kept in water where the appropriate quality can be maintained. Temporary hospital tanks or baths usually contain a relatively small volume of water and require regular and careful monitoring. Consideration should also be given to the opinion that koi appear less stressed if they are kept in a tank with at least one other fish.

Examination at the clinic – what to bring and how

Clearly, if the problem involves a solitary fish, that must be the one that is examined. If a number of fish are affected, the most representative one should be selected. The client should be warned that it might be advantageous to bring a dying fish to the clinic so that it can be sacrificed and a fresh postmortem examination performed. Recently dead fish may give some information, though rapid autolysis limits their value.

Transporting fish to the surgery poses a real practical problem. Water is very heavy, and the temporary container will not incorporate the normal equipment essential for maintaining the correct temperature, oxygen concentration or filtration. It is therefore important that the fish are kept in this container for the minimum time; thus there is an advantage in arranging a specific appointment for a quiet period.

The fish should be transported in enough of its tank or pond water to allow it to swim upright and turn around. About half of the container should contain air (enriched with oxygen, where possible). Clear strong plastic bags are ideal, as they can be sealed easily with rubber bands and they have the advantage that the fish can be observed through them. To reduce the risk of leaks, double-wrapping in a second bag is advisable. The plastic bag should then be covered in an opaque wrapping, and the whole thing placed in a picnic cooler or polystyrene box to provide temperature insulation. The client should be instructed to bring an equal amount of tank or pond water (bagged and insulated as above) to serve as recovery water if sedation or anaesthesia is performed. A small amount of this second sample can be used at the clinic for testing water quality, if required.

Prior to the transport of very large fish, it might be considered appropriate to add a tranquillizing dose of anaesthetic to the water. While this might help to reduce stress and prevent further trauma, it could also influence the findings of the clinical examination and reduce ectoparasite numbers.

Name:		Ref No: Date:
Address:		Tel:

Pond/Tank	Volume of water	
	Dimensions	
	Source of water	
	How long established	
	Frequency/method cleaning	
	Site within room/garden	
	Type of gravel/rocks	
	Pond/aquarium ornaments	
	Plants	
Water circulation	Pumps – types and capacity	
	Water changes – frequency/ proportion/source	
	Average water loss via leaks/ evaporation	
	Waterfalls/fountains/ air-stones	
	Material used in pipe manufacture	
Filtration	Types	
	Media used	
	Capacity	
	Flow rate	
	How long installed	
	Frequency/method of cleaning	
	UV filters – size, position and age of tube	
Heating	Types	
	Thermostats/monitoring	
Lighting	Natural/artificial	
	Types of tube	
Water quality	Parameters tested	
	Appearance of water	
	Frequency of testing	
Fish	Species	
	Numbers/size	
	Total bodyweight	
	Introduction of last fish	
	Quarantine procedure	
Nutrition	Type of food	
	Frequency/amount fed	
	Storage	
Prophylactic treatments	Medications used/dose	
	Frequency of use	
Health history	Disease problems in last 12 months	

Figure 9.1 Case record – management factors.

Name:		Ref No:
		Date:
Address:		Tel:

Numbers/species of fish affected	
Time scale	
Presenting signs	
Mortalities	

Possible changes in management acting as a trigger

Filter changes/cleaning		Introduction of new fish	
Pond/aquarium cleaning		Faulty heating/lighting/ pumping equipment	
Changes in feeding regime		Power failure	
Other			

Possible environmental changes acting as a trigger

Fluctuating ambient temperatures		Predators	
Algal blooms		Leaf fall	
New rocks, gravel or ornaments		Other (e.g. extreme weather conditions)	

Possible exposure to toxins

Metals		Biocides	
Gases		Therapeutic compounds	
Toxic organics		Other	

Self-medication

Compound used	Date used	Dose used
1.		
2.		
3.		

Figure 9.2 Case record – history of the current problem.

Client records

The examples of case records given in Figures 9.1 and 9.2 may be considered a useful way of keeping information for future use. If a client has a subsequent fish problem, the management details are already to hand and the veterinary surgeon can become familiar with the system before speaking to the client. This not only portrays an efficient and caring image, but also saves time, as it is only necessary to ask whether there have been any changes.

The treatment of a particular disease may involve the supply of 'prescription only' medicines. In the UK, the legislation limits this to 'animals in our care'. In situations where much of the information on the case is obtained by telephone, it is important that the records indicate that the veterinary surgeon is fully familiar with the case before medications are supplied.

Practice protocol

Veterinary surgeons prepared to tackle fish problems are relatively rare, and in a single practice there is usually only one with an interest. As this person will not be available at all times, a protocol should be agreed within the practice as to how best to deal with enquiries. The practice receptionists should be familiar with this protocol.

If a client is bringing a fish to the clinic, advice should be given as to the best way to transport the fish and what else to bring. The appointment should be made for a quiet period, to limit the time in the transport water. The practical difficulties of examining the fish will mean that the appointment will be relatively long and this too should be allowed for in the schedule (and costing).

Aquarium retailers – friends or competitors?

Many retail outlets have staff with a wealth of experience and knowledge. They are able to supply equipment and routine proprietary water treatments but not 'prescription only' medicines. Nor do they make money by providing advice. There is therefore no direct conflict of interest, and indeed there is much to be gained from developing a rapport with a good local retail outlet. Referral can be a two-way process, depending on the particular client needs. In the interests of cooperation, it is probably better if the veterinary surgeon avoids stocking a range of proprietary water treatments, but rather recommends clients to a particular retailer.

References

Stoskopf MK (ed.) (1988) Taking the history. In: *The Veterinary Clinics of North America: Small Animal Practice* **18** (2), 283–291. WB Saunders Company, Philadelphia

Wall T (1993) The veterinary approach to salmon farming in Scotland. In: *Aquaculture for Veterinarians*, ed. L Brown, pp. 193–222. Pergamon Press, Oxford

10

Examining the environment

Todd R. Cecil

Being unable to choose the environment in which they live, captive fish are dependent on the environment and quality of water that are provided. Optimal conditions vary according to species but must be correctly balanced to minimize stress and disease and to maintain health.

Fish coexist with many pathogens, whose presence is often of limited significance, but in many cases it is a deterioration or sudden change in water quality that precipitates a disease problem. Therefore, in addition to the use of specific medication, it is often essential to improve the environmental conditions so that fish may recover and recurrence of the disease may be avoided.

A thorough examination of the environment is time-consuming and is best performed before the fish are inspected. A methodical approach is required (a checklist similar to that in Chapter 9 is helpful) and the veterinarian needs to be familiar with the appropriate environmental conditions for the species under investigation. This information and descriptions of the various systems used in keeping ornamental fish are discussed in earlier chapters.

General considerations

Many species of fish are relatively easy to keep in captivity when correct environmental conditions are provided. Water quality parameters must be maintained within certain limits, as determined by the species. Freshwater fish are considered to be 'hardier' and able to endure wider fluctuations in water quality, temperature and nutrition; marine fish originate from large bodies of water (oceans) where temperature, water quality and nutrition rarely change and therefore these fish require more stable water conditions in captivity.

Large-capacity systems are more stable and resist changes in water quality more readily than small systems. In general, daily temperature and pH fluctuations are less dramatic and toxic waste products accumulate more slowly in a larger system. However, large systems take longer to clean and maintain, and routine maintenance will often become irregular and infrequent if it is labour-intensive.

In many cases, water quality problems are features of new ponds and tanks, hence the term 'new pond syndrome' or 'new tank syndrome'. This is often a consequence of an immature biological filter and the introduction of a large number of new fish from various sources. In addition, there are inevitably teething problems associated with new equipment, inexperience of the hobbyist, overzealous cleaning, overfeeding and inappropriate use of medications.

Mature systems (over 6 months old) with a stable population of fish have fewer problems related to water quality, unless the biological filter has been affected by excessive cleaning, pump failure or the use of antibacterial medications. Most health problems in these facilities follow the introduction of new fish (which are not quarantined) or overstocking due to substantial growth of the fish over several years.

> **TIP:** Ignore the fish initially and carry out a risk assessment of the environment from the fishes' point of view.

Examining ponds

Due to the size of some ponds and the complexity of their filtration systems, it is often difficult to inspect the facility in detail. Several features associated with the design and construction of a pond may indirectly affect water quality and consequently the health of the fish. In addition, exposure to climatic changes has a great effect on the conditions within the pond.

Position

Thoroughly examine the local environment around and above the pond. Look for signs of rainwater runoff from rockeries, patios and overhanging wooden structures that have been chemically treated (Figure 10.1). Overhanging plants and vegetation (Figure 10.2) may provide some shade and aesthetic appeal but poisonous sap, fruits, seeds and foliage may contaminate the water and prove lethal. The physical effects of a heavy leaf fall may cause other problems. In time, the overgrowth of vegetation (Figure 10.3) and roots of trees may cause damage to the pond structure. They may also provide access for predators.

Design

The shape of a pond influences the direction of water flow and currents. Intricate patterns, although aesthetically pleasing, often create areas of water stagnation.

The surface area must be sufficiently large to allow gas exchange: too small an area may lead to poor gas exchange and low dissolved oxygen levels.

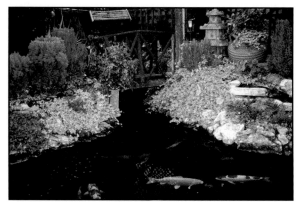

Figure 10.1 Outdoor pond with overgrowth of surrounding vegetation. Wood preservatives from various structures such as the wooden bridge and decking may run into the pond during heavy rainfall. Runoff from the soil may pollute the water with suspended solids and fertilizer. (© W.H. Wildgoose.)

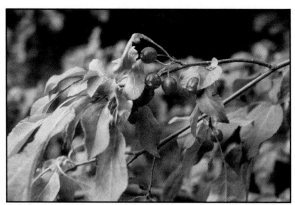

Figure 10.2 Overhanging tree with berries. Little is known about the harmful effects of many potentially poisonous plants in fish. The flowers and fruits are seasonal, and may not be present when visited by the veterinarian; some botanical knowledge is required. (© W.H. Wildgoose.)

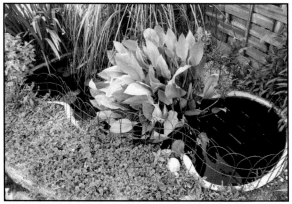

Figure 10.3 A badly neglected pond with serious overgrowth of plants. This preformed plastic pond was quite unsuitable for large koi and had an inadequate filter system. (© W.H. Wildgoose.)

Depth enables fish to escape from predators and provides a layer of warm water at the bottom of deep ponds in cold winter weather. Pumps that continuously circulate this warm water through the filter may create a chilling effect and cause hypothermia.

Construction

The materials used to construct the pond may leach harmful chemicals into the water column. Untreated concrete and fibreglass that has not cured correctly have been associated with high pH and styrene toxicity, respectively.

Objects within the pond ('furniture') such as structures of chemically treated wood and metal (copper, galvanized zinc and lead) (Figure 10.4) have been associated with health problems. It is not always possible to confirm that a substance is harmful to fish; in cases where there is doubt, all unnecessary objects should be removed and the pond stripped back to the bare essentials. Fish will live quite happily in a bare environment until the problem is resolved and the water quality improves. Occasionally the most innocuous-looking object is the cause of a problem (Figure 10.5).

With the expansion of koi keeping, local koi clubs have become useful sources of information on the design and construction of ponds and filtration systems.

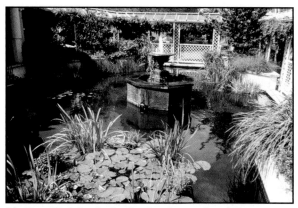

Figure 10.4 Aesthetically pleasing environments are not necessarily healthy ones for stocking with fish. Large metal fountains may pollute the water with toxic heavy metals. Large aquatic plants provide shelter from sunlight, predators and veterinarians. (© W.H. Wildgoose.)

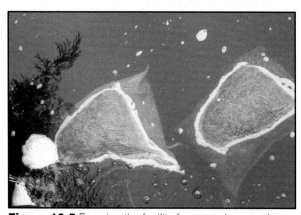

Figure 10.5 Examine the facility for any submerged objects. Some seemingly innocuous materials may leach harmful substances. Open-weave bags of barley straw are used to control algal growth in outdoor ponds but anaerobic decomposition of the straw can produce toxic by-products. (© W.H. Wildgoose.)

Examining aquaria

In contrast to ponds, the examination of aquaria is relatively uncomplicated because most are of a standard design and construction. Their small size also makes them easy to inspect. Most are situated indoors and are therefore in a more stable climatic environment, though they can be subjected to other disturbances such as noise, vibration, unnatural lighting patterns and excessive social activity. Pollution from toxic aerosols and other air-borne chemicals is also a potential hazard.

Water appearance

Many hobbyists assume that fish require pristine water conditions for good health but in reality the clarity of water is more for the viewing pleasure of the keeper. Algae are a normal component of aquatic ecosystems and serve many useful purposes: they produce oxygen by photosynthesis, provide a food source for herbivorous fish and can remove some toxins from the water column.

Excessive algal growth (Figure 10.6) can reduce dissolved oxygen levels at night and create environmental hypoxia in the hours just before daybreak. Algal accumulation on the surface is often termed 'scum' and, in excess, restricts photosynthesis by submerged plants and reduces gas exchange at the surface. Filters can become blocked and their biological efficiency reduced. Algal decomposition removes oxygen and may produce harmful substances such as hydrogen sulphide. Some species of algae, such as *Microcystis aeruginosa*, are capable of producing neuro- and hepatotoxins that are harmful to fish and mammals. Filamentous algae must be removed manually but unicellular (unattached) algae can be controlled by ultraviolet filter units.

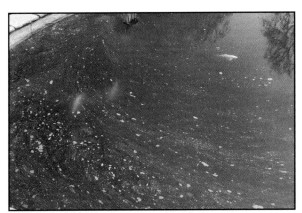

Figure 10.6 Algal bloom with proteinaceous scum and uneaten food on the surface. Poor visibility made it difficult to catch the fish or see into the water; a net was used to dredge the bottom for sediment. (© W.H. Wildgoose.)

Sludge and sediment comprise organic waste material and debris such as uneaten food, faecal matter and dead algae. Slow accumulation over prolonged periods is not of concern but sediment should be removed regularly to prevent the development of anaerobic zones during decomposition.

Suspended solids will alter the water's appearance and colour. The use of unwashed coral sand will produce a fine milky discoloration in a marine aquarium. Fine powdered clays (e.g. montmorillonite) have recently been used to add various minerals to the water in koi ponds. It is uncertain how beneficial these may be to the fish.

Aquatic plants

Adequate water depth is required in facilities with live plants but this should also allow sufficient light to penetrate to submerged plants. Deep ponds or 'show aquaria' (which are taller than standard tanks of the same volume) are unsuitable for plants unless additional lighting is provided. Poor growth of algae and aquatic plants in outdoor ponds can be an indication of poor water conditions related to the presence of harmful exogenous substances.

Live plants and their soil substrate may contain eggs of parasites such as fish lice or leeches. Therefore, before being introduced, new plants should be disinfected with a suitable proprietary product or dilute solution of potassium permanganate.

Large plants and shelves provide areas for fish to hide but also alter water flow and make it difficult to catch fish for examination. In addition, these items make it more difficult to clean the pond. Sometimes, minimal is better.

Filtration

Filtration systems are used to maintain good water quality. The variety of methods employed includes mechanical, chemical and biological filtration.

- Mechanical filters remove suspended solids and other debris. Many mechanical filters can be reused by rinsing or 'backwashing' the medium
- Chemical filters employ binding materials to remove compounds from the water. These include activated charcoal and zeolite, an ammonia-binding medium
- Biological filters function by encouraging various microorganisms to convert nitrogenous wastes into less toxic compounds.

No one type of filter provides perfect results and a combination of methods is often used. Examples of various materials and equipment are given in earlier chapters in this book. It is essential to have a basic understanding of the purpose and design of filtration systems, since their malfunction is often the cause of poor water quality. In many cases, it will be necessary for the veterinarian to suggest practical solutions to improve their function.

Pond filtration systems

To process effectively the substantial volume of water in a pond requires a large filtration system. Although some units are manufactured commercially, many are homemade; their construction is often an evolutionary process and different designs are constantly being developed and 'improved'. A pond with a low stocking density can be maintained with a simple gravel-bed filter but most enthusiasts want a heavily stocked pond with as many fish as possible. Therefore, filtration systems must be capable of handling a high biological load.

To inspect these systems thoroughly involves opening each chamber to see how they have been constructed. It is advisable to sketch a plan of the pipework and layout of the system to gain a better understanding of the design and function (Figure 10.7). Observing the flow of water through the different compartments will often reveal shortcomings in the construction and, on occasion, the fact that the water may completely bypass the filter media (Figures 10.8 and 10.9).

It is often necessary to remove some medium to determine the amount of organic debris that collects in the chambers and to assess the level of maintenance. There should be very little debris in a well maintained

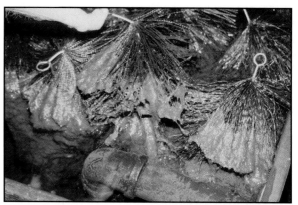

Figure 10.9 In multi-chambered filter systems, only the first chamber should contain debris. The black brushes act as a mechanical filter and remove suspended solids. They must be cleaned regularly to avoid becoming blocked with debris and algae. In this case, the water started to channel past the brushes and deposit debris in the subsequent biological chambers. (© W.H. Wildgoose.)

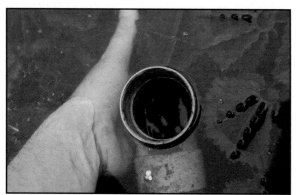

Figure 10.7 In some homemade systems it is difficult to appreciate the direction of flow of the water and see if sediment is collecting in the bottom of the filter chambers. It is often necessary to examine the pipework and chambers manually to assess the build-up of debris. (© W.H. Wildgoose.)

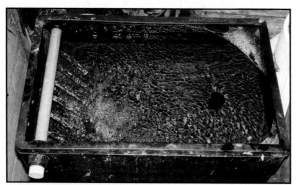

Figure 10.8 To inspect the filter system, take off the covers, identify the relevant pipework and assess its functionality. Single-chamber external filters such as this one have a layer of foam on the top, which frequently becomes blocked by sediment. This causes the water level to rise and drain through the overflow on the right hand side, bypassing all the filter medium below. The foam must be rinsed clean on a regular basis. (© W.H. Wildgoose.)

filter system. The design should allow any debris to accumulate in a void or separate chamber that is easily cleaned through a bottom drain. Unfortunately, this is rarely the case, and cleaning of multifunctional single-chambered units is often difficult and time-consuming. As a result, maintenance is often inadequate.

> **TIP:** Roll up your sleeve and scrape the bottom of the filter chamber with your hand to assess the depth of sediment.

Partially blocked pipes due to a build-up of sediment in the filtration system will reduce water flow significantly. It may be necessary to measure the flow rate through the filter using a bucket of known volume and a stopwatch. It should be noted that if sediment is disturbed and enters the pond, then not only does it reduce visibility and make it difficult to catch fish but it may also introduce toxic compounds resulting from anaerobic decomposition.

Aquarium filtration systems

The commercial filtration units used for aquaria are manufactured to a high standard and various sizes are available for different sizes of tank. Their compact size and construction make them easy to inspect and maintain. It is advised that the medium is examined to ensure that it is still porous and allows a good flow of water. Activated carbon should be changed at regular intervals to avoid the release of harmful substances that have been adsorbed.

Stocking conditions

Stocking density

A sparsely stocked pond or aquarium is usually more resistant to changes in water quality. Suitable stocking densities for different facilities are given in the appropriate chapters of this book.

Although a larger filtration system may permit a higher stocking density, it may also result in a catastrophe if there is any disturbance to the biological filter or water quality. It should be appreciated that growth of the fish over a period of a few years may result in an overstocked facility. Equally, this may occur following the successful hatching and rearing of fry within the tank or pond.

Compatibility

Behaviour
In a facility with several different species, considerable attention must be given to their compatibility. This mainly applies to tropical freshwater and marine fish. In general, herbivorous fish tend to cohabit better than carnivorous or piscivorous species. Size, sex, breeding status, stocking density and geography of origin also play significant roles in domination and tolerance. Ample hiding areas and multiple feeding stations should be provided for the benefit of less dominant species. New fish should be introduced slowly and a few at a time.

Water chemistry
If species are to be mixed, it is recommended that fish with similar tolerances of temperature, salinity and pH be kept together. Species that cohabit in the same geographical location tend to do well in captive systems when proper husbandry is provided.

Disease
It is inadvisable to mix species from different geographical origins: one species may be a subclinical carrier of a disease that could prove devastating to another naïve population.

Husbandry

The examination of husbandry practices is a routine component of fish health investigation. Detailed information about the system should be recorded methodically, together with maintenance procedures. Owners should be encouraged to keep their own records, since these are often helpful in the investigation of a health problem.

Some information about the standard of husbandry can be gleaned from the owner by detailed questioning but it is often necessary to look for evidence in the environment. Routine fish husbandry includes:

* Water quality testing
* Feeding
* Water changes and top-up
* Cleaning and disinfection
* Quarantine of fish and plants
* Use of chemical medications.

Water quality testing
The routine monitoring of water quality is an essential aspect of preventive medicine in fish keeping. A variety of water quality test kits is readily available from most aquatic retail outlets. They vary in their sensitivity but most are easy and quick to use. Basic test kits measure pH, ammonia, nitrite and nitrate. Other kits are available for measuring alkalinity, dissolved oxygen, chlorine, salinity, hardness and copper levels.

Regardless of the size of a filtration system, it is essential that water quality be tested routinely. As an absolute minimum, the metabolic wastes and their associated parameters should be measured (Figure 10.10). These include ammonia, nitrite, nitrate, temperature and pH but it may also be necessary to test for other parameters. The results from some tests may be influenced by various additional factors that must be taken into account; for example, dissolved oxygen levels will vary according to the time of day when the tests are performed and ionized ammonia will depend on temperature and pH.

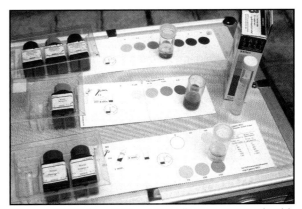

Figure 10.10 Standard water quality parameters should always be checked by the veterinarian. Regardless of the appearance and design of a filtration system, the result of its functionality is that it should be able to provide good water quality. (© W.H. Wildgoose.)

Inexpensive commercial colorimetric test kits are available in two forms: wet and dry. Both are sufficiently accurate for the hobbyist and for helping to identify problems. In wet chemistry tests, various liquids or powders are added to a small measured volume of water. The mixture is agitated and the parameter is quantified by comparing the colour change in the reagent with a colour chart. The dry test kit is used in a similar manner, adding a reagent tablet to the sample. Dry test kits have a longer shelf life but are slightly more expensive. Other equipment used to test water parameters is discussed in more detail in Chapter 13.

There is no standard recommended interval for testing water parameters and after the first few weeks testing is often performed infrequently unless there are health problems. It is advisable to test water quality daily for the first 3 weeks, then weekly for a month and every 2 weeks thereafter when the system has become stable. This guideline should be altered according to the introduction of new fish and whenever there are signs of disease.

TIP: The tests should always be performed personally by the veterinarian, if only to confirm the results obtained by the owner.

Feeding practices

Feeding methods vary greatly between species and systems. Fish should be given no more food than they can consume in 2–3 minutes, after which time any excess and uneaten food should be removed. Different species should be given an appropriate diet: surface-feeding species should be given a floating flake or pellet food; bottom-feeding species should receive a sinking pellet; some carnivorous fish will only eat live prey. If some fish are aggressive feeders, feeding at several locations will enable less dominant fish to feed.

It is recommend that all fish are fed a variety of foodstuffs to ensure adequate intake of essential nutrients. It is a false assumption that any one food item will provide a complete balanced diet: fish that will eat only a selective diet should be given a suitable vitamin and mineral supplement.

Water changes

Regular partial water changes are often required to remove or dilute nitrates and other substances in the water. The quantity and frequency of these changes will vary according to the system in question.

When adding water to the system, effort should be made to match temperature and pH. Complete (100%) water changes should never be performed, since the dramatic change in water chemistry may be physiologically stressful to the fish.

Ponds: Water changes are only performed as and when required and as dictated by the water quality.

Aquaria: Approximately 25–30% should be changed every 2 weeks in a stable system unless severe circumstances arise. For marine species, because of water lost by evaporation, freshwater should be added regularly to maintain the correct salinity.

Cleaning and disinfection

The bottom of the tank or pond and the filter chambers should be cleaned regularly to remove any debris or sediment. The frequency with which this is performed varies with the stocking density and organic load in the system. The cleaning of biological filtration systems should never be so thorough that the film of slime on the medium is removed. The nitrifying microorganisms that remove the ammonia and nitrite colonize all submerged surfaces in the system and overzealous cleaning will seriously affect the biological filter. Media should be rinsed gently in a bucket of water from the tank or pond; tap water may contain traces of chlorine, which may kill the nitrifying microorganisms.

Regular disinfection of equipment and nets is seldom performed by hobbyists, because the traces of some agents are harmful to fish. Mechanical cleaning and use of detergents followed by rinsing with clean fresh water is often considered adequate if the equipment is allowed to dry thoroughly.

Quarantine

The principles of quarantine and isolation of new fish are discussed elsewhere. It is advisable to examine the quarantine facility to ensure that it is of a suitable size and has adequate filtration. All new fish should be isolated for 4 weeks prior to introduction to the main facility. During this time, it may be appropriate to use medications to treat for various parasites, but it is not possible to exclude all pathogens.

Chemical medications

Inexperienced owners, who inevitably encounter health problems with their new facility, often resort to the use of chemical medications. They fail to recognize an underlying water quality problem and assume that the ensuing parasitic or bacterial disease will be resolved with the use of chemicals. Equally, some owners regularly medicate their ponds or tanks with various products on a prophylactic basis, assuming that this will provide some degree of protection. Neither of these activities is beneficial in the long term and may create further environmental stress.

The use of some antibacterial medications (e.g. methylene blue, antibiotics) as a permanent bath may also harm the biological filtration.

As mentioned above, husbandry practices will vary significantly with each individual system. Being consistent and diligent will enable hobbyists to monitor the smallest environmental changes and enable them to take prompt remedial action to maintain the health of their fish.

Further reading

Andrews C, Exell A and Carrington N (1988) *The Manual of Fish Health.* Tetra Press, Morris Plains, New Jersey

Bassleer G (1996) *Diseases in Marine Aquarium Fish: Causes – Symptoms – Treatment.* Bassleer Biofish n.v., Westmeerbeek, Belgium

Beleau MH (1988) Evaluating water problems. In: *The Veterinary Clinics of North America: Small Animal Practice: Tropical Fish Medicine,* ed. MK Stoskopf, **18**(2), 291–304. WB Saunders Company, Philadelphia, Pennsylvania

Burgess WE (1987) *Marine Aquariums: a Complete Introduction.* TFH Publications, Neptune City, New Jersey

Butcher RL (1993) The veterinary approach to ornamental fish. In: *Aquaculture for Veterinarians,* ed. L Brown, pp. 357–378. Pergamon Press, Oxford

Cecil TR (1999) Husbandry and husbandry-related diseases of ornamental fish. In: *The Veterinary Clinics of North America: Exotic Animal Practice: Husbandry and Nutrition,* ed. JR Jenkins, pp. 1–18. WB Saunders, Philadelphia, Pennsylvania

Johnson EL (1997) *Koi Health and Disease.* Reade Printers, Athens, Georgia

Moe MM Jr (1982) *The Marine Aquarium Handbook.* Green Turtle Publications, Plantation, Florida

Moyle PB and Cech JJ Jr (1988) *Fishes: An Introduction to Ichthyology,* 2nd edn. Prentice Hall, Englewood Cliffs, New Jersey

Post G (1987) *Textbook of Fish Health.* TFH Publications, Neptune City, New Jersey

Spotte S (1992) *Captive Seawater Fishes: Science and Technology.* John Wiley & Sons, New York

Stoskopf MK (1988) Taking the history. In: *The Veterinary Clinics of North America: Small Animal Practice: Tropical Fish Medicine,* ed. MK Stoskopf, **18**, 283–291. WB Saunders Company, Philadelphia, Pennsylvania

Stoskopf MK (1993) Environmental requirements and diseases of carp, koi, and goldfish. In: *Fish Medicine,* ed. MK Stoskopf, pp. 455–461. WB Saunders, Philadelphia, Pennsylvania

Winfree RA (1992) Nutrition and feeding tropical fish. In: *Aquariology, the Science of Fish Health Management,* eds JB Gratzek and JR Matthews, pp. 187–207. Tetra Press, Morris Plains, New Jersey

11

Restraint, anaesthesia and euthanasia

Lindsay G. Ross

Fish find all forms of handling stressful. They struggle during capture both in and out of their natural environment and can easily suffer significant damage to their epidermis (which is external to the scales). Once damaged, osmoregulatory and pathogenic problems follow. Therefore, fish need to be immobilized before attempts are made to perform many tasks. Sedation may be essential to minimize stress and physical damage during capture or handling.

There are many instances in which some form of calming technique will be required – for example, during handling and injection of dangerous species, paracentesis of abdominal fluids and radiography. In other cases, additional time may be needed to handle fish or perform a surgical procedure and then full surgical anaesthesia will be required.

Although there is some disagreement over the nature of pain perception in fish, it is now considered that fish have a high ability to feel pain (Erdmann, 1999; Gregory, 1999). Any invasive procedure seems certain to cause some degree of pain and steps must be taken to alleviate any consequent suffering.

Physical restraint

Fish can be handled without anaesthesia for simple procedures such as physical examination and injection, which can often be performed entirely underwater without causing harm. Similarly, careful but firm handling of broodstock fish can enable stripping of eggs and sperm without any sedation.

Handling is improved if the head and eyes are covered and any noise and other disturbances are minimized. Larger fish can be grasped by the caudal peduncle and then supported under the abdomen or in a manner similar to that shown in Figure 11.1. Moist cloths are occasionally used to protect the skin but care should be taken that these are not themselves abrasive. Some caution needs to be taken with species that have hard spines: even those on tilapia or catfish can be dangerous and painful, and some are poisonous.

Handling is easier if fish are gently crowded into an area of their enclosure from which they can be netted. These nets should be appropriate to the size of the fish and preferably of knotless material to minimize skin damage. Sock nets (Figure 11.2) are useful for carrying large fish for short distances. Placing a sock net over the head of a fish will calm it sufficiently to allow basic

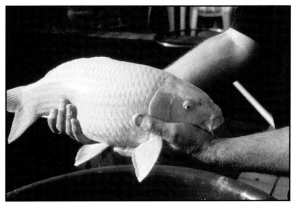

Figure 11.1 Manual restraint of large koi. Some placid fish can be held out of water for up to a minute, enabling close examination of the external surfaces. Not all koi can be handled in this way, and experience is required. (© W.H. Wildgoose.)

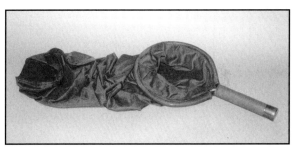

Figure 11.2 Sock nets (long tubular nets made of strong fabric and open at both ends) can be used to carry large fish by placing them in the middle and gripping both ends of the net before removing the fish from the water. (© W.H. Wildgoose.)

examination. Large pond fish should be netted into containers of clean water for movement or examination. Single smaller fish can be handled in a clear polythene bag, in which they can also be closely observed.

Sedation and anaesthesia

Sedation and general anaesthesia of fish are relative states on a continuum that provides various degrees of relaxation, analgesia, immobilization and unconsciousness. This may be achieved using chemical anaesthesia, hypothermia or exposure to an electric current.

Stages of anaesthesia depend on the combination of dose rate and length of exposure (Figures 11.3 and 11.4). In practice, there may not be clear conformity with every stage. At high concentrations, fish pass rapidly through all of the stages shown in Figure 11.3, while at lower concentrations a comparatively steady state may be maintained. Understanding the relationship between dose, exposure time and anaesthetic stage achieved is important in ensuring good control of a procedure.

Analgesia

Although assessment of analgesia is rarely made, the degree and nature of analgesia achieved are important. In most cases, analgesia has been assumed to be effective because the fish is immobilized, but this will not always be true.

Stage	Plane	Description	Physiological and behavioural signs
I	1	Light sedation	Responsive to stimuli but motion reduced, ventilation decreased
	2	Deep sedation	As above, but some analgesia, only receptive to gross stimulation
II	1	Light anaesthesia	Partial loss of equilibrium. Good analgesia
	2	Deeper anaesthesia	Total loss of muscle tone, total loss of equilibrium, respiration almost absent
III		Surgical anaesthesia	As above: total loss of reaction to even massive stimulation
IV		Medullary collapse	Respiration ceases, cardiac arrest, eventual death. Overdose

Figure 11.3 Stages of anaesthesia in fish (after McFarland, 1959).

Anaesthesia

The three obvious phases in practical fish anaesthesia are induction, maintenance and recovery. These vary in duration according to drug or method used, species and conditions. The many factors that can alter or mediate the efficacy of anaesthesia in fish are summarized in Figure 11.5. Perhaps the most important of these are species differences, health status and water temperature.

Preparation

During anaesthesia, it is not uncommon for some species to regurgitate food material, which may then irritate the gills. Similarly, fish often pass faeces during

Biological factors	Probable mechanism
Species	Differences in body design and habit Gill area to bodyweight ratio
Strain or genetic variance	Physiological variability Differences in enzymes?
Size and/or weight	Change in metabolic rate
Sex and sexual maturity	Lipid content? (Especially in gonads)
Lipid content	Lipophilic drugs? Oily fish or older specimens
Body condition	Exhausted animals, post-spawning
Health status and stress	Diseased or exhausted animals
Environmental factors	**Probable mechanism**
Temperature	Temperature quotient (Q_{10}) as in all ectotherms (poikilotherms)
pH	Effects on pKa (acid/base ionization constant) and ionization of molecules
Salinity	Buffering effects
Mineral content of environment	Calcium antagonism

Figure 11.5 Factors affecting the efficacy of anaesthetics for fish.

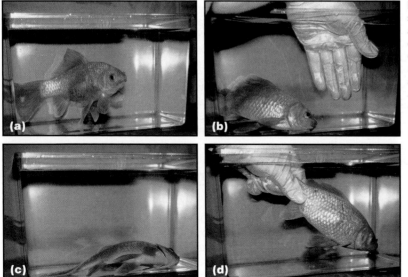

Figure 11.4 The most common stages of anaesthesia: (a) no anaesthetic is present and the goldfish demonstrates a normal posture; (b) light sedation, ataxia and reduced response to stimulation; (c) deep anaesthesia, with loss of muscle tone and total loss of equilibrium; (d) surgical anaesthesia, with lack of response to firm pressure on the peduncle. (© W.H. Wildgoose.)

induction and further pollute the water. Both events are minimized by starvation. Where possible, the patient should be starved for 12–24 hours prior to anaesthesia.

Induction
Induction should be rapid and fish will normally exhibit a succession of the signs described in Figure 11.3, notably ataxia and loss of the righting reflex, eventually passing into surgical anaesthesia with no reaction to any stimuli. Induction is often accompanied by hyper-activity, usually for only a few seconds, which is either a pharmacological side-effect or a reaction to slightly irritant properties of the drug.

Monitoring
For short procedures lasting no more than a few minutes, observation of respiratory rate (opercular movement) and response to manipulation will reflect the depth of anaesthesia. Respiration will usually be slow and regular, and there should be a minimal response to manual stimuli.

Effective monitoring of the lack of reflexes to assess the depth of anaesthesia may necessitate the use of either an electrocardiograph (ECG) or a Doppler pulse ultrasound probe, particularly during prolonged anaes-thesia. A routine ECG monitor or a simple bleeper triggered by the QRS complex can be used to detect heart rate. Electrodes are clamped lightly to the surface of the fins (the pectoral and anal fins are a good combination). The use of pulse oximetry has not proved particularly useful in fish.

Maintenance
Stable extension of an achieved stage can usually be maintained on a reduced drug dose. The environment of the anaesthetized fish and physiological needs such as the supply of oxygen and removal of carbon dioxide and metabolic wastes must be managed.

Recovery
Recovery should be quick and without altered behav-iour or other side-effects, though there will usually be some muscle trembling. Fish will attempt to right them-selves and begin to respond to noise or other sensory stimuli. Sympathetic handling and general good care are essential during this period, which may take any-thing from a few seconds to a few minutes.

Legislation
The legislation covering anaesthetic procedures and materials has been steadily improved and extended. Across the world it has many common features and all users of these drugs must comply with the relevant legislation for the country in which they operate. Treves-Brown (2000) gives a comprehensive overview of the current legal position in some countries.

In summary, an anaesthetic agent must satisfy various criteria:

- Safety (safe in storage and safe to the user, to the treated fish and to the environment)
- Quality (of an approved quality and free from harmful residues)
- Efficacy (effective for its intended purpose).

Consent forms
It is recommended that the risk to the patient is fully explained to the owner and that their written consent is obtained.

Health and safety
Few anaesthetic agents used in fish have been proved to be harmful to humans but it is recom-mended that operators should avoid direct contact with most chemicals and that goggles and protective gloves should be worn. Care should be taken to avoid splashes from fish during induction and hands should be washed afterwards.

Inhalation anaesthesia

This most widely used technique is analogous to gas-eous anaesthesia in terrestrial animals. The anaes-thetic drug in aqueous solution is ventilated by the fish, entering the bloodstream through the gills and passing rapidly to the central nervous system. On return to fresh water, drugs or their metabolites are excreted mostly via the gills, to a lesser extent via the kidney and to a small extent via the skin.

This technique is less predictable in air-breathers. For example, the snakehead is an obligate air-breather with much reduced gills and induction of anaesthesia is usually lengthy, unpredictable and frustrating. Eels and most catfishes are facultative air-breathers and have a similar response, often swimming violently around on the surface during induction. Care should be taken to avoid the fish jumping from the tank.

Inhalation anaesthetic agents
Figure 11.6 provides descriptions and dose rates for the most commonly used anaesthetic agents. When anaesthetizing an unfamiliar species, it is recommended that the drug of choice is one that has been used in other species most similar in structure, body design and habit to the subject. When using new anaesthetic agents, it is strongly recommended that the lowest dose rate be used initially on a few fish in order to monitor any adverse reaction. From this, a more appro-priate combination of dose and time can be selected for use with a good degree of confidence.

Preparation
Anaesthetic drugs for fish must be easily soluble in water or in a water-soluble solvent, which can be used as a vehicle. It is always preferable to use water from the fish's own tank or pond with which to make up the anaesthetic solution. For simple procedures, it is usually possible to immerse the fish directly in a suitable concentration of drug so that spontaneous ventilation is maintained. The required drug concentration is made up in an aerated container to which fish are transferred quickly but gently.

Anaesthetic solutions are most accurately made up using a measured volume of a standard stock solution (Figure 11.6). However, preparing stock solutions of expensive powdered anaesthetic agents such as MS222 may be uneconomical if used infrequently. In

Drug	Notes	Species	Dose
MS222 (Ethyl m-aminobenzoate, Tricaine methane sulphonate, Metacaine)	White crystalline powder; keeps well when dry Acidic in solution and irritant to fish Very soluble in fresh and sea water (up to 11% w/v) Stock solution (10 g/l) can be kept in sealed dark bottle for up to 3 months (eventually darkens and loses potency) Stock solutions or working solution can be buffered using sodium bicarbonate or Tris-buffer Good safety margin More potent in warm waters with low hardness Fat-soluble; slow recovery in older or gravid animals Currently not known to be toxic to humans at concentrations used Currently the only licensed fish anaesthetic in UK and USA	Carp Tench Grass carp Tilapia, adults Tilapia, fry Other species	20–85 mg/l 25–200 mg/l 75 mg/l 100–200 mg/l 60–70 mg/l 20–250 mg/l
Benzocaine (Ethyl-4-aminobenzoate)	White crystalline material; very similar to MS222 Almost totally insoluble in water (only 0.04% w/v) Must first be dissolved in acetone or ethanol Stock solution, usually 100 g/l; can be kept in sealed dark bottle for up to 1 year Regular use does not affect growth or reproduction Useful in freshwater, marine and tropical species (at higher doses) Good safety margin; less at higher temperatures Not affected by water hardness or pH Fat-soluble; slow recovery in older or gravid animals Not toxic to humans at the concentrations used	Tilapia Catfish Other species	100 mg/l 100 mg/l 25–200 mg/l
Quinaldine (2-4-methylquinoline) and Quinaldine sulphate	Quinaldine: yellowish oily liquid; limited water solubility; must first be dissolved in acetone or alcohol; unpleasant, irritant, insoluble and may cause corneal damage; low cost, therefore popular for collection of wild ornamental fishes Quinaldine sulphate: pale yellow water soluble powder; more costly than quinaldine and MS222 Solutions are acidic; usually buffered with sodium bicarbonate Stock solutions (10 g/l) can be kept in sealed dark bottles Less potent in soft water and more in warm water Ineffective below pH 5; more potent at higher pH Irritant and has unpleasant odour Not known to be carcinogenic	Cyprinids Grass carp Blenny Tropical marine Other species	12–37 mg/l 10–50 mg/l 2.5–20 mg/l 200 mg/l 2–150 mg/l
2-Phenoxyethanol (Phenoxethol, 2-PE)	Clear or straw-coloured oily liquid; slight aromatic odour Fairly soluble if vigorously mixed into water Working solution remains effective for at least 3 days Bactericidal and fungicidal in solution Relatively inexpensive Safer and more potent at lower temperatures	Carp Big head carp Grass carp Other species	0.1–0.5 ml/l 0.2 ml/l 0.2 ml/l 0.1–0.5 ml/l
Metomidate (Methoxymol, Marinil, Hypnodil, R7315)	Imidazole-based non-barbiturate hypnotic drug Variable results when used with some species Virtually no analgesia Darkening of skin in some species	Various species	0.5–10 mg/l
Etomidate (Hypnomidate, Amidate)	Imidazole-based non-barbiturate hypnotic drug Virtually no analgesia Used in aquarium species (danios, freshwater angelfish, platys)	Aquarium fish	2–4 mg/l
Clove oil	Koi Calm (NT Labs): Contains very wide range of turpenoid compounds; major consituent (70–90%) is the oil eugenol More soluble in hot water or 95% ethanol Stock solution (10 ml/l ethanol) remains effective for 3 months at room temperature Inexpensive; readily available without prescription Not unpleasant to handle Not known to be harmful to humans	Crucian carp Carp Channel catfish Other species	25–100 mg/l 25–100 mg/l 100–150 mg/l 20–100 mg/l
	Aqui-S: New, based on above compound, developed in New Zealand Contains 50% 2-methoxy-4-propenylphenol and 50% polysorbate 80 Generally regarded as safe for use in food fish by FDA More effective than clove oil Safe to fish and humans Inexpensive	All	6–17 mg/l
2-amino-4-phenylthiazole (APT, Phenthiazamine, Piscaine)	Used in Japan Probably acts by depression of the CNS Carp can be sedated (at low dose) for up to 72 hours	Carp Loach Other species	12–40 mg/l 50 mg/l 8–30 mg/l
Carbon dioxide	Effective in fish; questionable analgesia More control if oxygen levels also elevated Requires gas mixtures and monitoring equipment Also generated using acidified sodium bicarbonate (requires pH control) Released from Alka-Seltzer® tablets in water	Carp fry Other species	400 mg/l 120–150 mg/l
Lignocaine (Xylocaine, Lidocaine)	Widely used local and general analgesic Relatively cheap, easy to obtain Safe to humans at concentrations used with fish	Carp Other species	100 mg/l 100–150 mg/l
Fluorinated hydrocarbons (halothane, isoflurane)	Readily available in veterinary clinics Can be added direct to water by spraying into water through fine hypodermic needle (under surface) Can be vaporized and bubbled through water Difficult to control concentrations, due to insolubility Volatile agent hazardous to operators and difficult to scavenge Advisable only as last resort or for euthanasia	Carp Other species	0.4–0.75 ml/l 0.5–2 ml/l

Figure 11.6 Dose rates and notes for various inhalation anaesthetic agents (after Ross and Ross, 1999).

the absence of an accurate balance with which to weigh dry chemicals, it may be more practical to use a standard pharmaceutical scoop. As an example, a level 0.5 ml scoop, which holds approximately 400 mg of MS222.

Maintenance of water quality

Water quality needs to be carefully controlled during inhalation anaesthesia, particularly where many fish are being handled and where baths are being reused. The main problems are related to temperature, dissolved oxygen concentration, ammonia levels and build-up of faecal solids in the baths. If possible, anaesthetic baths and recovery vessels should use water from which the fish originated and at the same temperature. Small electrical heaters and coolers can be used (but will rarely be needed for short procedures) or cooling can be effected with ice packs. It is also important to ensure that fish do not become overheated or chilled while in air.

The holding tanks, anaesthetic bath and recovery vessel should be equipped with air-stones or, better, with fine bubble diffusers. Excreted solids are more problematic but water changes can be used and should be effected as often as needed.

Procedure

Induction should be rapid, handling time minimal and the fish should be transferred to clean, well aerated water within a few minutes following the required procedure. For adequate handling, it is not usually necessary to exceed stage 1 and plane 2 of McFarland's scheme (see Figure 11.3). Spontaneous ventilation of the gills is maintained and well aerated drug solution and recovery baths will ensure an adequate oxygen supply and no mortality. A scheme of work is useful to ensure that the welfare of the fish is maintained (Figures 11.7 and 11.8).

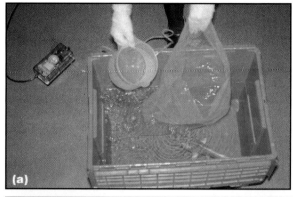
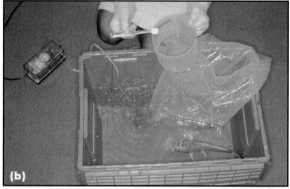
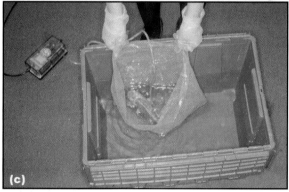

Figure 11.8 Practical anaesthesia of koi. (a) The koi is held in a large storage box containing water from the pond of origin. A stiff polythene bag is filled with a known volume of water (4 litres). Air-stones are present in the box and the bag. (b) A measured amount of anaesthetic agent is dissolved in a small amount of water and mixed with water in the bag. A level quarter-teaspoon measure (equivalent to 0.8 ml scoop) of MS222 contains approximately 650 mg and will produce a final concentration of 160 mg/l when mixed with 4 litres of water. (c) The fish is gently lifted by hand and placed in the anaesthetic solution in the bag until it reaches the desired plane of anaesthesia. This method requires a minimal amount of water and drug but care should be taken to ensure that the fish does not suffocate on the walls of the bag. (© W.H. Wildgoose.)

---

1. Prepare a stock solution of the anaesthetic agent. Store in a sealed dark bottle and refrigerate.

2. Prepare all relevant equipment for the intended procedure (e.g. nets, buckets, syringes, needles, injectable drugs).

3. Prepare the anaesthetic bath to the appropriate final concentration by slowly adding the anaesthetic agent to water, stirring thoroughly to disperse the drug and to prevent some drugs coming out of solution (e.g. benzocaine).

4. Prepare a recovery vessel of clean, well oxygenated water using air-stones or a bubble diffuser.

5. Adjust the pH and temperature in the anaesthetic bath and recovery tank to the same as that in the holding tank.

6. Gently net the fish and transfer it to the anaesthetic bath. Fish must not remain in the bath for extended periods.

7. Commence the procedure as soon as the fish can be handled gently and without struggling. This is usually achievable just before the fish lose equilibrium.

8. Immediately place the fish in the recovery tank. Substantial recovery will normally occur within 1 minute, though some species may require slightly longer. Avoid overstocking the recovery tank if several fish are being anaesthetized.

Figure 11.7 Scheme of work for using inhalation anaesthesia.

Direct application of inhalation agents

With large fish (e.g. sharks, groupers), where immersion is impractical or dangerous to the operators, drugs are sometimes applied directly to the gills. Inexpensive plastic spray bottles, widely available in garden centres, are ideal for this application. When used by divers underwater, the addition of a harmless dye such as food colouring helps to identify the distribution of the anaesthetic.

Artificial ventilation systems

In situations where prolonged surgical anaesthesia is required, a system of artificial ventilation can be used. These systems are also immensely useful for species that are slow to recover (e.g. debilitated fish and those under deep surgical anaesthesia). A supply of aerated anaesthetic solution at the correct temperature is simply delivered from a pipe or mouthpiece into the buccal cavity. The anaesthetic solution flows over gills and drains away. The following two systems are commonly used.

Non-recirculating system

An intravenous fluid bag and modified giving set (Figures 11.9 and 11.10) are used as the reservoir for the anaesthetic solution and delivery system. The bag is emptied and an opening is made at the top to allow filling with the anaesthetic solution and insertion of a small air-stone. The flow rate is controlled by the valve on the giving set. This system is suitable for small fish up to 250 g.

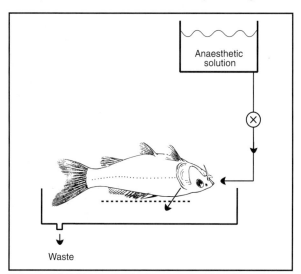

Figure 11.9 Non-recirculating system. A header tank contains a maintenance dose of anaesthetic solution that passes into the fish's mouth through a plastic tube. A valve mechanism ⊗ controls the rate of flow. Water passes out through the gills and drains away. Fresh anaesthetic solution is added to the header tank when required.

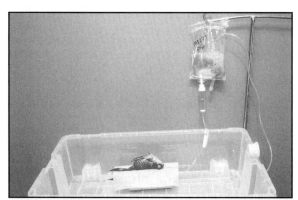

Figure 11.10 Working example of a non-recirculating anaesthetic system. An intravenous fluid bag contains the anaesthetic solution and an air-stone to aerate the water. A control valve regulates the water flow through a shortened giving set. Unrestricted flow will produce about 250 ml/min, enough for fish weighing up to 250 g. (© W.H. Wildgoose.)

Recirculating system

Several systems that enable the collection and recycling of the effluent anaesthetic solutions have been described in the literature (Brown, 1987; Lewbart *et al.*, 1995; Lewbart and Harms, 1999) (Figures 11.11 and 11.12). The flow rate is controlled by a valve on the tube leading to the mouth. Where submersible pumps are used, it is important to consider electrical safety for the operator. Due to the potential hazards of using 240 V electrical supplies in the UK, it is advisable to use a residual current device (RCD) or low-voltage (12 V) pumps.

Method: The anaesthetic should be maintained at the fish's acclimation temperature and should be aerated to ensure near-saturation of oxygen and to remove dissolved carbon dioxide.

1. Pre-sedated fish are transferred to a suitable fish holder, which can be made by slitting a block of foam plastic halfway through. When this block is opened, it will grip the fish lightly while allowing water or anaesthetic solution to flow across the gills.
2. The fish holder is covered with a surgical drape or waterproof tissue (Figure 11.13), which does not readily disintegrate. Wet surgical drapes may be used to protect the fish from the heat of lights.

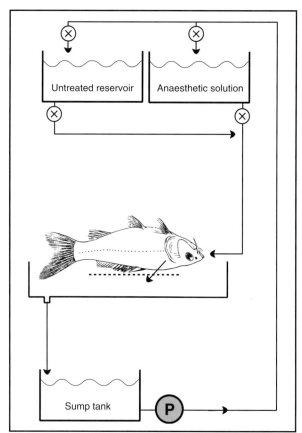

Figure 11.11 Simple recirculating anaesthesia system. Valves ⊗ control the flow rate and the choice of either anaesthetic solution or untreated water. This passes over the gills and drains from the trough into the sump tank for recirculating to the header tanks.

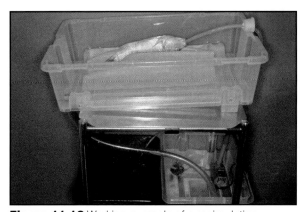

Figure 11.12 Working example of a recirculating anaesthetic system. The pump is a low-voltage pump for use in garden ponds. It has a valve that controls the output of water that enters the fish's mouth. Water drains back into the reservoir. To revive the fish, the pump and drain tube are moved into the blue reservoir on the left, which contains anaesthetic-free water. Air-stones are present in both reservoirs. (© W.H. Wildgoose.)

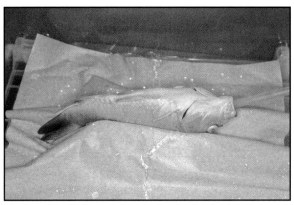

Figure 11.13 Restraining device for fish in dorsal recumbency. A block of foam is split half-way through and covered in a waterproof disposable drape. The fish should be positioned with the head free of the holder for the water to pass freely through the opercula. (© W.H. Wildgoose.)

3. The maintenance anaesthetic solution is usually at a lower concentration (half the induction dose) and is introduced into the buccal cavity from a plastic or rubber tube – silicon rubber is best.
4. The flow rate is adjusted so that a gentle flow of water passes over the gills. This varies according to the size of the fish: if the flow is too low, gas exchange will be poor; if it is too fast, gastric inflation or gill damage will result. Rates used in practice are between 1 and 3 l/minute per kilogram bodyweight.

Depending on the drugs used and assuming good environmental control, fish can be held in this state for several hours. Temperature control is important, as is prevention of drying of the skin, which can be alleviated by spraying with water at regular intervals from a small portable atomizer.

To terminate anaesthesia: the drug supply is stopped and clean drug-free water is passed over the gills until spontaneous ventilation returns.

Recovery

Anaesthesia is terminated by returning the fish to drug-free water but depth of anaesthesia may not be consistent using the bath technique, because drug dose and exposure time can act cumulatively. For example, levels of MS222 in brain and muscle continue to increase after blood levels have attained equilibrium. Therefore, a drug dose that is initially satisfactory can produce progressively deeper anaesthesia and eventual respiratory arrest. The resulting decline of water flow in the buccal cavity contributes to a reflex decline in heart rate and dorsal aortic blood pressure, producing a progressive hypoxia. No complications should occur during brief procedures, but lengthy exposure to a dissolved anaesthetic agent must be avoided.

Emergency resuscitation

Where a fish fails to recover spontaneous ventilation, the 'buccal flow/heart rate' reflex can be used to aid recovery. If the flow of water through the buccal cavity is increased, the heart rate will accelerate. The subsequent increased blood flow through the gills eliminates the drug more rapidly and hastens recovery.

In emergencies, this can be achieved by gently moving the fish through the water in a forward direction in the recovery bath. Alternatively, water can be passed through the buccal cavity from a narrow hose or using a modified rubber enema pump (Figure 11.14). Once the fish begins to ventilate spontaneously (this may take some time), it can be left to complete the process unattended. Respiration during recovery can often be very deep, with powerful regular movements of the opercula.

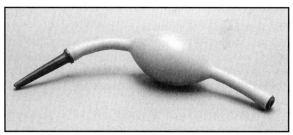

Figure 11.14 Modified Higginson rubber enema syringe for emergency resuscitation. The shortened ends contain one-way valves to ensure a unidirectional flow of water when the rubber bulb is squeezed. Gentle pressure is applied to the bulb to produce a flow of water appropriate to the size of the fish. (© W.H. Wildgoose.)

Parenteral anaesthesia

Although intravenous administration of anaesthetics is possible, in practice parenteral administration is usually given by intramuscular or intraperitoneal injection. This method of administration is more suited to larger fish in large aquaria where it is impractical to add the agent to the water. Injections are given by hand or using a pole syringe and the sites used are the same as those used for administering medicinal products (see Chapter 30). A list of suitable agents is given in Figure 11.15.

Drug	Notes	Species	Dose
Alphaxolone–alphadalone (Saffan)	Good anaesthesia but long duration Ventilation abolished at higher doses	Various species	12 mg/kg
Ketamine hydrochloride (Vetalar, Ketaset)	Good anaesthesia but long duration and prolonged recovery time Lower safety margin at higher temperatures	Bony fish Sharks and rays	66–68 mg/kg 12–20 mg/kg

Figure 11.15 Dose rates and notes for parenteral anaesthetic agents.

Non-chemical anaesthesia

There are two alternatives to the use of chemicals: hypothermia and electro-anaesthesia.

Hypothermia

Mild hypothermia will tranquillize or immobilize fish. It can be achieved by refrigeration, the addition of ice to the water or using dry ice (solidified carbon dioxide) in thermal contact with the water but physically and chemically isolated from it. Although there will be some immobilization and some reduction in sensitivity to stimulation, full analgesia will not be achieved.

Most fish have a relatively wide temperature tolerance but the amount of cooling that can be applied instantaneously depends on previous thermal history and current ambient temperature. If the temperature is lowered too far, or too quickly, death can ensue. Therefore, the main considerations are that the rate of cooling is carefully controlled and that the required low temperature can be easily maintained. In practice, gradual cooling is preferred because rapid chilling can produce osmoregulatory disruption and death. The technique has been used principally for transportation and minor surgery.

Temperate species can be cooled to about 4°C (depending on species and thermal history) to produce a deep narcosis from which recovery is rapid on return to the original temperature. Adult Atlantic salmon have been cooled to the temperature of iced water to produce a form of sedation that enables long-distance transportation of broodstock with no attendant mortalities. By contrast, some tropical species can only survive a limited instantaneous temperature decrease.

When hypothermia is used in conjunction with chemical anaesthesia, the normally effective dose of benzocaine could be reduced by about 30%. Overall, this technique has good calming properties for handling and transportation. When used alone, however, it is not suitable for any invasive work and almost certainly gives little analgesia.

Electro-anaesthesia

Direct current (DC) and alternating current (AC) with different waveforms have been used for anaesthesia and are commonly used in electro-fishing. All are capable of producing immobilization but their modes of action differ and only sine waves or chopped DC are fully effective in sea water. In general, the side-effects of electro-anaesthesia are no greater than those encountered using other methods but electrical stimulation can induce violent motor responses that can disfigure or even kill. The safety margin to the fish must be well understood and operator safety is of paramount importance but not easy to achieve in practice. While this technique has been used successfully, it is difficult to manage and its use in veterinary surgery is not recommended.

Sedation for transportation

The major concerns in transportation of fish are management of handling stress, temperature, dissolved oxygen levels and water quality. Sedation can be helpful in transporting fish, as it reduces metabolic rate and waste excretion. The simplest form of sedation is by cooling, using ice or dry ice, and this is routinely used in the aquaculture industry and for transportation of ornamental fish. In general, drugs can be used successfully at reduced dose rates and a wide range has been investigated, the most popular being MS222, benzocaine and 2-phenoxyethanol. Good results can be obtained when combined with moderate cooling, with 100% survival.

Euthanasia

It is sometimes necessary to kill fish humanely, either to avoid further suffering in a terminal case or to sacrifice a fish so that a postmortem examination can be performed. Euthanasia must be handled sensitively and with compassion. Some species will have little financial value but may have been owned for many years and be of great emotional value to their owners. Equally, owners may object to any mutilation of the body and wish to take their deceased pet home for burial. It is important that the chosen method of euthanasia is professional and causes an absolute minimum of physical and mental suffering. It is recommended that the procedure is fully explained to the owner and that their written consent is obtained.

Methods

Physical

Physical methods involve either dislocation of the neck or stunning with a sharp blow to the head using a club (called a priest). The latter technique is commonly used for farmed fish and is very effective, causing fatal damage to the brain tissues, but it requires skill and is unacceptable to most owners. It is also unsuitable if histological sampling of brain tissue is required.

Chemical

Chemical methods involve the use of an anaesthetic overdose, administered by either injection or immersion. As a guide, a dose of 5–10 times that used for anaesthesia will produce rapid and effective euthanasia. The immersion method is generally the most appropriate for pet fish, since it appears to cause minimal distress and is more acceptable to owners.

Where a chemical method is used, ensuring that death has occurred involves either pithing or the lethal injection of an additional anaesthetic drug (e.g. pentobarbitone).

Pithing ensures that the brain and anterior spinal cord are destroyed and should follow all chemical methods. Full pithing of a fish is carried out with a scalpel or sharp blade and a seeker or long needle. Typically, the spinal column is severed just behind the head and then a long needle or seeker is passed into the spinal cord and brain cavity with a number of lateral and vertical movements to destroy the nerve tissue. In practice, severing the spinal cord behind the head is usually sufficient. The technique should be practised on cadavers but, once mastered, the procedure is rapid and reliably ensures death.

Large fish such as adult koi have solid bones and a significant muscle mass behind the head, making it extremely difficult to sever the spine. In these cases, a lethal intravenous injection can be given into the caudal vein of the peduncle or the heart. In some large fish, veins are present on the dorsomedial aspect of the operculae and successful administration of the drug is easily achieved (Figure 11.16).

Fish that are too small to inject easily should be left in the strong anaesthetic solution for a minimum of an hour to ensure that they are dead. It should be noted that the heart will continue to contract for some minutes after the fish has died, and even when the heart is removed from the body.

Euthanasia by owners

There will be occasions when owners are unable or unwilling to bring a terminally sick fish to a veterinary practice for euthanasia. Owners who are also anglers will often use a physical stunning method to kill their fish. Others will want advice on suitable immersion agents that are common household chemicals or can be obtained without prescription. In this instance, the most appropriate agent to advise is clove oil, which can be obtained from local pharmacies. A minimum dose of

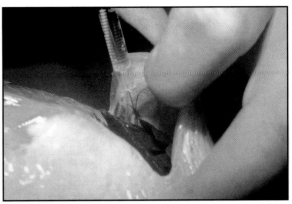

Figure 11.16 Veins present on the medial aspect of the opercula in koi. These are easily accessible with fine 25 gauge needles and provide good visibility for intravenous administration of lethal injections. (© W.H. Wildgoose.)

10 drops per litre should be used. The chemical must be mixed thoroughly into the water, using a whisk if necessary. Mixing the oil with a little hot water helps to disperse the agent, before adding it to the water containing the fish.

Further reading

Brown LA (1987) Recirculation anaesthesia for laboratory fish. *Laboratory Animals* **21**, 210–215

Erdmann Ch (1999) Schmerzempfinden unf Leidensfaehigkeit bei fishen. Eine Literaturubersicht. [The ability of fishes to feel pain and to suffer.] Dr. rer. Nat. thesis, Hanover

Gregory NG (1999) Do fish feel pain? *ANZCCART News* **12**, 1–3

Harms CA and Bakal RS (1995) Techniques in fish anaesthesia. *Journal of Small Exotic Animal Medicine* **3**, 21

Lewbart GA and Harms C (1999) Building a fish anaesthesia delivery system. *Exotic DVM* **1.2**, 25–28

Lewbart GA, Stone EA and Love NE (1995) Pneumocystectomy in a Midas cichlid. *Journal of the American Veterinary Association* **207**, 319–321

McFarland WN (1959) A study of the effects of anaesthetics on the behaviour and physiology of fishes. *Publications of the Institute of Marine Science* **6**, 22–55

Ross LG and Ross B (1999) *Anaesthetic and Sedative Techniques for Aquatic Animals*. Blackwell Science, Oxford

Stetter MD (2001) Fish and amphibian anaesthesia. In: *The Veterinary Clinics of North America: Exotic Animal Practice: Analgesia and Anaesthesia*, ed. DJ Heard, pp. 69–82. WB Saunders Company, Philadelphia

Treves-Brown KM (2000) *Applied Fish Pharmacology*. Kluwer Academic Publishers, Dordrecht

12

Clinical examination

Gregory A. Lewbart

The purpose of a clinical examination is to identify physical and behavioural abnormalities. Interpreting the clinical history and examining the environment will provide important background information that will enable the clinician to focus on specific aspects during a clinical examination. However, the whole fish should be inspected carefully and thoroughly. This chapter highlights key features that must be examined to assist in forming a differential diagnosis or direct the clinician to further procedures required for the confirmation of a diagnosis.

Preliminary examination

It is advisable to observe the fish in their aquatic environment before capturing or restraining them for a more detailed examination. Unfortunately, some fish may be moribund or even dead on presentation, which precludes this valuable preliminary examination.

Healthy fish will have clear bright coloration, move through the water column effortlessly, swim with conspecifics (if it is a schooling species) and lack any apparent lesions or gross abnormalities. Because of some marked species differences, the general features of sick fish should be compared with those of normal healthy fish of the same species. During this examination, the following points should be noted.

- Position in water column. Are fish at the surface or on the bottom? Note that some species are normally bottom- or surface-dwelling fish.
  Is their posture abnormal: are they in lateral or dorsal recumbency?
- Behaviour. Are fish huddled near a fountain, water inlet or aerator? Are they mouthing at the surface and does this vary during the day? This may suggest hypoxia.
- Swimming. Are the fin movements normal or are the fins clamped close to the body surface? Are there erratic movements or signs of irritation (e.g. rubbing on objects)?
- Appetite. Is food still present in the water and do the fish eat when it is offered?
- Gross lesions. Are there any spots, swellings, ulcers or areas of altered pigmentation? Are the fins inflamed or frayed at the edges?

Physical examination

Following observation of the fish in its own environment, it should be removed from the facility for a more detailed examination. A list of useful equipment is given in Figure 12.1.

Where possible, the fish should be inspected at close quarters while still in the water. The use of a clear plastic bag or aquarium will suffice. This provides an opportunity to note any subtle lesions or abnormalities,

Air pumps, tubing and airstones
Anaesthetic agent (MS222, clove oil)
Aquaria (assorted glass and plastic types)
Auroscope and various sized cones
Blood collection tubes (plain, heparin)
Camera
Catheters (assorted types and sizes)
Clear plastic bags (assorted sizes)
Dechlorinator (proprietary product)
Dissecting kit
Doppler pulse ultrasound probe
Electronic meter (pH, conductivity)
Endoscope
Filters (sponge/box type for aquaria)
Fluorescein strips
Gloves (latex, non-sterile, disposable)
Lubricating jelly
Magnifying glass/optical head loupe
Measuring cylinder/jug
Microscope, glass slides and coverslips
Needles and syringes
Nets (assorted types and sizes)
Ophthalmoscope
Oxygen supply
Pipettes (plastic)
Refractometer (for salinity and plasma protein)
Rubber bands (various sizes)
Ruler (metric)
Salt
Surgical pack(s)
Tongue depressors
Towels (cloth and disposable paper)
Water quality test kits
Water sample bottles (glass and plastic, 250 ml)
Weighing scales (1 g increments)

Figure 12.1 Equipment required for clinical examination of fish.

which may not have been evident during the preliminary examination. Certain skin parasites and other disease problems are more readily identified while the fish is still in water. The use of a magnifying lens or optical loupe is essential when examining small species. Maintaining photographic records of the fish and its environment is strongly recommended, since high quality colour images provide valuable information for future reference.

Following this 'in-water' examination, it may be necessary to sedate the patient and remove it from the water for closer examination. Where possible, the fish should be examined while held over water to minimize any damage if the fish is dropped or jumps out of the clinician's hands. Detailed clinical examinations may be limited by the size of the patient and are often restricted to visual examination of external surfaces. However, a routine and methodical approach should be developed. It is often best to start at the head and work towards the tail.

> **TIP:** There may be more than one clinical disease present at any one time and the clinician should avoid being distracted by obvious external lesions.

General appearance

When the patient has been sedated, it should be weighed on an accurate scale and the weight recorded (Figure 12.2). A general clinical impression of the fish's body condition should be noted at this time. If a fish is underweight, its head may appear 'too large' for its body and may also appear 'triangular' in cross-section due to decreased epaxial muscle mass and pronounced vertebral processes. Fish that appear swollen or abnormally large may be retaining fluid (ascites) (Figure 12.3), eggs or air, or have an intra-abdominal mass. Fish can become obese and accumulate large amounts of abdominal fat. For the medical record, a fish can simply be categorized as normal, underweight or overweight.

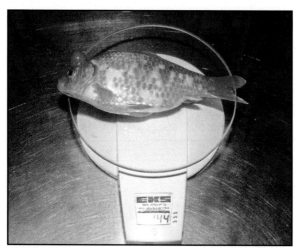

Figure 12.2 All fish should be weighed on accurate gram scales appropriate to the size of the fish. Convenient electronic digital kitchen scales are adequate in most cases. (© W.H. Wildgoose.)

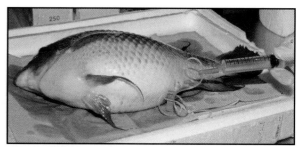

Figure 12.3 This Pearcii cichlid has a severely swollen abdomen. Ascitic fluid is being removed from the coelomic cavity with a butterfly catheter and syringe.

The total length (from the snout to the tip of the caudal fin) should be recorded. The length of the caudal fin can vary in some fancy goldfish or the edges may become damaged. Therefore, it is also advisable to record the standard length, from the snout to the base of the caudal fin. All lesions and abnormalities should be measured, recorded and marked on an outline sketch of the fish.

Skin

The skin is the largest organ on a fish's body. It is quite sensitive to injury and therefore physical contact should be kept to a minimum. Powder-free latex gloves should be worn while examining the fish. With an anaesthetized patient, all skin surfaces (dorsal, ventral, and lateral) should be examined thoroughly (Figure 12.4). The patient should be placed on a firm moist surface such as a wet, fine-weave towel or open-cell foam. The eyes should be shielded from the bright lights of the examination room and lubricated with ophthalmic ointment if the fish will be out of water for more than a few minutes. A large syringe can be used to moisten the fish's body with clean water if necessary.

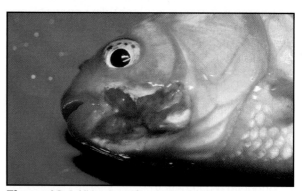

Figure 12.4 All body surfaces should be inspected thoroughly. This applies particularly to the ventral surfaces of pond fish, since this aspect is rarely visible unless the fish is restrained or removed from the water for examination. (© W.H. Wildgoose.)

Colour

Skin colour should appear normal when compared with conspecifics. Any areas of depigmentation, hyperpigmentation or fading should be noted. Some fish can change colour quickly when subjected to stress, poor handling and even anaesthesia. These extrinsic factors should be taken into account when recording any clinical findings.

Texture

The skin should appear uniformly smooth and mucus-covered. Any areas of oedema, haemorrhage, abrasion or ulceration should be noted. Many ectoparasites (e.g. fish lice, anchorworm, isopods) are grossly visible and will disrupt the normal texture of a fish's skin.

Scales

Scales are produced by osteogenic cells in the dermis and are an important mechanism of protection and defence for many fishes. It is important to be aware of normal variations in scale patterns: some fish, such as the doitsu variety of koi, possess scales only over certain parts of their body. Normal scales will appear even, lie flat against the body, and require some force to remove them. Scales that appear elevated, fall out easily or are covered with algal or fungal growth should be noted and examined more closely.

Fins

The fins are thin appendages used primarily for locomotion. They generally consist of supportive bony rays covered by a thin layer of sensitive epithelial tissue (Figure 12.5). Due to their transparent structure, lesions and parasites on the fins are often readily visible. A small biopsy may be taken from the fin for microscopic examination and inspection for parasites. It will usually regrow quickly if the biopsy is taken close to the distal edge of the fin.

Other appendages, such as the barbels, should be examined carefully for signs of injury, including inflammation, thickening or abnormal shortening.

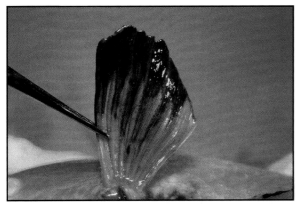

Figure 12.5 The fins should be examined carefully for signs of damage or colour change. The pelvic fin on this goldfish developed abnormal black pigmentation a few days after midline abdominal surgery. This resolved and returned to its original golden colour after a further 8 weeks. (© W.H. Wildgoose.)

Mouth

The mouth is easily examined in a sedated fish. A tongue depressor or blunt spatula can be used to inspect the oral cavity and examine for the presence of lesions or foreign bodies. Some fish have sharp teeth associated with the mandible and maxilla (Figure 12.6), while cyprinids such as goldfish and koi lack buccal teeth and have blunt molar-like pharyngeal teeth. An auroscope or endoscope can be used to inspect the mouth and pharynx.

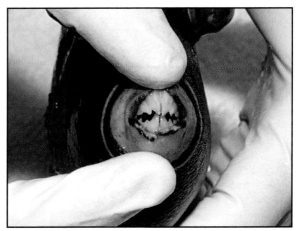

Figure 12.6 Care should be taken when examining the mouth of some fish. The sharp teeth of this anaesthetized triggerfish are capable of causing severe injury.

Olfactory openings

Most fish have bilateral olfactory openings or nostrils in the dorsal region of the head. These pores are symmetrical and easy to examine. In many species the opening is divided by a flap, which creates an inlet and outlet for water to flow over the olfactory laminae (Figure 12.7).

This area should be checked for haemorrhage, ulceration and other abnormalities.

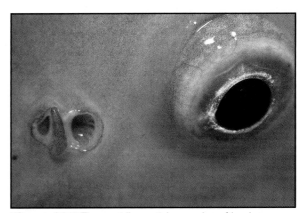

Figure 12.7 The nostrils contain a series of laminae which form the olfactory rosette. This delicate tissue is covered by the olfactory epithelium and prone to bacterial infection and ulceration. (© W.H. Wildgoose.)

Eyes

The eyes are readily examined on fish. The size and shape of the globes should be identical, particularly in some fancy goldfish that are intentionally bred with enlarged eyes. Any endophthalmos or exophthalmos should be noted, since this may be unilateral or bilateral (Figures 12.8 and 12.9). The corneas should be clear and bilaterally symmetrical. A portable ophthalmoscope can be used to examine the intra-ocular structures and retina. An ophthalmic slit lamp can provide even more ocular detail. Fluorescein dye may improve visualization of corneal ulcers, which are quite common in fish (see Chapter 18).

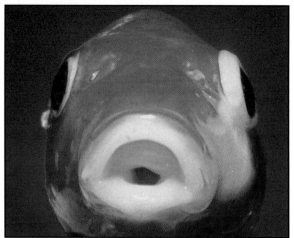

Figure 12.8 Exophthalmos is easiest to appreciate by comparing one eye with the other and viewing them from the front. This koi has a mild degree of unilateral exophthalmos affecting the left eye. (© W.H. Wildgoose.)

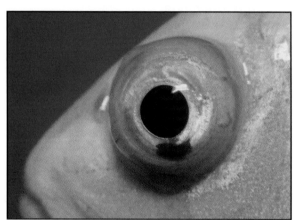

Figure 12.9 Each eye should be examined carefully. This koi has exophthalmos but also mild hyphaema, a clinical sign that is easily overlooked. (© W.H. Wildgoose.)

Opercular cavity

Both opercular cavities should be examined for lesions and abnormalities on both the external and internal surfaces. Opercular movements can be counted and recorded as the respiratory rate. This varies between species and is influenced by stress and dissolved oxygen levels but normal rates should be below 80 per minute.

Gills

The gill arches can be examined by gently deflecting the operculum (Figure 12.10). Most fish possess four gill arches on each side. At the base of each arch are gill rakers, which help to clear the opercular cavity of debris. The gill lamellae should be examined for overall integrity, colour, areas of pigmentation or depigmentation, haemorrhage and necrosis. Both sets of gills should be inspected before taking a lamellar biopsy (see Chapter 13). An auroscope or endoscope can be used to view the gills in species with small opercular openings (e.g. eels and puffers).

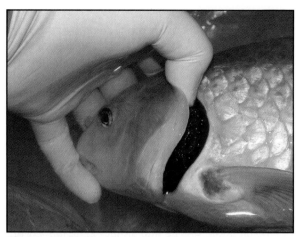

Figure 12.10 The gill can be examined briefly in a conscious fish by wedging a thumb under the dorsal part of the operculum. This will provide a rough impression of gill condition but anaesthesia is required for a more detailed inspection. (© W.H. Wildgoose.)

Heart

In some fish, the heart can be observed beating through the skin in the 'throat' (the midline area just posterior to the base of the opercula). In many fish, a Doppler pulse ultrasound probe (Figure 12.11) is a more reliable and accurate method of establishing heart rate. This varies between species and is influenced by stress and temperature but normal rates are often between 30 and 70 beats per minute. Standard stethoscopes used for terrestrial animals are of little use on fish patients.

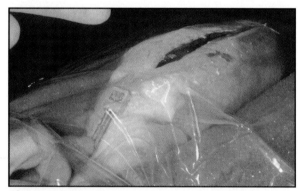

Figure 12.11 A Doppler pulse ultrasound probe is being used to monitor a patient's heart rate during intra-abdominal surgery.

Abdomen

In addition to visual inspection, the abdomen should be palpated and percussed, particularly if there is abnormal swelling. This enables detection of some firm internal masses or intra-abdominal fluid. Ballottement, a palpatory manoeuvre, can be used to identify a floating mass within a fluid-filled abdomen.

Vent

All fish have at least one external opening for the discharge of faecal and urinary waste and reproductive products. This opening should be examined for patency, and a small lubricated catheter or blunt probe can be inserted if in doubt (Figure 12.12). Many anaesthetized fish will defaecate shortly after induction, providing a valuable faecal sample. The vent should be inspected for signs of inflammation, swelling, protrusion, ulceration and the presence of endoparasites (e.g. *Camallanus*). Abnormally pale or trailing faeces may be associated with gastrointestinal disease.

Skeleton

While under anaesthesia, the body of the fish should be gently flexed and manipulated. Spinal flexibility varies considerably between species, and radiography may be required to provide more information. Abnormal rigidity of the spine can be due to severe bone disease.

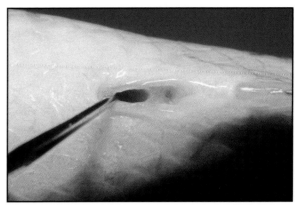

Figure 12.12 Examining a normal vent in a koi. The blunt seeker has been inserted into the anterior opening (on left), which leads to the rectum. The posterior depression is the opening into the bladder. (© W.H. Wildgoose.)

13

Laboratory techniques

Peter J. Southgate

Clinical signs exhibited by unhealthy fish are common to many diseases and pathological conditions. These signs are frequently limited to lethargy, anorexia and colour changes. Identifying specific disease conditions based on these presenting signs alone is very difficult and this is compounded by the problems associated with the clinical observation and examination of fish in an aquatic environment. These factors make a certain amount of laboratory analysis essential for the specific identification of fish diseases.

The extent of this analysis will vary with the number and value of the fish available, the value of the fish to the client and the nature of the problem under investigation. Some conditions, such as primary skin parasitism, may show obvious signs of colour changes, skin damage and irritation. Here the investigation may require only the identification of the parasite by examination of fresh skin preparations, though other causes of skin irritation due to water quality problems and toxic insult may also need to be ruled out. Clinical signs of ascites, haemorrhage and lethargy may need more detailed investigations, including bacterial and viral analysis, histopathology, toxicology and water quality tests.

Laboratory investigation often necessitates the sacrifice and sampling of individual fish. In some circumstances, due to the small number of specimens involved or the high value of the fish, it may only be possible to carry out a relatively limited investigation on a living (usually anaesthetized) specimen. Visual examination of gross lesions, microscopic examination of wet preparations from the gill and skin, together with blood and faecal sampling and some bacteriology may be all that is practical.

For a conclusive postmortem to be carried out, it is imperative that only fresh material is examined. This is particularly true when histopathology is required, since fish tissue degenerates so quickly that taking samples even 1 hour after death could give results that are of little diagnostic use. Ideally, living but obviously affected or moribund fish should be sacrificed for examination. Failing this, samples should be taken from a fish as soon after death as possible. Taking samples from frozen or refrigerated fish should usually be avoided, though these could be used for some virological or bacteriological procedures.

Submission to the laboratory

Although many investigations may be performed in a practice laboratory, some samples need to be sent to external laboratories. It is advisable to contact the laboratory for advice on specific packaging requirements and to inform them of the material being submitted. Postal regulations may vary between different countries but standard guidelines for posting pathological specimens must be followed. In general, the samples should be sealed in a leak-proof non-breakable container, suitably labelled. This should be packed in sufficient absorbent material to soak up all fluid in the event of leakage and then placed inside a further leak-proof rigid container. This outer container should be packed inside a padded bag with the laboratory submission form. The package should be labelled 'Pathological specimens' and 'Fragile – handle with care'.

Water quality

Water quality is critical to the health of fish, and changes in water quality can result directly in pathology or influence the impact of other disease factors. Regular water quality monitoring is often performed by the ornamental fish keeper and water analysis should be considered as part of an investigation into fish disease.

A wide range of water testing systems is available, from budget colour-change papers to highly sophisticated multi-test and electronic analysers. Most test kits (Figure 13.1) are based on colorimetric analysis, where colour changes on a test strip or within a solution are compared with standards. More sophisticated and accurate kits employ spectrophotometer techniques (Figure 13.2). The accuracy and sensitivity of commercial kits can vary enormously but good affordable kits are available for the range of parameters that are most important to the fish keeper.

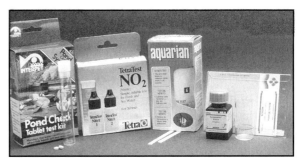

Figure 13.1 Some simple affordable test kits for monitoring water quality, based on the use of (from left to right) a dry tablet, liquid reagent, impregnated dipstick and dry powder reagent. (© W.H. Wildgoose.)

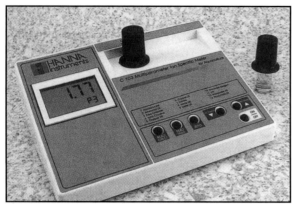

Figure 13.2 Multi-parameter ion-specific photometers are accurate and, for portability, some can operate on a 9 volt battery. The instrument is set to zero with a water sample, then reagents are added to produce a colour change that is measured by a photocell. (Courtesy of Hanna Instruments.)

For more sophisticated or esoteric investigation, such as cases where the presence of a toxin is suspected, it may be necessary to engage the services of a professional laboratory. The interrelationships between water quality parameters must also be considered, such as the relationship between free ammonia and pH. It is important that a sufficient number of parameters are examined to enable meaningful interpretation.

Sampling technique

Sampling water for toxicological analysis is outlined in Chapter 26. Although the standards for sampling for the basic water quality parameters may not be so critical in terms of chemical cleanliness, it is still important to use chemically inert containers and ensure that contamination is avoided. Some test kits provide their own sampling devices. General advice includes the following:

- Rinse the container, including the stopper, several times in the water to be analysed
- Ensure that the water sampled is representative: do not sample from the surface, where debris and other contaminants may be present
- Fill containers to the brim and replace stoppers under water to exclude air.

Analyse the water as soon as possible but, if necessary, the sample can be stored in a refrigerator for a few hours. If the sample is to be sent to a laboratory, then it should be transported on ice as soon as possible. It is recommended that more than one sample be taken, since replicates will help to overcome any error from one sample.

Basic water quality parameters

The main water quality parameters analysed for routine monitoring and disease investigation are:

- Temperature
- Dissolved oxygen
- Ammonia
- Nitrite

- Nitrate
- pH
- Hardness
- Chlorine/chloramine (to ensure suitable water supply).

Test kits are available for most of these and suitable multi-test colorimetric kits will cover all parameters of interest. Oxygen and temperature are frequently measured using suitable hand-held meters (Figure 13.3). If 'gas bubble disease' (supersaturation) is suspected, a total gas meter may be required.

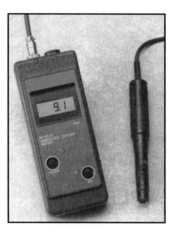

Figure 13.3 Portable dissolved oxygen meters can be calibrated in air for a percentage saturation value or in zero-oxygen solution for a measurement in milligrams per litre. The selective membranes that cover the polarographic probe require periodic replacement. (Courtesy of Hanna Instruments.)

In marine systems, salinity is measured (Figure 13.4), using a hydrometer to measure the specific gravity of the sea water. Alternatively, the refractive index of the sample can be determined using a salinometer (a hand-held refractometer designed for the measurement of salinity), calibrated in parts per thousand. Salinity can also be measured in terms of conductivity with the use of a conductivity meter or by chloride titration.

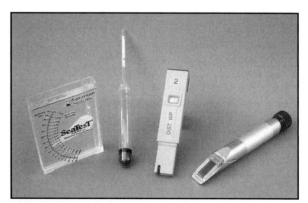

Figure 13.4 Salinity can be measured to varying degrees of accuracy, using (from left to right) a 'swing-needle' hydrometer, a floating hydrometer, a conductivity meter and a refractometer. (© W.H. Wildgoose.)

The measurement of redox potential in marine systems, particularly when first establishing an aquarium, is a convenient way of ensuring that biological filtration systems are functioning and is a useful alternative to monitoring ammonia and nitrite levels. Small redox meters are available for this purpose.

Marine systems employing ozone for water sterilization may also require ozone determination, using an electronic probe.

Portable electronic multi-test kits are commercially available and can be highly accurate (approaching laboratory standard) but great care must be used in their maintenance and calibration.

Clinical examination

The examination of fish for behavioural abnormalities and gross signs of disease is covered in Chapter 12. This chapter is devoted to more detailed clinical examination, using a variety of laboratory techniques.

Suitable affected specimens should be chosen for investigation. A limited amount of examination can be carried out on a conscious fish held in a net or a damp towel, but this can be stressful and damaging to the fish and frequently makes examination very difficult. If the fish is not to be sacrificed, it is advisable to anaesthetize it at this stage, though the anaesthetic agent may remove some of the ectoparasite burden from the fish.

Sick or moribund specimens should be killed for further examination by either an overdose of anaesthetic, or a sharp blow to the head (stunning), or severing the spinal cord behind the head. If blood samples are to be obtained, this should be performed either while the fish is anaesthetized or immediately after stunning. Very small fish should be killed by either anaesthetic overdose or decapitation.

Postmortem examination

As emphasized above, it is very important that a postmortem is performed and samples for histological and bacteriological examination are obtained as soon as possible after death. The extent of the postmortem will depend on the nature of the problem under investigation and the facilities available.

> **TIP:** Postmortem examination is best performed on freshly killed fish or within 1 hour of death.

The following is a logical series of procedures that cover all the basic requirements of fish disease investigation.

1. Carry out an external examination. Record the weight, the total length (from snout to tip of the tail) and the standard length (from snout to end of the peduncle). The fish should be examined for the presence of gross external abnormalities. Factors to consider include the following.
   - Skin:
     - Variation in colour
     - Excess mucus production
     - Gross lesions (e.g. ulceration, haemorrhage, scale loss)
     - Parasites – visible to the naked eye
     - Fungal infection
     - Tumours
   - Fins:
     - Loss of or eroded fin or tail
     - Haemorrhage (particularly at base of fins)
     - Fungal infection
     - Tumours
   - Eye:
     - Evidence of damage
     - Exophthalmos
     - Corneal opacity or ulceration
     - Cataract
     - Tumours
   - Other gross abnormalities (e.g. opercular damage, deformities, abdominal swelling, protruding haemorrhagic vent).

2. Examine gill and skin preparations for the presence of ectoparasites.

3. Take blood samples if required.

4. Carry out an internal examination. This applies mostly to fish large enough to examine, since gross examination of very small fish may be limited.
   (i) The abdomen is opened by cutting along the ventral midline, from between the pectoral fins, through the pelvis to the vent. Avoid opening the gut and spilling the intestinal contents – this is particularly important if bacteriological examination is to be carried out. Improved exposure of the abdominal contents may be achieved by removing the lateral abdominal wall (Figure 13.5), again taking care not to damage the viscera.

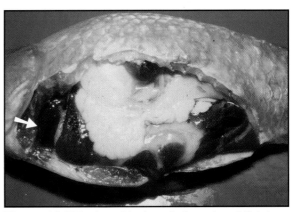

Figure 13.5 The lateral body wall of a male goldfish is removed to expose the internal organs during a postmortem examination. The pericardial sac is opened to reveal the heart (arrowed). (© W.H. Wildgoose.)

   (ii) The abdominal organs can be gently separated and moved ventrally to expose the swim-bladder and kidney (Figure 13.6). The viscera of most carp are strongly adherent and have fine adhesions to the body wall: this is considered normal.
   (iii) Note the consistency and colour of the liver and the presence and nature of any free abdominal fluid. Note any gross abnormality in the abdomen such as haemorrhage, parasitic cysts, tumours or swim-bladder abnormalities.

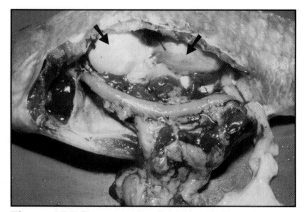

Figure 13.6 The gonad is reflected ventrally at the cloaca and the liver is resected to expose the bowel and white bilobed swim-bladder (arrows). The latter can be removed to allow more access to the posterior kidney situated on the dorsal aspect of the body cavity. (© W.H. Wildgoose.)

(iv) If bacteriological examination is to be carried out, it should be performed at this stage.

(v) The stomach and gut should be separated from the rest of the viscera and opened. Gut contents should be examined for evidence of feeding. Note the nature of the gut contents and presence of any parasites. Large gut parasites, such as tapeworms, can be removed for identification. A gut scrape should be prepared for microscopic examination and identification of any endoparasites.

(vi) Obtain tissue squashes and smears from the liver, kidney and spleen for parasitic and bacteriological examination.

(vii) Samples should now be taken for virological and histopathological examination.

Cases that may become the subject of legal proceedings should be carefully recorded with sufficient detail to enable identification of the fish. This should be supported by clear photographs of any external features or colour patterns and clinical lesions.

Ectoparasite examination

Some of the larger ectoparasites, such as *Lernaea* and *Argulus*, are visible to the naked eye but the majority of protozoan and metazoan ectoparasites can only be seen by microscopic examination of preparations of skin and gill tissue.

It is preferable to examine a number of fish, since the ectoparasites will not be evenly distributed throughout the fish population. Always ensure that the water in which the fish are being held prior to examination is well oxygenated, to maintain the viability of any parasites present.

Skin preparations

Skin scrapes enable the identification of ectoparasite infestation. Bacterial and fungal infection of the skin may also be detected using this technique.

1. Using a blunt scalpel blade or the edge of a slide, remove a small quantity of mucus from the skin. As parasites often concentrate in areas adjacent to fins, it is useful to take mucus scrapings from behind the pectoral fin (Figure 13.7) or parallel to the dorsal fin. When present, it is valuable to take scrapings from the edge of skin or fin lesions.

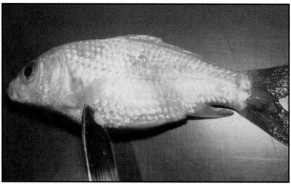

Figure 13.7 A skin scraping is taken from behind the pectoral fin, using a blunt scalpel. A small sample of opaque mucus is visible on the blade. (© W.H. Wildgoose.)

2. Transfer the mucus sample to the slide, add a drop of water and apply a cover slip (Figure 13.8). Always use water in which the fish have been kept; avoid tap water or distilled water, as the presence of chlorine or different osmotic pressure may destroy some parasites. Examine immediately so that motile parasites are easily visualized.

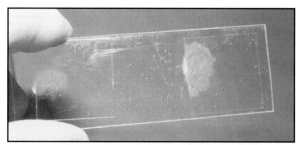

Figure 13.8 The mucus is transferred to a microscope slide and mounted with a drop of tank/pond water and a glass cover slip. (© W.H. Wildgoose.)

3. The majority of protozoan and metazoan parasites (Figure 13.9) can be seen using ×40 magnification (i.e. ×10 eyepiece and ×4 objective). Some of the smaller protozoans are more difficult to see and may require ×100 magnification. Many of these parasites are refractile to light and the use of phase-contrast often improves their visibility. If this is not available, lowering the condenser to adjust the level of illumination of the image is equally effective.

Skin preparations may be taken from live fish, using the same technique, but care must be taken not to damage the skin and it is preferable to take an impression smear, using a dry slide. A useful skin biopsy may

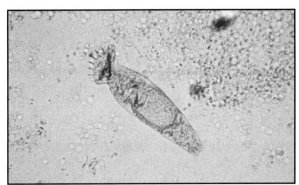

Figure 13.9 A skin fluke is visible under low-power magnification (×40 original magnification) among the cell debris and mucus. Most microscopic ectoparasites are motile, refractile to light and more visible with phase-contrast or a low condenser setting. (© W.H. Wildgoose.)

be obtained by clipping a small piece of fin, preferably from an area of fin damage but avoiding fin rays, and examining as for a standard skin scrape. These biopsies, together with needle biopsies of skin tumours, can also be fixed in 10% neutral buffered formalin for histological analysis.

Gill preparations

Wet mounts of gill tissue (gill squashes) are prepared in a very similar way to that for skin scrapes. They are useful in determining the presence of parasites, and may be of use in the assessment of general gill health and local bacterial and fungal infections. In a recently sacrificed fish the technique is as follows.

1. Expose the gill by lifting or removing the operculum.

2. Remove a small number of filaments from the gill arch (do not include any cartilage). It is best to avoid using the outermost arch, which is sometimes in poor condition and may give a false impression of the general health of the gill (Figure 13.10).

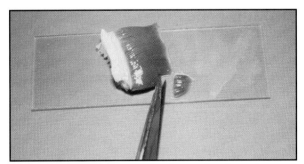

Figure 13.10 A gill biopsy is taken, using fine scissors to sample the tips of several gill filaments. (Reproduced with the permission of *In Practice*.)

3. Place the gill tissue on a microscope slide. Add a drop of water and apply a cover slip with sufficient pressure to allow the individual gill filaments to fan out (Figure 13.11).

4. Examine using the same technique as that described for skin preparations (Figure 13.12).

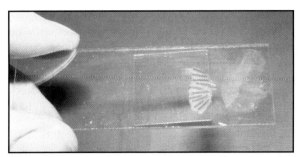

Figure 13.11 The filaments are separated in a drop of tank/pond water and a cover slip is applied lightly. (Reproduced with the permission of *In Practice*.)

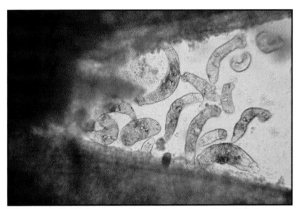

Figure 13.12 A severe infestation of motile gill flukes is visible between the gill filaments under low-power magnification (×40 original magnification). (© W.H. Wildgoose.)

In a live anaesthetized fish, an impression smear can be taken by gently pressing a dry slide on to the gill tissue; mucus and parasites will adhere to the slide, which can then be examined as above. It may be possible to do this in a conscious fish by restraining it in a wet towel, particularly if there is concern that anaesthetic agents will destroy some parasites.

A gill biopsy involves sampling a tiny amount of tissue from the tips of the gill filaments using fine scissors (e.g. iridectomy scissors) or lightly scraping with a blunt scalpel blade. Great care should be taken to avoid damage to the bulk of the gill and there should be minimal haemorrhage. The samples should be prepared and examined as above. Although this technique causes minimal damage, it is an awkward procedure to perform and should only be attempted on anaesthetized fish.

Interpretation of gill preparations

Some idea of gill health can be obtained by the examination of gill squashes. High levels of mucus production as a response to parasitic or water quality insult may be identified. Epithelial hyperplasia may be seen as apparent thickening and 'clubbing' at the tips of the gill filaments or fusion of adjacent areas of the gill. However, the assessment of gill health by means of fresh gill squashes must be viewed with caution as it relies heavily on the technique and experience of the operator. The appearance of a gill in a fresh preparation may often be contradicted by its histological appearance.

The presence of bacteria may also be determined in fresh gill preparations. These will frequently be found in cases of environmental gill disease and often accompany increased levels of mucus and particulate matter. When high levels of bacteria are present, they may grossly resemble 'cotton wool' on the gill. Smaller numbers can be seen in fresh preparations but it is often necessary to use higher magnification than that used for parasite screening (i.e. ×400 magnification).

Fungal infection of the gill, usually with *Saprolegnia*, may also be identified. The fungal hyphae are large enough to be easily identified with ×100 magnification. A small drop of methylene blue dye may help to visualize fungal elements in a wet preparation.

Blood sampling

Haematology and clinical chemistry have been underused in the investigation of fish disease because of the lack of baseline information, the wide variability in 'normal' values within species and the perceived differences between species. However, blood analysis is now being used more frequently in ornamental fish practice and is becoming a useful adjunct to other diagnostic techniques. This is particularly true where the sacrifice of specimens for examination is not possible and the range of other available diagnostic techniques is limited.

Baseline information is mostly available for farmed species of fish and for carp (Figure 13.13). Very few data are available for marine and freshwater tropical fish and it is not easy to extrapolate from one species to another. Replicate samples from a number of fish are helpful, as is taking additional samples from apparently 'normal' specimens or populations.

Haematocrit	33.4 ± 1.51%
Erythrocyte count	1.67 ± 0.08 million/μl
Haemoglobin	82 ± 3.6 g/l
Leucocyte count	37.8 ± 2.88 thousand/μl
Leucocrit	1.0%
Plasma sodium	130.3 ± 1.4 mEq/l
Plasma chloride	125.2 ± 1.8 mEq/l
Total plasma protein	25–35 g/l
Plasma albumin	7.6–8.5 g/l
Plasma glucose	1.7–2.6 mmol/l

Figure 13.13 Haematology and blood chemistry values for common carp. (After Groff and Zinkl, 1999.)

The range of apparently normal values is wide for most blood parameters and these vary with the age and physiological and nutritional status of the fish and with various environmental parameters. Additionally, general stress and the very act of obtaining samples may affect the results and it is usually advisable to anaesthetize the fish before sampling. If fish are to be sacrificed, then the blood should be obtained immediately after stunning the fish.

Obtaining blood samples

Blood may be withdrawn from a number of sites, including direct cardiac puncture, but the preferred site for most operators is the caudal vein, using either a lateral or a ventral approach. The site of entry of the needle is approximately halfway along the caudal peduncle. For the lateral approach, the needle is inserted just below the lateral line angled towards the head (Figure 13.14). When the bony vertebral column is encountered, the needle is angled slightly below to enter the caudal vein. For the ventral approach, the needle is inserted in the ventral midline alongside, or just caudal to, the anal fin. When the vertebral column is encountered, the needle is withdrawn slightly to enter the caudal vein. Haemolysis occurs readily with fish blood and as little vacuum should be put on the syringe as possible. For this reason, vacuum blood collection tubes are best avoided.

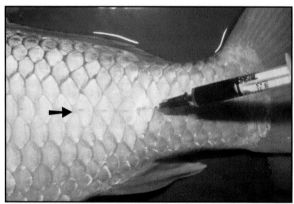

Figure 13.14 Taking a blood sample from the caudal vein of a koi using a lateral approach. A long needle is inserted under the scales of the peduncle at a point on or just below the lateral line (arrowed). (© W.H. Wildgoose.)

Blood can usually be obtained using this method in fish weighing over 25 g. In smaller fish that are to be sacrificed, it is possible to obtain a blood sample by cutting off the tail and exposing the caudal vein. Blood can then be withdrawn using a capillary tube, but care must be taken not to dilute or contaminate the sample. There is usually sufficient blood to perform a blood smear examination and haematocrit.

Heparin is the most useful anticoagulant. Since fish blood clots rapidly, all the equipment used (including needles and syringes) should be rinsed in heparin.

Changes to blood parameters occur very rapidly after sampling and analysis should be carried out as soon as possible. If plasma is required, the sample should be spun down immediately and the plasma withdrawn; this can then be frozen if necessary. Likewise, if a clotted sample is required then the serum should be drawn off as soon as possible, before significant haemolysis occurs.

Bacteriology

A number of factors must be taken into account if a meaningful result is to be obtained from the bacteriological examination of fish. The fish are naturally in intimate contact with the normal bacterial flora of their environment and although some of these bacteria are frequently implicated in fish disease, contamination of samples with clinically insignificant environmental bacteria is a problem. This is particularly true if samples are taken from skin lesions or gill tissue, where a certain amount of caution must be exercised in interpretation of results. Likewise, taking samples from dead fish should be avoided if possible, due to the rapid postmortem invasion of tissues with clinically insignificant organisms.

Sampling equipment

Several instruments are available for obtaining samples. Disposable sterile plastic loops, available in a variety of sizes are probably more practical for 'field' use than a wire loop or probe which needs to be flame-sterilized. The latter are used when a medium is being directly inoculated with a sample ('plated out').

If the sample is being submitted to a laboratory, it is more usual to use a sterile swab to obtain the inoculum, though competitive growth from contaminants is more likely than with direct plate inoculation. A variety of swabs is available and the small human nasal or ENT swabs are most practical. Swabs must be kept cool and should be plated on suitable media as soon as possible.

Transport medium helps to maintain the viability of the bacteria. Amies transport medium with charcoal is usually used for samples from fresh water. Specific marine transport agar containing some salt can be prepared on request by some companies (e.g. Technical Services Consultants Ltd, Heywood).

Delays and lack of temperature control with swabs submitted by post may cause organisms to die off or be overgrown with contaminants. As a result, it is preferable to use a rapid delivery service with some method of keeping the swabs cool, using proprietary cool-bags and freezer blocks. Inoculated plates can also be submitted by post, preferably sealed with a proprietary sealing tape. It is important to follow guidelines for the submission of infectious agents by post.

Sampling

As with other investigations, sampling should be performed on affected or moribund specimens. Skin, fin or gill lesions can be sampled but care should be taken to avoid contamination. The area should be seared with a hot scalpel before sampling within the lesion.

The kidney, because of its relatively protected position, is the most frequently sampled organ from which an uncontaminated inoculum may be obtained. Any organism causing a bacteraemia or septicaemia is likely to be recovered from this tissue, due to its highly vascular nature and phagocytic function.

Depending on the fish species involved, the kidney may be exposed by stripping away the swim-bladder. In goldfish and carp, the sample can be obtained from the kidney tissue lying between the chambers of the swim-bladder (Figure 13.15). In small fish, a sterile loop can be inserted directly into the kidney. In larger fish, the tough kidney capsule may need to be incised with a sterile scalpel prior to taking the sample. In very small fish, it may be easier to cut off the head to expose

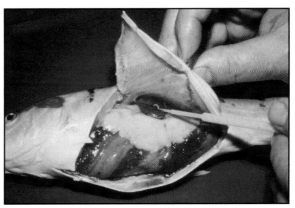

Figure 13.15 A bacteriological sample is taken using a sterile loop inserted into the posterior kidney of a koi. Care must be taken to avoid accidental contamination of the site during exposure of the organ. (© W.H. Wildgoose.)

the anterior end of the kidney, sear the end with a hot scalpel and obtain an inoculum by inserting a sterile wire into the exposed end of the kidney.

In live fish, samples can be taken by swabbing external lesions and by culturing blood and ascitic fluid samples but there is a risk of contamination in these cases.

Inoculation of culture plates

The inoculum on the loop or swab is plated out on a suitable medium by using a standard bacteriological technique of spreading the material on a segment of the plate and then, using a re-sterilized or new disposable sterile loop, streaking the sample on a second segment of the plate. This procedure is continued until the whole plate is used (Figure 13.16). This technique ensures that the inoculum is diluted over the plate and aids isolation of single bacterial colonies.

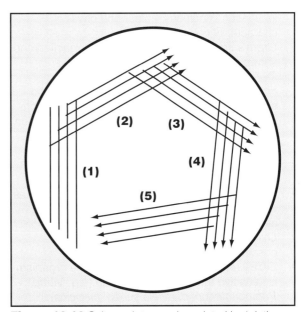

Figure 13.16 Culture plates are inoculated by 'plating out' to thin out the sample, using a series of three to four short strokes with a sterile loop.

Most bacterial pathogens of fish can be cultured on standard bacteriological media. Trypticase soy agar is the most frequently used, at a standard incubation temperature of 22°C. Some organisms are far more fastidious and require specialized media, culture conditions and prolonged incubation. For example, *Cytophaga*-like organisms and *Flavobacterium* require a low-nutrient agar and a lower incubation temperature: a specific medium, 'cytophaga agar', has been developed for this purpose. Mycobacteria are also more successfully cultured on specific mycobacterium media such as Löwenstein–Jensen medium and often require a prolonged incubation of several weeks.

Bacteriological identification

When any bacterial growth is obtained, it is vitally important that any identification and further action is focused on bacterial isolates that are considered to be significantly involved in the disease under investigation. It is easy to obtain a mixed growth of bacteria, particularly when sampling under less than ideal circumstances or sampling from contaminated lesions. The diluting effect of plating out to obtain single colonies helps in differentiating the organisms present and it may be necessary to examine all of these and determine their significance. If time allows, it helps to subculture each organism to ensure sufficient pure growth in order to carry out identification. If rapid identification is needed, this will need to be carried out on the primary culture and it is imperative that a pure growth of an apparently significant organism is used to do this.

Various bacteriological tests are carried out to establish the identity of the organism in question. There are specific texts on fish bacteriology for details of isolation and identification, but the standard procedures most frequently used include the following:

- *Growth characteristics* – medium used, incubation conditions, colour and physical character of colonies
- *Gram's stain* – categorizes by Gram reaction and shows morphology of the organism
- *Ziehl–Neelsen stain* – identifies acid-fast organisms such as *Mycobacterium*. A specific staining kit is available (e.g. BDH, Poole) which uses a modified cold staining method. In addition to Ziehl–Neelsen stain, mycobacteria can be identified using Auramine O fluorescent stain
- *Motility test* – differentiates motile from non-motile organisms
- *Oxidation/fermentation (O/F) test* – demonstrates whether the organisms break down glucose aerobically or anaerobically
- *Oxidase test* – indicates whether bacteria possess specific oxidase enzymes
- *O/129 reaction* – indicates whether the organism is sensitive to the vibriostat O/129 (e.g. *Vibrio*, *Photobacterium damsela* subsp. *piscicida*)
- *API test system* (Bio Merieux, Basingstoke) – a very useful system of identifying specific biochemical and metabolic activities of the

bacteria under investigation. The system consists of a strip of compartments holding reagents that react to the metabolic activity of the organism, usually by colour change (Figure 13.17). The organism is added to each of the compartments and the strip is incubated. The resultant series of colour changes is then compared with the known pattern for specific organisms. This system is very useful in helping to identify aquatic organisms, although it is not infallible. When used in concert with the other tests noted above, this should give an accurate identification of bacterial identity in the majority of cases.

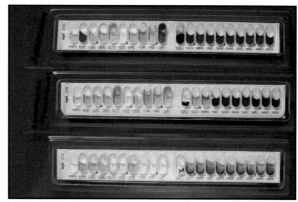

Figure 13.17 The API test system for identification of bacterial organisms. The lower strip is unused; the middle one has been inoculated with *Aeromonas salmonicida* and the top with *Vibrio anguillarum*. (© W.H. Wildgoose.)

Serology

In addition to the above, a number of commercial serological test kits are available for a limited number of common bacterial pathogens of fish. These are mostly aimed at the aquaculture market but some, notably for *Vibrio anguillarum* and *Aeromonas salmonicida* (e.g. Bionor, Norway), may be of use in ornamental fish. The test is based on the enzyme-linked immunosorbent assay (ELISA) technique, where the presence of a bacterial antigen is identified by visual agglutination with latex coated with specific antibody. Although highly accurate, auto-agglutination and false negative results can occur.

Antibiotic sensitivity testing

It is advisable to carry out antibiotic sensitivity testing in any case of bacterial disease. This will help to select an appropriate treatment and indicate if any antibacterial resistance is present. It must be emphasized that a pure culture of significant bacteria must be used for the test and it is preferable to subculture from original isolates to ensure the purity of the organisms involved. For rapid results, sensitivity testing is sometimes carried out on plates directly inoculated from sampled fish. Although this speeds up the process, there is a danger of obtaining a mixed bacterial culture and misleading results. If tests are carried out in this way, it is essential that follow-up tests on known pure subcultures be carried out to verify the results. The procedure is as follows.

1. Remove a bacterial colony from a pure culture using a sterile loop.

2. Suspend the bacteria in a small volume (0.5 ml) of sterile water in a sterile bijou bottle. Avoid touching the neck of the bottle with the loop or fingers. It is easier to suspend the bacteria by rubbing the loop on the inside of the bottle, replacing the cap and gently shaking the bottle.

3. Using a sterile pipette, place a few drops of this suspension on the surface of an agar plate. The agar used should be a specific one that allows the diffusion of the antibiotic through the medium and ensures an accurate representation of sensitivity. Sensitest agar and Mueller–Hinton medium are the most common.

4. Place antibiotic sensitivity discs on the surface of the agar, using an applicator or sterile forceps. Place the discs equidistant from each other and the edge of the plate (Figure 13.18). Appropriate discs are available from commercial laboratory supply companies. The strength of the discs should reflect the expected *in vivo* response of a sensitive organism to an antibiotic treatment. Those commonly employed in fish practice are:

- Amoxycillin (2 μg)
- Enrofloxacin (5 μg)
- Oxolinic acid (2 μg)
- Co-trimoxazole (25 μg)
- Oxytetracycline (30 μg)

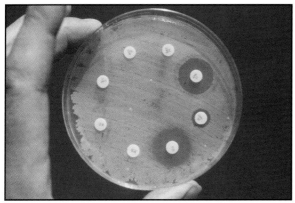

Figure 13.18 Antibiotic sensitivity test with *Aeromonas hydrophila* showing resistance to six out of eight antibiotics. Bacterial resistance to multiple antibiotics is common. (© W.H. Wildgoose.)

5. Invert the plate, medium uppermost, and incubate at an appropriate temperature.

6. When a good growth of bacteria is visible on the plate, the antibiotic sensitivity of the organism is shown by the absence of bacterial growth around the disc (the zone of inhibition). The size of this zone will reflect, to some extent, the degree of susceptibility of the bacterium to that antibiotic (the larger the zone, the more susceptible the

bacterium), and the drug of choice is likely to be that exhibiting the largest zone of inhibition. It must be borne in mind that this test does not replicate the true clinical conditions of fish receiving antibiotic treatment, but does help in deciding the most effective treatment to use. A more accurate method of testing antibiotic sensitivity is to determine the minimum inhibitory concentration (MIC) of a drug by carrying out serial dilutions of antibiotic, testing against a controlled sample of the bacteria and finding the lowest concentration of antibiotic that will stop bacterial growth. The treatment is then chosen based on its *in vivo* concentration being greater than the MIC (Figure 13.19). This method is less likely to be used in day-to-day sensitivity testing.

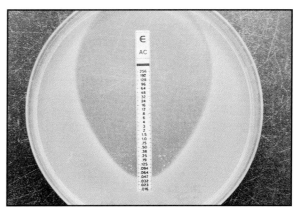

Figure 13.19 The minimum inhibitory concentration (MIC) determined using the 'E-test'. Here, a minimum *in vitro* concentration of 0.047 μg of ampicillin per kilogram bodyweight is required, to be effective against this strain of *Aeromonas hydrophila* from a goldfish. (Courtesy of G. Barker.)

Stained tissue smears

A technique that gives a rapid indication of bacterial infection is to make a direct smear from tissues. This technique is particularly useful in identifying infection with *Cytophaga*-like organisms or mycobacteria that are more difficult to culture. Impression smears can be made of gill tissue and stained to indicate the presence of *Cytophaga*. To make a smear of internal tissues, a small piece of kidney or spleen is first blotted dry to remove surface fluid and blood and the surface of the tissue is pressed a number of times along a dry slide. The slide should be carefully heat-fixed and stained with Gram's stain. If acid-fast organisms are suspected then smears should be stained with Ziehl–Neelsen stain. In this case, granulomata may be present and can be used for preparation of a smear.

Parasitology

The preparation of gill and skin squashes for the identification of ectoparasites is detailed above. Exactly the same technique can be used for the examination of kidney and liver tissue (e.g. for sporozoan parasites) and scrapes of the gut mucosa (e.g. for

Hexamita). If the presence of a parasite is suspected then squash preparations can be made of any tissue (e.g. gonad, eye, muscle). Impression smears of the kidney can also be stained with Giemsa stain and examined for the presence of sporozoans. A drop of blood can be examined for the presence of trypanoplasms and trypanosomes. Large metazoans, nematodes and cestodes can be preserved in 5% neutral buffered formalin or 70% ethanol for subsequent identification. In live fish, a faecal sample may be obtained by gentle abdominal massage or by flushing the rectum with sterile saline, using a catheter. Some fish may also pass faeces when anaesthetized. The sample can then be examined for evidence of nematode or cestode infestation.

Histopathology

Sampling tissue
Pieces of tissue no larger than 0.5 cm³ are taken from the following organs:

- Gill – cut out a section of gill arch. It is preferable to take the sample from an inner gill arch as the outer one is prone to damage and may give an unrepresentative histological appearance
- Heart
- Liver
- Spleen
- Intestine
- Kidney (avoid areas sampled for bacteriology)
- Skin/muscle – a block of skin/muscle removed across the lateral line gives a good representation of red and white muscle, and includes the fat body around the lateral line.

These are the principal organs that are screened for histopathological examination but if any gross abnormalities are noted in other tissues then these should also be included.

If small fish are submitted for examination it is rarely possible to sample individual organs. In general, a fish with a body depth of less than 1 cm would not be sampled in the above manner, but the body can be cut into 0.5 cm 'steaks' (transverse sections from head to tail) and all the sections fixed. An alternative technique for use in very small fish is to remove the lateral abdominal wall and tease out the viscera to ensure adequate fixative penetration. The operculae should also be removed, to ensure adequate fixation of the gills.

Fixatives
The standard fixative for fish histology is 10% neutral buffered formalin (Figure 13.20). Other fixatives, such as formal saline and Bouin's fluid can also be used. Regardless of which fixative is used, it is essential that there is a sufficient volume of fixative to ensure adequate fixation of the tissues: ideally, there must be at least 20 × volume of fixative to tissue.

TIP: To minimize autolysis of the tissues during the fixation process, use chilled fixative stored in the refrigerator.

- 100 ml 40% formaldehyde
- 900 ml tap/distilled water
- 4 g sodium dihydrogen phosphate (NaH₂PO₄H₂O)
- 6 g disodium hydrogen phosphate (Na₂HPO₄)

Figure 13.20 Formula for 10% neutral buffered formalin.

For ease of posting, it is acceptable to fix tissue in a large volume of formalin for 24 hours before reducing the volume of fixative and forwarding to the laboratory.

Histopathological examination
Standard histological processing is used to produce mounted tissue sections. These are usually stained with haematoxylin and eosin for examination. Specific stains can be used to demonstrate particular pathogens, such as Gram's stain for bacteria, Ziehl–Neelsen stain for acid-fast bacteria and silver stains for fungi. Immunohistochemistry is also used to demonstrate mycobacterial infection. Histopathological interpretation should be undertaken by experienced pathologists familiar with the unique microscopic characteristics of fish tissues (Figures 13.21, 13.22 and 13.23).

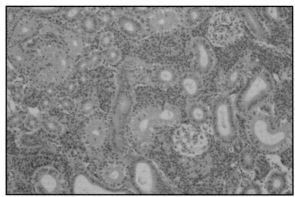

Figure 13.21 Normal histology of the posterior kidney from a koi. There is a substantial amount of normal haemopoietic tissue present in the interstitial tissue. This is occasionally misinterpreted as neoplastic by those not experienced in fish pathology. H&E stain, ×100 original magnification. (© W.H. Wildgoose.)

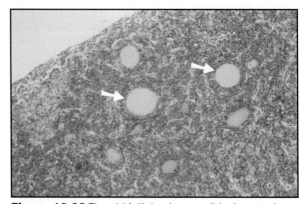

Figure 13.22 Thyroid follicles (arrowed) in the anterior kidney of a koi. In carp and goldfish, some thyroid tissue is found in many organs, including the heart, spleen and posterior kidney. H&E stain, ×100 original magnification.

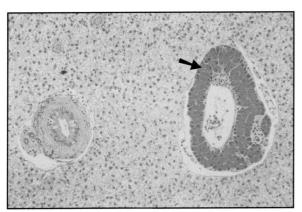

Figure 13.23 Hepatopancreas of a carp. The distinctive pancreatic tissue (arrowed) contains large eosinophilic zymogen granules and surrounds a blood vessel. H&E stain, ×100 original magnification. (© W.H. Wildgoose.)

Mycology

Most fungal infections are identified on gross inspection or by microscopic examination of fresh preparations taken from the gill and skin, and by histopathology. The principal freshwater fungal pathogen, *Saprolegnia*, is relatively easy to culture by sampling a portion of hyphae from an affected area, placing on a suitable medium such as corn meal or Sabouraud dextrose agar and incubating at room temperature. Subcultures may be required to eliminate bacterial contamination. Presumptive identification will be made on morphology of fungal hyphae, though specific diagnosis will depend on the production and identification of the zoosporangia.

> **TIP:** Commercial agar plates containing a modified Sabouraud agar (e.g. Dermafyt Test®, Kruuse) can be used to culture some aquatic fungi. These sealed plates are commonly used in general practice and have a 2-year shelf life.

Virology

Analysis of fish tissues for the presence of virus infection can only be carried out by specialized laboratories. If a virus infection is suspected, it is advisable to contact a competent laboratory to discuss the most appropriate sampling procedure. It is often possible to submit live fish but freshly dead or tissue samples submitted on ice (Figure 13.24) may be acceptable. If spring viraemia of carp virus (SVCV) is suspected, samples of kidney, spleen and liver (as large as possible) should be submitted on ice to arrive at the laboratory within 24 hours. SVCV can be identified by immunofluorescence and ELISA techniques but definitive diagnosis depends on virus isolation.

Virus particles may also be identified by using electron microscopy (EM). Although EM can be performed on formalin-fixed tissue, better results are obtained if

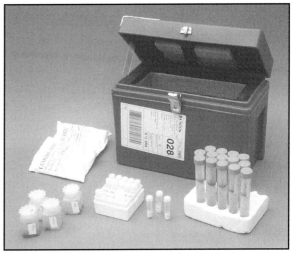

Figure 13.24 Packaging and cooling blocks for the submission of samples for virology. Various samples may be required, including some in (from left to right) neutral buffered 10% formalin, glutaraldehyde and transport medium. A courier service may be required to deliver the samples within 24 hours. (© W.H. Wildgoose.)

tissue is sampled specifically for EM. Tiny pieces of tissue, less than 1 mm^3, should be fixed in glutaraldehyde for an hour, rinsed repeatedly in phosphate buffer and submitted for processing and examination.

Toxicology samples

Samples required and method of sampling are discussed in Chapter 26.

Further reading

Groff JM and Zinkl JG (1999) Hematology and clinical chemistry of cyprinid fish. *Veterinary Clinics of North America: Exotic Animal Practice* **2**, 741–776

Inglis V, Roberts RJ and Bromage N (eds) (1993) *Bacterial Diseases of Fish*. Blackwell Scientific Publications, Oxford

Noga EJ (1996) *Fish Disease: Diagnosis and Treatment*. Mosby-Year Book Inc., St Louis, Missouri

Roberts RJ (ed.) (1989) *Fish Pathology*, 2nd edn. Baillière Tindall, London

Stoskopf MK (ed.) (1993) *Fish Medicine*. WB Saunders Company, Philadelphia, Pennsylvania

Takashima F and Hibiya T (eds) (1995) *An Atlas of Fish Histology*. Gustav Fischer Verlag, Stuttgart

Acknowledgements

The author would like to thank staff at the Fish Vet Group at Inverness and in particular David Cox, Iain McEwen and Marion Urquhart for their help and advice. He is also grateful to the Editor of *In Practice* for permission to reproduce some illustrations from an earlier article by the author (Southgate P, 1994, *In Practice* **16**, 252–255).

14

Diagnostic imaging and endoscopy

Mark D. Stetter

Diagnostic imaging can be an important clinical tool in the investigation of disease in ornamental fish. Radiography and ultrasonography are commonly performed by veterinarians, and the same basic techniques used in small animal medicine can be used with fish. Computed tomography (CT) and magnetic resonance imaging (MRI) can produce very high quality images, but are less commonly available. To interpret the images obtained accurately, some knowledge of the internal anatomy is required (Chapter 16).

For radiography, CT and MRI, the highest quality images are obtained by removing the patient from water. This is in contrast to ultrasonography, where the image is actually enhanced by leaving the patient in water. In most cases, fish must be sedated or anaesthetized in order to position them correctly for imaging. Various anaesthetic agents can be used and these are discussed in Chapter 11. Once immobilized, fish can be safely removed from the water for up to 4 minutes while being positioned for imaging.

Radiography

The same equipment and techniques used with domestic animals will apply to ornamental fish (Figure 14.1). Indications for radiography include routine disease screening and diagnostic evaluation of ill animals. Most commonly, radiography has proved useful in determining the aetiology of abdominal swelling or buoyancy problems in fish.

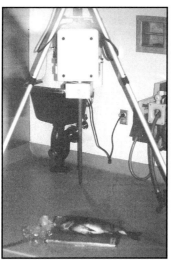

Figure 14.1
Radiography of a fish, using a portable equine X-ray unit. This enables radiographs to be taken on site, close to the fish's facility. The fish is in right lateral recumbency and the radiographic cassette is wrapped in a clear plastic bag to prevent damage from water and salt.

Equipment

The use of rare-earth intensifying screens and a suitable high definition film such as fine grain or mammography film can provide excellent images. The radiographic cassettes should be placed inside sealed plastic bags to prevent damage from ingress of water (Figure 14.1). The use of a grid to reduce scatter radiation is rarely required since the region under investigation is usually less than 10 cm thick.

During handling and positioning, the use of a perforated plastic bag to remove the animal from its water bath and position it on the cassette will minimize trauma to the skin.

Technique

As with other animals, it is best to obtain two views to improve interpretation of the radiographs. A standard lateral view should be taken with the fish in right lateral recumbency, using a vertical beam (Figure 14.2). Depending on the species, some fish can be positioned in ventral recumbency (with or without support) to provide a dorsoventral view. Other species may be difficult to position accurately and therefore a ventrodorsal view can be taken using a horizontal beam, with the fish in lateral recumbency. Flat fish may require only one view (perpendicular to their flat surface) to provide sufficient information.

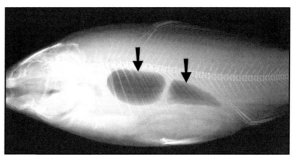

Figure 14.2 The normal radiographic anatomy of koi fish. The skeletal features are readily visible, as are the two chambers of the swim-bladder (arrowed). The coelomic organs occupy the poorly defined area below the swim-bladder. (© W.H. Wildgoose.)

Contrast studies

Contrast medium can be used to enhance soft tissue structures within the body cavity. In most cases, this is limited to a positive contrast study of the gastrointestinal tract, using either barium sulphate or a water-soluble agent such as iohexol. By outlining the gut, it is possible to improve visualization of the size and location of the other organs.

The volume of the agent used depends on the size of the patient and on the species (whether or not there is a stomach, for example) but 5 ml/kg bodyweight is commonly used. A small volume is less likely to be regurgitated, since the agent may irritate the gill tissues. It is administered using a soft rubber or plastic catheter of an appropriate size but metal stomach tubes may be required if the presence of pharyngeal teeth (as in carp) (Figure 14.3) makes it difficult to pass a catheter. The medium is best given when the fish is lightly sedated. Radiographs can be taken at various intervals following administration (Figures 14.4 and 14.5). The timing of these will vary according to the area under investigation and motility of the bowel, which may be temperature related. Total clearance of the agent from the bowel may take up to several days and a suitable holding facility may be required if serial radiographs are required over an extended period.

Although it is possible to use negative contrast media such as gas or air within the body cavity, the resulting disturbance to the fish's buoyancy will limit the usefulness of this technique. Free gas can be found in the body cavity following abdominal surgery or in rare cases with rupture of the swim-bladder (Figure 14.6).

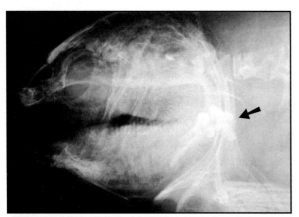

Figure 14.3 Lateral skull radiograph of a koi. Koi and some other cyprinids have pharyngeal teeth (arrowed), which are clearly visible on the radiograph.

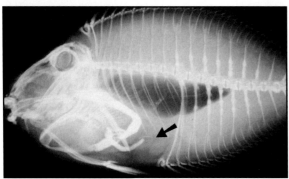

Figure 14.4 Lateral radiograph of a surgeonfish. Barium sulphate was administered by gavage to help to delineate the gastrointestinal tract. A thin linear radio-opaque piece of metal wire (arrowed) is present in the mid-caudal coelomic area. Following ingestion, this perforated the intestines and caused a coelomitis.

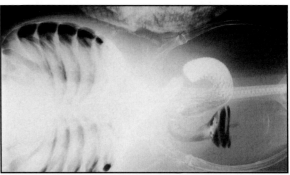

Figure 14.5 Ventrodorsal radiograph of a cownose ray. Barium sulphate was administered to outline the gastric mucosal folds. The air-filled spiral colon can also be visualized adjacent to the stomach.

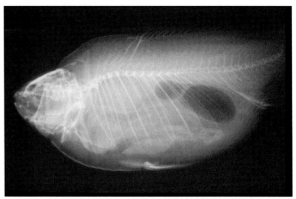

Figure 14.6 A goldfish with rupture of the posterior chamber of the swim-bladder. Free gas is present within the body cavity and caused significant buoyancy disturbance. The anterior chamber was full of fluid, which is visible as a homogeneous area, but the cause is unknown. (© W.H. Wildgoose.)

Equally, the air within the swim-bladder can act as a negative contrast medium and may help to outline the margin of other superimposed lesions within the body cavity.

Interpretation

From good quality radiographs, it should be possible to visualize the skeletal anatomy, the swim-bladder, and a homogeneous soft tissue area, which includes all the coelomic organs (Figure 14.2). Various skeletal abnormalities such as fractures and bone disease (Figure 14.7) are easily visualized. Due to the lack of visceral coelomic fat, individual soft tissue organs such as the heart, liver, spleen and kidney are not commonly identified. The presence of a space-occupying soft tissue mass within the body cavity may also be related to displacement or deformity of the swim-bladder (Figure 14.8). Due to some marked differences in anatomy, it is often helpful to compare radiographs with those of healthy fish of the same species (Figures 14.9 and 14.10).

Safety

The legislation controlling the use of ionizing radiations varies from country to country. This usually applies to the use of the equipment (X-ray generator and personal protection), supervised areas, personal dosimetry

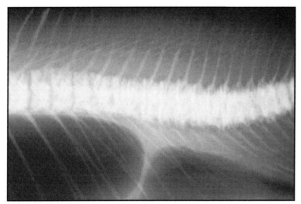

Figure 14.7 A koi with extensive pathological change in the vertebrae that caused a progressive rigidity of the spine. The cause was not identified but was suspected to be of a metabolic origin. (© W.H. Wildgoose.)

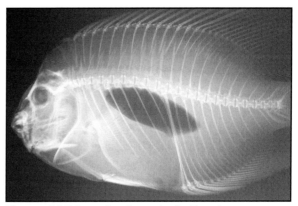

Figure 14.9 Lateral radiograph of a French angelfish. There is good detail of the skeletal anatomy and swim-bladder but a distinct lack of contrast of the soft tissue organs.

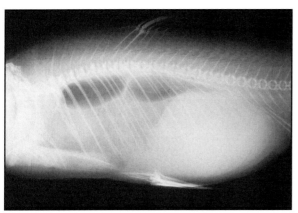

Figure 14.8 A koi with a large intracoelomic tumour. A large homogeneous tissue mass is visible in the caudal part of the body cavity and there is some displacement of the swim-bladder. (© W.H. Wildgoose.)

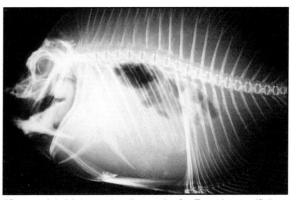

Figure 14.10 Lateral radiograph of a French angelfish that was exhibiting abnormal buoyancy. There is increased radio-opacity of the swim-bladder. A severe granulomatous disease of the swim-bladder and kidneys was found during the postmortem examination.

and record keeping. Although no additional measures are required for the radiography of fish, the safety of all staff involved must be considered, particularly when using portable equipment.

Ultrasonography

Ultrasound imaging provides an excellent complement to radiography in fish because it can differentiate various soft tissue structures and provide useful information about organ location, size and pathological changes.

Equipment

B-mode real-time ultrasound machines are most commonly used for examination of fish. Smaller species are best scanned using a 7.5 or 10.0 MHz transducer, while larger fish (over 3 kg) may be imaged using a 5.0 MHz probe. Very large patients (e.g. sharks, tuna, grouper) may need a 2.5–3.5 MHz transducer in order to acquire an adequate image.

Technique

For ultrasonography, fish are usually left in the water for imaging (Figure 14.11), therefore acoustic gel

as commonly used with terrestrial patients is not required. This is particularly useful with very small patients, where the water can act as an echolucent stand-off and provide acoustic enhancement. In most cases, there is no need for direct contact between the probe and the fish since the water acts as an acoustic coupling agent.

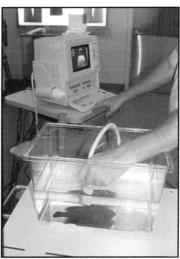

Figure 14.11
Ultrasound scanning of an African cichlid. The patient has been sedated and is held in a bath with a maintenance dose of anaesthetic agent. Due to the small size of the fish, the probe is held at some distance to the animal, thus allowing the water to act as an echolucent stand-off.

Positioning of the probe varies depending on the target organ and may need to be adapted according to the anatomy of the patient (Figures 14.12 and 14.13). Fish with very thick scales may be more difficult to scan due to poor ultrasound penetration (specular reflection), which may produce artefacts in the image. In larger patients, visceral organs can also be imaged by placing the ultrasound transducer down the oesophagus (Figure 14.14). This transoesophageal image often yields high quality images of the heart (Figure 14.15), liver, gastrointestinal tract and gonads.

Unlike other diagnostic modalities, ultrasound imaging and interpretation are greatly limited by the experience of the operator. Practitioners are encouraged to improve their diagnostic skills by taking every opportunity to correlate surgical and postmortem anatomy with ultrasound findings.

Interpretation

Depending upon the equipment, the size of the fish and the experience of the operator, ultrasonography can provide useful images of the soft tissues. It can be used to image the heart, liver, gall bladder, gastrointestinal tract, gonads, eye (Figure 14.16) and various muscles. However, due to the marked reverberation echoes, ultrasound is of little value in imaging air-filled structures such as the swim-bladder. In addition, due to the proximity of the kidney to the swim-bladder in most species, ultrasonography has limited value in identifying renal disorders. Pathologies that may be detected by ultrasound include neoplasia (Figure 14.17), granulomatous disease and abnormalities of the gonads. Conversely, normal tissue appearance can be demonstrated in circumstances where disease may be suspected.

Safety

The use of any electrical equipment in an environment where water may have potentially lethal consequences must be fully considered. A residual current device (RCD) should be used on all electrical equipment – particularly in the UK, where the mains supply is 240 volts.

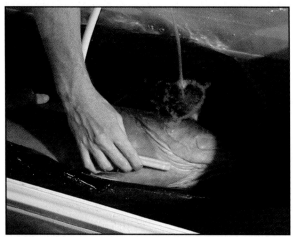

Figure 14.12 Cardiac ultrasound examination of a grouper. Percutaneous image acquired by placement of the probe on the ventral area, just between the base of the pectoral fin and the operculum.

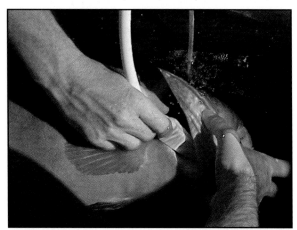

Figure 14.13 Cardiac ultrasound examination of a grouper. In species with very thick scales, a better cardiac image can be obtained by lifting the operculum and placing the probe just beneath the gill arches.

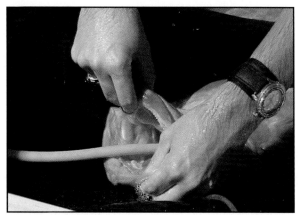

Figure 14.14 Trans-oesophageal ultrasound imaging provides excellent detail of the heart, liver, gastrointestinal tract and occasionally the gonads. A 5.0 MHz linear equine rectal probe is being used *per os* in this grouper.

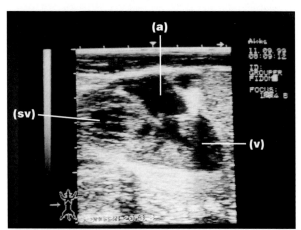

Figure 14.15 Cardiac ultrasound image in a grouper using the trans-oesophageal method. In this long axis view, the thin-walled atrium (a), the thick-walled ventricle (v) and the fibroelastic sinus venosis (sv) are clearly visible. In real time, the AV valve can be seen closing with each ventricular contraction.

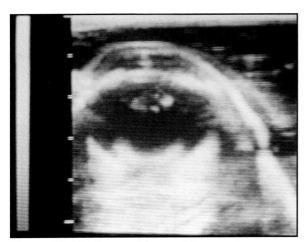

Figure 14.16 Ultrasound image of the eye of a grouper. From the top of the image to the bottom, the following structures can be identified: cornea, anterior chamber, iris, lens, vitreous humour and retina. Ultrasonography can be an excellent diagnostic tool for evaluating the causes and extent of exophthalmos in fish.

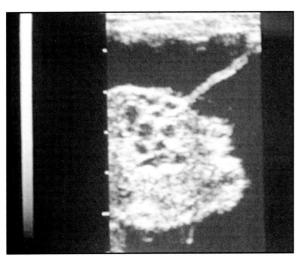

Figure 14.17 Ultrasound image of a koi with abdominal distension. A large amount of coelomic fluid with a polycystic mass attached to the body wall by a fibrin tag can be seen. Exploratory surgery revealed an undifferentiated carcinoma.

Advanced imaging techniques

Nuclear medicine (scintigraphy) involves the intravenous injection of radioactive-labelled agents that are taken up by specific tissues, depending on the agent used. As an example, technetium MDP is taken up into areas of bone where there is inflammation or osteoblast activity. A scintillation detector or gamma camera is used to view the areas where the isotope accumulates. The use of this technique has been described in fish (Bakal *et al.*, 1998) but the excretion of the radioisotope into the fish's environment requires considerable attention to various aspects of radiation safety.

CT and MRI offer the best anatomical detail of the patient. CT scanning is based on conventional radiography, where the X-ray tube rotates rapidly around the patient and the emergent X-ray beam is detected by electronic sensors (Figure 14.18). The signal is analysed and a cross-sectional image is produced (Figures 14.19 and 14.20). CT is most suited to the investigation of skeletal disease and its use in fish has been reported (Lewbart *et al.*, 1998; Tyson *et al.*, 1999). Contrast studies using conventional media can also be performed.

MRI produces an image by mapping out the location of protons (usually hydrogen nuclei) in body tissues using a combination of magnetism and radio waves. A computer generates a cross-sectional image of the patient. The scanning times are much longer than for CT and there must be no movement by the

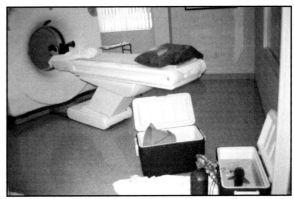

Figure 14.18 Facilities for CT scanning of fish. The patient was anaesthetized and placed in lateral recumbency on foam blocks within the container, which was partially filled with a maintenance dose of anaesthetic.

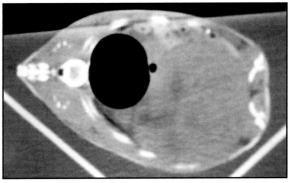

Figure 14.19 A mid-body cross-section CT image of a koi. The fish was scanned while part submerged in anaesthetic solution. This demonstrates the vertebral body, swim-bladder and a large coelomic mass. (Courtesy of Michele Miller and Don Neiffer.)

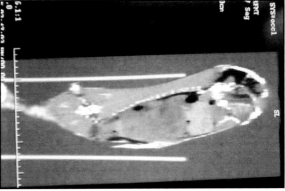

Figure 14.20 A sagittal plane image of the fish in Figure 14.19, showing that the mass occupies much of the body cavity. (Courtesy of Michele Miller and Don Neiffer.)

patient during this period. MRI is most suitable for imaging soft tissues and specialized contrast medium can be used for some studies (Bakal *et al.*, 1998; Blackband and Stoskopf, 1990; Tyson *et al.*, 1999).

The primary disadvantages of these imaging techniques include their availability, cost and need for longer anaesthesia. Veterinarians are using these techniques more often and, because the newer units provide faster and more detailed images, it is obvious that both CT and MRI will be used more commonly in the future.

Endoscopy

Endoscopy can be used for both diagnostic and therapeutic purposes. In addition to the gross visualization of organs, it is possible to collect tissue samples using biopsy forceps through the instrument channel. There is now a wide range of equipment available that is suitable for use in fish but, due to the size of most patients, the smallest diameter endoscopes should be used.

Technique

Endoscopes may be inserted into natural orifices such as the mouth and under the gill covers to view areas that may be otherwise difficult to inspect. It is possible to examine the buccal cavity, the pharynx, the gills and the proximal oesophagus, though this can be difficult in species with well developed pharyngeal teeth, such as carp. Entry through the genital pore of large fish will allow evaluation of the reproductive status of some species.

Examination of the internal organs requires a surgical approach and details of site preparation are found in Chapter 31. This may involve the use of skin disinfectants, application of surgical drapes and removal of a few scales. Due to the compact nature of the organs within the body cavity and limited elasticity of the body wall, insufflation with air or carbon dioxide will be required. This can be performed through the injection port of the sleeve or through a Veress needle inserted obliquely through a stab incision in the anterior midline. The telescope is often inserted in a midline position just anterior to the vent following a stab incision and blunt dissection with mosquito forceps, but other points of entry can be used according to the area under investigation (Figure 14.21). Care should be taken to avoid perforating the internal organs – particularly with gravid female fish, where the ovaries can occupy much of the body cavity.

This approach provides an adequate view of most organs, including the gonad, spleen, gastrointestinal tract and pericardial area. However, in koi and other carp, extensive adhesions between the viscera and body wall severely restrict the use of this technique.

Rigid laparoscopic examination is a very useful diagnostic technique to help to determine the aetiology of swim-bladder disease. The author initially uses radiography to determine the exact anatomical location of the swim-bladder and identify a point of entry with the telescope for maximum diagnostic sampling. Fluid and/or tissue can be collected for cytology, microbiology or histopathology. In some cases, it may be necessary to deflate the swim-bladder to allow the kidneys to be viewed.

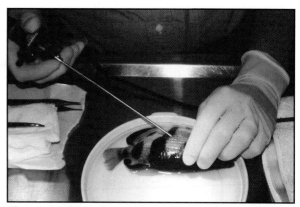

Figure 14.21 Endoscopic examination of an archerfish. In most cases, a midline ventral approach is used but here a lateral approach improves visualization of the swim-bladder and adjacent organs.

Although the gas will eventually be absorbed, as much gas as possible should be removed from the body cavity to prevent problems due to excessive positive buoyancy following the procedure. The entry sites can be closed using a simple suture or tissue adhesive.

Further reading and references

Anon. (1999) *The Ionising Radiations Regulations (1999)*. Statutory Instrument (1999) No. 3232. The Stationery Office Ltd, Norwich

Bakal RS, Love NE, Lewbart GA and Berry CR (1998) Imaging a spinal fracture in a kohaku koi (*Cyprinus carpio*): techniques and case history report. *Veterinary Radiology and Ultrasound* **39**, 318–321

Blackband S and Stoskopf M (1990) In vivo nuclear magnetic resonance imaging and spectroscopy of aquatic organisms. *Magnetic Resonance Imaging* **8**, 191–198

Goddard PJ (1995) Ultrasonic examination of fish. In: *Veterinary Ultrasonography*, ed. PJ Goddard, pp. 289–302. CAB International, Wallingford, Oxon

Lee R (ed.) (1995) *Manual of Small Animal Diagnostic Imaging*. British Small Animal Veterinary Association, Cheltenham, Glos

Lewbart GA, Spodnick G, Barlow N, Love NE, Geoly F and Bakal RS (1998) Surgical removal of an undifferentiated abdominal sarcoma from a koi carp (*Cyprinus carpio*). *The Veterinary Record* **143**, 556–558

Love NE and Lewbart GA (1997) Pet fish radiography: technique and case history reports. *Veterinary Radiology and Ultrasound* **38**, 24–29

Mattson NS (1991) A new method to determine sex and gonad size in live fishes by using ultrasonography. *Journal of Fish Biology* **39**, 673–677

Murray MJ (2000) Application of rigid endoscopy in fishes. *Exotic DVM* **2.3**, 29–33

National Radiological Protection Board and the Health and Safety Executive (1988) *Guidance Notes for the Protection of Persons Against Ionising Radiations Arising from Veterinary Use*. Her Majesty's Stationery Office, London

Nyland TG and Mattoon JS (eds) (1995) *Veterinary Diagnostic Ultrasound*. WB Saunders Company, Philadelphia, Pennsylvania

Sande RD and Poppe TT (1995) Diagnostic ultrasound examination and echocardiography in Atlantic salmon (*Salmo salar*). *Veterinary Radiology and Ultrasound* **36**, 551–558

Stetter MD, Raphael BL, Cook RA, Haramati N and Currie B (1996) Comparison of magnetic resonance imaging, computerized axial tomography, ultrasonography, and radiology for reptilian diagnostic imaging. *Proceedings of the American Association of Zoo Veterinarians*, pp. 450–453

Stoskopf M (1989) Clinical imaging in zoological medicine: a review. *Journal of Zoo and Wildlife Medicine* **20**, 396–412

Stoskopf MK (1993) Clinical examination and procedures. In: *Fish Medicine*, ed. MK Stoskopf, pp. 62–78. WB Saunders Company, Philadelphia, Pennsylvania

Stoskopf MK (1993) Surgery. In: *Fish Medicine*, ed. MK Stoskopf, pp. 91–97. WB Saunders Company, Philadelphia, Pennsylvania

Tyson R, Love NE, Lewbart G, and Bakal R. (1999) Techniques in advanced imaging of fish. *Proceedings of the American Association of Zoo Veterinarians*, pp. 201–202

15

Skin disease

William H. Wildgoose

CHAPTER PLAN:
Anatomy
Investigations
A systematic approach
Colour change
Inflammation: generalized
    Septicaemia (e.g. Gram-negative)
    Spring viraemia of carp
Inflammation: localized
    Parasites (e.g. *Argulus, Lernaea*)
    Bacteria (e.g. Gram-negative)
    Sunburn
Loss of colour
    Management problems (e.g. poor water quality)
    Mycobacteriosis (tuberculosis)
    Neon tetra disease (e.g. *P. hyphessobryconis*)
    Excess mucus (e.g. ectoparasites)
    Epidermal hyperplasia
Bruising
    Trauma
    Bacteria (e.g. Gram-negative)
Visible parasites
Parasites (e.g. *Argulus, Lernaea*, leeches)
Fungi
    Saprolegnia
    Dermocystidium koi
Spots
Nuptial tubercles
White-spot (e.g. *Ichthyophthirius, Cryptocaryon*)
Velvet (e.g. *Amyloodinium, Piscinoodinium*)
Black spot
Epitheliocystis
Swellings
Nodular lesions
    Bacteria (e.g. *Mycobacteria, Nocardia*)
    Parasites
        Myxozoa (e.g. *Henneguya, Myxobolus*)
        Microsporeans (e.g. *Glugea*)
        'Yellow grub'

    Fungi (e.g. *Ichthyophonus*)
    Lymphocystis
    Gas bubble disease
Neoplasia
    Carp pox
    Papilloma
    Pigment cell tumours
    Fibroma
Others
    Dermocystidium
    Subcutaneous fluid-filled cavity
Ulcerations
Bacterial ulcers (e.g. Gram-negative)
Hole-in-the-head (e.g. *Spironucleus?, Edwardsiella*)
Head and lateral line erosion
Mouth fungus (e.g. *Flavobacterium, Cytophaga*)
Trauma
Texture changes
Excess mucus
    Ectoparasites (e.g. *Ichthyophirius, Ichthyobodo*)
    Tet disease (e.g. *Tetrahymena corlissi, Uronema*)
    Bacteria (e.g. *Flavobacterium*)
    Poor water quality
Lack of mucus
    Chronic irritation
    Detergents
    Skin lesions
Raised scales
    Dropsy
Fin lesions
Fin rot (e.g. *Flavobacterium*)
Carp pox
Lymphocystis
Epidermal hyperplasia
White-spot
Lernaea
Hyperaemia (e.g. septicaemia, stress)
Tumours (e.g. carp pox, fibromas)
Nuptial tubercles

The skin of a fish provides a barrier and first line of defence against infection, osmotic pressure and mechanical injury. Being the most visible part of the fish, it is where disease is often first seen.

Owners frequently treat fish diseases symptomatically without establishing a diagnosis. As a result, many cases seen in veterinary practice are those that do not appear to respond to proprietary medicines, and these often require simple investigations in order to reach a diagnosis.

Fish diseases usually arise from a complex interaction of a variety of factors. The majority of problems affecting ornamental fish involve stress due to poor husbandry. Consequently, fish may be debilitated and susceptible to several opportunistic pathogens that are ubiquitous in the aquatic environment.

The skin is the primary target organ for a number of common infectious agents. Its importance in maintaining internal homeostasis is a major reason why skin damage can kill fish. In addition, skin lesions may reflect systemic disease processes.

While it is not possible to show examples of all skin diseases as they appear on different species of fish, it is hoped that this chapter will be a useful aid to diagnosis and direct the reader towards an appropriate course of action.

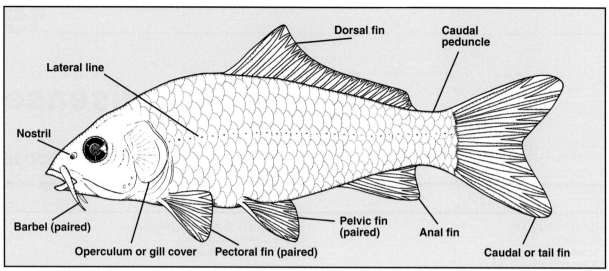

Figure 15.1 The external anatomy of a fish.

Anatomy

External features

The body form and external features of fish vary greatly between species as an adaptation to their individual habitats and behaviour. The main features are illustrated in Figure 15.1.

- Barbels are paired structures situated near the mouth, serving as tactile and taste organs. The shape, length and number vary between different species: some catfish have four pairs whereas koi have two pairs of different length
- The nostrils are paired pouches with olfactory receptors that are used for long-range detection (smell) of food and other objects
- There is no external ear but sound is detected by the swim-bladder and bones that are connected to the inner ear or labyrinth

- The operculum or gill cover is a hard bony plate that protects the delicate gill tissues and is actively involved in the mechanics of respiration
- The lateral line is a sensory organ consisting of a canal system with mechanoreceptors that detect sound and pressure changes. The canals are punctuated by a series of small pores, which are visible along the flanks and extend on to the head in some species
- The vent consists of separate openings to the anus, the genital pores and the urinary papilla or bladder
- The caudal peduncle is the area of the body that tapers towards the tail or caudal fin.

Histological structure

Appreciation of the histological structure (Figure 15.2) of fish skin allows a better understanding of many diseases.

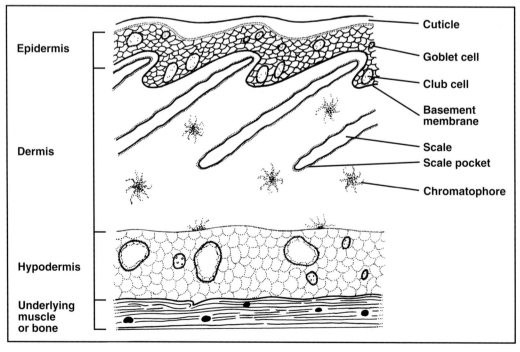

Figure 15.2 Histological structure of fish skin.

Cuticle

The cuticle (the outermost layer) allows the fish to move smoothly through water. It is about 1 µm thick and consists of mucus and cell debris. It also contains antibodies (IgM) and lysozymes that have anti-bacterial and antifungal properties. This layer is usually lost during the routine processing of samples for histopathology.

Epidermis

The epidermis consists mainly of fibrous malpighian cells; together with the cuticle, it forms a waterproof barrier. The thickness of the epidermis varies with species, age and site on the body. Mucus-secreting 'goblet cells' are located in the epidermis; in some species, 'club cells' secrete a potent alarm substance when the skin is damaged.

Unlike mammals, in fish the epidermal cells at all levels are capable of mitotic division, but this occurs mostly at the deepest level, near the basement membrane. During wound healing, there is a loss of the intercellular attachments and the cells migrate rapidly to cover the defect and provide some waterproof integrity. This leads to a reduction in the thickness of the surrounding epidermis and produces a thin layer of epidermis at least one cell thick over the wound. This process occurs independently of water temperature but is inhibited by the presence of pathogens and necrotic tissue. Later, these malpighian cells undergo cell division to restore the epidermal layer. This is a slower process and is dependent on ambient temperature.

Dermis

The dermis consists of two layers:

- The upper layer contains collagen and reticulin, which form a supportive network
- The lower, deeper layer is a more compact mass of collagen fibres that provides the main structural strength of the skin.

The scales are flexible bony plates that develop in scale pockets in the upper loose connective tissue. They are not shed regularly but grow with the rest of the body. Some fish do not have scales and the epidermis is often thicker in these species.

The dermis may also contain pigment cells called chromatophores. These produce different colorations when acting individually or in combination, and by the reflection and refraction of light. The pigment cells found in fish are:

- Melanophore (black)
- Xanthophore (yellow)
- Erythrophore (orange/red)
- Leucophore (white)
- Iridophore (reflective/iridescent).

Hypodermis

The hypodermis is the deepest layer of the skin and consists of loose fatty tissue connecting the skin to the underlying structures. Due to its design and good blood supply, bacterial diseases spread rapidly along this layer.

Investigations

It is important to know the normal features of the species under investigation. Colour changes and other features, such as nuptial tubercles on goldfish, can develop during normal breeding activity. Some exotic varieties of goldfish, such as orandas, are deliberately bred with verrucose masses around the head.

Skin disease may affect single or multiple fish; it can be irritant or non-irritant and often (but not always) compromises the health of the patient. Observation of abnormal behaviour such as 'flashing' (the fish swims rapidly in an arc to rub its body against a rough surface) may suggest irritation of the fish. Irritant diseases can result from infestation with ectoparasites or from environmental chemicals or pollutants. Some species may jump more frequently, though frequent jumping can be a normal behaviour in certain pond fish.

Laboratory tests

The laboratory diagnosis of fish disease is discussed in Chapter 13 and only brief comments will be made here in relation to skin diseases. The most important procedures used to investigate disease in ornamental fish are outlined below; some or all of these tests may be required to confirm a diagnosis.

Water quality analysis

Routine investigation should involve checking levels of ammonia, nitrite, nitrate and pH; additional parameters such as hardness and dissolved oxygen may be required in some circumstances. The effects of environmental factors such as high levels of nitrite and extremes of pH can cause skin irritation and damage, with increased mucus production.

Skin scrape examination

Examination of skin scrapings by light microscopy is a routine procedure in fish health management. Many fish pathogens are opportunists and these may complicate primary disease. Low numbers of parasites are normal and are tolerated by fish but stress factors and illness allow multiplication to a level where signs of disease are seen. Therefore, improving environmental conditions is an essential part of therapy.

Scrapings of body mucus are usually taken (using a blunt scalpel blade) from behind a pectoral fin or the operculum – sites where parasites are most likely to be found. This may necessitate the use of an anaesthetic for some active fish, though it is claimed that this may reduce the numbers of ectoparasites. Alternatively, light manual restraint may allow a scraping to be taken from close to the dorsal fin. Samples should be taken from two or three different sites on each fish and, where possible, from several fish in the same group to obtain a better overall impression of the level of ectoparasite infestation.

Most ectoparasites can be seen under low-power magnification ($\times$ 40) but, since many are refractile, they are more visible using phase contrast or with the condenser racked down. Small protozoans such as *Ichthyobodo* are better seen at medium power magnification ($\times$ 100), as are the 'haystack formations' of *Flavobacterium columnare* colonies. The latter are most visible at the edge of the mucus sample, where they are silhouetted against a plain background.

Gill sample examination
Under light anaesthesia, mucus and the tips of a few gill lamellae can be sampled for microscopy by performing a light scrape over the gill surface. Skin parasites found here in significant numbers may reflect the scale of the infestation and can affect the prognosis if there is extensive damage to the gill.

Postmortem examination
A postmortem examination should be performed as soon as possible, preferably within 1 hour of death since autolysis of tissues is often rapid. Refrigeration may extend the interval to a few hours but the results should be interpreted with care. Gross examination may reveal sufficient information but bacterial and histological samples are usually taken at this time.

Bacteriology
Swabs of superficial lesions are invariably contaminated with environmental bacteria. Swabs taken from the kidney at postmortem examination therefore provide a better source of samples in cases when a systemic bacterial infection is present. The culture and identification of pathogens and interpretation of the results is best performed by laboratories familiar with fish diseases. However, as discussed above, some species of bacteria can be difficult to culture and diagnosis of *Flavobacterium columnare* infections is best achieved by microscopic examination of a scraping from the lesion.

Other bacteria associated with skin disease in fish include Gram-negative species such as aeromonads, pseudomonads, vibrios and occasionally mycobacteria and nocardiae.

Histopathology
Histological examination of fish tissues plays an important role in routine disease investigations. Gill, heart, liver, spleen, bowel and anterior and posterior kidney are routinely sampled at postmortem examination and a section of skin and underlying muscle (containing both red and white muscle fibres) is usually taken from close to the lateral line. Other obvious lesions, such as tumours and ulcers, should also be sampled at the junction with normal tissues. Although the primary interest here may be a skin lesion, all tissues should be sampled to assess their role in the disease process. In live fish, biopsy samples can be taken from proliferative lesions but this procedure is more invasive and may predispose the patient to secondary wound infections.

A systematic approach

It is difficult to categorize all skin diseases into a simple list and so a systematic approach has been adopted based on the following presenting clinical signs:

- Colour change
- Visible pathogens
- Spots
- Swellings
- Ulcerations
- Texture changes
- Fin lesions.

Inevitably, there is a certain degree of overlap and the distinction between some groups may not always be particularly clear. As with many other fish diseases, one disease will often result in a multitude of secondary infections because the effects of stress produce a general depression in the natural defence mechanisms. Therefore, it is possible that an initial problem, such as poor water quality, will stress the fish and allow parasite numbers to increase, producing physical damage to the skin that may then become further infected by bacteria and fungi.

Colour change

Changes in the coloration of fish can sometimes be due to normal camouflage behaviour or sexual responses. The skin colour of some species, such as discus, darkens when ill or in poor water conditions. Pigment cells in the dermis are under neurological control and therefore any damage or irritation to the nerve supply may cause colour changes (Figure 15.3). Pigment cell tumours may present as a discrete plaque or raised mass of abnormal coloration (see Figures 15.21 and 15.22).

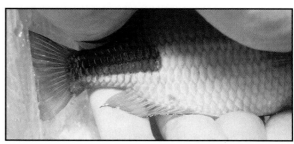

Figure 15.3 This fish, a characin, developed a discrete purple-blue coloration on its caudal peduncle following local injection of an antibiotic to treat the ulceration between its anal and caudal fins. The dramatic colour change, due to irritation of the nerves, developed in seconds but took several weeks to resolve. (By permission of *In Practice.*)

Inflammation: generalized

Septicaemia
Septicaemia may result in a widespread reddening, visible as hyperaemia of the fins and other non-pigmented areas of the body (Figure 15.4). Many cases are caused by Gram-negative bacteria such as aeromonads, pseudomonads and vibrios. Goldfish may also develop patches of brown pigmentation (Figure 15.5) that disappear with successful antibiotic treatment.

Spring viraemia of carp
Spring viraemia of carp (SVC) is caused by *Rhabdovirus carpio*. It affects carp, goldfish, orfe, pike, roach, rudd, tench and Wels catfish, producing various clinical signs that include abdominal swelling, exophthalmos, petechial haemorrhages and darkening of the skin. There are no pathognomonic signs for the disease, which is notifiable in the UK, but a history of recent introductions, rising springtime water temperatures,

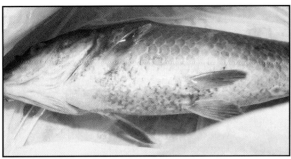

Figure 15.4 Petechiation and ecchymosis are most visible on the ventral surface and pale or white areas of fish. The generalized septicaemia in this koi was confirmed by isolation of *Aeromonas* from an ulcer near its mouth, as well as from the kidney. (By permission of *In Practice*.)

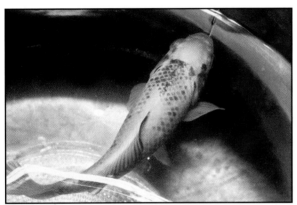

Figure 15.5 Septicaemia in goldfish often produces patches of brown pigmentation in the skin and fins, which may be localized or widespread. Following successful antibiotic treatment, these disappear and the gold coloration returns. (By permission of *In Practice*.)

known outbreaks or multiple deaths may be suggestive. Any suspicion of the disease is notifiable in the UK under the Diseases of Fish Acts (1937 and 1983) and European Community legislation.

Inflammation: localized

Parasites
Fish lice, *Argulus* (see Figure 15.9), use a stylet near their mouth to penetrate the skin and inject digestive enzymes into the host tissues. The female of the anchor worm, *Lernaea* (see Figure 15.10), attaches to the host with a large penetrating cephalic process. Both parasites infest freshwater fish and produce a localized inflammatory reaction and skin damage, which is then susceptible to secondary bacterial infection.

Bacteria
Petechiation and ecchymosis can result from bacteraemia, producing localized areas of redness (Figure 15.6).

Sunburn
Sunburn causes petechiation and patches of erythema on white and non-pigmented dorsal surfaces of exposed fish. This often occurs in shallow ponds where there is no shade and the water is exceptionally clear.

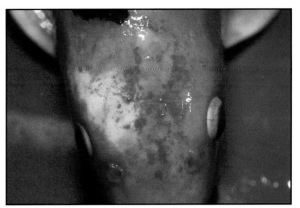

Figure 15.6 Local ecchymosis and petechiation on the head of a koi, which were assumed to be due to bacteraemia since the fish also had a small body ulcer. An injectable antibiotic was administered and the cranial discoloration resolved within 7 days. (By permission of *In Practice*.)

Loss of colour
Albinism is a general term used to describe a number of genetic defects that affect the pigment cell system. True albino fish are cream to white in colour with red eyes and are often selectively bred for these characteristics.

Management problems
Poor water quality can affect the colour of delicate aquarium fish, such as discus, which require very specific water conditions. A lack of dietary pigments and chronic nutritional deficiencies can also result in dull coloration of some species. Indoor fish that are not exposed to natural sunlight or specific fluorescent lighting tend to be pale and less vibrant in colour.

Mycobacteriosis (tuberculosis)
Various species of mycobacteria infect fish, producing non-specific clinical signs such as loss of colour, emaciation and non-healing ulcerations. It is thought that there may be a high incidence of mycobacteriosis (Figure 15.7) in aquarium fish that goes undetected. Owners should be advised about the implications of this disease following its confirmation by histopathology and bacteriology.

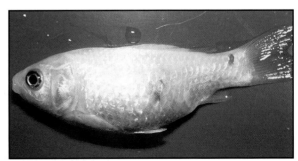

Figure 15.7 This is the same goldfish as in Figure 15.5, on presentation 6 years later when it had abdominal swelling and body ulcers with a caseous discharge. Its original gold colour had disappeared completely except for a small localized area on its caudal peduncle. Postmortem examination revealed extensive internal granulomas due to mycobacteria. (By permission of *In Practice*.)

Neon tetra disease

'Neon tetra disease' is caused by a microsporean parasite, *Pleistophora hyphessobryconis*, that infects the muscle tissue of various aquarium fish such as tetras, barbs, danios and goldfish. It produces focal areas of colour loss and grey or white patches due to muscle necrosis, particularly along the dorsum.

Excess mucus

Excess mucus production is caused by various factors (see later section on texture changes) and is sometimes called 'slime disease'. The associated thickening of the cuticle dulls the colours of fish and gives the skin a light grey appearance.

Epidermal hyperplasia

Epidermal hyperplasia is common, particularly in pond fish. In some species, it is due to a viral infection of epidermal cells and may be associated with cyprinid herpesvirus infection, the causative agent of carp pox (see later). Lesions appear as smooth milky-white plaques, about 1 mm thick and up to several centimetres across (Figure 15.8). They are more visible on the dark pigmented areas of the body and can be differentiated from diseases producing excess mucus by the fact that the lesions cannot be scraped off easily.

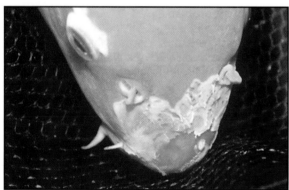

Figure 15.8 Epidermal hyperplasia, common in koi, is seen as discrete smooth milky white plaques. The hyperplastic tissue will often slough periodically after several months, as was the case with the lesion on this koi's snout. (By permission of *In Practice*.)

Bruising

Trauma

Damage to the skin because of poor handling and netting may produce bruising. Injection sites in pale coloured fish commonly develop a bruise that may persist for several days. Predatory birds such as herons can cause a range of lesions, including bruising, lacerations and deep puncture wounds (see Figure 15.28). Frogs grIp the head and opercula of pond fish during the frog-breeding season in early spring, causing localized bruising.

Bacteria

Prior to ulceration, infection with Gram-negative bacteria (e.g. aeromonads and pseudomonads) may appear as a localized area of inflammation, which then darkens like a bruise, due to the enzymatic effect of bacterial toxins in the dermal tissues.

Visible pathogens

Parasites

Some microscopic ectoparasites and the tissue reaction that they produce may be grossly visible as small spots (see later). Larger parasites that are visible to the naked eye include:

- Fish louse, *Argulus* (Figure 15.9)
- Anchor worm, *Lernaea* (Figure 15.10)
- Leech, *Piscicola* (Figure 15.11).

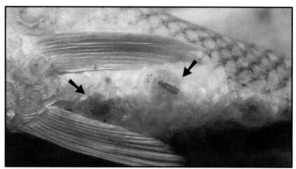

Figure 15.9 The crustacean parasite *Argulus* (arrowed) can measure up to 7 mm and can be difficult to see on fish, due to its semi-transparent body. The parasites move over the surface of the fish but can swim freely in the water, laying eggs in the environment.

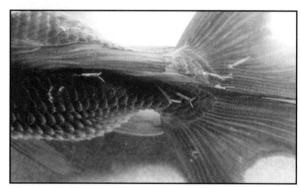

Figure 15.10 *Lernaea* is a freshwater copepod that attaches to the host with a large cephalic process and can measure up to 15 mm in length. Only the female is parasitic and she can be recognized by a pair of trailing egg sacs, which are more easily recognized while in water. (By permission of *In Practice*.)

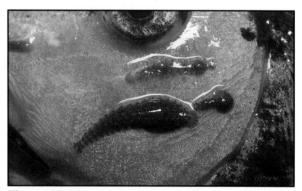

Figure 15.11 Leeches attach to the host by a large suction pad and move around with a characteristic contractile action. A common leech, *Piscicola geometra*, can measure up to 4 cm in length. (By permission of *In Practice*.)

Large flabelliferan isopods (up to 60 mm) can occasionally be found on the skin or in the buccal cavity of marine fish. Although not a skin parasite, the intestinal nematode *Camallanus* is a red thread-like worm that can be seen protruding from the anus of some tropical aquarium fish such as mollies and platys.

Fungi

Saprolegnia

Saprolegnia is a fungus or water mould that commonly infects damaged skin and gills of freshwater fish. It resembles white cotton-wool (Figure 15.12), though in pond fish it may appear green, due to trapped algae.

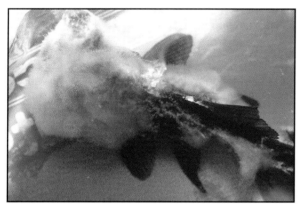

Figure 15.12 Infection with a *Saprolegnia* fungus. The delicate fungal structure resembles cotton-wool but collapses into a slimy mass when removed from the water. Fish with extensive lesions, such as this black moor goldfish, are unlikely to recover, due to loss of osmoregulatory control. (By permission of *In Practice*.)

Saprolegnia is often a secondary invader of skin wounds and infects fish with concurrent diseases. It is a reflection of serious underlying husbandry problems and poor water quality. It is important to distinguish this organism from 'mouth fungus' and 'peduncle disease', which look similar but are caused by *Flavobacterium columnare*, a bacterium that usually infects the mouth or the root of the tail, respectively (see Figure 15.31).

Dermocystidium koi

Dermocystidium koi infects the dermal tissues in koi, producing a smooth raised swelling which later ulcerates to reveal a mass of hyphae (see Figure 15.24 and section on swellings).

Spots

Spots that form part of the natural coloration of some fish are usually bilaterally symmetrical and should be differentiated from pathological lesions. In this chapter, the distinction between large spots and small swellings is based on size and both sections may apply to the same lesion.

Nuptial tubercles

'Nuptial tubercles' are raised multicellular keratinous nodules (1–2 mm in diameter). They are usually found on the opercula (Figure 15.13) and leading edge of the pectoral fins of male goldfish and are more visible in the breeding season. Although they resemble 'white spot' parasites, routine scraping does not dislodge them.

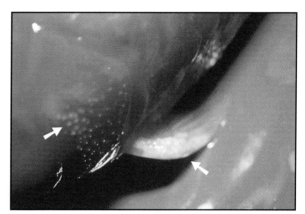

Figure 15.13 Nuptial tubercles are multicellular keratinous nodules, visible as spots on the operculum and pectoral fin of this male goldfish (arrowed). During the breeding season, they become larger and can measure up to 2 mm.

White spot

'White spot', also known as 'ich', is a protozoan parasite infection which in freshwater fish is caused by *Ichthyophthirius multifiliis* (Figure 15.14). The mature parasites can measure up to 1 mm in size. They are more easily seen on the dark areas of the body but in large pond fish it can be difficult to see these parasites until considerable damage has been done to the skin. Initially there may be an excess of mucus and thickening of the epithelium, producing a grey sheen to the skin. Although this common disease is often regarded as a minor problem (since it is easily treated with proprietary medicines), these parasites can cause extensive damage to gill tissue if treatment is delayed.

Cryptocaryon irritans produces a similar disease in marine fish (Figure 15.15).

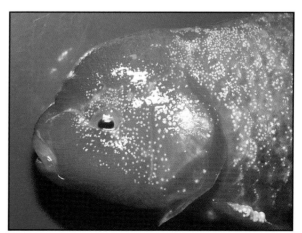

Figure 15.14 'White spot' is caused by small white protozoan parasites (measuring up to 1 mm) that are more visible on the dark-coloured areas of the body.

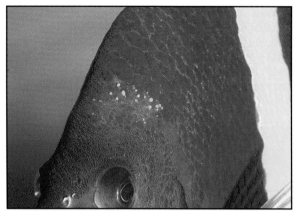

Figure 15.15 'Marine white spot' is caused by infection with a ciliate protozoan, *Cryptocaryon irritans*. A small number of maturing parasites (trophonts) can be seen above the head of this purple moon angelfish. (By permission of *In Practice*.)

Velvet

A dinoflagellate, *Piscinoodinium*, is the cause of 'velvet' (also known as 'rust disease' or 'gold dust disease') in tropical freshwater fish. The parasites can be seen as very fine spots on the skin and produce a gold- or rust-coloured velvet-like layer over affected areas. The organisms sometimes cluster together to form larger spots.

The marine counterpart, also called 'coral fish disease', is caused by *Amyloodinium*.

Black spot

Metacercariae of digenean flukes (*Neascus*) migrate to the skin and cause a reaction in the dermis, stimulating melanocytes around the parasitic cyst to produce 'black spot' (Figure 15.16). Affected fish are intermediate hosts in the life cycle and the lesions can measure up to 0.5 mm.

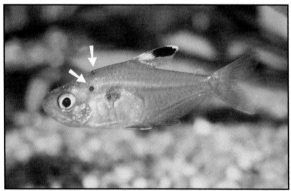

Figure 15.16 'Black spot'. The two dark spots behind and above the head of this small characin are caused by the intermediate stage of a digenean fluke. The cluster of very small spots near the middle of the body is an area of natural pigmentation. (By permission of *In Practice*.)

Epitheliocystis

Epitheliocystis is caused by a chlamydia-like organism, which infects epithelial cells of the gills and, less commonly, the skin. The hypertrophied cells produce small white nodules up to 1 mm in size.

Swellings

It should be possible to differentiate between superficial raised masses on the surface of fish and underlying internal swellings. Disruption of the scales will indicate that a lesion lies in the lower compact dermis, whereas epidermal lesions are superficial to the scales. Some swellings can be identified easily on gross inspection but confirmation may require histological examination.

Nodular lesions

Nodular lesions tend to be small discrete masses that may cluster to form a large cauliflower-like mass.

Bacteria

Infection with mycobacteria and nocardiae produces granulomas in the dermis and other tissues. Lesions vary in size and can affect all species but are more common in aquarium fish.

Parasites

Myxozoan parasites (e.g. *Henneguya* and *Myxobolus*) produce pseudocysts that enlarge slowly in various tissues and are usually found in wild-caught fish.

Microsporeans are intracellular parasites. *Glugea* can produce large hypertrophied cells or xenomas, white nodular structures several millimetres in size.

'Yellow grub', characterized by cystic lesions up to 5 mm in diameter, is caused by infection with the metacercariae of *Clinostomum*. This digenean trematode encysts in the musculature of fish and can result in ulceration if near the skin.

Fungi

Ichthyophonus hoferi is a fungus-like organism that causes a chronic systemic granulomatous disease and mainly affects marine fish. Dark raised dermal granulomas, up to 1 mm in size, give the skin a rough sandpaper-like feel, due to loss of the overlying epithelium.

Vesicles

Small, discrete raised vesicles or bullae measuring up to 4 mm in diameter have been found on koi with body ulcers (Figure 15.17). This may be an unusual epidermal response to bacterial infection.

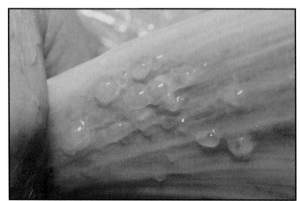

Figure 15.17 Vesicles, measuring up to 4 mm, on the caudal fin of a koi with a body ulcer. Following injection with an antibiotic, the lesion resolved within 48 hours.

Lymphocystis

Lymphocystis is a chronic disease caused by an iridovirus, which mainly affects tropical marine fish, producing massive enlargement of dermal fibroblasts (Figure 15.18). These measure about 1 mm but often cluster to form larger nodules up to 1 cm across. The disease has a low mortality rate; affected fish may recover if the cause of stress is corrected and environmental conditions improved.

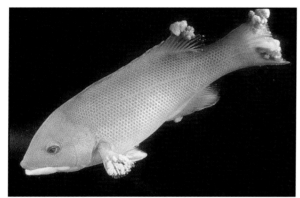

Figure 15.18 *Lymphocystis* affecting the fins of an immature California sheepshead, a coldwater marine fish. The lesions developed shortly after arrival at a public aquarium but resolved within 6 weeks without the need for medication. (Courtesy of the National Aquarium in Baltimore.)

Gas bubble disease

Supersaturation of the water with dissolved gases, particularly nitrogen, results in so-called 'gas bubble disease': emphysema of the tissues, including the skin and gills. A variety of environmental factors that act to draw air into solution under pressure (e.g. leaking water pumps; venturis), heavy algal growth and the use of borehole water predispose fish to this disease.

Neoplasia

Several types of skin tumour have been recorded in fish, the most common of which are described below. These are larger masses and are often solitary well circumscribed lesions, which can affect any area of the body. Fish can live for a long time with many neoplasms. Some can be removed successfully under general anaesthesia, although many will recur.

Carp pox

Carp pox is an infection of epidermal cells with cyprinid herpesvirus 1 and is technically described as a papilloma. It commonly affects carp but is also found in other coldwater and tropical fish. It manifests as drops of 'candle wax' on the body and fins (Figure 15.19), which are often grey or white, though these lesions may contain some pigment. It is caused by a viral infection but only a few fish exhibit lesions at any one time. Carp pox (and other papillomas – see below) often regress spontaneously after several months but may reappear. Some individuals can be affected with extensive lesions for many years.

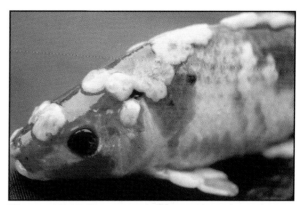

Figure 15.19 Carp pox, a benign epidermal neoplasm, produces a characteristic smooth raised lesion that resembles drops of candle wax. It can affect any area of the body, and ranges from discrete masses measuring a few millimetres in size to large extensive plaques.

Papilloma

Papillomas are the most common skin neoplasm of fish and are usually found on individual fish (Figure 15.20). They vary considerably in size and appearance: they may be smooth or verrucose, sessile or pedunculate, localized or extensive, single or multiple. Papillomas can be found on most external sites but rarely cause clinical problems unless they interfere with the mouth or operculae. Occasionally several fish may be affected, particularly when there is a viral aetiology (see carp pox section, above). Papillomas have been found in association with squamous cell carcinoma and epidermal hyperplasia in some species.

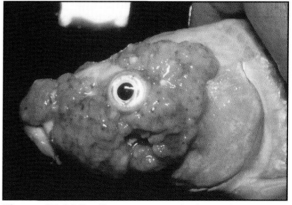

Figure 15.20 Papillomas can vary in size and appearance. This mature koi has a large lesion on its head that sloughed completely on several occasions. There is epidermal hyperplasia, seen as a darker area extending over the operculum and behind the head. (Reproduced with the permission of *Veterinary Record.*)

Pigment cell tumours

Melanomas are the most common type of pigment cell tumour. Erythrophoromas (Figures 15.21 and 15.22) also appear to be relatively common but rarely cause clinical problems. Confirmation requires pigment analysis but diagnosis is often based on gross coloration. It is thought that there may be a genetic predisposition among fish for these tumours, since they are found in some hybrid species, such as swordtail × platy.

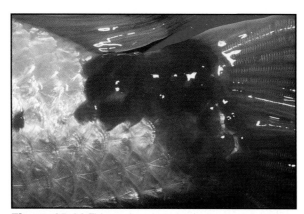

Figure 15.21 This erythrophoroma (red pigment cell tumour) developed as an extensive plaque over the caudal peduncle of this goldfish. The lesion had been present for a few years but did not cause any clinical problems. (By permission of *In Practice*.)

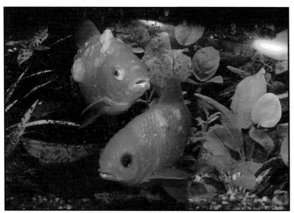

Figure 15.22 These two goldfish had been isolated for several years before erythrophoromas developed spontaneously on one fish and then 12 months later on the other. Due to their extensive nature, surgical treatment was not possible. One fish survived for more than 4 years, though some lesions increased in size. (By permission of *In Practice*.)

Fibroma

Fibromas (Figure 15.23) are less common and superficially may clinically resemble papillomas. Histologically, they may be confused with some pigment cell tumours.

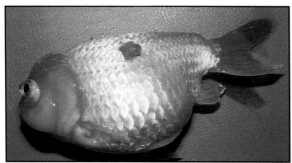

Figure 15.23 A fibroma on the dorsum of a lionhead goldfish. This discrete raised mass developed over a few weeks. Following surgical excision, the fish lived for a further 3 years before dying from an unrelated problem. (By permission of *In Practice*.)

Other swellings

Dermocystidium infection

Dermocystidium is a group of fungal-like organisms that infect many species of fish. *D. koi* produces a smooth raised lesion with a uniform colour (Figure 15.24) in the dermis of koi. The lesions rupture as they reach about 1 cm in size and the exposed hyphae release thousands of characteristic spores (6–15 µm) that are easily identified by microscopy. Usually one or two fish are affected with a few lesions. Surgical removal is possible but some lesions may heal spontaneously after eruption. The mode of transmission is unknown.

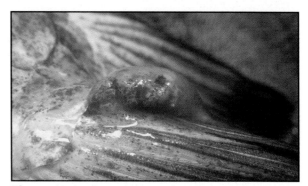

Figure 15.24 *Dermocystidium koi* lesion on the tail fin of a koi. Small lesions may resemble carp pox, but as these grow they become quite distinctive and white hyphae become visible through the epidermis. The lesions eventually rupture when they are about 1 cm in size. (By permission of *In Practice*.)

Subcutaneous fluid-filled cavity

Adverse reactions to long-acting oxytetracycline injections can produce large collections of sterile tissue fluid at the injection site. The serosanguineous fluid should be aspirated to avoid ulceration of the overlying skin. Occasionally, purulent fluid may collect at subcutaneous sites following localized bacterial infection.

Ulcerations

Most ulcerations have a similar gross appearance. They are often caused by bacteria, although fungi may be involved in secondary infections. Lesions may occur on any area of the body surface but some diseases are localized to the lateral line.

Ulcers

Ulcers may be punctate lesions on the head, where the skin is in direct contact with the skull, or deep and invasive lesions on the body, which expose underlying muscle (Figure 15.25) and may penetrate the body cavity.

Superficial ulcers are a common problem in koi and other coldwater fish. Atypical *Aeromonas salmonicida* has been shown to be a primary cause of this disease in goldfish but frequently several species of bacteria may be isolated from these lesions, including other Gram-negative bacteria such as aeromonads, pseudomonads and *Cytophaga – Flexibacter – Flavobacterium* genera. Several fish may be affected and

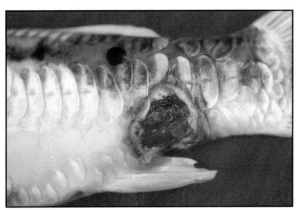

Figure 15.25 Body ulcer on a koi. Early lesions start as a localized area of inflammation, which later darkens like a bruise and eventually ulcerates, exposing the underlying tissue. They are often caused by bacterial infection but they may become further infected by *Saprolegnia*. (By permission of *In Practice*.)

the disease can spread to all fish in a pond, causing considerable mortality. Poor water quality and poor husbandry are common underlying problems, which must be improved to assist recovery.

Mycobacteriosis can also produce chronic ulcerative lesions in aquarium fish (see Figure 15.7) and vibrios are found in ulcers on marine fish.

Hole-in-the-head

In cichlids such as discus and oscars, 'hole-in-the-head' presents as shallow ulcerations on the head (Figure 15.26) and along the flanks. This is a common problem in these fish and several factors may precipitate clinical disease.

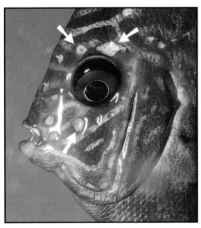

Figure 15.26 'Hole-in-the-head' disease in a discus. Small ulcers (arrowed) that develop in the sensory pits on the head gradually expand and may coalesce into large lesions. (By permission of *In Practice*.)

It has been suggested that the disease is due to *Spironucleus*, a flagellate protozoan that causes enteritis, but it may also involve a nutritional component, environmental stress or a superficial bacterial infection. The mortality rate is low but the disease is disfiguring. Hobbyists often use metronidazole in the food and in the water but the disease frequently recurs and other systemic antibiotics may be required.

In catfish, systemic infection with *Edwardsiella ictaluri* may produce ulcers on the head and dorsum. The chronic form of the disease produces an erosion on the top of the skull in some species.

Head and lateral line erosion

'Head and lateral line erosion' is a syndrome, recognized in tropical marine angelfish and tangs, that presents as chronic ulceration of the head and lateral line (Figure 15.27). Fish continue to eat but can develop secondary complications. The lesions vary in size and depth, and may develop over many months.

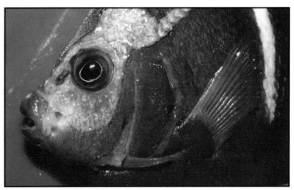

Figure 15.27 Extensive ulceration in a passer angelfish due to 'head and lateral line erosion'. Also known as 'marine hole-in-the-head', this syndrome often starts soon after captivity. (By permission of *In Practice*.)

Poor nutrition, stress and viral infection are suggested causes of this disease, which is associated with a low mortality rate. Due to the selective feeding habits and natural diets of some species, there may be a nutritional component to the disease. It does not respond to copper-based treatments and there is no known cure, though exposure to natural light may prevent the disease and help some lesions to heal.

Mouth fungus

'Mouth fungus' is a term used in the hobby literature to describe an erosion of the mouth in tropical aquarium fish caused by *Flavobacterium columnare* and other related bacteria. The same species produce fin rot (see Figure 15.31) and other skin lesions. Poor water quality, overstocking, high temperatures and stress predispose fish to this disease.

Trauma

Poor handling and netting can cause a variety of skin lesions such as lacerations, punctures and erosions. Similar injuries occur less commonly, from fighting and from attack by predators such as carnivorous fish, fish-eating birds (Figure 15.28) and mammals.

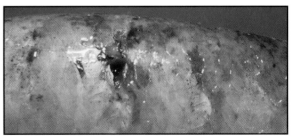

Figure 15.28 This small puncture wound on the body of an orfe was the result of an attack by a grey heron (*Ardea cinerea*) and penetrated deep into the dorsal musculature of the fish, fracturing the spinous processes of some vertebrae. (By permission of *In Practice*.)

Texture changes

Some 'textural' conditions are difficult to detect visually and hence to demonstrate photographically. The use of bare hands when examining fish may allow a better appreciation of these skin lesions.

Excess mucus

The quantity and consistency of the normal cuticle varies between species. Some fish, such as oscars and discus, are particularly slimy and this mucus is ingested as the first food for fry in these species.

The non-specific term 'slime disease' is used to describe the condition where abnormal and excessive amounts of mucus are produced by fish in response to the irritant effect of a variety of agents. Excess mucus dulls some colours and gives the skin a greyish sheen.

These cases are best observed using indirect lighting as the fish moves around in the water. Microscopic examination of skin scrapings is usually required to identify ectoparasitic causes of the condition so that successful treatment can be carried out.

Parasites

Many species of parasite irritate the skin and stimulate mucus production (Figure 15.29). These include protozoans such as *Ichthyophthirius*, *Ichthyobodo* (*Costia*) and *Chilodonella* and trichodinids such as *Trichodina* and *Trichodinella*. The metazoan skin fluke, *Gyrodactylus*, also produces skin disease. In marine fish, similar protozoans (*Cryptocaryon* and *Brooklynella*) and skin flukes (*Benedenia* and *Neobenedenia*) can be found.

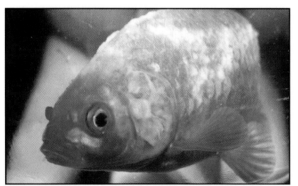

Figure 15.29 Excess mucus ('slime disease') gives the skin a patchy grey-white appearance. In this goldfish, a severe 'white spot' and *Ichthyobodo* infestation was identified on microscopic examination of a skin scraping.

Tet disease

Tetrahymena corlissi, a ciliate protozoan ectoparasite, infests freshwater tank fish, including guppies. 'Tet disease' (occasionally called 'guppy killer') produces discrete pale white patches, due to excess mucus and focal necrosis, particularly around the eyes. Mortalities occur because of invasion of the muscle and deeper tissues.

Uronema, the marine counterpart of this parasite, causes similar pathology but ulceration is a feature in the later stages of disease.

Bacteria

Infection with *Flavobacterium columnare*, often referred to as 'columnaris disease', causes localized grey patches

of mucus on the skin. The same organism is a cause of 'fin rot' (see Figure 15.31), 'mouth fungus' and 'peduncle disease', according to its location on the body.

Poor water quality

The irritant effect of some chemicals and extremes of pH (too acidic or too alkaline) can affect the mucus cells or change the quality and consistency of the cuticle.

Lack of mucus

A lack of mucus is normal in some fish, particularly some marine species.

Chronic irritation

Prolonged irritation by pathogens or poor water conditions, as described above, will eventually exhaust the mucus-secreting cells, producing a rough dry texture to the skin surface.

Detergents

Some medications, such as benzalkonium chloride, can remove much of the cuticle.

Skin lesions

Damage and erosion of the epithelium by pathogens and the dermal granulomas produced by *Ichthyophonus* cause the skin to feel rough, like sandpaper.

Raised scales

'Dropsy' is a non-specific term used to describe oedematous conditions in fish. It can apply to both abdominal distension (ascites) and cutaneous oedema. The latter causes the scales to protrude and may be either localized around skin lesions or generalized; it is occasionally called 'pine-cone disease', due to its gross appearance (Figure 15.30). Exophthalmos due to retrobulbar effusion occasionally accompanies dropsy and may be unilateral or bilateral.

Any condition that affects osmoregulation, such as gill or kidney disease, can produce tissue oedema. In goldfish, dropsy is often due to kidney disease and some fish may respond to antibiotics. However, many have asymmetrical abdominal distension due to polycystic lesions in the kidneys. In contrast, large old koi have a high incidence of abdominal neoplasia and consequently many affected carp either deteriorate and die or require euthanasia.

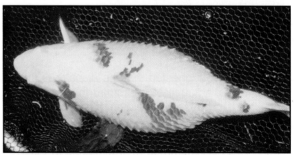

Figure 15.30 'Dropsy' in a 10-year-old koi with protrusion of the scales. The fish displayed both abdominal distension and cutaneous oedema for several months and required euthanasia due to its deteriorating health. Postmortem examination revealed severe ascites, a fluid-filled gonad and a large hepatic tumour.
(By permission of *In Practice*.)

Fin lesions

The normal shape and position of the fins varies considerably between different species. Some of this variation is due to the natural requirements of the fish but some is the result of deliberate breeding, as found in the many varieties of fancy goldfish. The pectoral and pelvic fins are paired and connected to bony girdles embedded in the body musculature. All other fins are unpaired. The fins consist of webbed structures supported by fin rays, which are either spiny or soft. The former are simple single bones; the latter are segmented and formed by two identical cartilaginous components. In some species, such as guppies, the anal fin in the male fish is modified and known as a gonopodium. It is used for internal fertilization, to insert sperm into the genital opening of female fish.

Examination of the fins is aided by viewing them against a dark background using indirect lighting and magnification. Some diseases, such as carp pox, lymphocystis, epidermal hyperplasia and some ectoparasites, are more visible on the fins due to their translucent structure. The microscopic examination of a fin clip can be used to identify some lesions and pathogens. This involves clipping a small piece from the edge of the fin with a pair of sharp scissors and preparing the sample as described for a skin scraping.

A common sign of illness in freshwater fish is when the fins are clamped or held against the body. This is a behaviour change rather than a specific disease of the fins. In contrast, this behaviour is normal in some marine fish.

Many diseases of the skin can affect the fins, some of which start as lesions on the fins. 'Fin rot', for example, in which the delicate fin tissue literally rots away (Figure 15.31), is caused by infection with *Flavobacterium columnare* and other related species of bacteria. This may progress on to the body from the tail fin to produce 'peduncle disease'. This disease often affects debilitated fish that have been exposed to poor water quality and stressful conditions such as transportation. Similar necrosis of the fins, together with marked inflammation, can be found in fish with body ulcerations due to infection with Gram-negative bacteria.

Hyperaemia of the fins is readily visible in many species and may be caused by septicaemic infections. Systemic bacterial infections in goldfish may produce small localized patches of brown pigmentation on the fins. In long-finned fish, pronounced blood vessels (Figure 15.32) are an indication of stress (e.g. overcrowding, poor water quality) and often resolve when the stressor is removed. Very long fins are also susceptible to damage through contact with the substrate and are often attacked by aggressive cohabitants ('fin nipping'), as exemplified by Siamese fighting fish.

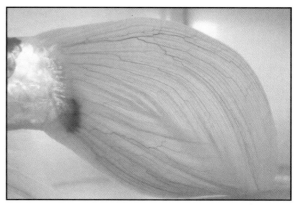

Figure 15.32 Hyperaemia in fish with long delicate fins is often an indication of stress. The prominent blood vessels are easier to see when the fish is in the water and viewed against a light background.

Tumours such as papillomas (including carp pox) and fibromas may also be localized on the fins. Nuptial tubercles, described earlier in the section on spots, occasionally appear hypertrophied as large verrucose masses, up to 1 cm in size, close to the body on both pectoral fins (Figure 15.33). On close inspection, there may be other signs of localized epithelial hyperplasia, but they should not be mistaken for neoplasms and they rarely cause problems to the fish.

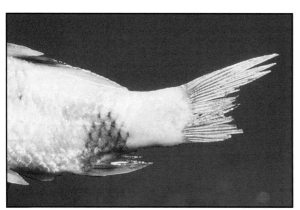

Figure 15.31 'Fin rot' due to bacterial infection with *Flavobacterium columnare*. In this young koi, the caudal fin is severely eroded and the disease has progressed on to the caudal peduncle, visible as a grey-white plaque posterior to the anal fin. (By permission of *In Practice*.)

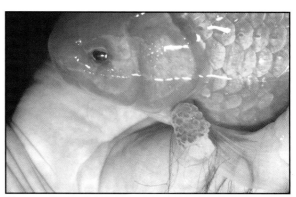

Figure 15.33 Nuptial tubercles occasionally become hyperplastic and develop into large verrucose masses on both pectoral fins. These lesions rarely affect the health of the fish, though they may trap strands of filamentous blanket weed in outdoor ponds. (By permission of *In Practice*.)

The treatment of fin lesions often involves the successful treatment of a generalized skin disease. However, localized lesions on the fins can be trimmed or excised and treated topically. In some cases, it may be necessary to excise exposed fin rays close to the body surface to improve wound healing. With time, some damaged fins can regrow substantially.

Further reading

Groff JM (2001) Cutaneous biology and diseases of fish. In: *The Veterinary Clinics of North America: Exotic Animal Practice: Dermatology*, ed. R Schmidt, pp. 321–411. WB Saunders Company, Philadelphia

Murphy KM and Lewbart GA (1995) Aquarium fish dermatologic diseases. *Seminar in Avian and Exotic Pet Medicine* **4**, 220–233

Paul-Murphy J and Moriello K (1995) Skin diseases of pet fish. In: *Small Animal Dermatology*, eds K Moriello and I Mason, pp. 213–218. Elsevier Science, Oxford

Stuart N (1988) Common skin diseases of farmed and pet fish. *In Practice* **10**, 47–53

Acknowledgements

The author is grateful to: the *Veterinary Record* and *In Practice* for permission to publish illustrations and text based on an original article by the author (Wildgoose WH, 1998, *In Practice* **20**, 226–243); and to the National Aquarium in Baltimore for the use of Figure 15.18.

16

Internal disorders

William H. Wildgoose

CHAPTER PLAN:
Anatomy
Investigations
A systematic approach
Oral lesions
Ulceration
  Trauma
  Bacterial
Obstruction
  Peri-oral
    Epidermal hyperplasia
    Neoplasia
    Dental overgrowth
  Intra-oral
    Swelling
    Foreign body
    Parasites
Deformity
Abnormal body shape
Body wall lesions
  Parasitic cysts
    Myxozoa
    Microsporeans
    Metacercariae
  Neoplasia
  Abscesses
  Granulomas
  Goitre

Subcutaneous fluid-filled cavity
  Haematoma
Spinal lesions
  Congenital
  Acquired
    Physical
    Infection
    Nutritional deficiency
    Chemicals
Abdominal enlargement
  Neoplasia
  Swim-bladder disorders
  Polycystic kidneys
  Gastric foreign body
  Obesity
  Ascites
  Blood
  Ovarian disorders
  Intestinal obstruction
  Parasites
Disease of the vent
Abnormal faeces
Visible parasites
Inflammation
Protrusion
Emaciation
Starvation
Chronic disease

In contrast to those of farmed fish, internal disorders of ornamental fish have long been overlooked. Much of the early literature was written with an emphasis on identification of external diseases and occasional speculation about internal disorders. This is partly due to the limited investigations previously carried out and the need for specialized procedures such as histopathology and diagnostic imaging. As a result, some common disorders remain unresolved, such as the buoyancy problems of fancy goldfish.

Pathology is frequently present in the absence of any obvious clinical signs and can be difficult to attribute to any specific cause. Affected fish may be presented with non-specific signs of illness, such as lethargy and anorexia. Unfortunately, the low financial value of some ornamental fish often limits the scale of investigations and their size frequently makes some methods impractical.

While this chapter presents an overview of internal disorders, it is by no means complete and only lists conditions commonly found in a few species. However, it is hoped that cases presented here will highlight the range of disorders that exist and encourage readers to investigate this aspect of fish health in more detail.

Anatomy

The great diversity among ornamental species makes it impossible to give a detailed account of their anatomy and physiology. The following is a brief outline of the major systems (Figure 16.1).

Musculoskeletal system

Skeletal features are used to classify fish broadly into those with a bony skeleton (teleosts, higher members of the Class Osteichthyes) and those with a cartilaginous skeleton (elasmobranchs, the major group of the Class Chondrichthyes). There is no bone marrow and most haematopoiesis is carried out in other organs. The vertebral column normally follows a slightly curved path from the back of the skull to the root of the caudal fin. Even within the same species, the number of vertebrae varies and is affected by environmental conditions during larval development.

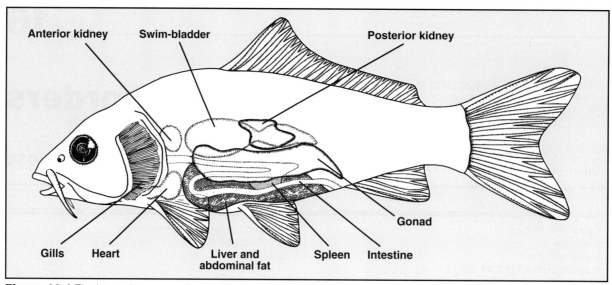

Figure 16.1 The internal anatomy of a carp.

Most of the axial musculature on each side consists of 'white' muscle fibres, which contract rapidly for sprint swimming but have little stamina and soon become exhausted, as they are poorly vascularized and anaerobic. The less numerous 'red' fibres found near the lateral line contract more slowly but are highly vascularized and aerobic, allowing the fish to swim for long periods of time.

Body cavity

This is a true coelomic cavity but is often referred to as the abdominal cavity. Ribs support the muscular lateral walls. The heart and anterior part of the kidney lie at the cranial end of the cavity and are separated from the other organs by a fine transverse septum. Most of the body cavity is occupied by the other organs, which are covered with a peritoneal membrane and a small quantity of serous exudate. In carp, it is normal to find many fine adhesions between the abdominal organs and the body wall (Figure 16.2).

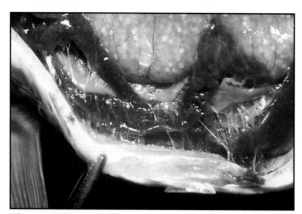

Figure 16.2 Many fine peritoneal adhesions are found in normal koi and other carp.

Digestive system

The digestive tract varies between different species according to their wide range of feeding habits and diets. Fish may be omnivores, herbivores or carnivores. Predators have well developed grasping teeth, a distinct stomach with acidic secretions and a relatively short intestine. Herbivorous fish have teeth within the oral cavity, a poorly defined stomach and a long intestinal tract.

Oral cavity

The shape of the mouth is modified according to the feeding habits of the fish. The oral cavity contains the tongue and teeth; there are no salivary glands. In some cyprinids, such as carp and goldfish, the teeth develop from the last gill arch and are found at the entrance to the oesophagus. The latter is a short muscular passage. In some tropical fish, such as pufferfish, there are oesophageal sacs that can be filled with water or air, inflating the body and acting as a defence mechanism.

Stomach and intestinal tract

The stomach varies in size with species, and may be entirely absent in some, such as carp. In some species, such as the salmonids, blind-ending sacs (caeca) are found in the pyloric region of the stomach, where fat digestion and some absorption takes place. The number of these caeca, if present, varies between species.

The length and shape of the intestinal tract also vary according to diet. In most cases it is a simple digestive tube but in elasmobranchs and primitive teleosts, such as sterlets, the lower part forms the spiral colon or spiral valve, which has a large surface area that enables greater absorption of nutrients. The posterior intestine or rectum terminates at the anus or vent in teleosts. In sharks and rays the rectal gland, a short blind-ending thick-walled tube, opens into the intestine near the cloaca and is thought to be involved in salt excretion.

Liver

The liver is a large organ and varies in colour from reddish-brown to light brown or off-white, depending on the diet of the fish. It may be a discrete organ found in the anterior body cavity or extend between the loops of the intestine. In some species, it is a compound organ and forms a hepatopancreas; in others, the pancreas is a separate organ. The gall bladder is connected to the liver, and contains greenish bile that empties into the intestine through the common bile duct.

Body fat levels can be assessed by noting fat deposits found within the body cavity. Emaciated fish often have no visible body fat, whereas overfeeding results in large deposits and subsequent fatty damage to the liver.

Swim-bladder

The swim-bladder (gas-bladder) is a large gas-filled organ that is derived from the digestive system. It consists of one, two or three interconnected chambers and is linked to the oesophagus by the pneumatic duct. This duct is patent in some fish (physostomes) and allows air to be swallowed to inflate the swim-bladder. In other species (physoclists), the duct is closed and complex capillary beds (rete mirabile) in the wall of each chamber control the gas content. This vascular area is also found in many physostomes, and gas exchange is controlled by various muscles and the overlying epithelium.

The swim-bladder is involved in maintaining buoyancy and is often reduced in size or absent in bottom-dwelling fish and elasmobranchs. It may also play some role in perception of sound waves, respiration and sound production.

Cardiovascular system

The fish heart is a two-chambered organ with four distinct regions and it lies within the pericardial sac. Venous blood enters the thin-walled sinus venosus and flows into the thicker atrium. It is then pumped into the muscular ventricle and exits through the bulbus arteriosus, which consists of elastic connective tissue and smooth muscle. Blood then passes through the gills and then directly into the systemic circulation. There are several different vascular patterns found in fish and most have well developed renal or hepatic portal systems. In addition to its vascular function, the heart has a phagocytic endothelium in some species.

Fish have an extensive lymphatic system but there are no lymph nodes. Most haematopoietic tissue is found in the kidney and spleen where, in some species, characteristic phagocytic melano-macrophage centres are formed in conjunction with the white cell system.

The spleen is a dark red or blackish elongate organ found close to the stomach or among the intestinal loops. It is involved in haematopoiesis, phagocytosis and may contain pancreatic tissue.

Urinary system

The kidneys of fish vary considerably and are found in a retroperitoneal position, dorsal to the swim-bladder. The organ has two distinct parts: the anterior or 'head' kidney and the posterior or 'tail' kidney. They may form one continuous organ or may remain distinctly separate. The anterior kidney is involved in haematopoiesis and phagocytosis, whereas the posterior kidney, in addition to containing haematopoietic tissue, contains the excretory components responsible for some osmo-regulation and excretion of nitrogenous waste. The structure of the nephron varies considerably, but the urine is excreted through ureters to a urinary papilla, and in some cases a urinary bladder.

Reproductive system

There is also a great diversity in the reproductive systems of fish. Some produce eggs and sperm for external fertilization while others copulate, with the discharge of either fertilized eggs or young fish. The testes are paired smooth white organs found adjacent to the swim-bladder. The ovary varies from a simple cluster of ovarian follicles to a complex organ similar to a uterus in viviparous species. Mature ovaries represent up to 70% of the total bodyweight. Eggs pass either through an oviduct to the outside (e.g. perches and some cyprinids) or into the abdominal cavity and are then evacuated through a genital opening (e.g. in salmonids).

Endocrine system

There are many endocrine glands and these differ considerably from their mammalian counterparts in structure and location. For example, thyroid tissue in goldfish and carp is distributed throughout many organs, including the heart, spleen and kidney. With the exception of thyroid hyperplasia, internal disorders that specifically affect the endocrine system are uncommon in fish and few at present have any clinical significance. Consequently, the reader is referred to the specialist texts for more comprehensive details.

Investigations

All disease investigations in fish should involve inspection of the environment, measuring water quality, and microscopic examination of skin and gill mucus samples. In addition, several techniques can provide more useful information about internal disorders.

Clinical examination

The size and shape of most ornamental fish preclude detailed internal examination. Despite this, it is possible to gather some information from a visual inspection and observation of unusual behaviour.

Gentle palpation may allow detection and appreciation of the nature of abnormal swellings: these may be firm or soft fluid-filled, and they may be discrete or diffuse. Examination may be performed on conscious fish but some species may require sedation to permit a detailed inspection. Anaesthesia may also be safer and less stressful to both fish and handler when examining dangerous or venomous species. Abnormal or restricted flexion of the spine is best appreciated under general anaesthesia.

Ballottement (a method of palpation used to detect a floating object within a body cavity) may allow the detection of an internal mass in a large fish with a swollen abdomen. Some non-pigmented tropical aquarium fish have relatively transparent bodies that allow visualization of the internal organs, and this can be enhanced by transillumination.

Radiography

Several features can be seen readily on radiographs but it is essential to be familiar with the normal internal anatomy of the species under examination. Spinal lesions such as fractures and abnormal curvature are common, but other bone deformities and periosteal disease may also be detected. Disorders of the swim-bladder such as collapse, over-inflation and displacement are often visible. Gas and radiopaque food debris are commonly seen in the bowel and foreign bodies are occasionally found.

Inserting a radiopaque tube in the stomach prior to exposure will help to distinguish between gas in the stomach and that in the swim-bladder. Contrast studies using barium sulphate or other media, such as iohexol, often help to determine motility and identify radiolucent foreign bodies in the gastrointestinal tract, and partial or complete obstruction. Internal masses can sometimes be identified by their uniform texture and the displacement of other organs, such as the intestinal tract and chambers of the swim-bladder.

Ultrasonography

Ultrasound can be used to differentiate soft tissue abnormalities and is used routinely to check the development of gonads in farmed fish. However, the resolution limits of the equipment make it impossible to detect organs or lesions smaller than 4 mm.

Other imaging technology

The use of computed tomography (CT scanning), magnetic resonance imaging (MRI) and nuclear scanning have been reported in a few cases. As the experience and equipment for these specialized techniques become more readily available, their application to fish will continue to expand.

Endoscopy and laparotomy

In fish of a suitable size, endoscopes can be used to inspect the oral cavity and proximal oesophagus. Where the internal anatomy permits, they are also useful for laparoscopic visualization and biopsy of the internal organs through a small incision in the body wall. Unfortunately, this is of limited use in carp because of their extensive peritoneal adhesions (see Figure 16.2). Endoscopes can be used to examine, biopsy and culture the swim-bladder.

Laparotomy is an invasive surgical approach that can be used in large fish. However, the potential complications and attendant risks may outweigh the benefits, and other imaging methods may prove safer in most cases.

Electrocardiography

Cardiac lesions are often found in ornamental fish on histological examination and are occasionally visible during an autopsy. Collection of an electrocardiogram (ECG) in fish is possible using electrodes lightly clamped to the skin at the base of the pectoral fins and the anal fin. Although P, QRS and T waves can be identified, interpretation of clinical abnormalities still requires further study.

Laboratory samples

Faecal samples enable the identification of various endoparasites of the alimentary tract. Unfortunately, saprophytic organisms from the environment rapidly contaminate faecal samples at the bottom of a tank. Unlike freshwater species, marine fish do not have formed faeces. Fish often defecate when immersed in anaesthetic solution, but otherwise fresh faecal samples can be obtained by aspiration using a small catheter passed through the anus under anaesthesia.

Other than in a few species, there is little published information about clinical pathology in ornamental fish. The usefulness of haematology and biochemistry is limited by the present lack of suitable comparative data.

Cytological examination of fine needle aspirates and ascitic fluid obtained by paracentesis can provide useful information. In some cases, small samples of urine can be obtained from the bladder and examined for the presence of parasitic spores.

A stomach wash can be collected by using a suitably sized catheter and sterile saline. Parasites (such as flagellates) that cause life-threatening disease in marine angelfish are easily seen in the stomach contents by light microscopy.

A systematic approach

Internal disorders can be grouped according to the following presenting signs:

- Oral lesions
- Abnormal body shape
- Diseases of the vent
- Emaciation.

Oral lesions

The mouth varies in shape and function according to feeding habits. Constant mechanical movement makes this area prone to injury and secondary infection. Lesions will not only affect the fish's ability to eat but also interfere with respiratory function.

Ulceration

Trauma

Ulceration as a result of constant trauma is often seen on the chin or snout of large fish kept in aquaria that are too small or that encourage patterned swimming. Other traumatic lesions may arise following rough handling and accidents. Mouth-fighting in some tropical fish, such as cichlids, can result in damage to the lips and jaw.

Bacterial

Fish are vulnerable to infection by various species, including Gram-negative bacteria such as aeromonads, pseudomonads and vibrios. These usually produce raw ulcerative lesions, similar to those found on other areas of the body, and the condition is commonly referred to as 'mouth rot' (Figure 16.3). In tropical freshwater fish, *Flavobacterium columnare* produces a feathery lesion around the mouth that is commonly called 'mouth fungus' or 'cotton-wool disease' since it resembles infection with *Saprolegnia*.

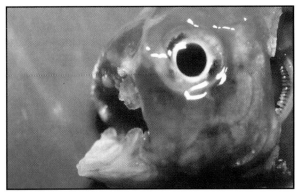

Figure 16.3 Severe 'mouth rot' due to bacterial infection in a goldfish. There is extensive necrosis of the soft tissues and exposure of the facial bones.

Obstruction

Oral obstructions arise from lesions that occur both around and inside the mouth.

Peri-oral

Epidermal hyperplasia: Localized areas of epidermal hyperplasia have been found around the mouth of koi. This rarely becomes extensive or causes complete obstruction but has been associated with the formation of papillomas. Carp pox infection (cyprinid herpesvirus) or minor abrasion due to bottom-feeding habits may predispose this area to hyperplasia.

Neoplasia: Papillomas and other tumours may develop around the mouth (Figure 16.4). Some may become so large that they cause obstruction and require surgical removal. Depending on the location and nature of the tumour, complete excision is rarely possible but debulking the lesion will be effective in most cases.

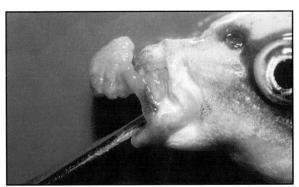

Figure 16.4 A papilloma on the lip of a 3-year-old carp that was kept in an indoor aquarium. Most of the tumour was surgically removed but localized epidermal hyperplasia remained around the mouth.

Dental overgrowth: The front teeth of pufferfish are fused together and are used to remove food from rocks. In captivity, these fish are often given inappropriate food that is seldom hard enough to keep the teeth worn down. The resulting dental overgrowth may require physical trimming under general anaesthesia. In the long term, the provision of corals and harder molluscs, such as clams and snails, should maintain normal dental wear.

Intra-oral

Mouth-brooding is a normal reproductive behaviour in some species of cichlids and catfish. The eggs or fry are held in the mouth as protection from predators.

Some aquarium fish, such as red-tailed catfish, occasionally regurgitate their meal. This is thought to be due to environmental stress or unsuitable diet. Some fish will regurgitate their stomach contents when recovering from anaesthesia.

Swelling: Pus-like fluid-filled swellings and granulomas have been found in the pharynx and may have arisen from penetration by sharp food materials (Figure 16.5). If severe, there may also be external submandibular or facial swelling.

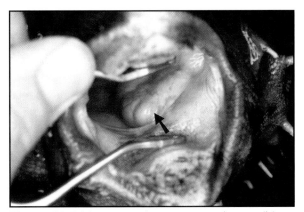

Figure 16.5 A large granulomatous mass (arrowed) in the pharynx of a porcupine pufferfish. The lesion also contained liquid pus and was thought to be due to penetration by prawn exoskeleton in the diet.

Neoplasia within the oral cavity has been recorded and surgical removal has occasionally been successful, though access is often restricted.

Rarely, lymphocystis (iridovirus infection) may cause the formation of nodules in the oropharynx that may prevent small fish from swallowing their food.

Foreign body: Some aquarium fish may ingest foreign objects, to identify edibility and remove food particles from the surface. Goldfish occasionally present with pieces of gravel lodged in their mouth. In many cases, they will successfully spit out the gravel, but in a few cases manual removal may be required.

Parasites: Flabelliferan isopods are large crustacean parasites measuring up to 60 mm in length. They are occasionally found on the head or in the oral cavity of tropical marine fish.

Deformity

In some species, several cartilaginous bones around the mouth form an extending tube that enables the fish to search for food items at the bottom of ponds. Damage to any part of this structure will result in varying degrees of deformity and occlusion of the mouth (Figure 16.6). This may follow ulceration or traumatic injury but may also be due to a congenital defect.

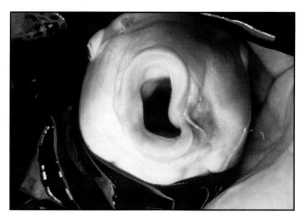

Figure 16.6 Dislocation of the bones on the left side of the mouth in this adult koi caused partial obstruction and poor closure. The fish had difficulty eating a pellet diet and had laboured respiration. The cause was unknown.

Various other deformities have been recorded, including abnormal shortening of the maxilla and mandible and deviation of some facial bones. Neoplastic growths of bone, cartilage and fibrous and dental tissues have also been reported.

Abnormal body shape

This section describes swellings that develop beneath the scales, in or below the dermis. Other, more superficial swellings are described in Chapter 15.

New World cichlids such as the Midas cichlid are sexually dimorphic and mature males have a pronounced swelling in the dorsal cranial area (cephalic hump), which is normal for many in this family.

Most diseases that cause abnormal swelling involve lesions in the body wall, the spine or the body cavity. These produce either unilateral or bilateral swelling, which may be symmetrical or asymmetrical. Gentle physical palpation will reveal if the swelling is soft or firm, diffuse or localized. Other clinical signs, such as buoyancy disorders or skin lesions, may provide more information about the nature of the swelling. Further procedures will be required to help to identify the underlying cause.

Body wall lesions

Oedema of the skin can result from several different pathologies and causes the scales to rise, due to fluid collection in the scale pockets. This may be local or generalized and is discussed under texture changes of the skin (Chapter 15).

Parasitic cysts

Several parasites produce cystic swellings in ornamental fish. Myxozoan parasites such as *Henneguya* and *Myxobolus* produce pseudocysts, which enlarge slowly in various tissues; these are usually found in wild-caught fish.

The microsporean *Pleistophora hyphessobryconis* causes 'neon tetra disease' and infects muscle tissue of various aquarium fish such as tetras, barbs, danios and goldfish. It produces focal areas of swelling due to muscle necrosis, particularly along the dorsum.

The metacercariae of the digenean trematode *Clinostomum* produce cystic lesions measuring up to 5 mm in diameter. The parasite encysts in the musculature of fish and is commonly called 'yellow grub'.

Neoplasia

Tumours of the muscle, fibrous tissues or pigment cells (Figure 16.7) have been found in ornamental fish. Others have resulted from invasion by underlying intra-abdominal tumours.

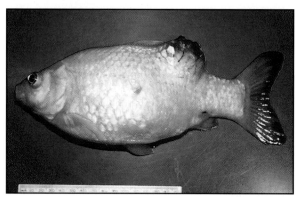

Figure 16.7 A 14-year-old goldfish that had a large tumour on its dorsal surface for 3 years. Histological examination identified this deeply invasive mass as a melanoma.

Abscesses

It is uncommon to find pus-like fluid-filled swellings in fish but these may result from infection with Gram-negative bacteria such as aeromonads or pseudomonads, or acid-fast mycobacteria.

Granulomas

Infection with mycobacteria and nocardiae may produce granulomas in the dermis and deeper tissues. Lesions vary in size and can affect all species.

Ichthyophonus hoferi is a fungus-like organism that produces small dark raised granulomas throughout the deep tissues and affects mainly marine fish.

Goitre

Thyroid hyperplasia (goitre) is commonly seen in fish living in large recirculating systems and fed on inappropriate diets that are deficient in iodine or that contain goitrogenic substances. Bilateral swellings can be seen at the base of the gill arches of teleosts and on the throat of elasmobranchs. The disorder is corrected by adding potassium iodide or calcium iodate to the food or water.

Subcutaneous fluid-filled cavity

Adverse reactions to long-acting oxytetracycline injections can produce large collections of sterile serosanguineous fluid at the injection site.

Haematoma

A haematoma of the body wall and its successful surgical treatment has been described in an ornamental cichlid (Harms *et al.*, 1995). The cause of the lesion was unknown.

Spinal lesions

Spinal injuries have been widely reported in many species and have several aetiologies. Species with long slender bodies, such as orfe, appear more vulnerable to spinal damage. Lesions may be congenital or acquired, presenting as visible deformity and abnormal posture. They may be produced by vertebral fracture or luxation, and result in abnormal curvature of the spine with varying degrees of kyphosis, lordosis and scoliosis.

Congenital

Inherited lesions may follow the transfer of genetic defects. Developmental injury may result from damage, such as temperature shock, to the eggs during critical stages of the incubation period (Figure 16.8).

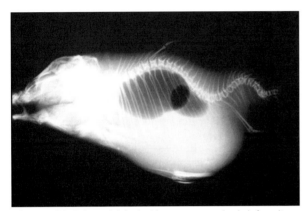

Figure 16.8 An adult koi with a severe spinal deformity that was thought to be congenital in origin. There is also a large tumour causing distension of the posterior abdomen and displacement of the swim-bladder.

Acquired

There are undoubtedly many cases that are not investigated but the following is a guide to the commonest reported causes of spinal problems.

Physical: Traumatic injury may result from poor handling during netting or manual restraint. Vertebral fractures have been caused by stray current from unearthed electrical equipment such as pumps and lights (Figure 16.9), or by lightning strike and during electronarcosis. Tumours of the bone or cartilage are uncommon but other locally invasive tumours may cause pathological fractures.

Infection: Bacterial infection with *Aeromonas hydrophila* and granulomas produced by mycobacteria and nocardiae have caused spinal deformity in some fish. Fungal granulomas of *Ichthyophonus hoferi* may also cause spinal lesions. Spinal compression and fusion of the vertebrae in some freshwater fish have been associated with cysts produced by the myxosporean, *Myxobolus ellipsoides.*

Nutritional deficiency: Phosphorus and the essential amino acid tryptophan must be present in the diet for correct bone formation. Vitamin C (ascorbic acid) deficiency has been shown to affect the growth and development of bone and cartilage in fish.

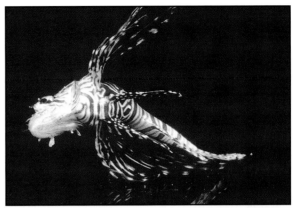

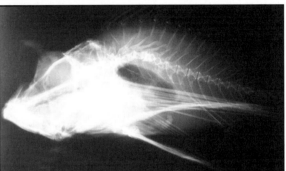

Figure 16.9 A lionfish with a fractured spine. The injury is thought to have developed following an electric shock from a faulty water heater. A dorsoventral radiograph revealed fracture and displacement of the vertebral column. The injury produced a marked scoliosis, debilitating the fish to a degree where euthanasia was required. (© National Aquarium in Baltimore.)

Chemicals: Overdose with organophosphates and carbamate insecticides can cause violent muscle spasm and subsequent spinal deformity due to vertebral fracture. Some fish are more sensitive than others to these chemicals and there is a greater potential toxicity in some species of characins, cyprinids and elasmobranchs. Overdosing with formalin has caused similar fractures in young orfe (Figure 16.10). Although rarely used now, organochlorines accumulate slowly in the body and interfere with collagen formation, causing spinal deformity.

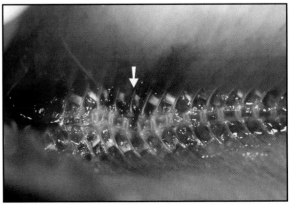

Figure 16.10 Vertebral fracture (arrowed) in a young orfe following bath treatment with an overdose of a proprietary medicine containing formalin. There is lateral deviation and haemorrhage at the fracture site.

The herbicide trifluralin causes fluorosis, the result of chronic accumulation of fluoride. This produces hyperplasia of bone cells and irregular bone growth.

Heavy metals such as lead, zinc and cadmium are soluble to varying degrees under certain water conditions. They accumulate in some tissues and cause damage that may result in vertebral fracture and deformity.

Abdominal enlargement

Some varieties of fancy goldfish are intentionally bred with a swollen abdomen and detection of abnormal swelling can be difficult in these fish.

In some species, gravid females may appear more swollen than male fish. However, in the absence of any other characteristic, this is rarely a useful method of determining sex. Similarly, livebearers and most sharks will show substantial abdominal enlargement during gestation. As an exception, male seahorses incubate fertilized eggs in an abdominal brood pouch and may develop a distended abdomen prior to release of their young.

Pufferfish and porcupinefish can inflate their bodies by filling oesophageal sacs with air or water as a defence against predators.

Neoplasia

Ornamental fish are often kept in captivity for many years. Consequently, they are prone to age-related diseases, and neoplasia is a common cause of abdominal swelling. Due to their relatively inactive lifestyle, most fish survive for a considerable time, with the result that many of these tumours become enormous (Figure 16.11). Some lesions consist of poorly differentiated solid tissue; others may have large cystic areas and produce substantial volumes of ascitic fluid. The tissues of all organs may undergo neoplastic change but those found most commonly originate from the gonad, liver and bowel. Renal tumours appear to be common in oscars. However, in many cases it is not possible to identify the tissue of origin accurately.

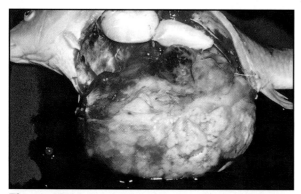

Figure 16.11 An adult koi with a massive gonadal tumour that accounted for one-third of its bodyweight.

Swim-bladder disorders

It is rarely possible to determine the cause of these abnormalities in live fish, but laparoscopic examination can be used where abnormalities of the swim-bladder are suspected. A fine needle aspirate or wash using sterile saline may also provide diagnostic information.

Abnormal fluid accumulation in the swim-bladder will cause loss of buoyancy and in severe cases will produce abdominal swelling (Figure 16.12). This may be due to bacterial, fungal or myxosporean infection. Affected fish are unable to maintain neutral buoyancy and sink to the bottom, where prolonged contact eventually causes inflammation and ulceration of the body surfaces in contact with the substrate.

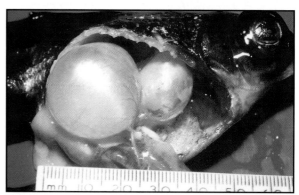

Figure 16.12 A fancy goldfish with abdominal swelling due to abnormal fluid collection in the swim-bladder. A mixed infection of pseudomonads and *Aeromonas hydrophila* was isolated from the translucent yellow fluid.

Over-inflation will produce abnormal positive buoyancy, causing the fish to float on the surface when at rest (Figure 16.13). This is common in fancy varieties of goldfish: many cases are of sudden onset, with no specific preceding event. Affected fish often float on one side, and part of the swim-bladder may deviate from its normal midline position. The degree of inflation and the position of the swim-bladder can be assessed radiographically (Figure 16.14).

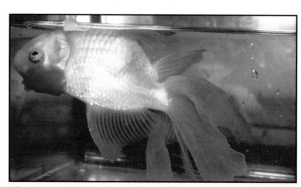

Figure 16.13 Abdominal swelling in a fancy goldfish that developed excessive positive buoyancy.

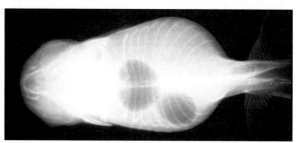

Figure 16.14 Dorsoventral radiograph of the goldfish in Figure 16.13, showing displacement of the posterior chamber of the swim-bladder and some unilateral abdominal swelling on the opposite side.

In some cases, freshwater fish will recover spontaneously after a short period of starvation, a change of water temperature and addition of salt. Others have responded to being fed a single green pea (canned or cooked and lightly crushed) once daily. Cases that fail to recover following this environmental manipulation occasionally improve by aspiration of some air using a syringe and hypodermic needle inserted through the body wall. There are hazards using this blind technique and many cases will relapse within a few days. Carbonic anhydrase inhibitors such as acetazolamide may also be useful in preventing the continued production of gas within the swim-bladder.

Continued exposure of the skin to air produces desiccation of the affected epidermal tissues. In addition to the subsequent skin necrosis and secondary infection, other systemic effects due to the over-inflation usually prove fatal.

Herniation of the swim-bladder through the body wall has been recorded in a cichlid with long-standing abdominal swelling. The fish recovered following successful surgical repair (Lewbart *et al.*, 1995).

Polycystic kidneys
This condition commonly affects goldfish and is known as kidney enlargement disease. Affected fish have varying degrees of cystic change (Figure 16.15) and in severe cases the kidneys may occupy most of the abdominal cavity.

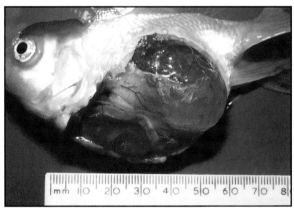

Figure 16.15 Polycystic lesions in the kidneys of the goldfish in Figure 16.13. The kidneys in severe cases may occupy up to 90% of the abdominal cavity.

This is a chronic disease and produces massive abdominal enlargement, which is often asymmetrical. The swim-bladder is often displaced or compressed, and the two chambers may appear further apart on radiography. Some cysts may have a genetic origin but kidney enlargement disease is thought to be due to infection with a myxosporean, *Hoferellus carassii*. Histological examination reveals massively dilated tubules but parasites are rarely found. Although there is no known treatment, affected fish may survive for many months.

Gastric foreign body
Red-tailed catfish often swallow foreign bodies (Figure 16.16); this is thought to be a territorial behaviour in this

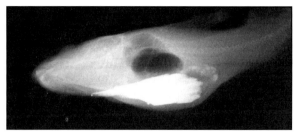

Figure 16.16 A young red-tailed catfish that swallowed an irregularly shaped piece of slate. The sharp anterior end penetrated the body wall but was removed successfully through the mouth while under anaesthesia.

species. The fish regurgitate most objects within a few days but in some cases manual removal through the mouth may be required, while under anaesthesia. Species such as giant gouramis have also been known to swallow gravel and other small objects. Depending on the size of the foreign body, there may be some abdominal distension, loss of appetite, poor buoyancy control or complications from obstruction.

Obesity
Overfeeding and the use of inappropriate diets with a high fat content will result in obesity with large collections of intra-abdominal fat and fatty damage to the liver.

Ascites
Many disorders result in the collection of substantial volumes of ascitic fluid in the body cavity. Any disease that disrupts normal osmoregulation will potentially produce ascites, with or without cutaneous oedema. This includes diseases affecting the gills, liver, kidney and heart. In addition to chronic organ failure, neoplasia is commonly found in older fish (Figure 16.17) whereas ascites in younger fish is often due to acute bacterial disease.

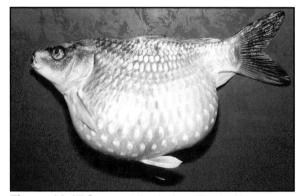

Figure 16.17 Severe abdominal swelling in this 12-year-old koi had been present for 1 year. Half of its bodyweight was due to intra-abdominal fluid and there were two cystic neoplastic masses.

The resulting abdominal swelling is often called 'dropsy' and may occur in conjunction with exophthalmos and cutaneous oedema (Chapter 15). Aspiration of some fluid may provide information about the underlying cause, but complete drainage has limited benefit since the fluid will usually reappear within a few days.

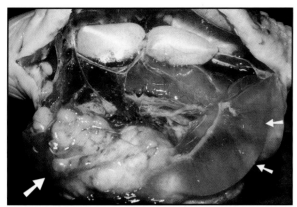

Figure 16.18 An adult koi with abdominal swelling for 6 months. In addition to a large liver tumour (large arrow), the bilobed sacks of the gonad (small arrows) were filled with translucent yellow fluid.

In some female fish, large quantities of ascitic fluid will collect in the ovaries (Figure 16.18) and this may drain through the genital pores when the fish is removed from the water. Excess fluid is often found in the pericardial sac.

Blood
Free blood is rarely found within the body cavity and is unlikely to cause noticeable abdominal swelling. However, blood-tinged ascitic fluid can result from acute systemic bacterial infection with aeromonads and pseudomonads. In carp and related species, this may also be associated with the notifiable disease, spring viraemia of carp.

Ovarian disorders
Rupture of the ovary, with subsequent peritonitis and adhesions, has been found in a few fancy goldfish with abdominal swelling (Figure 16.19). It has not been possible to identify the underlying cause.

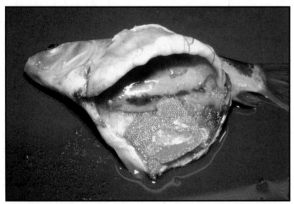

Figure 16.19 Ruptured ovary in a common goldfish that had severe abdominal enlargement for several months. A large volume of ascitic fluid and degenerating eggs were present in the abdominal cavity.

'Egg-bound' is a term occasionally used to describe female fish that have large numbers of mature eggs in the ovary and are unable to release them. There is speculation about the aetiology but it may involve a lack of suitable egg-laying sites in the environment. It

is questionable if this produces ill health in affected fish, since eggs can potentially be reabsorbed. It is unlikely that the administration of a mammalian or synthetic pituitary extract will be of any benefit in most fish.

Dystocia has been reported in elasmobranchs and some cases have been treated successfully by surgical intervention (Lewbart, 1998).

Intestinal obstruction
Complete obstruction of the intestine is uncommon but may be caused by a foreign body or intestinal parasites in some fish. The adult stage of the cestode *Bothriocephalus* infects carp and when present in sufficient numbers can cause lethargy, emaciation and abdominal swelling.

Parasites
Various parasites may be found within the body cavity or gastrointestinal tract. Few of these produce abdominal swelling but this may occur because of associated tissue pathology.

Infestation with the flagellate *Cryptobia* produces granulomas in the stomach of cichlids and is commonly called 'Malawi bloat' or 'cichlid bloat'.

The plerocercoid stage of the cestode *Ligula* is found free within the body cavity. It can measure up to 20 cm and be present in large numbers in cyprinids, particularly roach, gudgeon and bream.

Diseases of the vent

Abnormal faeces
Normal faeces are dark green or brown in colour but often vary according to the species of fish and the diet. The faeces of many freshwater fish have a regular diameter and break off soon after emerging from the vent, while the faeces of many marine fish are not formed and tend to disperse in the water.

Abnormal faeces may be pale, white, yellow or mucoid in appearance (Figure 16.20). These are usually described as long and stringy, with a tendency to trail from the vent. Occasionally, they may contain fat or gas and float at the surface. In severe forms of enteritis, blood may be present.

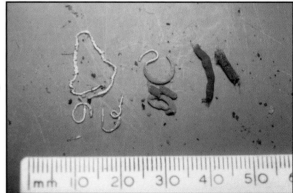

Figure 16.20 In freshwater fish, abnormal faeces may be long, white and stringy (left) or pale in colour (centre). Normal faeces from a goldfish are dark coloured and found in short fragments (right).

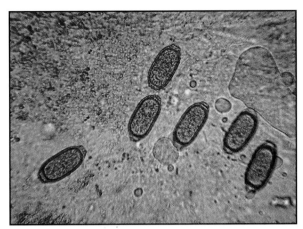

Figure 16.21 Ova of *Capillaria* with characteristic bipolar 'plugs', in a faecal sample from freshwater angelfish experiencing chronic mortalities in a breeding unit.

Microscopic examination of fresh faecal samples allows identification of several common pathogens. These include parasitic adults and ova of *Capillaria* (Figure 16.21) in freshwater angelfish, flagellate protozoans such as *Spironucleus* and *Hexamita* in cichlids, and coccidians in a wide range of species. Bacteria and some virus infections may also cause enteritis.

Visible parasites

The endoparasite *Camallanus* is typically found in livebearers and is seen as a red adult nematode protruding from the anus (Figure 16.22).

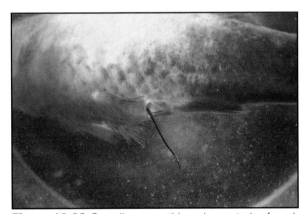

Figure 16.22 *Camallanus* are thin red nematodes found commonly in livebearers such as this platy. The parasites are only visible when protruding from the anus to release their live larvae.

Inflammation

Local trauma and bacterial infection occasionally cause inflammation and ulceration of the vent and anal fin. Reddening around the vent, with or without a bloody exudate, can be seen in some systemic bacterial diseases.

Protrusion

Any condition causing abdominal swelling may potentially cause protrusion of the vent, due to increased intra-abdominal pressure.

Prolapse of ovarian and intestinal tissue through the genital pore or anus has been recorded in fish. Some cases have been successfully treated by surgical excision of the exteriorized tissue (Lewbart, 1998).

Emaciation

Unless fish are weighed regularly, identifying weight loss is difficult since disease processes are often well advanced before clinical signs are visible. Some fish may not become lethargic until they are close to death. The shape of some fish makes it difficult to assess emaciation but indications include:

*   Loss of muscle mass along the back (Figure 16.23)
*   Hollow appearance to the abdomen
*   Sunken eyes.

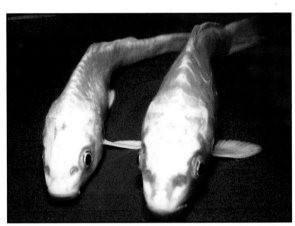

Figure 16.23 Juvenile koi with wasting of the dorsal musculature. Both fish are affected but the one on the left exhibits severe weight loss. Atrophic pancreatic cells thought to be a result of chronic malnutrition were found on histological examination. The other similarly affected fish in the group recovered on an improved diet.

Starvation

It is rare for ornamental fish to suffer from starvation but nutritional deficiencies or feeding an inappropriate diet may cause weight loss or poor growth rates. Due to their particular dietary requirements, wild-caught marine fish may starve to death from being offered unsuitable food. Competitive feeding and aggression may limit the access of some fish to food. Physical obstructions in and around the mouth may prevent affected fish from eating.

Mouth-brooding species of fish do not feed during brood care and may lose a substantial amount of bodyweight during this period.

Chronic disease

In many cases, there will be other clinical signs of longstanding disease. Granulomatous lesions caused by mycobacteria, nocardiae and *Ichthyophonus* often result in damage to major organs. Intestinal parasites such as cestodes, nematodes and protozoans reduce the availability of nutrients to the host. Non-intestinal parasites and neoplasia may cause weight loss due to damage to vital organs or systemic effects. Other forms of chronic organ failure that affect the liver and kidneys, in particular, are occasionally identified on routine histological examination and may account for some unidentified causes of weight loss.

References

Harms CA, Bakal RS, Khoo LH, Spaulding KA and Lewbart GA (1995) Microsurgical excision of an abdominal mass in a gourami. *Journal of the American Veterinary Medical Association* **207**, 1215–1217

Lewbart GA (1998) *Self-Assessment Colour Review of Ornamental Fish*. Manson Publishing, London

Lewbart GA, Stone EA and Love NE (1995) Pneumatocystectomy in a Midas cichlid. *Journal of the American Veterinary Medical Association* **207**, 319–321

Acknowledgements

The author is very grateful to Edward Branson, Bernice Brewster, Ruth Francis-Floyd and Brent Whitaker for their assistance and advice with the text; and to the National Aquarium in Baltimore for the use of their photographs in Figure 16.9.

17

Respiratory disease

Sara Childs and Brent R. Whitaker

CHAPTER PLAN:
Anatomy
Physiology
Clinical signs
Investigations
A systematic approach

Normal gross appearance
Environmental hypoxia
Toxins
    Ammonia
    Organic compounds
    Chlorine
    Ozone
Virus
    Koi herpesvirus

Colour change
Pallor: generalized
    Anaemia
        Haemoparasites
    Excess mucus
        Toxins
        Ectoparasites
    Hyperplasia and hypertrophy
        Toxins (e.g. copper)
        Suspended solids
        Ectoparasites
        Nutritional imbalance
Pallor: localized
    Necrosis
        Bacteria
            Flavobacterium branchiophilum
        Fungi
            Saprolegnia
            Branchiomyces
        Parasites
            Sanguinicola
Brown coloration
    Methaemoglobinaemia
        Nitrite toxicity

Visible ectoparasites
White spot
    Ichthyophthirius/ Cryptocaryon
Dinoflagellates
    Amyloodinium/ Piscinoodinium
Gill flukes
Leeches
Isopods
Copepods

Swellings
Nodular lesions
    Parasites
        Glochidia
        Myxosporeans (e.g. *Henneguya, Sphaerospora*)
        Microsporeans (e.g. *Glugea*)
        Metacercaria
    Epitheliocystis
    Lymphocystis
    Hyperplasia and hypertrophy
    Telangiectasis
Large swellings
    Neoplasia
        Papilloma
        Squamous cell carcinoma
        Branchioblastoma
        Chondroma
        Thyroid neoplasia
    Goitre

Miscellaneous
Haemorrhage
    Necrosis
    Spontaneous
Foreign bodies
Opercular deformity
    Congenital/genetic
    Nutritional imbalance
        Vitamin A deficiency
        Vitamin C deficiency

The anatomy and physiology of the respiratory system of fish differs markedly from those of mammals, birds or reptiles. Clinical signs of respiratory disease in fish species are often non-specific.

Various features of the fish respiratory system predispose to disease. The gills are located externally, providing constant exposure to the aqueous environment for gas and ion exchange but also to toxins and other irritants that may be present. The substantial branchial blood supply is attractive and accessible to parasitic organisms, which may be partially concealed and protected by the operculum. In addition, the fragil-ity of the thin respiratory epithelium renders it vulnerable to invasion by a variety of pathogenic organisms.

Anatomy

With few exceptions, the major respiratory organs of fish are the gills. Embryonically, the gills arise within the walls of the pharyngeal pouches, which are paired evaginations of the embryonic pharynx. These pouches are separated from ectodermal invaginations by a thin membrane (branchial plate), which subsequently ruptures and establishes a pathway for water to flow from the pharynx to the exterior of the animal. The external surface of the gills of most fish is protected by a bony opercular flap, which is anchored at the hyoid arch and extends caudally.

The branchial region of the fish is composed of four or more gill arches on either side of the pharynx. Their associated gill rakers and pharyngeal teeth are located medially. The evenly spaced gill rakers enable the fish to separate food particles efficiently from the water as it flows in through the mouth and out over the gills. Several bones, the basibranchial, hypobranchial, ceratobranchial, epibranchial and pharyngobranchial form a typical gill arch. The arches are attached dorsally to the pharyngeal roof and ventrally to the hyoid apparatus. Two rows of gill filaments, referred to as primary lamellae, project from the lateral surface of each gill arch. Each primary lamella has rows of secondary lamellae that extend perpendicularly to its axis (Figure 17.1).

Each secondary lamella consists of two layers of epithelial cells surrounding a vascular space. The epithelium rests on a basement membrane, which overlies a network of pillar cells that provides the supporting framework for the vascular space. Within the vascular space lies both an afferent and an efferent artery, which are connected by a capillary plexus. This arrangement of the secondary lamellae and their blood supply allows for the counter-current mechanism of gas exchange.

The act of respiration results in a unidirectional flow of water over the gills. With the mouth open and the operculum closed, the pharyngeal floor is lowered, drawing water into the pharynx. The mouth is then closed, the opercula opened and the pharyngeal floor

raised, forcing water to the exterior through the opercular cleft. Under normal conditions, these actions occur rhythmically, providing a nearly continuous flow of water over the gills.

Unlike most teleosts, the anabantids (a small group of ornamental fish) have an accessory organ of respiration called the labyrinth or suprabranchial organ, which lies within the first epibranchial chamber located in the roof of the mouth behind the eyes. It consists of many epithelium-covered bony plates, which are modified lamellae from the first functional gill arch. These fish, which include the gourami and *Betta*, are able to utilize atmospheric oxygen by obtaining air at the water surface and compressing it into the labyrinth chamber. Blood diverted from the gill filaments then passes through the rich vascular supply of the suprabranchial epithelium, where gas exchange can occur.

Physiology

The primary function of the gill is respiration. It has three other major functions: excretion of nitrogenous waste products, acid–base balance and osmoregulation.

Respiration

There are important challenges to respiring in an aquatic environment. Firstly, there is relatively little oxygen in water (0–14 mg/l) compared with air (260 mg/l). Secondly, water is very dense in comparison with air, requiring greater energy expenditure to move it over the respiratory epithelium.

The ventral aorta collects unoxygenated waste-filled blood from the tissues and divides into the afferent branchial arteries, which supply each gill arch.

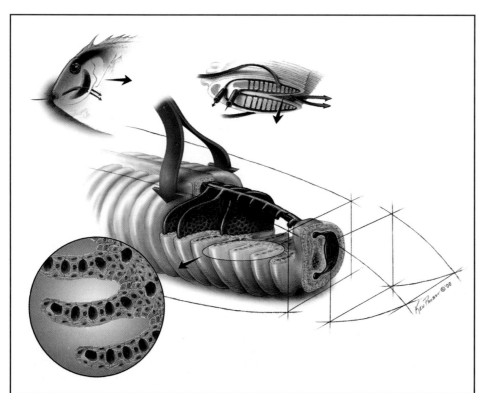

Figure 17.1 Anatomy of the teleost gill. Water flows in through the mouth and over the primary and secondary lamellae. A vascular plexus providing a counter-current mechanism for gas exchange connects efferent and afferent blood vessels within the lamellae. Histologically, secondary lamellae are only a few cell layers thick, facilitating gaseous exchange and the elimination of metabolic wastes. (© Ken Probst, Johns Hopkins Art as Applied to Medicine.)

These vessels ultimately form afferent and efferent filament arteries and capillary networks in the secondary lamellae. Laminar flow of water across the gill filaments parallels the secondary lamellae. Therefore, as unoxygenated blood flows through the secondary lamellae it encounters fresh, oxygenated water flowing in the opposite direction. This counter-current mechanism is so efficient that almost all of the oxygen is removed from the water as it passes over the gills. Oxygenated blood then enters the dorsal aorta and is distributed to the tissues of the body. Similar principles govern the exchange of carbon dioxide, which is produced in the tissues and diffuses through the gill epithelium into the aquatic environment. The exchange of gases at epithelial and endothelial interfaces is mediated by haemoglobin in the blood, much as in mammals, birds and reptiles.

Nitrogenous waste excretion

In addition to the elimination of carbon dioxide, the gills play a vital role in the excretion of other metabolic wastes. Both active and passive methods are utilized to transport ammonia (a product of protein metabolism) across the gill epithelium. In some fish, 75% or more of nitrogenous waste is excreted via the gills.

Acid–base balance

Acid–base balance is maintained by exchange of bicarbonate for water and chloride ions by specialized chloride cells in the gill epithelium.

Osmotic control

The ionic composition of most aquatic environments differs markedly from the tissue fluid of fish. Most fish are therefore at constant risk of electrolyte imbalance as internal and external fluids attempt to reach equilibrium. The abundant exposed epithelium provided by the gills for gas exchange also supplies a large surface area of semi-permeable membrane across which ions can diffuse.

Freshwater and marine fish are exposed to very different environments, and thus face different osmotic challenges. The tissue fluids of freshwater fish are hypertonic relative to the external environment; thus water tends to diffuse across the gill epithelium into the fish. In marine fish, the environment is hypertonic relative to the tissue fluids, promoting efflux of water from the body into the external environment with a concurrent influx of ions into the fish.

Specialized chloride cells located in the gill epithelium contribute significantly to the maintenance of osmotic balance. These cells are found primarily at the base of the secondary lamellae, occurring in high concentrations in marine fish and in low concentrations in freshwater fish. Although the exact mechanisms by which the process occurs are unknown, the most common theories support the active transport of ions through these cells. Ion pumps located in the cell membrane utilize energy in the form of adenosine triphosphate (ATP) to transport ions across the gill epithelium against their concentration gradient.

For every molecule that is transported across the epithelium, another ion must be exchanged. For example, in freshwater fish, inward movement of sodium is coupled with the outward movement of hydrogen and ammonium ions. The inward movement of chloride is coupled with the outward movement of bicarbonate. Thus, osmotic regulation is closely intertwined with the processes of waste excretion and acid–base balance.

Because freshwater fish are constantly faced with the influx of water into their tissues, they transport sodium chloride into their tissue fluid across the gill epithelium. Excess chloride is excreted primarily by the kidneys. The reverse process occurs in marine fish: water diffuses out through their gills and salts diffuse in. These species replace water lost to the environment through their gills by drinking up to 35% of their bodyweight in sea water per day. This adds to the salt content of their blood as well as that which diffuses in across the gills. Chloride cells actively transport most of the excess sodium and chloride across the gill epithelium and out of the fish. In contrast to freshwater fish, the counter-ion for sodium in the ATPase ion pump is potassium rather than hydrogen or ammonia.

Clinical signs

Occasionally, a specific clinical sign suggests a particular respiratory disease in fish, but more often clinical signs are ambiguous and represent a variety of conditions. For example, fish may be hypoxic due to low levels of dissolved oxygen in the water or because of excess mucus production stimulated by ectoparasites. In both cases, the fish will appear depressed and lethargic, with increased movement of the opercula.

- *Tachypnoea and dyspnoea* are common indicators of respiratory compromise. The normal fish appears to put little effort into respiration. Increases in the degree of buccal and opercular movement in each respiratory cycle, as well as an increase in ventilatory frequency, are important signs as they represent a response to hypoxia
- *Hovering or piping* (gulping air) near the air/water interface is abnormal for most species. Fish continuously performing this action are seeking the higher concentrations of oxygen often found in the uppermost few millimetres of water. In cases of hypoxia, fish may also attempt to gasp for air at the surface. The exposure of the lamellae to air results in their collapse, reducing surface area and compounding respiratory compromise. Fish may also gather at the sides of tanks or in areas of water inflow where oxygen levels may be higher or water flow more rapid. It is important to appreciate that the anabantids have adapted to poorly oxygenated waters and may normally obtain air at the water surface
- *Intermittently or permanently flared opercula* may be a sign of severe or impending respiratory distress. It may precede or be a sign of an agonal response in which the mouth may also be held open. Flared opercula are more easily assessed when viewing the fish from above

- *Unilateral respiration* is rare but can arise due to the obstruction of one operculum. This may occur, for example, due to the presence of a space-occupying lesion
- *'Flashing'* is the act of rubbing the skin or gills on solid objects in the environment. This behaviour is an attempt by the fish to rid the skin or gills of an irritant, and often indicates the presence of ectoparasites
- Occasionally fish will exhibit a *'cough' reflex*, which temporarily interrupts their ventilation cycle and sends a back flush of water over the gills. The purpose of this in the normal fish is to clear the gills and gill rakers of accumulated sediment and food debris. In the diseased animal, coughing may be an attempt to remove parasites or excess mucus from the gills.

Fish in respiratory distress, regardless of the cause, require immediate provision of additional oxygen. Gradual cooling of the water (if possible) may also be useful by increasing the dissolved oxygen capacity of the water. Diagnostic procedures and handling should be minimized until the critically hypoxic patient is stabilized.

Investigations

A thorough diagnostic approach is essential to the accurate interpretation of a clinical problem, establishing a concise list of differentials and ultimately reaching a diagnosis.

If fish are to be transported to the clinic for evaluation (see Chapter 9), the owner should be instructed to provide additional aeration by a battery-powered air pump during transport, especially for fish with respiratory difficulty. A sample of water should be brought for water quality analysis and should be of sufficient volume in which to anaesthetize the fish for diagnostic procedures if necessary.

Ideally, the patient should be brought for examination while it is still alive since tissue autolysis occurs rapidly in fish following death. Gill epithelium can show artefactual changes within 5 minutes of death and tissues must be placed in a fixative as soon as possible. Neutral buffered formalin is used in most situations but Bouin's is ideal for the gills, a select few other organs, or for whole small fish.

Clinical history

A detailed history is an indispensable component of a complete diagnostic approach. Various aspects of fish behaviour, fish husbandry and time scale of the disease should be examined, in addition to clinical signs. Many factors may affect the function of the respiratory system; therefore information about all aspects of care is necessary.

Observation

If the fish has been transported to the clinic without aeration, an air-stone should be placed into the water immediately. Then, prior to any handling, the fish should be observed.

- Record any abnormal behaviour and clinical signs such as flashing, piping, flared opercula or tachypnoea
- Note the fish's level of activity and location within the water column
- View the interaction of the fish with other system inhabitants and observe other fish for early or advanced signs of disease
- Examine for signs of trauma or any other abnormal external features such as parasites, swellings or other lesions.

In some cases, these observations may be easier to make if the fish is placed into a small clear container such as an aquarium or glass bowl. If the fish is in its normal habitat, examine the system and its environment.

Physical examination

During examination, powder-free latex gloves should be worn to prevent damage to the fish's skin and protective mucus layer, and also to protect the handler from potentially zoonotic pathogens. In some cases, a conscious non-venomous fish can be supported and examined with one side submerged in the water. This allows respiration to continue on one side, prolongs available examination time and may reduce the stress of the procedure for both fish and clinician. Depending on the length of the examination, the fish may need to be released briefly and periodically to breathe.

- The outer surface of the opercula should be examined for discolorations, evidence of trauma or petechial haemorrhages
- The gills are inspected by gently lifting the operculum. They should be bright red in colour with a smooth and symmetrical caudal edge. The striations due to the primary lamellae should be clearly visible (Figure 17.2). Pale pink gills in the live fish are indicative of anaemia, while pale brown gills suggest methaemoglobinaemia
- The outer surface of the gills must be inspected for excessive mucus, growths, white or yellow spots, haemorrhage, erosions or parasites

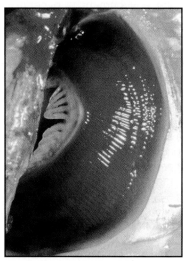

Figure 17.2 The normal gill of a koi. The tissue is bright red and the primary lamellae should be clearly visible on close inspection. (© W.H. Wildgoose.)

- All gill arches must be carefully examined, since many parasites will attach between the last two arches (where they are less likely to be expelled by the fish)
- A magnifying glass may be useful in the examination. The small opercular cleft in some species such as puffers, eels and some sharks makes it difficult to examine the gills without the aid of an endoscope or auroscope.

Laboratory tests

Equipment required to investigate respiratory disease in fish includes fine forceps and scissors and basic microscopic facilities. Suitable fish anaesthetics can be obtained from veterinary drug suppliers and easy-to-use water quality test kits are available from aquatic retailers.

Gill scrape examination

A wet mount preparation is one of the most useful diagnostic tools for investigation of fish diseases. The sample is placed in a drop of water from the tank or pond on a glass slide. If necessary, dechlorinated tap water can be used for samples from freshwater fish, but only salt water should be used for marine specimens. The sample is collected, placed on the water on the glass slide, gently mounted under a cover slip and viewed under both low and high power.

The inner opercular surface, which is a protected area that may harbour a variety of parasitic organisms, can be swabbed and the sample obtained applied to a wet mount. Gill smears, particularly of grossly visible lesions, may also be viewed on a wet mount preparation.

Biopsy examination

Gill biopsy is a vital component of a diagnostic evaluation of the respiratory system (Figure 17.3).

- The fish should be anaesthetized since it may otherwise struggle, resulting in gill damage and possibly life-threatening haemorrhage
- The operculum is lifted and the tip of a pair of fine scissors is inserted into the gill chamber
- The distal tips of three or four primary lamellae are carefully removed
- The biopsy sample is transferred immediately to a wet mount preparation for microscopic examination.

Removal of excess tissue can result in significant haemorrhage. Haemostasis (if necessary) can be achieved by gently crimping the ends of the cut lamellae with a pair of artery forceps. The primary lamellae of normal gill tissue are evenly tapered and secondary lamellae will be visible unless there are extensive pathological changes. A second biopsy may be taken for histological evaluation.

When disease is present, excess mucus accumulations or parasites may be observed under low power ($\times$ 40–100). Higher power ($\times$ 200–1000) can be used to inspect for smaller parasites, bacterial colonies or fungal hyphae. Various other pathological changes may also be identified. Tissue that appears grossly normal may still be functionally impaired. Changes not visible on fresh preparations may be more easily recognized on histological examination.

Postmortem examination

During this procedure, larger samples can be taken. An entire gill arch should be removed and viewed on a wet mount: gill parasites located at the base of primary filaments can be missed if only the tips are examined. A larger sample is ideal for histological examination but the preparation is thick and opaque, and certain pathogens may easily be missed on wet mount examination.

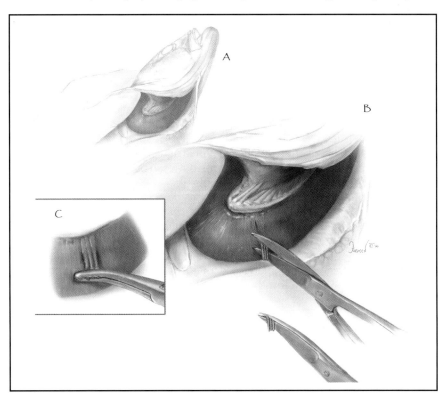

Figure 17.3 Taking a gill biopsy. (A) The fish is held firmly and the operculum is lifted to expose the lamellae. (B) A small amount of lamellar tissue is cut, using scissors. (C) Artery forceps are used gently to crimp the cut tissue if haemorrhage occurs. (© Farheen Rahman, Johns Hopkins Art as Applied to Medicine.)

Therefore, a sample of the lamellar tips should still be examined under high power.

As gill biopsies or scrapings are often not practical for smaller fish, one or more fish should be sacrificed if disease is present in a population and tissues should be collected for a complete gross and histological examination. Immediately after sacrificing the fish, one or more gill arches should be prepared and examined as a wet mount.

Bacteriology

Bacterial samples are easily obtained by gently rolling a sterile swab or loop along the gill surface. Results must be interpreted with caution, as pathogens may be difficult to distinguish from the normal flora present in gill chamber and mucus. Pure growth of a particular organism may be indicative of a bacterial infection.

A systematic approach

Many infectious and non-infectious agents can cause respiratory disease. This section attempts to categorize these based on clinical appearance:

- Normal gross appearance
- Colour change
- Visible ectoparasites
- Swellings
- Miscellaneous.

Normal gross appearance

A lack of visible changes to the gills does not exclude the possibility of gill disease. The acute onset of severe toxic and hypoxic conditions may result in sudden death with little visible gill pathology, whereas less severe conditions may produce changes that are more visible. Therefore, environmental investigation and histological examination of the gill are essential to assess gill function fully.

Environmental hypoxia

This is a common cause of morbidity in fish. In an aquarium system, it is usually the result of poor husbandry practices (e.g. overpopulation, poor aeration, high temperature, overfeeding). In ornamental ponds, algae and plant overgrowth, overcrowding of fish and dramatic variations in temperature can produce marked fluctuations in dissolved oxygen levels.

- Clinical signs include lethargy, anorexia, piping and tachypnoea
- Although not pathognomonic, fish dying from acute hypoxia commonly have flared opercula and a wide-open mouth
- Larger fish have a higher oxygen requirement and are usually affected first
- Some species, such as goldfish and the anabantids, are quite resistant to environmental hypoxia; therefore selective survival of these species may indicate low levels of dissolved oxygen

- Other species are particularly sensitive; in elasmobranchs, hypoxia may lead to renal lesions followed by death several days later
- Other diseases or environmental factors affecting the gill epithelium may render fish susceptible to even minor decreases in dissolved oxygen levels.

Toxins

Ammonia

Excessive levels of ammonia in the water are common in new facilities.

- Smaller fish are more susceptible to ammonia and are usually affected first
- Exposure to low levels of ammonia can cause gill irritation, whereas chronic exposure can result in hyperplasia and hypertrophy of the gill epithelium
- Dyspnoea and irregular respiratory patterns are often seen in affected fish, and sudden death can occur at high levels.

Organic compounds

Malachite green acts as a respiratory poison. Clinical signs of toxicity are similar to those caused by environmental hypoxia but increased aeration has no benefit and there is no antidote.

Volatile organic components of paints and sealers can cause congestion with telangiectasis of the gills and subsequent mortality. Proper curing of paints, sealers and PVC glues, together with repeated flushing of new systems with copious amounts of water, greatly reduces the risk of toxicity.

Chlorine

Chlorine is used in municipal water supplies as a disinfectant to ensure that the water is fit for human consumption. It is very toxic to fish and can cause acute gill necrosis with excess mucus production causing dyspnoea and sudden mortality.

Ozone

Ozone is used as a sterilizing agent in aquaria but is toxic at relatively low concentrations. Residual levels should be kept below 0.002 mg/l. Clinical signs of toxicity include agitation, respiratory distress and sudden death. Electronic equipment is available to measure residual ozone but it can be detected by the human nose at toxic levels.

Virus

Pathogenic koi herpesvirus causes high morbidity and mortality. Pathological changes in the gills may only be evident on histological examination but more visible pathology is is found in fish that survive for more than a few days (see Chapter 24).

Colour change

Altered gill coloration is a common clinical finding. Pallor may be generalized or focal. Small focal lesions may extend gradually to affect the whole gill.

Pallor: generalized

Anaemia

Although this is not a disease of the gills, affected fish can show signs of respiratory distress and pallor is more easily assessed by examining the gills (Figure 17.4).

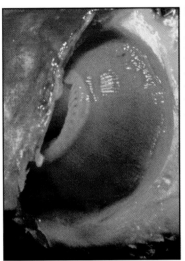

Figure 17.4 The pale coloration of the gill in this koi is due to severe anaemia. The packed cell volume was 4%, whereas the normal value is about 30–35%. (© W.H. Wildgoose.)

- *Haemolytic anaemia* is due to increased destruction of the erythrocytes as may occur in bacterial disease or infection with haemoparasites
- *Hypoplastic anaemia* is due to poor production of erythrocytes as a result of damage to the haematopoietic tissues, or vitamin or mineral deficiencies
- *Haemorrhagic anaemia* is from blood loss through physical injury and occasionally acute systemic disease (e.g. spring viraemia of carp).

Haemoparasites, when present in large numbers, can contribute to anaemia and, subsequently, respiratory distress. They can be found on a fresh gill biopsy or blood smear. They are also commonly observed in healthy animals and treatment is not recommended unless a life-threatening anaemia is present.

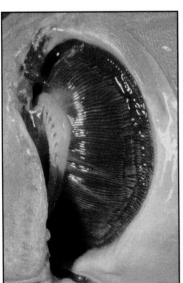

Figure 17.5 Excess mucus in the gill is produced in response to many irritant agents. Unless severe, it is difficult to appreciate visually but produces a grey sheen on the filaments, as seen in the ventral part of this gill. (© W.H. Wildgoose.)

Excess mucus

The lamellar epithelium of the normal fish contains a plethora of goblet cells, especially at the cranial and caudal edges as well as at the base of the lamellae. Increased mucus production (Figure 17.5) occurs in response to chronic irritation by various parasites or toxins. The mucus covers the epithelial surface and increases the distance through which gases and ions must pass.

Ectoparasites: Many parasites can infest and damage the gills (Figure 17.6). Protozoal infestations are a common cause of respiratory compromise, osmoregulatory failure and death.

Phylum and Class	Freshwater	Marine
Protozoa		
Ciliata	*Ichthyophthirius multifiliis* *Tetrahymena* spp. *Chilodonella* spp. Trichodinids *Trichophrya* spp.	*Cryptocaryon irritans* *Uronema* spp. *Brooklynella hostilis* Trichodinids
Flagellata	*Ichthyobodo necator* *Cryptobia* spp.	
Dinoflagellata	*Piscinoodinium* spp.	*Amyloodinium ocellatum*
Metazoa		
Monogenea	*Gyrodactylus* spp. *Dactylogyrus* spp.	*Gyrodactylus* spp. *Microcotyle* spp.
Copepoda	*Ergasilus* spp. *Salmincola* spp.	*Ergasilus* spp.

Figure 17.6 Parasites affecting the gills of freshwater and marine fish.

- 'White spot' (see under Visible ectoparasites) is one of the most serious ectoparasites and excess mucus is often the only clinical sign: by the time the characteristic white spots are visible, extensive tissue damage will have occurred (Figure 17.7)
- Trichodinids are ciliated protozoans that infest the skin and gills of freshwater and marine fish,

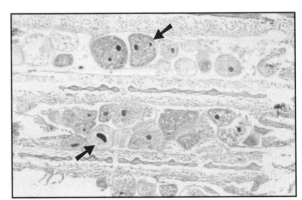

Figure 17.7 Histological section illustrating damage caused by a severe infestation of white spot. There is extensive destruction of the gill, with loss of secondary lamellae. The parasites (arrowed) are packed between the remnants of the primary lamellae. (× 100 original magnification. H&E stain.) (© W.H. Wildgoose.)

often in water with a high organic load
- *Ichthyobodo*, the flagellate previously known as *Costia*, infects freshwater fish, often after transportation. Affected fish are depressed and commonly exhibit respiratory distress.

Hyperplasia and hypertrophy

The response of the gill epithelial cells to irritation, whether from environmental toxins, suspended solids or infectious organisms, is to increase in number or size. Hyperplasia and hypertrophy thus result in increased thickness of the epithelium, which reduces its functional efficiency (Figures 17.8 and 17.9). Similar effects result from invasion by inflammatory cells in response to an infectious agent. These changes may be evident on wet mount preparations; if severe, they result in the fusion of adjacent secondary lamellae, thereby reducing the surface area.

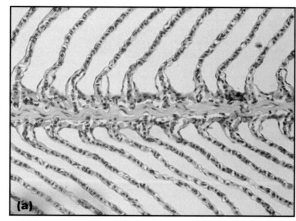

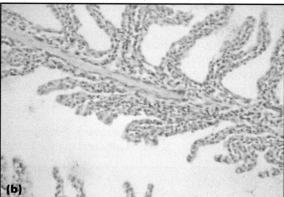

Figure 17.8 (a) Histological section of the gill showing normal primary and secondary lamellae. (b) Hypertrophy of the primary and secondary lamellae is seen in response to exposure to high levels of copper. (× 400 original magnification. H&E stain.) (© Brent Whitaker.)

- Nutritional imbalances, such as pantothenic acid deficiency, can also cause epithelial hyperplasia and lamellar fusion
- Long-term exposure to copper, commonly used to treat ectoparasites in marine fish, will cause gill hyperplasia and hypertrophy. The toxic effects can be minimized by continuously adding small amounts of copper, thus avoiding the high concentration 'spikes' that occur with bolus administration.

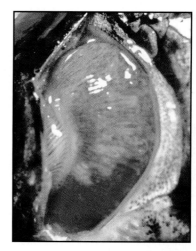

Figure 17.9 Extensive epithelial hyperplasia is visible as pale mottled areas in the dorsal part of the gill in this goldfish. Areas that are less severely affected are seen ventrally. (© W.H. Wildgoose.)

Pallor: localized

Necrosis

Necrosis of the gill epithelium results in increased water flow through the gills, causing disruption of normal homoeostatic mechanisms. The semi-permeable membranes of necrotic cells become damaged and fully permeable, allowing unregulated influx and efflux of fluids. In addition, disruption of the epithelial barrier enables secondary bacterial and fungal invasion.

Bacteria: Bacteria commonly found in gill disease include those in the *Cytophaga*, *Flavobacterium* and *Flexibacter* group. *Flavobacterium branchiophilum* can produce infection and disintegration of gill filaments, with affected areas appearing blanched and necrotic (Figure 17.10). Infection (and subsequent necrosis) begins at the lamellar tips and in severe cases extends to the gill arch. *Flavobacterium* is the primary cause of 'bacterial gill disease' and is frequently associated with stress. Clinical signs include lethargy, dyspnoea, coughing, and flared opercula.

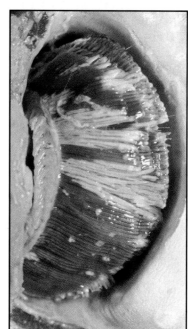

Figure 17.10 Severe necrosis due to bacterial gill disease in a koi. The characteristic blanched areas contained extremely high numbers of the filamentous bacteria, *Flavobacterium*. (© W.H. Wildgoose.)

Fungi: Fungal infections of the gills are common and usually the result of secondary infection. Intact epithelial layers and antibody-rich mucus normally inhibit growth of fungal spores in healthy fish. When host defences are compromised, fungal spores germinate and hyphae penetrate through the epithelium.

- In freshwater species, *Saprolegnia* is the most common fungal infection and presents as cotton-like growths on the skin or gills (Figure 17.11)
- *Branchiomyces* spp. are the causative agent of 'gill rot', a disease that primarily affects freshwater fish. The fungal spores concentrate in areas of high oxygen tension within the gills, resulting in growth of fungal hyphae throughout the lamellar capillaries. Obstruction of the vessels results in thrombosis and ischaemia within portions of the gill, causing areas of necrosis.

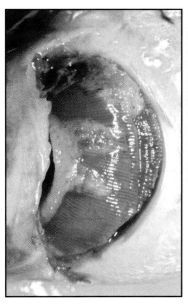

Figure 17.11
Saprolegnia infection in the gill. The collapsed fungal mass has a gelatinous appearance when the fish is out of water. Unicellular algae trapped among the hyphae give the lesion a green appearance. (© W.H. Wildgoose.)

Parasites: Digenetic trematodes of the genus *Sanguinicola* are known as 'bloodworms', due to their location in the circulatory system. Infected lamellae become swollen and ischaemic, then necrotic. In addition to blood vessels, adult parasites may also be found in the heart or peritoneal cavity. Their eggs lodge in the branchial capillaries, causing the lamellae to become swollen and ischaemic. Diagnosis is made by finding the eggs or first-stage larvae in the gills.

Brown coloration

Methaemoglobinaemia
This is not a disease of the gills but a clinical sign that is easily identified by examining the colour of the gills. Haemoglobin is oxidized to methaemoglobin, which cannot transport oxygen so efficiently. Consequently, severely affected fish are dyspnoeic in the presence of adequate dissolved oxygen levels. Other clinical signs include lethargy, gasping at the surface and sudden death. Nitrite toxicity is the commonest cause of methaemoglobinaemia in fish.

Visible ectoparasites

White spot
'White spot' is caused by *Ichthyophthirius multifiliis* in freshwater fish and *Cryptocaryon irritans* in marine species. Although the predominant clinical finding is small white spots on the fish's body, infestation can be limited to the gills, where white spots measuring up to 1 mm in diameter may be accompanied by petechiation. Affected fish may show loss of appetite, flashing and dyspnoea. Gill pathology can be severe, with extensive necrosis, epithelial hyperplasia, lamellar fusion and excess mucus production.

Dinoflagellates
The dinoflagellates that commonly cause gill disease are *Amyloodinium ocellatum* ('coral fish disease') and *Piscinoodinium* spp. ('velvet disease') in marine and freshwater fishes, respectively. Unlike most parasites of teleosts, *Amyloodinium* also infects elasmobranchs. The gills may exhibit very small dust-like white spots, which may be visible in a wet mount preparation as pear-shaped parasitic cysts attached to the lamellae. Respiratory distress may be followed by rapid spread of the organism and death of the host within 2–3 days. Affected fish may flash and exhibit tachypnoea and dyspnoea, but heavy infestation of the gills can result in death without any obvious clinical signs.

Gill flukes
Monogenetic trematodes referred to as 'gill flukes' commonly cause gill damage and disease. Hooks on the opisthohaptor of monopisthocotyle monogeneans (e.g. *Dactylogyrus*) cause physical damage to the gills whereas polyopisthocotyle monogeneans (e.g. *Microcotyle*) attach using many small suckers, effectively reducing the functional surface area of the gill (Figure 17.12). The larger gill flukes can measure up to 2 mm in length and are commonly found in most species of aquarium and pond fish. Clinical signs include tachypnoea, flashing, lethargy and death.

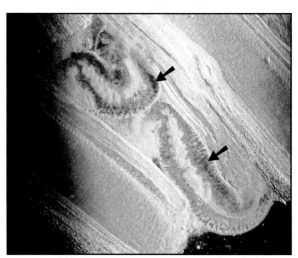

Figure 17.12 Polyopisthocotyle monogeneans (arrowed) use many suckers to attach to the gills. In large numbers these parasites can cover the lamellae, preventing normal gill function. (× 20 original magnification. Wet mount preparation.) (© National Aquarium in Baltimore.)

Leeches

Leeches are occasionally found attached to the gills of pond fish but are more commonly found on the external body surfaces.

Isopods

Isopods such as flabelliferans and gnathiids are large crustacean parasites measuring up to 6 cm in length. They are sometimes found in the gill cavity of tropical marine fish and less frequently on freshwater fish.

Copepods

Several freshwater and marine copepods attach to the gill arches and are usually an incidental finding, though large numbers can cause erosion or ulceration of the lamellae. *Ergasilus* spp. measure up to 2 mm, have paired trailing egg sacs and attach to the gills by large claspers, which can cause severe focal damage.

Swellings

Nodular lesions

Parasites

*   Glochidia are the infective larvae of freshwater bivalve molluscs. They may infect fish kept in outdoor ponds that are fed by natural streams or rivers. The larvae incite a marked hyperplastic response in the gill epithelium and small white nodular lesions up to 1 mm may be visible in infected fish.
*   Various species of myxozoan parasites (e.g. *Henneguya* and *Sphaerospora*) may produce pseudocysts that enlarge slowly. The whitish nodules located in the gill filaments may measure up to 4 mm
*   Microsporean parasites (e.g. *Glugea*) can produce hypertrophied cells or xenomas within the gill lamellae. These small white lesions, up to 2 mm in diameter, can provoke marked pathological changes in the gills
*   Metacercaria, the intermediate stage in the life cycle of digenetic trematodes, encyst in many tissues. Some species that encyst in the gills can provoke marked tissue reactions, including chondrodysplasia. The hyperplastic nodular lesions may measure up to 2 mm in diameter.

Epitheliocystis

The chlamydia-like organism that is thought to cause epitheliocystis infects the skin and gills of freshwater and marine fish. Transparent or white cysts measuring up to 1 mm in diameter may be seen on the gill lamellae (Figure 17.13). The infection is often benign but proliferative gill lesions can become severe and cause death.

Lymphocystis

Lymphocystis is a viral disease of freshwater and marine fish that stimulates marked hypertrophy of epithelial cells. The resultant nodular growths, which are usually cream in colour, are unsightly but rarely

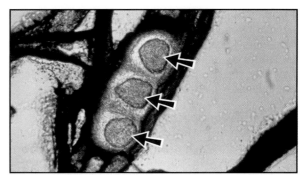

Figure 17.13 Epithelial cells of the gill are greatly enlarged (arrowed) due to infection by epitheliocystis in a flame angelfish. (× 20 original magnification. Wet mount preparation.) (© National Aquarium in Baltimore.)

cause fatality. If large lesions occur in the buccal or opercular cavities, respiration may be compromised.

Hyperplasia and hypertrophy

In severe cases of gill disease, hyperplastic changes may become so extensive that exuberant proliferation of the epithelium may extend from the tips of the primary lamellae, which may form nodules of epithelial tissue (Figures 17.14 and 17.15). In addition to many infectious and toxic agents, nutritional pantothenic acid deficiency may cause epithelial hyperplasia resulting in a clubbed appearance.

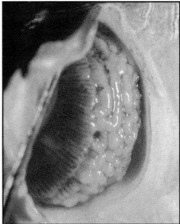

Figure 17.14 A severe hyperplastic response on the tips of primary lamellae produced a nodular appearance. This was thought to be due to nutritional deficiency since the young koi were reared on a homemade diet. (© W.H. Wildgoose.)

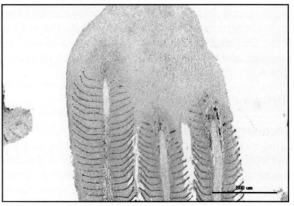

Figure 17.15 A histological section of the gill in Figure 17.14, revealing the extreme chronic hyperplastic change with consolidation and fusion of tips of adjacent primary lamellae. (× 40 original magnification. Bar = 500 μm. H&E.) (Courtesy of CEFAS, Weymouth.)

Telangiectasis

Dilatation of capillaries in the secondary lamellae occurs in response to a variety of chemical or physical injuries. This 'ballooning' of the small vessels results from the rupture of pillar cells and pooling of blood. These lesions are visible on a wet mount and may be visible grossly as small red spots on the lamellae. They often thrombose, fibrose and are then reabsorbed. Telangiectasis can be caused iatrogenically in gill biopsies, due to the action of cutting a sample, which results in a sudden increase in capillary pressure.

Large swellings

Neoplasia

Gill tumours are relatively rare. All tissue components of the gill may become neoplastic, in addition to the epidermis within the opercular cavity. The effect on the fish and the degree of mechanical interference with normal respiration depends on the size and location of the neoplasia.

- Papillomas are common in many species of fish and occasionally occur in the opercular cavity or cleft
- Squamous cell carcinomas have been reported less frequently in fish and can develop from pre-existing papillomas. They may be locally invasive and cause significant interference with normal respiration (Figure 17.16)
- Branchioblastomas (Figure 17.17) are benign tumours of blast cells thought to originate from mesenchymal blastema, which normally produces all the connective tissue components of the gills. These may originate spontaneously but have been experimentally induced by exposure to various carcinogens
- Chrondromas of the gills have been reported in fish and some have been associated with the metacercariae of a trematode
- Thyroid neoplasia, especially adenomas, is common in many species and may be visible on the lower posterior aspect of the opercular cavity. When severe, enlarged thyroid tissue will impair movement of the operculum and physically interfere with gill function.

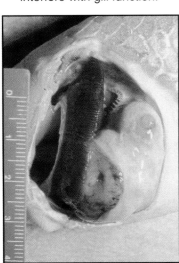

Figure 17.16
Squamous cell carcinoma. This koi was also affected with multiple papillomas on its head. The deeply invasive and proliferative tumour caused severe respiratory compromise. (Reprinted by permission of *Veterinary Record*.)

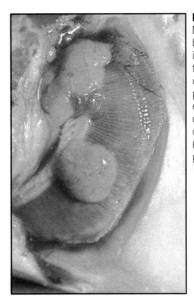

Figure 17.17
Multiple branchioblastomas in an adult koi. The tumours were found during a routine postmortem examination and caused no obvious clinical signs. (Reprinted by permission of *Veterinary Record*.)

Goitre

Thyroid hyperplasia or hypertrophy resulting in goitre is seen in both elasmobranchs and teleosts. The enlarged thyroid glands may physically interfere with normal respiration. Treatment with iodine in the food or water may reverse the condition in early cases.

Miscellaneous

Haemorrhage

Frank blood can occasionally be found in the opercular cavity. This usually results from necrosis of the gill tissue or physical trauma. Occasionally, some koi may haemorrhage spontaneously from the gills when caught for examination. The haemorrhage only lasts for one or two minutes and has no lasting effect. There is rarely any visible pathology present in these fish but a urine dipstick can be used to detect traces of blood in the water.

Foreign bodies

Substrate material such as gravel or small rocks may become accidentally lodged in the oral cavity of bottom feeders, restricting normal respiration.

Debris such as silt and unicellular and filamentous algae can become trapped among fungal hyphae and necrotic areas of the gills. This debris can also be found following agonal respiration of dying fish lying at the bottom of outdoor ponds.

Opercular deformity

Physical deformity of one operculum or both (Figure 17.18) can compromise normal respiratory movements as well as predispose the gills to infectious diseases or parasitism. Deformities may be due to:

- Congenital or genetic defects resulting from inbreeding or crossbreeding of certain fish strains
- Environmental parameters such as pollution or unsuitable temperatures, which may adversely influence the development of eggs and fry

- Nutritional imbalances (common carp and salmonids have developed deformed gill opercula following experimentally induced vitamin A and C deficiency).

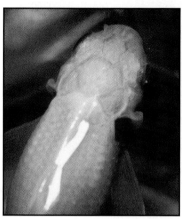

Figure 17.18 This opercular deformity was present in this goldfish when purchased 2 years earlier. The curled free edges of both operculae exposed the underlying gill tissue but caused no clinical problems. (© W.H. Wildgoose.)

Further reading

Ellis AE, Roberts RJ and Tytler P (1978) The anatomy and physiology of teleosts. In: *Fish Pathology*, ed. RJ Roberts, pp. 13–55. Baillière Tindall, London

Evans HE (1992) Anatomy of tropical fishes. In: *Aquariology*, eds JB Gratzek and JR Matthews, pp. 71–93. Tetra Press, Morris Plains

Ferguson HW (1989) *Systemic Pathology of Fish: A Text and Atlas of Comparative Tissue Response in Diseases of Teleosts*. Iowa State University Press, Ames, Iowa

Gilmour KM (1998) Gas exchange. In: *The Physiology of Fishes*, ed. DH Evans, pp. 101–128. CRC Press, Boca Raton

Goven BA, Gilvert JP and Gratzek JB (1980) Apparent drug resistance to the organophosphate dimethyl (2,2,2-trichloro-1-hydroxyethyl) phosphonate by monogenetic trematodes. *Journal of Wildlife Disease* **16**(3), 343–346

Herman RL and Meade JW (1985) Gill lamellar dilatations (telangiectasis) related to sampling techniques. In: *Transactions of the American Fisheries Society* **114**, 911–913

Karnaky KJ (1998) Osmotic and ionic regulation. In: *The Physiology of Fishes*, ed. DH Evans, pp. 101–128. CRC Press, Boca Raton

Oestmenn DJ (1985) Environmental and disease problems in ornamental marine aquariums. *Compendium on Continuing Education for Practicing Veterinarians* **7**(8), 656–668

Rasmussen JM, Garner MM and Petrini KR (2000) Presumptive volatile organic compound intoxication of sharks and teleost fish in a newly constructed aquarium: why fish and paint fumes just don't mix. In: *Proceedings of the American Association of Zoo Veterinarians, International Association for Aquatic Animal Medicine*, September 17–21, New Orleans, pp. 367–368

Wildgoose WH (1992) Papilloma and squamous cell carcinoma in koi carp (*Cyprinus carpio*). *Veterinary Record* 130, 153–157

Wildgoose WH and Bucke D (1995) Spontaneous branchioblastoma in a koi carp (*Cyprinus carpio*). *Veterinary Record* 136, 418–419

Acknowledgements

The authors thank Valerie Lounsbury, Nathan Yates and Michele Martin for their constructive review of this chapter and Susie Ridenour, librarian at the National Aquarium in Baltimore, for her assistance in obtaining our reference materials. We are also grateful to the editor of the *Veterinary Record* for permission to reproduce Figures 17.16 and 17.17. Lastly, we thank Farheen Rahman and Ken Probst, students of the Johns Hopkins Art as Applied to Medicine program, for their wonderful illustrations.

18

Ocular disorders

Brent R. Whitaker

Ocular disorders are commonly observed in both elasmobranch and teleost fishes. Even the novice fish hobbyist will readily discern a discoloured, cloudy, ulcerated or disproportionate eye. Veterinarians comfortable with the assessment and diagnosis of ophthalmic disease in terrestrial species will find that working with fish can be quite rewarding. Once the clinician is at ease with anaesthetizing and handling the fish (Chapter 11), a thorough examination of the eye can readily be accomplished.

In some cases, lesions are subtle and require knowledge of the non-diseased eye for the species. Anatomical variation is great among species; this is readily noted in the shape of the pupil and coloration of the iris. The clinician should take every opportunity to observe the eyes of healthy fish and an ophthalmic examination should be part of every physical examination.

Ocular abnormalities found in fish include uveitis, corneal ulceration, cataracts and bi- or unilateral exophthalmos. Many of these lesions accompany systemic disease while others, such as some cases of gaseous exophthalmos, arise for unknown reasons. Rapid diagnosis and treatment of ocular conditions can prevent suffering and loss of vision or even life.

Treatment options for ornamental fish are limited only by the skill of the clinician and cooperation of the client. In some public display facilities, the loss of an eye may result in the removal of an otherwise healthy fish from the exhibit. In these cases, the placement of a prosthesis may benefit the fish and provide an interesting challenge for the clinician.

Anatomy

Represented by over 20,000 species, fish comprise a diverse group of animals that have evolved visual adaptations for life in a wide range of environments. Figure 18.1 illustrates the general anatomy of the teleost eye; Figure 18.2 summarizes several notable anatomical differences between the eyes of elasmobranchs and teleosts. Although teleosts lack eyelids, many have a membrane that covers the cornea, or folds of tissue around the eye. Three pairs of extraocular muscles are present, enabling the eyes of most teleosts to move independently of each other. This movement is involuntary and

so following objects using vision requires the fish to change position in the water – as seen readily in many triggerfish. Placement of the eyes on each side of the head provides most species with a binocular field of vision.

Globe

The globe is a flattened ellipse that is well protected by the cranium of some species, such as the cowfish, and fully exposed to injury in others, such as the cownose ray. Many nocturnal fish, such as the bigeye, have large eyes that enable them to hunt in low light levels. Some varieties of fancy goldfish are intentionally bred to have large eyes where fluid causes excessive distension of the periorbital skin (Figure 18.3).

Cornea

The refractive index of the cornea is similar to that of water and does not aid in focusing. Structurally, the cornea is like that of terrestrial animals, although slightly thicker. It consists of an epithelial layer (which is responsible for maintaining hydration), a superficial and deep stroma, the corneal endothelium and Descemet's membrane. Peripherally, the corneal endothelium thickens to form the annular ligament, which attaches to the anterior iris.

Sclera

A ring of cartilage within the anterior sclera and variably supplemented scleral ossicles give strength and structure to the globe. Below the sclera lies the argentea, a silvery yellow layer of guanine-containing cells that extends over the anterior iris and contributes to the colour and iridescence of the iris. The argentea is frequently present in fish larvae but less so in adults.

Choroid

The choroid gland, located in the posterior choroid, is found only in fish that possess pseudobranchs (accessory gills that are remnants of the first gill arch). Unique to teleosts, this gland contains a highly vascular choroid rete that forms a horseshoe-shaped structure around the optic nerve and is thought to provide nutrients, including oxygen, to the avascular retina.

Retina

The teleost retina may also derive nutrients from the falciform process, comprising an inward folding of the choroid through a foetal fissure into the

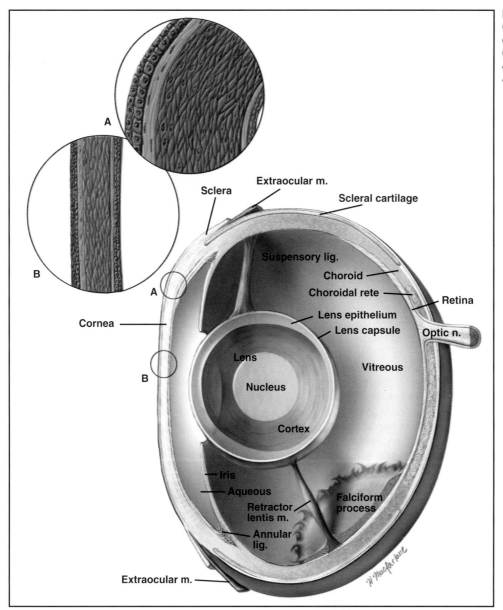

Figure 18.1
General anatomy of the teleost eye. (© Helen MacFarlane, Johns Hopkins Art as Applied to Medicine.)

Elasmobranch	Teleost
Fibrous choroidal tapetum	No choroidal tapetum
Eyelids present in sharks; absent in rays and skates	Most teleosts lack eyelids
Choroid gland absent	Many have choroid gland
Choriocapillaris provides nutrients to eye	Falciform process or tunica vasculosa retinae provides nutrition to eye
Iridial sphincter and dilatory muscles present	Iridial muscles absent
Protractor lentis muscle moves eye during accommodation	Retractor lentis muscle moves eye during accommodation

Figure 18.2 Comparative anatomy of the elasmobranch and teleost eye.

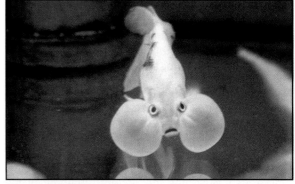

Figure 18.3 The bubble-eye variety of fancy goldfish has very bulbous eyes due to fluid in the periorbital area. (© W.H. Wildgoose.)

vitreous humour, or from a membrane (the tunica vasculosa retinae) that lies anterior to the retina and originates from a branch of the internal ophthalmic artery. Elasmobranchs lack a choroid gland but have a choriocapillaris – a collection of choroidal vessels and a capillary system, which is supplied by a single artery and drained by a dorsal and ventral vein. Most elasmobranchs have a fibrous choroidal tapetum; teleosts lack this structure.

Iris

The fish pupil varies greatly in size and shape among species. The iris of most teleosts contains little or no skeletal or smooth muscle; sphincter and dilator muscles are rudimentary or absent, except in elasmobranchs. The iris is attached to the cornea and is fixed in place by the annular ligament. If present, the ciliary body is undeveloped; ciliary processes and a ciliary epithelium are absent. Aqueous production may be from the root of the iris. The iridocorneal angle is filled with a mesh of mesenchymal-appearing cells and is separated from the anterior chamber by the annular ligament. There is incomplete separation of vitreous and aqueous humours, and the drainage of aqueous humour is not well understood.

Lens

The anterior portion of the large spherical lens protrudes past the iris, providing teleosts with wide-angle vision. The lens consists of a hyaline lens capsule surrounding the lens epithelium, cortex and nucleus. It is suspended by the suspensory ligament. Further support is provided by a posterior retractor lentis muscle in teleosts or an anterior protractor lentis muscle in elasmobranchs. Unlike the pliable mammalian lens, the fish lens is inflexible and accommodation is achieved by using these muscles to change its position within the globe.

Retina

The optic nerve enters the eye through either one or several optic discs posterior to the falciform process. Retinal anatomy is similar to that of other animals but receptor type and morphology vary among species. Deep-dwelling and nocturnal fish, for example, have a retina that is dominated by rods, while diurnal reef or shallow-water species are 'cone-rich'.

Light response

Without eyelids or the ability to decrease pupil size rapidly, fish rely on one of two methods to protect photoreceptors from bright light. The first is to retract the rods or cones into the retinal pigment epithelium. The second is to increase the amount of pigment in the retinal epithelial processes that surround stationary receptors. Both processes are slow and may take up to 2 hours to achieve complete protection. Therefore, a fish exposed to sudden and intense light may suffer retinal damage.

Investigations

Before the fish is handled, it should be observed swimming. Fish transported in containers that are opaque or that produce optical distortion can be placed in a clean glass tank for viewing. Asymmetry, opacity of the cornea or lens, corneal ulceration, periorbital or ocular gas and rupture of the eye are easily seen. Unilateral exophthalmos, for example, is often indicative of a localized infection, while bilateral exophthalmos suggests systemic involvement. Increased respiration, erythematous fins, abnormal posture and behaviour also suggest systemic disease. Most fish with compromised vision will keep the most affected eye away from the viewer. Small nets or other objects placed adjacent to the fish usually elicit a visually mediated behavioural response and can help the clinician to position the fish for viewing both eyes. With this method, some fish will clearly show a loss of vision; others may be difficult to assess due to cues from non-visual sensory systems. Digital cameras are useful to document the progression of ocular disease and the response to treatment.

Fish should be anaesthetized for safe handling. An aerated solution of buffered tricaine methane sulphonate delivered at 50–200 mg/l is recommended. Once anaesthetized, the fish should be placed gently in a lateral position on a non-abrasive, moistened plastic surface. This will help to prevent injury to the eye that is in contact with the surface. Anaesthesia can be maintained by passing the solution through the fish's mouth and over the gills using a syringe or other system, as described in Chapter 11.

A systematic ocular examination can be made using a direct ophthalmoscope, but a slit lamp is superior because it gives excellent magnification and allows a detailed evaluation of the depth of lesions in the cornea, anterior chamber, iris and lens. The fundus is best examined using indirect ophthalmoscopy (Figure 18.4). A pupillary light response is not easily observed in most fish and is therefore rarely useful. Once the initial examination has been made, the fish can be returned to either the anaesthetic solution or recovery water while preparations are made to conduct any further clinical tests. Ultrasound scanning of the eye using a 10 MHz probe is useful for investigating ocular disorders in large fish.

Systemic disease is often accompanied by conjunctival, corneal, iridal, lenticular or other changes in the eye. Corneal scrapings, using the blunt edge of a scalpel blade, or impression smears are easily collected for cytological examination.

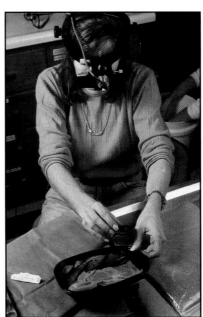

Figure 18.4
The fundus is best examined using indirect ophthalmoscopy. (© National Aquarium in Baltimore.)

Corneal ulceration or damage to the corneal epithelium can be assessed by staining with fluorescein or rose bengal stain. In cases of uveitis and panophthalmitis, a sample of vitreous or aqueous humour can be collected for cytology and aerobic, anaerobic and fungal culture using a 0.3 mm diameter needle. The site of penetration at the limbus is first cleansed using a topical disinfectant such as diluted chlorhexidine. The needle is then gently advanced into the eye, being careful not to damage any structures. Once the needle has been withdrawn, a small drop of cyanomethacrylate glue is used to seal the site.

Uveitis and panophthalmitis in fish can result from systemic conditions. Therefore, a complete physical examination is recommended for all fish presenting with ocular disease.

A systematic approach

The clinical signs of diseases of the eye can be grouped into:

- Scleral infections
- Keratitis
- Corneal ulceration
- Cataracts
- Lenticulopathy
- Uveitis
- Retinopathy
- Exophthalmos
- Gas accumulation.

Scleral infections
The sclera is rarely the site of infection, but *Myxobolus hoffmani* and *M. scleroperca* have been found in freshwater fish.

Keratitis
Superficial keratitis is seen grossly as corneal opacity. As the condition worsens, the cornea becomes more opaque and neovascularization may be observed. Punctate staining with fluorescein is indicative of epithelial damage. Interstitial keratitis is often associated with uveitis and involves the stroma and endothelium. Increased cloudiness of the cornea occurs due to corneal oedema, cellular infiltrates and fibroplasia. Actinic keratitis may result from excessive exposure to ultraviolet radiation. Nutritional causes of keratitis include deficiencies of vitamin A, riboflavin, or thiamine.

Parasites frequently cause damage to the cornea. Parasitic cysts within the cornea (such as those of the myxosporean *Myxobolus heterospora*) are rare, while damage caused by external parasites is common. Protozoa, including *Tetrahymena*, *Cryptocaryon*, *Ichthyophthirius*, *Henneguya* and *Glugea*, typically infect the skin and gills of fish and can also cause keratitis. Monogenetic trematodes (e.g. *Neobenedenia*), turbellarians and copepods, including *Lernaea* (anchorworm) and *Argulus* (fish lice), may cause serious damage, leading to ulcerative keratitis if treatment is not administered quickly. The diagnosis of many parasitic conditions requires microscopic examination of a corneal scraping, though some metazoa are easily recognized using a magnifying glass and a bright light. Bacterial and fungal keratitis are best diagnosed with impression smears or corneal scrapings prepared with Gram and Wright–Giemsa stains. Treatment must be specific for the organism identified.

Corneal ulceration
Ulcerative keratitis is common in ornamental fish and often results from trauma received during shipping, from aggressive tank mates, or from handling. Parasitic trematodes such as *Neobenedenia* are notorious for causing damage to the corneal epithelium that leads to ulceration. Vacuolation and swelling of the endothelium may also result in ulcerative keratitis. This condition is suspected when fish develop acute corneal opacity with or without evidence of a crater-like defect (Figure 18.5). The diagnosis is confirmed during examination of the eye by the retention of fluorescein stain (Figure 18.6), which fluoresces under cobalt blue light.

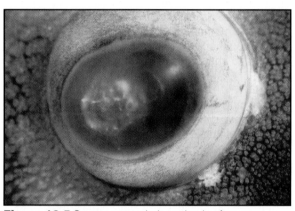

Figure 18.5 Severe corneal ulceration is often seen without the aid of special stains. This cornea is opaque due to oedema. (© National Aquarium in Baltimore.)

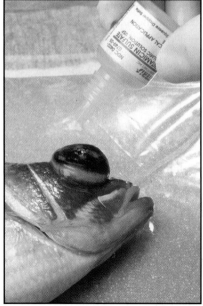

Figure 18.6 Exophthalmos and a severe corneal ulcer are being treated with ophthalmic gentamicin sulphate in this squirrelfish. The fluorescent green coloration of the cornea is due to retention of fluorescein dye. (© National Aquarium in Baltimore.)

In order to determine the course of treatment, it is important to know the extent of the corneal ulcer. Superficial ulcers enter only the superficial stroma, while deep ulcers affect the deep stroma and approach the corneal endothelium. A descemetocele results when only Descemet's membrane and the corneal endothelium remain intact. Descemet's membrane does not retain fluorescein, therefore only the walls of the ulcer fluoresce when examined with cobalt blue light. A descemetocele requires emergency treatment if rupture of the eye is to be prevented.

Fish treated for ulcerative keratitis should be separated from tank mates. Water quality must be excellent in order to minimize contamination by microorganisms, since nitrogenous wastes and other organic materials enhance the production of bacteria and fungi that can cause rapid progression of superficial ulcers. Salt may be added to a freshwater fish tank in order to reduce corneal oedema. Long-term antimicrobial baths are recommended. The author has had good success using Furazone Green, a commercial product containing nitrofurazone, furazolidone and methylene blue. It is used at the rate of 0.017 g/l of tank water for 10–14 days. If bacterial uveitis is present, injectable antibiotics are recommended.

Cyanoacrylate ophthalmic adhesive can be used to provide a waterproof patch for up to 10 days, allowing time for the corneal epithelium to heal. It can take less than 15 minutes to place a glue patch on the cornea. After the fish is anaesthetized, the ulcer is dried using sterile cotton swabs and flooded with a mixture of ophthalmic tobramycin and chloramphenicol. The swabs are then used to debride loose and necrotic corneal tissue. Additional antibiotic solution is placed on the lesion and allowed to soak for up to 1 minute before drying with sterile cotton swabs. A thin layer of cyanoacrylate adhesive is applied using a tuberculin syringe. Formaldehyde released from the glue as it cures provides additional antimicrobial protection. The repair is more likely to be successful with superficial ulcers. Deep corneal ulcers may benefit from the addition of a collagen shield.

Cataracts

Cataracts are common in ornamental fish. Fish owners readily notice when their pet's eye becomes opaque, and occasionally when there is loss of vision in one or both eyes (Figure 18.7). Lenticular opacities occur due to pathological changes, including hydropic swelling, lens fibre lysis, and epithelial hyperplasia resulting from trauma, malnutrition, toxic insult or infectious disease. Cataracts are defined by location and the quality and severity of the lesion.

Nutritional deficiency of zinc, riboflavin, methionine and tryptophan have been implicated in the development of cataracts in aquaculture species, and it is likely that they play a role in ornamental fishes. Ultraviolet (UV) radiation exposure can also cause cataracts and should be considered when ornamental pond fish develop cataracts. Most UV light is removed in the first 45 cm of water; therefore, providing sections of the pond with greater depths may be preventive.

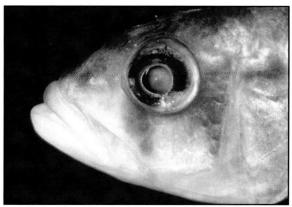

Figure 18.7 Hypermature cataract in a red-eyed guarti. (© National Aquarium in Baltimore.)

Cataracts can also be osmotically induced. Corneal ulceration leading to corneal oedema can cause the formation of cataracts due to dilution of the aqueous humour. These temporary cataracts resolve when water quality is improved or the ulceration heals. Most other cataracts are permanent.

Metacercariae of digenetic trematodes, including several species of *Diplostomum*, are reported to cause cataracts in aquaculture species as they migrate into the anterior segment of the lens. Three treatments, one every 5 days with a 2-hour bath of 2 mg praziquantel per litre, may reduce the number of parasites but does not diminish tissue reaction to dead metacercaria. Snails, which serve as the secondary host for digenetic trematodes, should be removed from the environment.

Cataracts can be differentiated from corneal disease and characterized using a slit lamp to define the location of the lesion. Most ornamental fish, especially those in small tanks and eating dead, pelleted or flake foods, are not severely affected by immature cataracts. Treatment of individuals with mature bilateral cataracts is accomplished by surgical removal of the lens (Figures 18.8 and 18.9). Unlike mammals, a fish lens affected by a cataract is extremely hard and phacoemulsification has not proved effective. Therefore surgical excision is required but should only be performed by those with proper training and equipment.

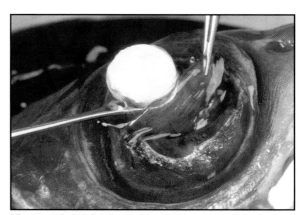

Figure 18.8 A fish lens affected by a cataract is extremely hard and must be removed completely, as seen in this squirrelfish. (© National Aquarium in Baltimore.)

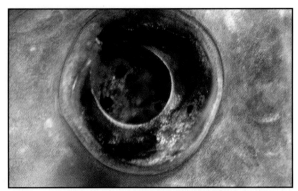

Figure 18.9 A guarti 3 weeks after removal of the lens. A small amount of corneal opacity remains at the site of the incision. (© National Aquarium in Baltimore.)

Lenticulopathy

Lens detachment and rupture of the hyaline capsule can occur. Release of lens proteins into the vitreous humour causes uveitis or endophthalmitis, which may result in rupture of the cornea or sclera and consequent phthisis bulbi. Rupture of the eye can also result in loss of the lens. Lenticular swelling leading to permanent damage is seen when fish are exposed to certain toxins, including crude oil.

Uveitis

Many diseases of the eye can cause inflammation of the uvea (the vascular coat of the eye comprising the iris and choroid). Diseases affecting the choroid include gas bubble disease, septicaemia, and myxozoan and microsporean infection. Systemic disease, metazoal migration and trauma can also cause uveitis. Non-specific sources of inflammation may include waterborne toxins.

Clinical signs include hyphaema, hyperaemia, hypopyon and aqueous flare (Figure 18.10). When uveitis is suspected, a complete examination of the fish, including blood culture, should be performed. If the infection is localized to one eye, an intraocular tap for bacterial and fungal culture is recommended as well as cytology. Treatment must be appropriate for the agents isolated and is likely to include antibiotics, antifungals and anti-inflammatory drugs. Water quality must be excellent in order to reduce the risk of further damage by non-specific inflammatory agents.

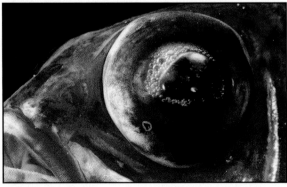

Figure 18.10 Uveitis in a squirrelfish. Hyphaema and gas are also present within the eye. (© National Aquarium in Baltimore.)

Retinopathy

Pathology of the retina is uncommon in fish, though vacuolation, cyst formation, hypertrophy, atrophy, necrosis, oedema, detachment and metaplasia of various layers have been reported. Metazoan parasites can cause necrosis of the neural retina. Other reported conditions include retinopathy associated with spontaneous diabetes, retinoblastomas and adenocarcinoma in the retinal pigment epithelium. Nutritional imbalances and toxins may also affect the retina.

Exophthalmos

Commonly referred to as 'pop eye', exophthalmos typically occurs due to the formation of retrobulbar oedema, which pushes the eye outward. Gas in or behind the eye, and other conditions, such as a retrobulbar mass, can also be causes. Exophthalmos has been associated with gas supersaturation ('gas bubble disease'), infectious agents including viruses, bacteria, parasites and fungi, and neoplasia. Although unilateral exophthalmos is indicative of localized infection, the condition is more frequently bilateral (Figure 18.11), which is indicative of systemic disease. In severe cases of exophthalmos, stretching of the optic nerve may result in blindness.

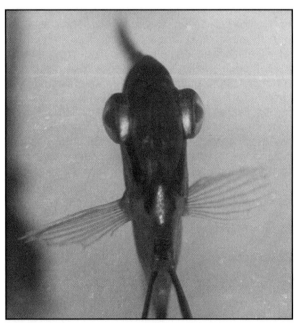

Figure 18.11 Bilateral exophthalmos in a freshwater angelfish with systemic infection. Unilateral exophthalmos is often suggestive of localized disease. (© Brent Whitaker)

The successful treatment of exophthalmos depends on identification and resolution of the underlying cause. Water quality parameters must be examined and a complete diagnostic work-up of the patient carried out. Empirical treatment with antibiotics and periorbital steroids has rarely been successful.

Gas accumulation

Intraocular and periocular gas (Figure 18.12) is commonly observed in marine fish and occasionally in freshwater species. Supersaturation of the water with gas or infection of the fish with gas-producing bacteria can cause this condition; however, in many cases the aetiology remains unidentified. The problem is most frequently seen in recently collected large-eyed marine teleosts such as the squirrelfish and the highhat. The decrease in atmospheric pressure from the fish's oceanic environment to the surface, and then again during transport by plane, may contribute to this condition.

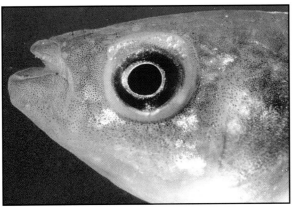

Figure 18.12 Periorbital gas is easily visible in this mummichog. The condition is caused by supersaturation of the water with air. (© National Aquarium in Baltimore.)

The accumulations of intraocular or periorbital gas that often accompany exophthalmos may cause tissue damage. This can lead to various pathological changes, including panophthalmitis, synechia formation, uveal oedema and congestion, spongiosis and suppuration of the cornea. Hydropic degeneration of the cornea, suppurative perineuritis of the optic nerve, rupture of the lens, cataract formation and thrombosis of the retinal artery leading to ischaemic necrosis of the globe may also occur. A diagnosis of supersaturation or gas bubble disease is easily made by finding gas bubbles in or around the eye, as well as in fin and gill clips examined under the microscope. More than one fish is usually affected. Diagnosis of other causes of gas accumulation may require an intraocular or periocular tap. This procedure can be used to reduce the amount of gas (and therefore the pressure) in the eye while collecting a small amount of aqueous humour for culture and cytology.

Treatment of fish with gas bubble disease is supportive and includes removing excess gas from the water by agitation and administering steroids and antibiotics to the fish, as appropriate. Treatment of chronic gas accumulation without an identified aetiology may benefit from the use of a carbonic anhydrase inhibitor such as acetazolamide at 6–10 mg/kg by a subconjunctival or peribulbar route once and then repeated as needed. Sygnathids (sea horses) are treated at a reduced dosage of 2–3 mg/kg by intramuscular or intracoelomic injection. This will, in some cases, reduce the production of new gas by the choroid gland. Removal of the pseudobranch may be helpful in cases that recur after initial response to a carbonic anhydrase inhibitor.

Causative agents

Infectious organisms

Bacteria, fungi, viruses, parasites and other infectious organisms can cause generalized infection of the globe and periocular tissues. Bilateral exophthalmos, endophthalmos, uveitis and opacity of ocular tissues are suggestive of systemic disease, while unilateral conditions are suggestive of localized infection. Ocular lesions are often readily apparent to the owner and the reason for visiting the veterinarian; however, the veterinarian should always complete a full physical examination in order to rule out systemic disease.

Parasites

Many parasites infect the eye. In addition to lenticular lesions and cataracts, digenetic trematodes can cause exophthalmos, lens dislocation, capsular rupture and subsequent uveitis, retinal cysts and retinal detachment. Although rare in ornamental species, helminth infections can also cause serious damage to the eye, including haemorrhagic uveitis, cataract formation, lens rupture, retinal detachment and rupture of the globe. External parasites, including monogenetic trematodes and crustaceans (*Lernaea* and *Argulus*), are capable of piercing the eye and initiating infection that often leads to damage of the cornea, lens and other ocular tissues. External protozoal parasites primarily infect the skin but can also damage the cornea.

Diagnosis of an external parasitic infection is made by taking a corneal scraping and finding the organisms in a wet mount. Some trematodes and copepods are large enough to identify grossly.

An accurate identification of the parasite and its life cycle is necessary to provide a proper treatment regime. Before therapy, a large water change (50% or more) is recommended to dilute the parasite burden. Details of specific antiparasitic medications can be found in Chapter 30.

In some cases, osmotic shock can be helpful for removing external parasites. For example, placing a shark in a freshwater bath for up to 5 minutes, or a teleost in a bath for 3–15 minutes, causes the trematodes to become opaque. Those that do not fall off can be removed manually. Similarly, freshwater fish can be given a saltwater bath (10–30 g/l). Unfortunately, many trematodes will recover once returned to their natural habitat.

Bacteria

Ocular lesions frequently accompany bacterial infections. In addition to increased respiration, poor body posture, erythematous and haemorrhagic skin and fins, septic fish may have uveitis, corneal opacity, or panophthalmitis (Figure 18.13). While the corneal lesions are often the result of trauma from lying on the bottom of the tank or being attacked by tank mates while debilitated, most of the lesions are due to the effects of circulating bacteria such as *Staphylococcus*, *Streptococcus*, *Aeromonas*, *Pseudomonas* and *Vibrio* species. Panophthalmitis may be accompanied by granulomatous lesions caused by *Mycobacteria*, *Nocardia* and *Flavobacterium*.

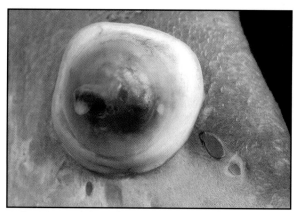

Figure 18.13 Panophthalmitis secondary to the rupture of a corneal ulcer and subsequent infection with opportunistic bacteria in a blue angelfish. (© National Aquarium in Baltimore.)

In cases of septicaemia, diagnosis is achieved by aseptically collecting blood for culture and cytology. In more localized infections, an intraocular tap may be required. Bacteria observed in these samples can be classified as Gram positive or negative, allowing the clinician to initiate treatment while cultures are pending. Granulomatous lesions caused by acid-fast bacteria are usually diagnosed histologically.

Fungi
Intraocular fungal disease is rare, while corneal invasion by fungi such as *Saprolegnia* in fish living in systems with poor water quality is more common. *Saprolegnia* are secondary invaders of corneal ulcers and other wounds. Cotton wool-like growths and corneal opacities are visible on the fish when it is in water. Once removed from water, the fungal mats collapse and may be difficult to see.

Diagnosis of external infection is made by observing the fungal hyphae on a corneal scraping. Intraocular infections require an intraocular tap followed by culture and cytology.

Treatment for external infections includes malachite green or formalin baths. Intraocular infections must be treated with a systemic pharmaceutical agent such as itraconazole. Doses are empirical but the author has had success at 10 mg/kg orally once daily for 30 days.

Viruses
A few viruses have been associated with ocular lesions. Exophthalmos may accompany viral diseases and has been associated with retrovirus and hepatic herpesvirus infections in salmon. Retinal vacuolation due to a nodavirus in flounder and a picornavirus in grouper has also been reported.

Lymphocystis, usually a self-limiting condition caused by an iridovirus, is common in ornamental fish and can sometimes affect corneal, iridal, choroidal, retrobulbar and optic nerve tissues. Lymphocystis is diagnosed by using light microscopy to find typical hypertrophied cells in a wet mount of a biopsy from the affected areas. Supportive care is the only treatment for viral infections.

Trauma
Ocular trauma can result in damage to all structures of the eye and rupture of the globe. These lesions are frequently seen in fish such as the cownose ray, whose anatomy provides little protection from the environment. They are also commonly observed in fish that have been recently collected or shipped. Periorbital abrasion with corneal ulceration, and occasionally hyphaema, are suggestive of trauma, which can result in loss of vision, uveitis, cataract and the formation of anterior or posterior synechiae.

Neoplasia
Primary neoplasia of the eye is rare, though a medulloepithelioma of the ciliary body has been diagnosed in a goldfish. As captive fish live longer, the likelihood of diagnosing neoplasia will increase.

Malnutrition
The effects of poor nutrition have been well studied in aquaculture species. Malnutrition of ornamental species is likely to produce similar effects. Rainbow trout fed riboflavin-deficient diets develop keratitis, corneal opacity and cataracts. Fusion of the anterior lens and corneal endothelium may also occur. Experimentally induced hypovitaminosis A produces pitting of the cornea similar to that in other animals fed vitamin A-deficient diets. This may lead to exophthalmos (which is seen with fluorescein as punctate staining) and uveitis, followed by retinal vacuolization and degeneration.

Further reading

Dukes TW (1975) Ophthalmic pathology of fishes. In: *The Pathology of Fishes*, ed. WW Ribelin and G Migaki, pp. 383–398. University of Wisconsin Press, Madison, Wisconsin

Hargis WJ (1991) Disorders of the eye in finfish. *Annual Review of Fish Diseases* **1**, 95–117

Kern TJ (1998) Exotic animal ophthalmology. In: *Veterinary Ophthalmology*, ed. KN Gelatt, pp. 1273–1306. Lippincott Williams and Wilkins, Baltimore, Maryland

Whitaker BR (1993) The diagnosis and treatment of corneal ulcers in fish. *Proceedings of the American Association of Zoo Veterinarians*, pp. 92–95. St Louis, Missouri

Wilcock BP and Dukes TW (1989) The eye. In: *Systemic Pathology of Fish*, ed. H Ferguson, pp. 168–194. Iowa State University Press, Ames, Iowa

Williams CR and Whitaker BR (1997) The evaluation and treatment of common ocular disorders in teleosts. *Seminars in Avian and Exotic Pet Medicine* **6:3**, 160–169

Acknowledgements

I thank Valerie Lounsbury, Nathan Yates and Angie Lawrence for their constructive review of this chapter. In addition, I extend my sincere gratitude to Susie Ridenour, librarian at the National Aquarium in Baltimore, whose perseverance made it possible to receive several needed references in a timely manner. Lastly, I thank Don Nichols, pathologist at the National Zoological Park, for his assistance with the histological anatomy of the fish eye and Helen MacFarlane, a student of the Johns Hopkins Art as Applied to Medicine program, who illustrated it.

19

Behavioural changes

Ruth Francis-Floyd and William H. Wildgoose

CHAPTER PLAN:
Feeding behaviour
Anorexia
    Ammonia
    Adverse pH
    Parasites
    Bacteria
    Dehydration
    Predation
Dysphagia
    Foreign body
    Neoplasia
Pica

Swimming behaviour
Abnormal schooling
Spinning, surfing or disorientation
    Ammonia
    Bacteria
        Streptococcus
        Edwardsiella ictaluri
    Viruses
    Toxins
        Organophosphates
        Flubendazole
    Parasites
        Myxobolus cerebralis
Piping
    Hypoxia
    Nitrite toxicity
    Gill disease
        Parasites
        Bacteria
    Anaemia
Abnormal buoyancy
    Excess positive buoyancy

Swim-bladder disorder
Gastrointestinal disease
    Edwardsiella tarda
Excess negative buoyancy
    Collapsed swim-bladder
    Gastric foreign body
Listing
Abnormal pitch
    Edwardsiella tarda
    Swim-bladder rupture
    Swim-bladder collapse
    Swim-bladder fluid
    CNS disease
Hanging or drifting
Flashing
    Ectoparasites
    Poor water quality
Jumping
    Hypoxia
    Inappropriate pH
    Waterborne irritant
Coughing
Clamped fins

Reproductive behaviour
Lip-lock
Spawning

Aggressive behaviour
Chasing and fin nipping
Territorial behaviour

Colour change
Courtship
Camouflage
Disease

Behavioural changes are often the first indication that there may be a health problem with a group of fish. Observant aquarists who are attuned to the normal behaviour of their pets may recognize when they are ill several days before fish actually begin to die. As in most aspects of veterinary medicine, an owner's observations should carry considerable weight with the clinician when assessing a situation. Teaching clients to observe their fish daily is an important educational tool.

Observation of behaviour in pond fish can be difficult, especially if an algal bloom is present. Often, it is only possible to observe fish at feeding times, and this may provide inadequate information unless the behavioural change is truly extreme – such as sudden cessation of all feeding activity. Careful observers might detect more subtle changes in the behaviour of pond fish and this level of acuity should be encouraged. By contrast, observation of fish in aquaria is much easier. Owners should pay attention to feeding behaviour, swimming behaviour and interactions between individuals. Specific behaviours and their possible significance can be classified into:

- Feeding behaviour
- Swimming behaviour
- Reproductive behaviour
- Aggressive behaviour
- Colour change.

Feeding behaviour

Changes in feeding behaviour are often the first indication of ill health. The most common changes are complete anorexia or decreased food consumption, an apparent inability to swallow food and occasionally, pica. A full health assessment of fish with changed feeding patterns is strongly recommended. The fish should be observed as closely as possible and any individuals that appear unwell should be removed to a separate facility for observation. Some medications can only be administered in the feed, therefore early detection of disease is essential for a successful outcome.

Anorexia

Anorexia in fish is a non-specific sign and can be due to various causes, including handling stress, adverse environmental conditions and infectious disease. A sudden cessation of feeding activity is cause for concern in any population of fish. Changes in water quality such as a sudden decrease in temperature, high ammonia or inappropriate pH may cause fish to stop feeding. Specific water quality parameters that may lead to anorexia are difficult to define due to species-specific requirements and adaptation to different environments.

Occasionally, fish become anorexic for no obvious reason. In the absence of an obvious abnormality, tube feeding with high calorie dietary supplements may stimulate the appetite. A thorough diagnostic evaluation, including a faecal examination and survey radiographs, is indicated before tube feeding. Large piscivores in public aquaria may develop prolonged anorexia for up to one month and occasionally force-feeding these fish will stimulate their appetite.

Ammonia

Many fish stop eating when ammonia levels are high. However, channel catfish that have lived in a high ammonia environment are able to adapt to it and may continue to feed despite extremely high concentrations of toxic un-ionized ammonia (> 2 mg/l).

pH

For freshwater fish, pH extremes that may lead to anorexia may be < 5.5 or > 10, but this varies considerably with species. For many freshwater species, pH extremes of < 4.0 or > 11.0 are lethal. Marine fish are generally less tolerant of pH extremes and their preferred pH is usually from 8.0 to 8.3, though some species may tolerate 7.5–7.8.

Parasites

Fish with heavy ectoparasite burdens will often start eating again, or more voraciously, when the parasites have been removed. Intestinal flagellate infections (e.g. *Spironucleus*) can be treated with metronidazole. Initially, therapy can be delivered by immersion and then changed to a medicated feed as the appetite improves.

Bacteria

If anorexia is due to bacterial infection, it is possible to initiate antimicrobial therapy either by injection or by immersion, and then change to an oral route when feeding resumes.

Dehydration

It is advisable to assess hydration status in anorexic marine species. In some cases, the use of freshwater or similar physiological fluid can be administered by gastric intubation to treat dehydration.

Predation

The first step in the investigation of anorexia in pond fish is to confirm that the fish are still present. Owners may not be aware of predators entering their pond, particularly if there is poor visibility. The lack or reduction of visible feeding activity is sometimes the only evidence that fish are no longer present. Signs of predation may not always be seen but the presence of piscivorous birds, certain animal tracks or some geographical locations may suggest that predation is possible. Fish most susceptible to predation are brightly coloured varieties such as goldfish or koi, or those that are frequently at the surface, as may occur with oxygen depletion. Deterring predators from small ponds includes the use of nets and bird-wire strung across the top of the pond. Electrified wire strung 30 cm above the ground around the perimeter of the pond may deter otters.

Dysphagia

Occasionally, a fish may be seen taking food particles into its mouth but allowing the food to float out again a few seconds later. Examination of the mouth and pharynx is essential, since fish may be thin and debilitated by the time they are presented and may not have eaten for several weeks.

Foreign bodies

Some fish, particularly red-tailed catfish, will swallow rocks, sand or other foreign bodies from the tank. These may cause obstruction and make it impossible for the fish to swallow. Careful examination of the mouth and pharyngeal area is strongly recommended – particularly in fish that have been collected by hook and line, since these occasionally have fishing tackle lodged in the pharynx.

Neoplasia

Oral neoplasia may occur in old fish and is discussed in Chapter 16. Pharyngeal obstruction in African cichlids due to goitre has been recorded (Wolf *et al.*, 1998) but concurrent *Mycobacterium* infection was present.

Pica

Pica is not fully understood in fish and in many instances is difficult or impossible to observe. Some species, most notably cichlids, frequently rearrange their environment by moving rocks and other objects around the tank. This behaviour is probably not harmful but intestinal impaction with sand or gravel has been reported, particularly in elasmobranchs in public aquaria. Diagnosis is usually confirmed by radiography. Treatment has included gastric intubation with lubricant. Early detection can be difficult and many of these cases are not recognized until postmortem examination. Impaction or foreign body ingestion should be considered in cases with anorexia, weight loss and lethargy, especially if fish are known to ingest objects from their environment.

Swimming behaviour

Abnormal or unusual swimming behaviour is often an early sign of disease in captive fish. These changes are more easily observed in fish kept in aquaria rather than ponds but observant owners quickly note subtle changes in swimming behaviour.

Abnormal schooling

Schooling is a social characteristic displayed by some species that swim in large numbers as an aggregate unit. Schooling fish can be differentiated from other fish that live in close proximity to conspecifics by the uniform geometric orientation maintained by the school. The fish may disperse when startled or during feeding. Lack of the behaviour in fish that normally school may be a sign of disease, particularly if only one fish is affected, or an environmental problem if the entire population behaves abnormally. Affected individuals should be removed and, depending on their value, should be thoroughly examined or, if debilitated, sacrificed for a full postmortem examination. Blindness should be ruled out as a cause of the change.

Spinning, surfing and disorientation

Spinning, surfing and general disorientation may be signs of neurological disease in fish. Extreme examples are obvious but the signs may be subtle and may only be noticed when fish are startled.

Ammonia

Acute ammonia toxicity is a well recognized cause of neurological disease in fish. This can result from a sudden increase in total ammonia, as might occur with 'new tank syndrome'. Alternatively, increased levels of toxic un-ionized ammonia may arise following a sudden increase in pH due to algal bloom in the presence of lower levels of ammonia. Where possible, frequent water changes (up to 50% daily) may be required to reduce ammonia levels. However, if the total ammonia concentration is high and pH is low, then water changes should be performed with caution. It is possible to precipitate a catastrophic fish kill by raising the pH before the ammonia has been eliminated from the system, resulting in a sudden and possibly lethal increase in the level of toxic un-ionized ammonia.

Bacteria

Bacterial infections known to cause neurological signs in fish include *Streptococcus* (e.g. *S. iniae*) and *Edwardsiella ictaluri*. Streptococcal infections have been reported in both freshwater and saltwater fish but they may be more severe in brackish and marine environments. Although *E. ictaluri* is primarily a problem in channel catfish, the organism has been described as a cause of meningitis in non-ictalurid fish. Samples from the brain of any fish showing neurological signs, particularly spinning, should be cultured.

Viruses

Spinning or other neurological signs are possible indications of viral diseases. Wolf (1988) and Plumb (1999) provided excellent reviews of viral diseases, including presenting signs for various species. Viral investigations are often pursued after more obvious causes have been ruled out.

Toxins

Toxins may also affect normal behaviour. Organophosphate toxicity may result in slow spinning or spiralling before death. The anthelmintic flubendazole has caused severe jaundice in discus fish, with quivering in the corner of the tank followed by uncontrollable spinning for several seconds (Francis-Floyd, 1994); the concentration of flubendazole used was not known and it was not possible to reproduce the same clinical signs.

Parasites

Whirling disease in salmonids is due to infection of fry with *Myxobolus cerebralis*. Fish under 6 months of age reared in earth ponds ingest the parasite in an intermediate host (e.g. *Tubifex* worm), which migrates to the cartilages of the skull. Damage and deformity caused to the auditory capsule and vertebrae result in a characteristic swimming abnormality of affected fish ('tail chasing'), particularly when they are fed or disturbed.

Piping

Gulping air at the surface is frequently referred to as 'piping'. It is often associated with hypoxia but can be normal behaviour in some fish. Air-breathing fish such as lungfish, labyrinth fish and some eels can utilize atmospheric oxygen and frequently gulp air from the surface. Surface-dwelling fish such as leaf-fish spend prolonged intervals at the surface. Siamese fighting fish and some gouramis build nests of bubbles for egg laying.

Abnormal behaviour is most obvious when the fish are startled: they will swim down into the water column briefly, but will return to the surface almost immediately. Piping represents an effort by the fish to utilize oxygen from a thin surface layer of water that is saturated with dissolved atmospheric oxygen.

If fish are severely stressed, aeration should be provided immediately. Affected fish may not tolerate a normal chemical treatment and so extreme care is recommended if any medications are used. Gill tissue will recover quickly when the cause of damage is removed.

Hypoxia

Low levels of dissolved oxygen are the commonest cause of piping. It is important to collect a water sample for measurement of dissolved oxygen. Confirming a diagnosis is often difficult, unless the water is tested while the fish are showing clinical signs. Dissolved oxygen levels vary significantly during the day.

Nitrite toxicity

High nitrite levels cause methaemoglobinaemia. Affected fish become dyspnoeic and the gills turn chocolate-brown in colour. Although possible, it is not always practical to measure methaemoglobin levels in blood and diagnosis is based on water quality tests and clinical signs.

Gill disease

Many types of gill disease result in clinical hypoxia. This includes parasitic infestations, bacterial infection and gill damage caused by over-treatment with caustic chemicals (e.g. formalin, potassium permanganate).

Parasites: Ichthyophthirius multifiliis infection is sometimes restricted to gill tissue and can cause catastrophic damage. The classical white spots that characterize these infections may not be visible but examination of gill tissue will reveal pale swollen filaments with massive numbers of parasites on wet mounts. Proliferative gill disease of channel catfish, caused by the myxozoan *Aurantiactinomyxon ictaluri*, is a well recognized cause of mortality.

Bacteria: Columnaris disease can cause significant destruction of gill tissue and is caused by bacteria of the genera *Flavobacterium*, *Cytophaga* and *Flexibacter*. Diagnosis can be made following gross examination and biopsy of affected tissue.

Anaemia

Anaemic fish may develop clinical hypoxia. The fish swim at the surface and may exhibit piping and increased respiratory rates. Anaemia can be confirmed by observing very pale or white gills and a low haemocrit in a blood sample. The causes of anaemia in fish are varied and not fully understood but include nutritional disease (vitamin deficiency), environmental disease (chronic exposure to low levels of nitrite) and infectious disease such as blood parasites (e.g. trypanosomes). Further details can be found in Chapter 17.

Abnormal buoyancy

Buoyancy abnormalities are relatively common in ornamental fish and can vary in severity according to the underlying aetiology. Some subtle cases may only be detected when the fish is at rest, since many will actively swim to compensate for any abnormality. Buoyancy disorders are discussed in Chapter 16 and are grouped into:

- Excess positive buoyancy ('floating')
- Excess negative buoyancy ('bottom sitting')
- Listing
- Abnormal pitch.

In most cases, radiography is required to visualize the distribution of gas in the body and help to identify the cause. Both lateral and dorsoventral views are required. Manual repositioning of the fish in the water will also indicate if a unilateral lesion is present: fish will rotate or return to the original abnormal position.

Excess positive buoyancy

Excessive amounts of gas within the body cause the fish to rise to the surface. This usually affects the swim-bladder but may also be due to gas within the gastro-intestinal tract or a gas-filled subcutaneous lesion, as sometimes occurs with *Edwardsiella tarda* infections.

Swim-bladder disorder: Over-inflated swim-bladders are common problems in certain fancy varieties of goldfish, particularly orandas (Figure 19.1). In many cases the cause is unknown and affected fish are often presented several days (if not months) after onset. Fish frequently list to one side or are completely upside-down. Many fish remain active and continue to eat, often swimming under objects to prevent themselves from floating to the surface. Management of these cases is difficult and not very rewarding. Air can be removed from the swim-bladder by paracentesis but fish often reinflate. New surgical procedures may improve the prognosis for some of these cases.

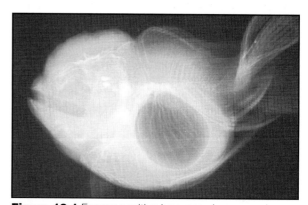

Figure 19.1 Excess positive buoyancy in an oranda (a fancy variety of goldfish) due to a grossly dilated swim-bladder. The problem had been present for 6 months and appeared to be associated with an excessively short body. Only one swim-bladder chamber is visible on the radiograph. (© W.H. Wildgoose.)

Gastrointestinal disease: Excessive gas in the bowel may cause fish to float to the surface (Figure 19.2). Freshwater angelfish with severe *Spironucleus* infestations may float at the surface but continue to eat. Examination of a fresh faecal sample may confirm the presence of large numbers of flagellates. Treatment with metronidazole, either in the food or as a bath, can be used and dramatic improvement should be noted within 24–48 hours.

Bacterial infection of the gut may also cause excessive gas production but these fish are often extremely ill and have no interest in food. A faecal culture may be useful and help to select an appropriate antibiotic.

Edwardsiella tarda: Infections may result in large gas-filled lesions between the dermis and skeletal muscle. Early infections may be readily visible along the lateral body wall and peduncle of the fish but these eventually burst, releasing gas with a foul odour. The organism usually responds quickly to appropriate antibiotic therapy and the mortality rate is usually low.

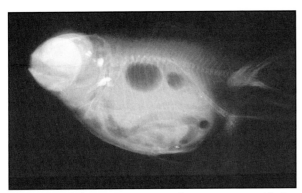

Figure 19.2 An excess amount of gas was present in the bowel of this fancy goldfish. This resulted in the fish floating at the surface when at rest, with the vent and anal fin above the surface of the water. The fish could regain its normal posture by intermittent active swimming, which also enabled it to feed. (© W.H. Wildgoose.)

Excess negative buoyancy

Resting on the bottom is normal behaviour for sedentary species and fish that are asleep. Sedentary species include *Plecostomus*, lungfish, algae eaters and some of the slower catfish. These fish are frequently hidden and move around very little unless stirred into activity by some external stimulus. Fish that are asleep lie on the bottom during periods of darkness and may initially be sluggish when roused or when the lights are switched on.

Excess negative buoyancy in normally active fish is due to loss of gas within the swim-bladder. This can be caused by rupture, filling with fluid or sometimes by pressure from intracoelomic space-occupying lesions. Occasionally, heavy gastric foreign bodies may make it difficult for the fish to swim to the surface.

Listing

Abnormal rotation along the longitudinal axis results in leaning over to one side (Figure 19.3). This can be associated with several disorders, some of which also cause either abnormal positive or negative buoyancy and are described above.

Abnormal pitch

This describes the relative position of the body in relation to its longitudinal axis and can be with head either up or down. It is often accompanied by some degree of listing. Many disorders that cause excess positive and negative buoyancy also cause abnormal pitch.

'Head standing' is also described as 'head-down', 'tail-up' or 'tail waving'. This is normal camouflage behaviour in some species such as shrimpfish, and is seen in many others while being attended by 'cleaner' fish. In diseased fish, head standing may be caused by:

- Large gas-filled lesions in the peduncle due to *Edwardsiella tarda*
- Rupture of the swim-bladder
- Collapse (Figure 19.4) or fluid filling of the anterior chamber in species with bilobed swim-bladders
- Degenerative changes in the central nervous system (Figure 19.5) or an abscess in the brain (Figure 19.6).

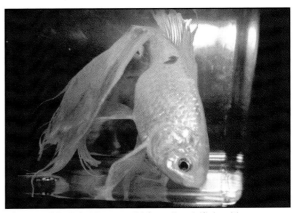

Figure 19.4 A 15-year-old fantail goldfish with a disorder that caused 'head standing' for over 7 years. Radiography revealed a collapsed anterior chamber of the swim-bladder, which was associated with a fibroma. In addition, a large granuloma was found in the cerebellum. (© W.H. Wildgoose.)

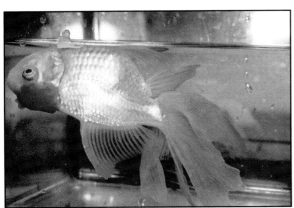

Figure 19.3 Excess positive buoyancy in a fancy goldfish. Abdominal swelling due to polycystic lesions in the kidney displaced the posterior chamber of the swim-bladder, which resulted in it consistently floating on one side. (© W.H. Wildgoose.)

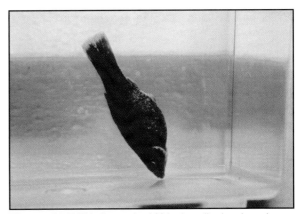

Figure 19.5 This 9-month-old black molly developed an abnormal 'head-standing' posture, which deteriorated over the course of one week. The same disorder had affected the parent and another offspring. Histopathological examination revealed vacuolation and degenerative changes in the mesencephalon. (© W.H. Wildgoose.)

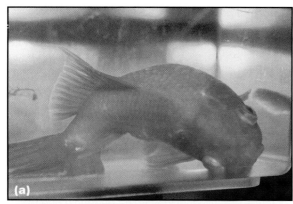

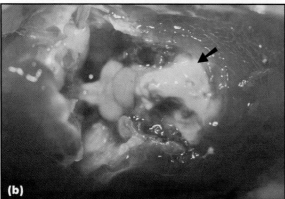

Figure 19.6 (a) A 7-year-old fantail goldfish that developed a sudden-onset loss of balance and incoordination. The fish lay on the bottom of the aquarium in an arched position and tended to revert to the same side when physically repositioned in the water. (b) A large granuloma (arrowed) found in the cranial cavity of the same goldfish. There were multiple granulomas in other organs, including the heart, spleen and kidney. Acid-fast bacilli were found in several of these lesions. (© W.H. Wildgoose.)

Hanging or drifting

In contrast to buoyancy problems, fish that are truly hanging in the water column do not float up to the surface. These fish are often extremely weak and listless and usually have no interest in feeding. They may be buffeted by currents, creating the illusion that there is some swimming activity. Unless the cause of illness can be identified and corrected quickly, the prognosis is often poor.

Flashing

'Flashing' describes a scratching behaviour exhibited by fish. The 'flash' results from brief exposure of the pale belly when the fish rolls over to scratch its back or flank on the bottom surface or on some object. The behaviour is generally considered a sign of irritation, with ectoparasitic infestation being a primary cause, though poor water quality may also be a factor.

Jumping

Jumping may be an exaggerated form of darting or it may be an attempt to escape. Some species are more likely to jump as a normal activity and therefore it is important to keep the tank or pond covered with a lid or netting. Normal fish of any species may break the surface of the water when startled or chased by a predator. However, in many cases it is an attempt to escape from adverse environmental conditions such as low dissolved oxygen, inappropriate pH or the presence of a waterborne irritant.

Coughing

'Coughing' is a behaviour in which the fish essentially back-flushes water across the gills. This is thought to be an effort to dislodge debris from the gills, or indicates irritation from ectoparasites.

Clamped fins

Fish with clamped fins are usually lethargic and hold their fins close to the body. This is often a non-specific sign associated with ill health but it is a normal posture for many marine fish.

Reproductive behaviour

Reproductive or courtship behaviour can be easy to recognize, but there may be unusual species-specific activities that are only associated with reproduction. Many of these include establishing and maintaining a territory as well as attracting a mate. Some species may be very aggressive in this regard and compatibility is an important consideration.

Lip-lock

Cichlids in particular may be observed grabbing and holding on to the mouthparts of a mate during courtship. Occasionally abrasions may result. Lip fibromas have been observed in angelfish and trauma from lip-locking has been considered as a possible contributing factor. Viral particles have been found in these fibromas, which can be surgically removed with good results.

Spawning

Some species may spawn in captivity, even though this may not always be desirable. Koi in particular become quite active and may be observed rolling on the surface. Milt may foul the water and the uninformed owner may suspect that some chemical or pollutant has been introduced. In most cases, the behaviour is transient and seasonal.

Angelfish that spawn may take over a large portion of their tank and essentially restrict the other fish to one corner. Careful observation may reveal that the pair has laid eggs on some object (perhaps a plant or even a piece of pipework). Angelfish and other cichlids do provide a significant amount of parental care and this behaviour may continue for several weeks. Separating the breeding pair from other fish is recommended where possible.

African cichlids are mouth brooders. When females are incubating eggs or fry they become anorexic and they have the appearance of 'puffy cheeks'. To determine whether reproductive activity is the cause of their odd appearance, the fish can be gently restrained and the mouth opened. Eggs may be visible, or fry (if present) may be seen swimming in and out of the female's mouth. Fry left with the female may not survive unless plenty of cover is provided. Commercial producers remove fry from females and rear them in separate aquaria, since cichlids are prone to consuming fry when parental care is discontinued.

Aggressive behaviour

Some fish are aggressive by nature and can cause serious problems if placed with inappropriate species in a community tank. The most extreme form of aggression is cannibalism of tank mates. Inappropriate choice of species may result in survival of the fittest, with one very large fish emerging from a group of smaller ones. Aggressive behaviour can result in chronic stress and predispose fish to opportunistic infections.

Chasing and fin nipping
Chasing and fin nipping are signs of aggression and indicate that the species involved may not be compatible. Fish likely to engage in chasing and fin nipping include tiger barbs, angelfish and some loaches – species that are frequently recommended for community tanks. Chronic problems can occur if these species are placed with fish that are passive or have long flowing fins. Wounds that result from aggression may develop secondary infection. Providing adequate cover such as plants or rocks may reduce aggression but sometimes the only solution is to separate the incompatible fish.

Territorial behaviour
Some species are strongly territorial by nature. They will establish a territory and vigorously defend it if other fish venture into the area, as exhibited by many cichlids and reef fish. Offering enough habitats so that all contenders can establish their own space may reduce territorial problems in a home aquarium. Alternatively, fish can be crowded so that no individual is able to establish its own territory, a method commonly used for the commercial production of tilapia.

Colour change

Fish have a tremendous capacity to change colour and this may be associated with courtship displays, camouflage or illness.

Courtship
Colour change associated with reproductive activity is usually associated with brilliant hues – as exhibited by male African cichlids, which become extremely colourful when sexually active.

Camouflage
Colour change due to camouflage may be identified by changing the environment and observing for colour changes in the fish. For example, channel catfish placed in a white bucket become very pale, but will assume the more normal dark dorsal coloration when returned to a natural environment.

Disease
Colour change associated with illness is likely to be observed in an animal with other behavioural signs of malaise, including lethargy and poor appetite. The causes of skin colour change are discussed in Chapter 15. Discus fish become very dark (or even black) when ill or chilled. Standard water quality parameters and temperature should be examined before conducting a detailed health investigation. Extreme darkening has been observed in gouramis infected with iridovirus, and death often follows within 24–48 hours.

References and further reading

Francis-Floyd R, Bolon B and Reed P (1994) Flubendazole toxicity in discus (*Symphysodon* sp.). *Proceedings of the International Association for Aquatic Animal Medicine* **25**, 61

Plumb JA (1999) *Health Maintenance and Principal Microbial Diseases of Cultured Fishes*. Iowa State University Press, Ames, Iowa, 328 pp.

Wolf JC, Ginn PE and Francis-Floyd R (1998) Goiter in a colony of African cichlids. *Journal of Fish Disease* **21**, 139–143

Wolf K (1988) *Fish Viruses and Fish Viral Diseases*. Cornell University Press, Ithaca, New York, 476 pp.

20

Sudden death

William H. Wildgoose

CHAPTER PLAN:	
Investigations	Gas bubble disease
A systematic approach	Hyperthermia
Environmental effects	Noxious algae
Hypoxia	**Infection**
Reduced oxygen saturation levels	**Accident**
Restricted gas exchange	Escape
Reduced photosynthesis	Electrocution
Increased consumption	Water loss
Toxins	Asphyxia
	Predation

In many cases, mortality is the first sign of a health problem. While these fish may appear to have died suddenly, owners have often overlooked the subtle signs of illness, particularly where there are many fish present in the same facility. This may reflect the owner's lack of experience and powers of observation. Fish remain unattended for several hours per day, during which time they may show signs of disease and die rapidly. Some fish may be overlooked while hiding among the plants and furniture in the tank or pond prior to being found dead.

The death of a single fish is a common event but it is not uncommon to receive a call from a distressed owner who has had most or all of their fish die suddenly, overnight. Similarly, owners may request a postmortem examination on a favourite or valuable fish that was found dead in the morning, having been healthy and feeding the previous evening. Extreme events such as these are challenging cases to investigate and require a methodical approach. Although it will be difficult to find the cause of mortality in many cases, it is important to show compassion and investigate the case as far as is practicable.

This chapter encompasses some of the common events that result in sudden and rapid mortality. It is hoped that it will assist in the diagnosis of cases where fish are found dead or dying with few signs of clinical disease.

Investigations

The investigation of these cases is often unrewarding but by necessity must be performed as soon as possible. In some cases, there may be legal or insurance aspects to consider, particularly where there are multiple deaths of valuable fish. Since much of the evidence in these instances can deteriorate rapidly, it is essential to keep accurate detailed records, both written and photographic. This may include keeping substantial samples of water in appropriate containers and the frozen carcasses of all the dead fish.

Clinical history

It is essential to take a detailed clinical history and note any changes leading up to the fatal event. Some problems, such as hypoxia, can only be determined from a clinical history since there is rarely any pathognomonic pathology. Particular attention should be paid to all recent events and where new fish have been introduced. Significant changes in management, such as excessive cleaning or switching off power to the biological filter, and the use of chemicals in and around the tank or pond must also be noted. Some features in the clinical history may suggest an underlying aetiology (Figure 20.1).

Clinical History	Possible Causes
All species, sudden onset	Waterborne toxin Accident
Few species, increasing numbers	Infectious disease
Solitary fish	Non-infectious disease Accident

Figure 20.1 Morbidity patterns.

Clinical examination

Detailed clinical examination of any survivors should be performed. Early signs of disease or lesions may be identified in subclinical cases and this may provide some clues as to the nature of the problem. The subtle signs of respiratory disease and internal disorders may not be grossly evident, particularly in small species. Due to the concealed location of the gill, fish may suffer severe gill damage before their respiration is compromised.

Water samples

Although accidental or malicious poisoning of garden ponds by neighbours is often suspected, it is usually very difficult to confirm unless there is supporting evidence. Substantial quantities of water should be kept frozen for specific toxicological analysis, as suggested in Chapter 26. Despite this, routine water quality tests should not be overlooked since these may reveal significant abnormalities. Due to the potential hazard to other aquatic life, water from these ponds should be disposed of carefully and after discussion with the relevant local water authority.

Postmortem examination

In many cases, the fish will have been dead for several hours and tissue autolysis will be advanced, particularly in warm weather. The cadaver should be placed in a sealed polyethylene bag and refrigerated or packed in ice until a postmortem examination is performed. Many motile protozoan parasites will have died, making their identification difficult, and there may be invasion by saprophytic organisms. It is still possible to recognize larger metazoan parasites by microscopy, even several hours after death.

Histopathology

Interpretation of tissue pathology may be inconclusive where postmortem change has occurred. Despite a sudden death, significant pathology in the major organs may suggest that disease was more longstanding than initially suspected.

Bacteriology

Samples from external surfaces will be of limited value due to contamination with commensals. In cases of peracute septicaemia, only swabs from the kidney may provide meaningful information.

Virology

Samples may be taken from autolysed tissues but subsequent virus culture may prove difficult and less reliable.

Toxicology

Frozen tissue samples may allow confirmation of poisoning in some cases but the laboratory should be contacted in advance for details of sample collection and preservation.

Radiography

Few lesions that cause sudden death will be visible on a radiograph. However, significant spinal fractures and dislocation may be present.

A systematic approach

Sudden death may affect one or more fish of the same species and may, in rare circumstances, affect all fish of different species in a facility. Most problems can be grouped according to aetiology:

• Environmental effects
• Infection
• Accident
• Predation.

Environmental effects

In most cases, environmental factors usually affect all those of the same species. Different species vary in their tolerance to adverse water conditions and more 'delicate' species in a mixed population may die while others remain unaffected.

Hypoxia

Hypoxic conditions may affect several fish of the same species, several different species or, in extreme cases, all fish. Larger fish have a greater oxygen demand and are often the first to die from hypoxia (Figure 20.2). In some cases, dead fish may be found with open mouths and flared opercula. Anaemia and gill disease such as hyperplasia and excess mucus will also reduce oxygen uptake by the fish. In many cases, the dissolved oxygen levels will have returned to normal before the investigation takes place, making it difficult to confirm hypoxia as the cause of death. However, supporting evidence may be revealed in a detailed clinical history.

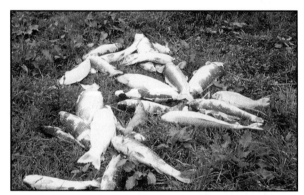

Figure 20.2 Sudden death of several large koi from a pond. The lack of any sign of disease and a clinical history of overnight mortality suggests death from hypoxia. (Courtesy of B. Brewster.)

In outdoor ponds, low oxygen levels occur just before sunrise when algal and aquatic plant respiration is at a peak. The level of dissolved oxygen is influenced by several factors, as follows.

Reduced oxygen saturation levels

The solubility of oxygen in water is reduced as the temperature and salinity increase.

Restricted gas exchange

Mechanical breakdown of water and air pumps or power failures may reduce oxygen levels by limiting gas exchange at the surface. Excessive growth of surface-living plants such as duckweed, lilies and floating iris will reduce the surface area and limit gas exchange at the air/water interface (Figure 20.3).

Reduced photosynthesis

Photosynthesis by aquatic plants and algae is reduced in cloudy weather and where there is excessive shade from surface plants. This will reduce oxygen production during the daytime and can affect the total dissolved oxygen level.

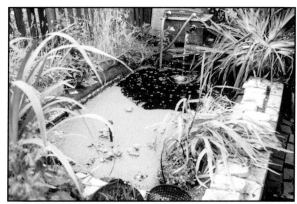

Figure 20.3 The heavy growth of surface plants in outdoor ponds restricts gas exchange at the air/water interface and reduces photosynthesis by limiting light penetration.

Increased consumption

This may occur due to overstocking, increased aerobic bacterial activity, algal blooms or use of oxygen-depleting chemicals such as formalin.

Toxins

Most toxic agents are not selective in their effect (Chapter 26). In many cases, most fish of all species will be affected. The deaths of amphibians and air-breathing fish in outdoor ponds may confirm the presence of noxious chemicals in the water rather than oxygen deficiency. Similarly, poor growth or death of plants and algae may suggest the presence of an environmental toxin that affects both flora and fauna.

The environment should be examined carefully for additional evidence of possible poisoning, such as a build-up of sludge in the filter unit, and any unusual smells, such as hydrogen sulphide and those associated with decaying organic matter. In new ponds, toxins leaching from pond finishes (for example, styrene leaching from newly applied fibreglass) may occur. The content of chlorine and chloramines in municipal water supplies varies considerably but may produce acute toxicity and death following excessive freshwater changes. Following heavy rain, water runoff from rockeries and overhanging chemically treated woodwork may wash fertilizer and chemicals into ponds. The toxic leaves, fruits or sap of some overhanging plants may also be responsible for sudden deaths. Unusual cases of poisoning have resulted from the release of tetrodotoxin from pufferfish and of mercury from broken thermometers.

Gas bubble disease

Faulty pumps, excessive photosynthesis by submerged plants and the use of borehole or spring water can cause supersaturation of water with nitrogen and other gases. This may produce fatal gas emboli in the blood and vital organs.

Hyperthermia

Faulty thermostats may result in overheating and mortality due to temperature stress. Aquaria exposed to the sun in hot summer weather may require shade or cooling systems to maintain optimal water temperatures for the species involved.

Noxious algae

Although uncommon, some noxious algae are associated with toxicoses to fish. In these cases, there are acute to chronic mortalities with respiratory and equilibrium problems. These signs are associated with water that is coloured red, green or brown and the suspended algae found in large numbers in gill and skin biopsies. Samples of algae should be taken for identification.

Infection

There are few infectious agents that cause sudden death in more than a few fish. In most cases, other in-contact fish will exhibit mild signs of disease when examined carefully. However, during the hot summer months in the UK, heavy mortalities have occurred in koi due to severe gill necrosis. In some instances up to 100% mortality has been experienced and has often followed the introduction of new fish. This may be due to pathogenic koi herpesvirus.

Infection by mycobacteria is usually regarded as a chronic disease but in small tropical species it is not uncommon to have sudden death following a failure to identify obvious signs of illness.

Fish suffering from chronic internal disease such as neoplasia may also be found dead as a result of a secondary bacterial infection. This may account for some cases that are assumed to be a result of 'old age'.

Accident

Many types of accident cause death and these include being trapped in plants, tank or pond decor, filter inlets and the pump intake (Figure 20.4).

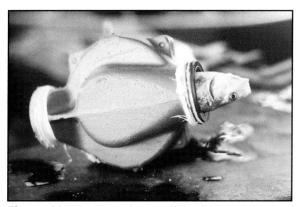

Figure 20.4 An unusual cause of death but one that could have been prevented by using a suitable grid over the inlet pipework. (Courtesy of B. Brewster.)

Escape

Aquaria should be covered, because some species commonly attempt to escape. These fish may sustain severe injury, concussion and death. Pond fish such as koi and goldfish are also known to jump out, particularly from shallow ponds and isolation facilities. There are anecdotal reports of fish being found several hours later, with dried skin, and then being returned to the water and making a full and uneventful recovery. Netting stretched across the pond can prevent these escapes.

Electrocution

This is a serious hazard to both the fish and the owner. Great care must be taken when switching off the electrical circuits. Depending on the duration and nature of the shock, some fish will recover and survive the incident, having been 'anaesthetized' by the stray current.

Water loss

Occasionally the outflow pipe from the pump may loosen and detach, resulting in large volumes of water being accidentally pumped out of the pond or tank. This is a particular problem when water is pumped to an external filter chamber.

Asphyxia

Gill obstruction from an oral foreign body, and even by frogs clasping a fish's head and operculae during the mating season, can result in suffocation.

Predation

Inappropriate mixing of some species, particularly in tropical aquaria, can result in predation by carnivorous species. Aggression from other fish is one of the commonest causes of injury in aquarium fish and may result in death. This is often regarded as a form of predation or territorial behaviour. Most marine fish are highly territorial and may even show aggression towards members of their own species. This problem can be prevented by the correct choice of species; recommendations can be found in most books for the hobbyist.

Fish in outdoor ponds are vulnerable to attack from piscivorous birds (cormorants, herons), reptiles (alligators, aquatic snakes) and mammals (cats, foxes, racoons, opossums and otters). Predated fish usually go missing but some may be found dead with characteristic external injuries. Suitable barriers should be erected and areas for fish to hide must be provided. Herons can be deterred by building steep pond sides that prevent access by wading, fixing wires or monofilament nylon around the pond, and installing decoys such as artificial predatory animals or herons.

Acknowledgement

The author is very grateful to Ian Walker, Todd Cecil and Frank Prince-Isles for their helpful comments with early drafts of the text and to Bernice Brewster for supplying some photographs.

21

Parasitic diseases

Matt Longshaw and Stephen W. Feist

Many of the huge number of parasites that have been recorded from fish are capable of inducing significant mortalities among captive and wild stocks. Accurate identification of parasites is important, in order that a build-up of parasite numbers can be prevented.

Information about transmission requirements and potential intermediate hosts is often crucial to selection of the most appropriate management action to reduce or eliminate the problem. While the greatest threat to fish is from organisms that do not require an intermediate host (including metazoan as well as protistan parasites), myxozoans, which do need intermediate hosts, are common fish parasites and several species are serious pathogens of ornamental fish. Helminth parasites can also cause significant pathology. Since the normal host–parasite relationship is very sensitive to environmental changes and to the immunocompetence of the host, reduction of environmental stress will enhance the fish's ability to cope with the presence of parasites.

Protistan parasites

Protistan parasites include representatives from five phyla and they may infect almost any organ or tissues of the host. Figure 21.1 provides a classification for protistan parasites, including all major groups of significance for ornamental fish.

Flagellates

Parasitic flagellates are amongst the most important protistan parasites of fish and can occur in both freshwater and marine habitats. Some have a direct life cycle; others utilize a leech vector in transmission. They are typically parasitic on the skin and fins and in the bloodstream. All possess flagella during at least one stage in the life cycle.

Oodinids

The two main oodinids of importance in captive fish are *Amyloodinium ocellatum*, the causative agent of 'velvet disease' or amyloodiniosis in marine fish, and *Piscinoodinium pillulare* in freshwater. (The old name '*Oodinium*' for freshwater representatives of this group is incorrect but may be found in some texts and is widely used by aquarium hobbyists.)

The parasitic stage (trophont) is around 150 μm in length, though some are larger. This feeding stage is attached to the host by a disc embedded in the host

Group and genus	Disease	Site of infection	Marine/ freshwater
FLAGELLATA (flagellates)			
Oodinidae			
Amyloodinium	'Marine velvet'	Gills; skin; fins	Marine
Piscinoodinium	'Velvet'	Gills; skin; fins	Freshwater
Trypanosomatidae			
Trypanosoma	Trypanosomiasis	Blood	Both
Bodonidae			
Cryptobia	Cryptobiosis	Gills	Freshwater
Ichthyobodo	Costiosis	Skin; gills	Freshwater
Trypanoplasma	Trypanosomiasis	Blood	Both
Hexamitidae			
Spironucleus		Systemic	Both
CILIATA (ciliates)			
Sessile			
Apiosoma		Skin; gills	Freshwater
Capriniana		Skin; gills	Freshwater
Epistylis		Skin; gills	Freshwater
Motile			
Brooklynella		Gills	Marine
Chilodonella		Skin; gills	Freshwater
Cryptocaryon	'Marine white spot'	Skin	Marine
Ichthyophthirius	'Ich', 'white spot'	Skin	Freshwater
Tetrahymena	'Tet disease'	Systemic	Freshwater
Trichodina	Trichodinosis	Skin; gills	Both
Trichodinella		Skin; gills	Both
Uronema		Systemic	Marine
RHIZOPODA (amoebae)			
Acanthamoebae	Amoebiasis	Systemic	Freshwater
Hartmanella	Amoebiasis	Systemic	Freshwater
Paramoeba	Amoebiasis	Gills	Marine
Thecamoeba	Amoebiasis	Gills	Freshwater
Vahlkampfia	Amoebiasis	Systemic; gills	Both
Vexillifera	Amoebiasis	Internal organs	Freshwater
APICOMPLEXA			
subclass Coccidia (coccidians)			
Eimeria	Coccidiosis	Various organs	Both
Goussia	Coccidiosis	Various organs	Both
MICROSPORA (microsporeans)			
Glugea	Microsporidiosis	Various organs	Both
Heterosporis	Microsporidiosis	Various organs	Both
Pleistophora	Microsporidiosis	Various organs	Both

Figure 21.1 Classification of protistan parasites of fish.

epithelium. Its body is sac-like. *A. ocellatum* does not survive below 17°C, and has an optimal temperature range of 23–27°C.

Life cycle: The life cycle is direct. The trophont detaches from the host, encysts and undergoes a series of divisions to produce the free-swimming infective stage. The length of time for development at each stage is temperature dependent: as a general rule, the higher the temperature, the faster the reproductive rate.

Pathology: *A. ocellatum* appears to be non-host-specific and may infect freshwater fish at low salinities. It is mainly found in the gills but in heavy infections may be found on the skin and fins and in the gastrointestinal tract.

P. pillulare is also non-host-specific, though some fish species appear refractory to the parasite. It is particularly a problem in tropical species but may occur in temperate fish species. The gills, skin and fins are most frequently affected.

Both species are highly pathogenic to the fish host and infections can be fatal. Infected fish show general signs of discomfort, including increased flashing and reduced feeding. In heavy infections, a velvety or gold appearance due to the presence of large numbers of parasites may be apparent. Gills may be hyperplastic and inflamed with concurrent haemorrhaging.

Diagnosis: General disease symptoms and the presence of the parasite in skin and gill scrapings are indicative.

Treatment and control: Copper sulphate is generally used to treat infections (but caution must be exercised in marine systems). Ultraviolet light is effective in killing free-swimming stages and the complete absence of light for a minimum of 30 hours will kill the tomite stages of *P. pillulare*. Avoidance of overcrowding may reduce the possibility of fatalities.

Trypanosomes

Although generally rare, some trypanosomes in marine and freshwater systems may be pathogenic under certain conditions. Fish trypanosomes (Figure 21.2) possess a single flagellum, either attached to the body or extending free. The average length of most trypanosomes is 40–50 μm (though some species are over 100 μm long). They occur within the blood. Data on host specificity is lacking and it may be that some species have a wide host range.

Life cycle: Fish trypanosomes are transmitted by a leech vector – typically *Piscicola geometra* or *Hemiclepsis marginata* in freshwater.

Pathology: Following infection, there is a prepatent period of up to 9 days when no trypanosomes will be detected in the blood. After this, rapid division of the parasite can lead to large numbers of parasites in the blood. Due to an immune response by the fish host, numbers often decline and disease symptoms subside.

Trypanosoma carassii is pathogenic to juvenile carp and in some cases death may result. It is probable that juvenile fish are more susceptible to infection and fish with prior exposure to trypanosomes are immune to reinfection. Infected fish show anaemia and histopathological changes to the liver, kidney and spleen.

Diagnosis: Infection is indicated by the presence of typical trypanosomes in the blood, which can be determined at necropsy or by taking a blood sample.

Treatment and control: There are no known treatments for trypanosomes. Avoidance of leech vectors in the system will ensure that the parasite is not transmitted between fish.

Bodonids

The genera *Ichthyobodo*, *Cryptobia* and *Trypanoplasma* are parasitic in fish. Within the genus *Ichthyobodo*, the only parasitic species is *I. necator* (Figure 21.3), previously known as *Costia*. It occurs in freshwater but may be able to tolerate transfer to salt water, and it has a temperature range of 2–30°C.

Ten species of *Cryptobia* have been described from fish and most are not considered highly pathogenic. They have two flagella and attach to the host via the posterior or recurrent flagellum. They are more elongate than *Ichthyobodo* and are less firmly attached to the host.

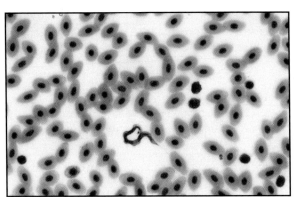

Figure 21.2 An example of a *Trypanosoma* sp. can be seen amongst the nucleated erythrocytes in this stained blood smear. (May-Grünwald–Giemsa stain.)

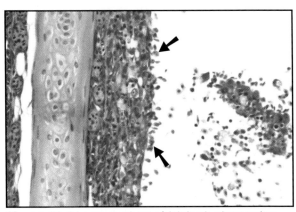

Figure 21.3 Large numbers of *Ichthyobodo* parasites (arrowed) attached to the surface of the gill. (H&E stain.)

There is some debate as to the taxonomic position of *Trypanoplasma*: some workers claim that the organisms are blood stages of *Cryptobia* and this is supported by recent molecular evidence. Around 35 species have been described from freshwater fish, the most important being *T. borrelli* in cyprinids and *T. salmositica* in salmonids. *T. bullocki* has been described from a number of marine fish hosts.

Life cycle: The life cycle of *I. necator* is direct, with transmission from fish to fish through the water. The attached parasitic phase is pyriform and capable of detaching and re-attaching to the fish host. The flat free-swimming stage is around 10–20 µm long and may have two pairs of flagella; it reproduces by binary fission.

Pathology: In general, infected fish show excess mucus production, increased flashing and possibly scraping behaviour.

I. necator is typically found on skin and gills but may attack all epithelial surfaces. It tends to cause mortalities in juvenile and debilitated fish. Symptoms are typical of external parasitism, with increased mucus production giving rise to a bluish sheen on the fish. Destruction of the epithelial cells with subsequent sloughing of these cells, and in some cases hyperplasia, may be noted. The parasite may be able to form cysts under adverse environmental conditions but this has yet to be confirmed.

Cryptobia are found attached either to the gills or within the gastrointestinal tract. Two forms occur in the gills: the more common *C. branchialis*, parasitic on a wide range of hosts worldwide, and the smaller *C. agitans*. Fish infected with gill *Cryptobia* show symptoms typical of protistan ectoparasite infestations, which may include anorexia and emaciation. Only one intestinal form, *C. iubilans*, is considered pathogenic in freshwater; it is parasitic in cichlid fish. *C. iubilans* infections in cichlids are commonly called 'Malawi bloat' and typically lead to gastrointestinal granulomas, which may also be found eventually in most tissues.

Trypanoplasma are found mainly in the bloodstream but also in other tissues. Disease symptoms include anaemia, exophthalmos, ascites and concurrent abdominal distension. Fish may also be lethargic, with a reduced appetite.

Diagnosis: Attached forms of *I. necator* are difficult to detect in skin or gill scrapes, though the flagellated forms may be seen. The free-swimming stages swim in an erratic, spiral manner. *Cryptobia* species are readily identifiable in gill or gut scrapes and the blood stages (*Trypanoplasma*) can be seen in blood samples.

Treatment and control: General treatments for parasites or the use of formalin baths may be effective. Elimination or avoidance of the leech vector will prevent transfer between fish hosts for those species utilizing a vector. For *I. necator* infections, either a potassium permanganate bath or raising the water temperature to above 32°C may be efficacious. Isolation of infected fish in clean water may prevent transfer to susceptible hosts.

Hexamitids

This family contains two genera of importance in wild and captive fish: *Hexamita* and *Spironucleus* (Figure 21.4). Differentiating between the two is difficult. Both have three pairs of anterior flagella and one pair of posterior flagella. *Hexamita* species are generally round to pyriform, whilst *Spironucleus* is more elongate.

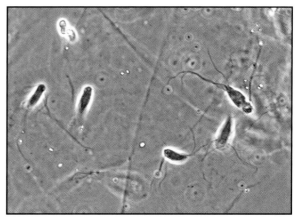

Figure 21.4 *Spironucleus* observed by phase contrast. Note the elongate body and presence of flagella. (Wet mount preparation.)

Life cycle: Hexamitids are assumed to have a direct life cycle, with transmission from fish to fish via the water. However, it is known that *Hexamita* spp. can transmit via free-swimming trophozoites or by hatching from resistant cysts.

Pathology: Both genera can be found in healthy fish and it is believed that stress plays a role in disease outbreaks. Recent work has implicated *Spironucleus vortens* in hole-in-the-head disease in angelfish and other aquarium fish (G.C. Paull, personal communication) whereas previous authors had suggested that *Hexamita* was involved and even responsible for this condition. It is possible that the disease is compounded by poor husbandry and immunosuppressed fish.

Most infections with hexamitids are innocuous and the parasites may be classed as endocommensals. In heavy infections, haemorrhaging, peritonitis and death may be noted. In *S. vortens* infections in angelfish and discus, the appearance of typical 'hole-in-the-head' disease is apparent.

Diagnosis: Presence of the parasite in scrapes or smears and general disease symptoms indicate an infection, including lateral line and head erosion.

Treatment and control: Treatment with dimetridazole or furazolidone (amongst others) may kill the organisms and an improvement in the general husbandry should assist in minimizing the disease.

Ciliates

Ciliates are typically ectoparasitic and are found in both marine and freshwater environments. They may be sessile or motile and their life cycles range from simple binary fission (producing identical offspring) to the production of free-swimming, ciliated infective stages.

Sessile ciliates need to be identified when still alive. They are generally flask-shaped and firmly attached to the host. *Capriniana* spp. are readily distinguished from other ciliates by the presence of numerous tentacles at the apical end. *Epistylis* and *Apiosoma* spp. are non-contractile and possess a ring of cilia around the apical end. *Epistylis* spp. are normally colonial whilst *Apiosoma* spp. are solitary. The most important sessile ciliates on freshwater fish include *Capriniana piscium*, *Apiosoma piscicolum* and *Epistylis lwoffi*.

Diagnosis
The major clinical signs of external protozoan infections include excess mucus production, ragged fins, increased flashing behaviour (rubbing) and, in some cases, lethargy. Diagnosis is by the presence of the parasites in skin, gill or internal body scrapes and smears. All parasites in this group contain cilia, which are visible by light microscopy.

Treatment and control
For most of the external stages of ciliates, general treatments for parasites are effective, along with formalin baths and freshwater/saline baths. Prolonged immersion in a potassium permanganate or copper solution may be effective in reducing or killing the parasites. The more specific treatment of 'white spot' is described below.

Tetrahymena corlissi
Tetrahymena corlissi resembles the theront stage of 'white spot' (described below), being pear-shaped and around $60\,\mu m \times 30\,\mu m$. The marine equivalent, *Uronema marinum*, is 30–50 µm in length. The life cycle of both species is direct.

T. corlissi has been implicated as the causative agent in 'Tet disease' ('slime disease') in guppies and other live-bearers. It is typically found in the skin, muscle and internal organs and infected fish can die within 24 hours of symptoms appearing. *U. marinum* may become systemic; it causes gill and skin lesions.

There is some dispute as to the true pathogenic potential of these parasites and it is possible that other factors, such as bacterial infections or poor water quality, may predispose fish to disease. Infections are generally recognized as small whitish patches on the skin, often around the eye; sloughing of the outer layers of the skin may be apparent in later stages. 'Dropsy' is often present. In *U. marinum* infections, fish can appear listless and usually die of respiratory failure due to high numbers of parasites on the gills.

Chilodonella
Chilodonella spp. are found worldwide and infect a wide range of freshwater fish. They are highly motile, flattened, heart-shaped and around 30–70 µm in length. The two main free-living species affecting fish are *C. hexasticha* and *C. piscicola*, found on the skin and gills (Figure 21.5). Both are considered highly pathogenic, due to their wide temperature tolerance and ability to survive in brackish water. They are able to form persistent cysts. The marine equivalent,

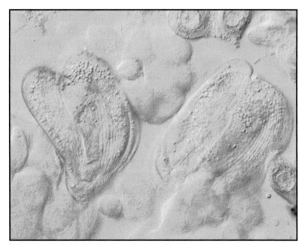

Figure 21.5 *Chilodonella* sp. The heart-shaped organism and its longitudinal striations are visible. (Wet mount preparation, DIC microscopy.)

Brooklynella hostilis is a recognized pathogen in aquarium fish and has a similar size range of 35–85 µm in length. Infections with these parasites result in necrosis of the epithelial layers of the skin and gills and may result in mortalities if not treated.

Trichodinids
These disc-shaped ciliates have internal blades, or denticles, the morphology of which is an important feature in species differentiation. They reproduce by binary fission and can readily attach and detach from the fish host. They occur in freshwater and marine environments; most are ectoparasitic on the skin and gills but a few are found internally.

The most important genera in fish are *Trichodina* (Figure 21.6) and *Trichodinella*. Most trichodinid species are capable of inducing disease in fish; amongst those recorded as pathogens are *Trichodinella epizootica* on a wide range of freshwater hosts and *Trichodina truttae* on salmonids.

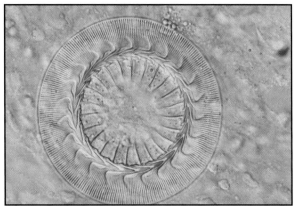

Figure 21.6 Example of *Trichodina* sp. The radial denticles used in species differentiation can be seen clearly. (Wet mount preparation, DIC microscopy.)

Ichthyophthirius multifiliis
I. multifiliis (Figure 21.7) is the causative agent of 'white spot' or 'Ich'. It is able to tolerate a wide range of water temperatures and can infest both coldwater and tropical fish species.

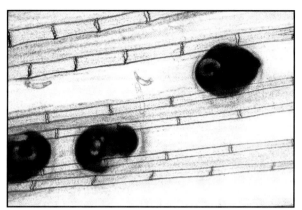

Figure 21.7 Three *Ichthyophthirius multifiliis* trophonts on the fin of a goldfish. Note the presence of a horseshoe-shaped nucleus in the trophont. Some monogeneans *Gyrodactylus* sp. are also present in this sample. (Wet mount preparation.)

Life cycle: The life cycle is direct and numbers can build up rapidly in aquaria. The free-swimming infective stage (theront) is ciliated, pear-shaped and around 30–45 μm in length; it dies if it fails to find a host within about 48 hours at 24–26°C. On locating a host, it penetrates the epidermis and develops into a ciliated trophont, typically seen on the skin as a white spot up to 1 mm in diameter, with a large horseshoe-shaped nucleus and visible to the naked eye. The trophont breaks through the epidermis and becomes an encysted tomont, which attaches to an inanimate substrate, divides and then releases infective theronts. The life cycle can be completed in around 15 days at 15°C, 10 days at 20°C and 6 days at 27°C. The marine equivalent, *Cryptocaryon irritans*, has an identical life cycle.

Pathology: In 'white spot' infections, the presence of the parasite can lead to epithelial hyperplasia and in some cases necrotic changes. The release of the trophont stage from the host causes disruption of the epidermal layers and osmotic disturbance and can lead to secondary bacterial infections. The pathology and disease associated with *C. irritans* are identical to those caused by *I. multifiliis*.

Treatment and control: If 'white spot' is identified before the infective stages are released, infected fish should be removed from the system and quarantined. It should be noted that only the free-swimming (theront) stage is susceptible to chemical treatment and thus three repeat treatments should be given when this stage is off the host. Treatment intervals are temperature dependent and should be as follows: 5-day intervals above 16°C; 7-day intervals at 10–16°C; and 14-day intervals under 10°C. Due to the vigorous immune response of fish to *I. multifiliis*, it is realistic that a vaccine would be effective.

Amoebae

Amoebae are recognized as serious pathogens in some aquaculture facilities, especially in cyprinids. It is likely that they may also constitute a hazard for fish in captivity due to their mode of transmission and ability to increase rapidly in numbers on debilitated fish.

Amoebae are typified by their highly organized internal structure and movement by protoplasmic flow or by pseudopodia. They reproduce by binary fission and some species may form resistant cyst stages. Those that infect fish are normally found free-living in the environment. Most do not cause disease unless the fish are immunosuppressed or there is an environmental imbalance.

Pathology: Excessive levels of bacteria on the fish or in the environment may facilitate growth of the amoebae. A number of species have been implicated in mortalities of fish, predominantly in salmonid aquaculture and some cultured flatfish. They include *Thecamoeba hoffmani* and *Paramoeba pemaquidensis* from the gills of salmonids (Figure 21.8), *Vexillifera bacillipedes* in lesions of the internal organs of rainbow trout and a systemic infection of *Acanthamoeba polyphaga* in tilapia.

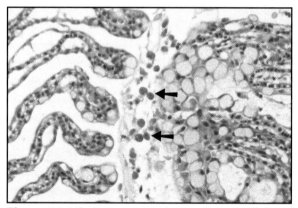

Figure 21.8 Typical amoebae (arrowed) present in loose association with the tips of the gill filaments. (H&E.)

Typical clinical signs include respiratory distress and lethargy. *V. bacillipedes* infections are characterized by 'dropsy', anaemia, nodules on the visceral organs and enlarged kidney and spleen. Histologically, in the gills there may be lamellar hyperplasia and hypertrophy, cellular infiltration and necrosis.

Diagnosis: Amoebae are readily visualized in wet mounts of affected tissues, though speciation is problematic. Some amoebae can be cultured using various agars (e.g. cerophyl–seawater agar, Difco Bactoagar) to allow further study.

Treatment and control: Good hygiene and husbandry should aid in reducing the possibility of amoebae becoming a problem. Some amoebic infections have been treated by saltwater or formalin baths but this may require prolonged exposure.

Coccidians

Over 200 parasitic coccidian species have been recorded in fish but many of them have low pathogenicity and do not appear to induce significant disease. The main species likely to be encountered in ornamental fish belong to the genera *Eimeria* and *Goussia* (Figure 21.9).

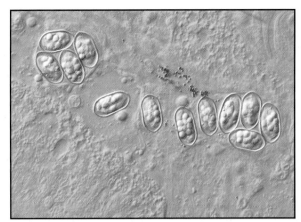

Figure 21.9 Squash preparation of *Goussia metchnikovi* in kidney tissue from a gudgeon. (Wet mount preparation, DIC microscopy.)

Life cycle: Having been ingested by a host fish – either directly, or via a paratenic host (a transport host in which no parasite development occurs) or other vector – mature infective oocysts release sporozoites, which invade host tissues. After several stages of development within host cells, sporocysts containing infective oocysts are released via host faeces to continue the cycle.

Pathology: Coccidian parasites usually affect the epithelial linings and tissues of the gastrointestinal tract (Figure 21.10). In some cases, other organs such as the liver and spleen may be the focus of infection.

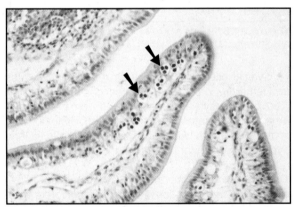

Figure 21.10 Coccidia (arrowed) are present in the epithelial cells of the intestine in this histological section. (ZN stain.)

To date, few infections have been described from ornamental fish species. The two main forms of coccidiosis in carp are diffuse coccidiosis, caused by *Goussia carpelli*, and nodular coccidiosis, a serious disease caused by *G. subepithelialis*. Other parasites, such as *G. sinensis* and *G. aurata*, are recognized pathogens of silver carp and goldfish, respectively. *Eimeria* spp. appear to be less problematic but some, such as *E. rutili* and *E. anguillae*, can induce pathogenic changes in their hosts (roach and eels, respectively).

Clinical signs generally include lethargy, poor feeding, emaciation and the presence of mucus strands protruding from the anus, but most infections do not produce clinical signs and will usually be detected as incidental findings in general health examinations. *G. subepithelialis* induces a characteristic nodular appearance to the intestine, in which much of the normal structure is replaced by parasite stages. Cases of diffuse coccidiosis may be recognized by reddening (haemorrhaging) of the intestinal wall.

Diagnosis: Suspicion of coccidial infections will be based on the presence of mucus strands in the faeces or intestinal haemorrhaging. Confirmation requires the examination of faeces or caecal scrapes for the presence of characteristic coccidial oocysts. Tissue smears using Ziehl–Neelsen or Giemsa stains are especially effective for detecting these. Infections are also readily detected in histological sections, where all stages may be visualized. Species identification requires careful measurement of the various stages and is primarily based on the organization and structure of the oocysts and sporozoites.

Treatment and control: There are no recommended treatments for coccidial infections. As for other protistan infections, careful monitoring and good husbandry, with removal of fish exhibiting clinical signs of infection, offer the best method for reducing the impact of disease caused by these organisms.

Microsporeans

Microsporeans are relatively common intracellular parasites of fish and certain species may have a wide host range in wild and captive fish stocks.

Life cycle: The life cycle is direct and infections are transmitted by ingestion of spores, either as 'free' spores or via crustacean vectors such as brine shrimp or *Daphnia* spp. After ingestion, infective sporoplasms are released and enter the target host cell, where the parasite undergoes vegetative development. Large numbers of spores are produced and released from the host cell on the death of the host (naturally or by predation) or on rupture of xenomas situated in epithelial tissues, releasing spores directly to the environment.

Pathology: Depending on the specific parasite, large xenomas may be formed in various organs (Figure 21.11) or, in the case of certain *Pleistophora* and

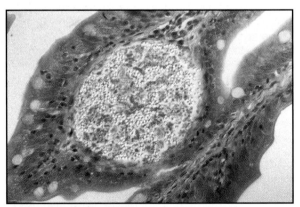

Figure 21.11 A microsporean xenoma in a histological section of the gastrointestinal tract. Note the presence of numerous refractile spores within the xenoma. (H&E stain.)

Heterosporis spp., invasion of skeletal muscle cells can result in destruction of the musculature. Other species infect oocytes.

Most infections with microsporean parasites have the potential to cause significant disease and may result in mortality in severe infections. Cyst-forming species may impair organ function; gill infections may result in respiratory impairment; and gonadal infections clearly have the potential to reduce reproductive capacity and spawning success significantly.

The most commonly encountered infections in ornamental fish species are likely to be those infecting the musculature.

- *Glugea* spp. can infect multiple organs and affect many different fish species. Diseased fish may exhibit large boil-like lesions, easily visible to the naked eye. Rupture of these produces open wounds and may result in secondary infections with opportunistic bacteria.
- Neon tetra disease, caused by *Pleistophora hyphessobryconis*, results in mortality in a number of species. Affected fish are lethargic and may exhibit infected muscle segments, which are visible as greyish or whitish patches under the skin.
- *Heterosporis finki* and *H. schuberti* infect the musculature of ornamental fish. Although clinical signs appear to be uncommon in freshwater angelfish infected with *H. finki*, significant mortalities have been reported among cichlids infected with *H. schuberti*.

Diagnosis: Microsporean infections can only be identified by microscopic examination. Careful examination and measurement of fresh spores will generally allow identification to genus. Stained smears from infected tissues will reveal the characteristic spores and developmental stages. Histological sections will also reveal these and provide valuable information on the extent and severity of the infection to be assessed. Species identification requires electron microscopy.

Treatment and control: There are no recommended treatments for microsporean infections. Several experimental studies have demonstrated the efficacy of fumagillin, an antimicrobial that has been used for the treatment of the microsporean *Nosema* in honey bees. Prevention is difficult, since the spores are long-lived and not reliant on intermediate hosts for transmission. Good hygiene precautions and effective quarantine regimes offer the best chance of minimizing the risk of introduction of microsporean parasites.

Myxozoan parasites

Myxosporeans
Myxosporeans (phylum Myxozoa) are common parasites of fish and almost any organ and tissue can be infected (Figure 21.12). For most of their life cycle they are multicellular but, because of their small size, diagnostic methods for their detection are principally those used for protistan parasites.

Group and genus	Disease	Site of infection	Marine/ freshwater
MYXOZOA (myxozoans)			
Chloromyxum	Myxosporidiosis	Kidney; gall bladder	Both
Henneguya	Myxosporidiosis	Various organs	Both
Hoferellus	KED	Kidney	Freshwater
Kudoa	Myxosporidiosis	Musculature	Marine
Myxidium	Myxosporidiosis	Kidney; gall bladder	Both
Myxobolus (=*Myxosoma*)	Myxosporidiosis	Most organs	Both
Sphaerospora	Myxosporidiosis	Kidney	Both
Tetracapsula	PKD	Kidney; spleen	Freshwater

Figure 21.12 Classification of myxozoan parasites of fish.

Several species are responsible for major disease conditions affecting commercially important fish species, and several genera are known to be parasites of ornamental fish. *Myxidium*, *Sphaerospora*, *Chloromyxum* and *Myxobolus* (= *Myxosoma*) may be commonly encountered in a variety of organs and tissues. Other genera, such as *Ceratomyxa*, *Parvicapsula*, *Ortholinea* and *Kudoa*, mostly known as marine parasites, display a wide range of spore shape. The recently erected taxon *Tetracapsula bryosalmonae* (Myxozoa: Malacosporea) is the parasite that causes proliferative kidney disease in salmonids.

Life cycle: Myxosporeans have a complex life cycle involving intermediate or alternate hosts (oligochaetes, polychaetes and bryozoans). The requirement for intermediate hosts provides the possibility for control of infection by removal of these hosts or even preventing their introduction in highly controlled environments such as aquaria.

Pathology: The clinical signs of infection vary greatly, depending in particular on the site of infection. Most infections elicit only minimal host response, unless the parasite develops in atypical tissues.

- Most cyst-forming histozoic species, such as *Myxobolus cyprini*, *M. koi* and the majority of *Kudoa* species, do not cause significant pathology unless (rarely) infections are particularly severe and affect organ function. Rupture of cysts exposes spores and developmental stages of the parasite to the host's immune system and an inflammatory response ensues. For *M. cyprini* and *Kudoa* spp. this results in muscle necrosis. For certain marine fish, infections with *Kudoa* and other muscle-invading genera such as *Unicapsula* and *Hexacapsula* can result in dramatic enzymatic degeneration of the muscle after death. In aquaria, affected fish may not exhibit clinical signs.
- Most *Myxidium* and *Sphaerospora* species are coelozoic and are typically encountered in the gall bladder and urinary system (Figure 21.13), respectively, where a localized pathological response may occur. Both genera contain important pathogens – particularly *Sphaerospora*, which has extrasporogonic proliferative stages,

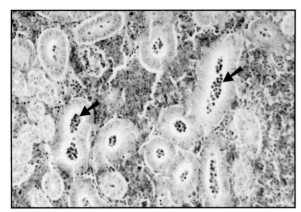

Figure 21.13 *Sphaerospora renicola* spores (arrowed) in the kidney tubules of carp. Compared with uninfected renal tubules, parasitized tubules are greatly dilated. (Giemsa stain.)

which in the case of *S. renicola* cause swim-bladder inflammation and degenerative changes in the kidney of carp. *S. molnari* causes significant dysfunction of the gills in carp and other cyprinids. The parasite provokes a marked hyperplasia of the respiratory epithelium, resulting in fusion of the lamellae.

- 'Kidney enlargement disease' (KED) is a relatively common disease of goldfish and common carp (including koi). Affected fish may be oedematous and listless but the main presenting feature is of gross abdominal swelling caused by renal hypertrophy. On dissection, in severe cases, the kidney has a polycystic appearance with the majority of cysts containing fluid. The causative agents, *Hoferellus carassii* (in goldfish) and *H. cyprini* (in carp), induce a marked dilation of the renal tubules with hyperplasia of the tubule epithelium (Figure 21.14). Some parasite stages are intracellular but diagnosis is usually based on the clinical signs and the observation of spores with characteristic caudal projections in the lumen of tubules. Some cases of KED are considered to be the result of a developmental anomaly (see Chapter 27).

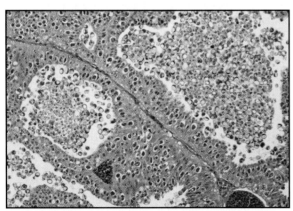

Figure 21.14 Histological section of the kidney from a goldfish with kidney enlargement disease. Massive numbers of parasites are present within the lumen and hyperplastic epithelial cells of the renal tubules. (H&E stain.)

- Infections with *Chloromyxum* are usually located in the gall bladder but plasmodial stages of the parasite can in some cases pass through the bile duct and cause localized hepatitis and focal necrosis of the hepatic parenchyma. Renal infections with *Chloromyxum* may be encountered but do not usually induce a significant host response.

- *Tetracapsula bryosalmonae* (formerly known as PKX) is a parasite of salmonid fishes and also uses a number of bryozoan species as hosts. Proliferative kidney disease (PKD) has been well described in salmonids and the severity of the clinical signs is related to the intense inflammatory response to the proliferative stages of *T. bryosalmonae* in the kidney and spleen in particular. Similar stages have been detected in the gills of carp and the detection of *Tetracapsula* infections in other fish species (including ornamental fish) seems likely. The fish host for the only other described species (*T. bryozoides*) is currently unknown but it is possible that *Tetracapsula* spp. can complete their life cycle in the bryozoan host without the need for a fish host.

Diagnosis: The main method for diagnosis is by careful examination and measurement of fresh (unfixed) mature spores (Figure 21.15) (Lom and Arthur, 1988). However, it is important to realize that it is sometimes the proliferative 'extrasporogonic' stages that induce the vigorous host response.

Pre-spore stages will often be encountered in fresh preparations and these should be photographed if possible. Preserved material in the form of tissue

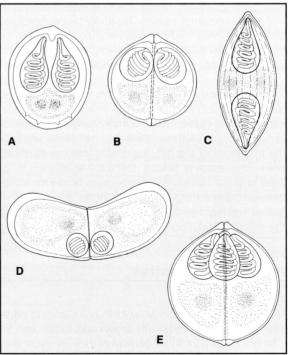

Figure 21.15 Examples of myxozoan parasites. (a) *Myxobolus*; (b) *Sphaerospora*; (c) *Myxidium*; (d) *Ceratomyxa*; (e) *Chloromyxum*.

impression smears, air dried, fixed in acetic methanol (glacial acetic acid and methanol) or a similar fixative and stained with Giemsa or tissues prepared for histological examination may be essential for accurate diagnosis. More sophisticated methods are available for certain parasites such as *Tetracapsula* (e.g. labelling with specific antibodies or detection using molecular techniques).

Treatment and control: There are no recommended treatments for the prevention of myxosporean infections but there is some experimental evidence that fumagillin may be effective in reducing infections of *S. renicola*, *T. bryosalmonae* and *Myxobolus cerebralis* (the causative agent of salmonid whirling disease). Prevention should be based on good husbandry, avoidance of possible intermediate hosts and removal of clinically affected fish to prevent the release of spores.

Malachite green has been used effectively to treat PKD in salmonids but is not licensed for use in food-producing species. Under experimental conditions fumagillin and toltrazuril have been shown to be effective against KED in goldfish due to infection by *H. carassii* (Yokayama *et al.*, 1990).

Metazoan parasites

Figure 21.16 provides a classification of the metazoan parasites, including representatives within each group found in ornamental fish. The two main groups known to be able to reproduce readily in aquaria and which cause most problems are the monogeneans and the crustaceans. Most of the other groups, whilst not able to complete their life cycle without utilizing other hosts, can in some cases cause disease or render the host unsightly.

In common with most ectothermic animals, metazoan reproduction is temperature dependent. Generally, the closer to the maximum temperature range of the parasite, the higher the reproductive rate will be. There are no clinical signs common to all the groups but general signs such as increased flashing, abnormal behaviour or excess mucus production may be noted.

In general, good husbandry and quarantining of new fish can prevent the problems that occur with these parasites. Removal of infected fish to a quarantine tank, disinfection of affected aquaria and avoidance of intermediate hosts (either in live food or within the system) are appropriate for all metazoan infections.

Monogeneans

Monogenean flukes are ubiquitous in marine and freshwater systems and are predominantly parasites of fish. Whilst most are host-specific, some can infect a number of different hosts and in captive environments can rapidly build up to high levels, causing direct mortality or allowing the invasion of secondary infectious agents. Further information on monogeneans in captive fish, including therapeutants, is discussed in Thoney and Hargis (1991).

Group and genus	Common name	Site of infection	Marine/ freshwater
MONOGENEA (monogeneans)	**Flukes**		
Benedenia	Capsalids	Skin	Marine
Dactylogyrus	Flukes	Gills	Freshwater
Dermophthirius	Capsalids	Skin	Marine
Gyrodactylus	Skin flukes	Skin; fins	Both
Microcotyle		Gills	Marine
Neobenedenia	Capsalids	Skin	Marine
DIGENEA (digeneans)	**Flukes**		
Bucephalus		Muscle	Freshwater
Clinostomum	'Yellow/white grub'	Skin	Freshwater
Diplostomum	Eye flukes	Eye	Both
Neascus	'Black spot'	Skin	Freshwater
Posthodiplostomum	'Black spot'	Skin	Freshwater
Sanguinicola	Blood flukes	Blood	Freshwater
CESTODA (cestodes)	**Tapeworms**		
Atractolytocestus		Gut	Freshwater
Bothriocephalus	Asian tapeworm	Gut	Freshwater
Diphyllobothrium		Viscera, muscle	Both
Khawia		Gut	Freshwater
Ligula		Viscera, muscle	Freshwater
Triaenophorus		Viscera, muscle	Freshwater
NEMATODA (nematodes)	**Roundworms**		
Anisakis		Viscera, muscle	Marine
Camallanus	'Red worm'	Gut	Freshwater
Capillaria		Gut	Freshwater
Eustrongylides	'Red worm'	Viscera, muscle	Freshwater
Hysterothylacium		Gut	Marine
Philometra	'Blood worm'	Viscera, muscle	Freshwater
ACANTHOCEPHALA	**Spiny-headed worms**		
Echinorhynchus		Gut	Both
Pomphorhynchus		Gut	Both
ANNELIDA (annelids)	**Leeches**		
Myzobdella		Skin	Marine
Piscicola		Skin	Freshwater
MOLLUSCA (molluscs)			
Unioida family (glochidia)			Freshwater
CRUSTACEA (crustaceans)			
Copepeda (copepods)			
Caligus	Sea lice	Skin	Marine
Ergasilus	Gill maggots	Gills	Both
Lepeophtheirus	Sea lice	Skin	Marine
Lernaea	Anchor worm	Skin	Freshwater
Lernaeenicus		Skin	Marine
Salmincola		Gills	Freshwater
Branchiura			
Argulus	Fish lice	Skin	Freshwater
Isopoda (isopods)			
Flabellifera (suborder)		Skin	Marine
Gnathiidae (suborder)	Gnathia	Skin	Marine

Figure 21.16 Classification of the major groups of metazoan parasites, with examples of common genera within each group.

Monogeneans are generally found on the skin or gills of fish and each type is adapted specifically for these habitats. Some can be found within the visceral cavity of elasmobranchs. Typically, they range in size from 0.5 mm to 2 mm, though some can be up to 5 cm long. They are characterized by a contractile body with a holdfast or opisthohaptor at the posterior end.

The two major monogenean groups, the Polyopisthocotylea and Monopisthocotylea, differ in the structure of the opisthohaptor. Monopisthocotyleans have a single haptor with large central anchor hooks or haptors and several smaller marginal hooks around its edge; they typically feed on skin and mucus and are whitish in colour. Polyopisthocotyleans have muscular finger-like projections on the opisthohaptor, with clamps or suckers instead of hooks; generally they feed on host blood and are dark brown. Monogenean taxonomy is based on the mode of reproduction and the arrangement and shape of the hooks or clamps.

The most important monogeneans in captive environments are *Gyrodactylus* spp. (Figure 21.17). These monopisthocotyleans are typified by their small size (less than 1 mm in length), two large central anchors and 16 marginal hooks on the opisthohaptor. They do not have eyespots and juveniles can often be seen in the uterus of adults. Most marine and freshwater fish species can be infected.

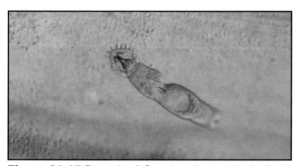

Figure 21.17 Example of *Gyrodactylus* sp. attached to the fin of a goldfish. The parasite is firmly attached by the opisthohaptor. The uterus contains a juvenile and is clearly visible in the middle of the body. (Wet mount preparation, DIC microscopy.)

Other monopisthocotyleans of concern are *Dactylogyrus* spp., infecting mainly cyprinids. They are usually found on the gills and are similar in size to *Gyrodactylus* spp. but reproduce oviparously and have four eyespots on the anterior end.

Examples of monogeneans in marine aquaria include the capsalids, typified by a large circular opisthohaptor on the posterior end and two smaller suckers on the anterior end. This group includes species of *Benedenia* (Figures 21.18 and 21.19) and *Neobenedenia*, which infect a wide range of tropical marine fish, and *Dermophthirius*, a parasite of elasmobranchs.

Most polyopisthocotyleans do not cause major problems in enclosed systems but there are reports of species that do, including *Discocotyle sagittata* (Figure 21.20) in cultured salmonids and *Pseudanthocotyloides heterocotyle* in herring. There have also been mortalities associated with *Erpocotyle laevis* in the gills of cold-water smoothhounds (Longshaw and Feist, unpublished data).

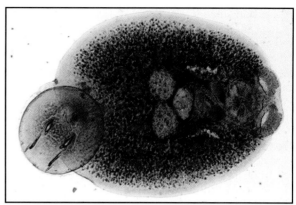

Figure 21.18 *Benedenia* sp. removed from the skin of a marine fish. The round opisthohaptor, typical in capsalid monogeneans, is used to secure the parasite to the host. (Wet mount preparation.)

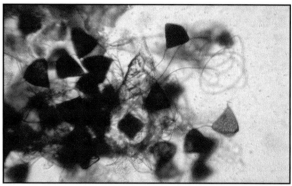

Figure 21.19 Characteristic tetrahedral *Benedenia* eggs with fine threads used for attachment to fish and other objects. (Wet mount preparation) (© W.H. Wildgoose.)

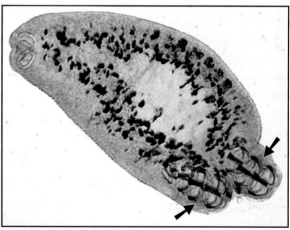

Figure 21.20 *Discocotyle sagittata*, a polyopisthocotylean monogenean, isolated from the gills of trout. Unlike the adult forms, this immature specimen contains three pairs of clamps (arrowed), rather than four. Breakdown products of host blood can be seen as dark deposits at the periphery of the parasite. (Wet mount preparation.)

Life cycles: Monogeneans are either oviparous (egg laying) or viviparous (giving birth to live young) (Figure 21.21). Transmission is direct in each case. The eggs of oviparous monogeneans settle on a substrate, or in bunches on gill filaments in the case of some capsalids. Upon hatching, a free-swimming stage

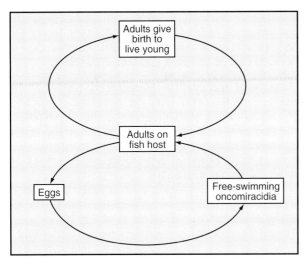

Figure 21.21 Typical species-dependent life cycle of monogeneans, showing the two alternative pathways.

(oncomiracidium) will seek out a suitable fish host, attach and develop into an adult.

Viviparous monogeneans are potentially more harmful as their mode of reproduction can allow numbers to build rapidly in favourable conditions, such as fish debility or increased water temperatures. It is possible for some of the daughter parasites within the uterus to contain a developing embryo, thus allowing a rapid increase in the population.

Pathology: The site of infection determines clinical signs, though in general infections are typified by excessive mucus production, increased flashing (rubbing), lethargy and anorexia. At the site of infection there can be focal haemorrhaging and noticeable grey areas associated with excess mucus. The feeding behaviour of monogeneans invariably means that there is destruction of the epithelium, resulting in osmoregulatory failure and invasion by secondary pathogens.

Diagnosis: Diagnosis is by clinical signs and presence of the parasite in skin or gill scrapes. In histological sections, presence of sclerotized clamps or hooks associated with host tissue and the body of the parasite can sometimes be seen.

Treatment and control: Monogenean infections are often associated with poor husbandry and water conditions, and it is imperative that conditions are improved prior to further treatments. Chemical treatment is determined by the type of reproduction and varies according to species. It is important to monitor the situation closely and attempt different remedies until the problem is cured. General treatments for genera such as *Gyrodactylus* and *Dactylogyrus* include the use of formalin and methylene blue. If these treatments fail, it is possible to use organophosphates, and in some cases the use of mebendazole and praziquantel has been successful. Marine species may be treated by freshwater dips using purified water derived by reverse osmosis. In the case of oviparous species, repeat treatments and disinfection of the system may be required.

Digeneans

Digenean flukes are generally found in the gastro-intestinal tract or the musculature, depending on their stage of development. Invariably, wild-caught or pond-reared fish in contact with infected alternative hosts will harbour infections but, due to their complex life cycles, digeneans are generally not considered to be of concern in aquarium systems since they cannot complete their cycles. They can appear as unsightly or dark nodules under the skin when they occur in the musculature.

Digeneans occur in almost all species of fish, both marine and freshwater. Metacercarial stages of some digeneans found in wild-caught or pond-reared fish produce raised nodules on the surface of the fish and are better known by the colour of these cysts; for example, 'black spot' is formed as a result of hyperpigmentation by the host reaction to *Neascus* sp. and *Posthodiplostomum* sp., while yellow and white grubs (*Clinostomum* spp.) form yellow or white nodules. *Diplostomum* spp. are generally found in the lens, though in minnows they are found in the cranial cavity.

The blood fluke *Sanguinicola* spp. is a potentially serious problem in cyprinids (Kirk and Lewis, 1994). On infecting fish, the cercarial stages migrate around the body via the blood, reaching the heart and then the gills. Here, they release eggs that can become systemic within the heart, kidney and gills. After hatching within the fish hosts, the miracidia leave the host, causing disruption to the areas through which they migrate.

Digeneans are dorsoventrally flattened, 0.5–5 cm in length, and possess a simple gut and an anterior and a ventral sucker (Figure 21.22). In some species these suckers can be much reduced or vestigial. Some digeneans possess a ring of circumoral spines around the anterior sucker.

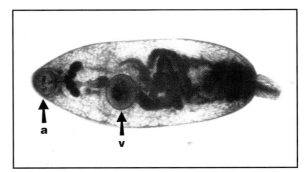

Figure 21.22 A typical digenean. Note the presence of an apical (a) and a ventral (v) sucker (arrowed). (Wet mount preparation.)

Life cycle: Aquatic digenean life cycles (Figure 21.23) are complex and use at least two hosts: a fish as second intermediate or final host and, usually, a snail as primary host. The adults are hermaphroditic.

Pathology: There are no clinical signs common to digenean infections. There may be alteration in behaviour, inability to swim and find food, and in some cases localized necrosis or haemorrhage caused by entry or

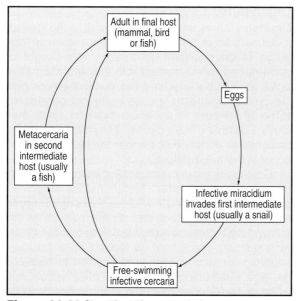

Figure 21.23 Simplified life cycle of digenean parasites.

exit of the parasite. Digeneans residing in the gastrointestinal tract do not normally elicit a host response, unlike those found in other tissues or organs. In small fish, invasion by large numbers of cercaria can lead to osmotic failure and allow secondary infections to occur. Migrations by the parasite through the host tissues can cause localized damage, inflammation and haemorrhage. In the case of infections by *Sanguinicola* spp., fish can be lethargic, emaciated and show exophthalmos. 'Black spot', 'yellow grub' and 'white grub' are characterized by localized swelling, usually close to the skin surface. Eye infection by *Diplostomum* spp. can cause blindness and altered behaviour; also, due to the reduced ability to visualize food, some fish may become emaciated. Fatalities due to digeneans are uncommon in aquaria.

Diagnosis: Detection of the presence of the parasite in tissues (either by dissection or in tissue sections) will allow diagnosis. Removal and dissection of raised nodules or cysts on the skin surface will demonstrate the presence of metacercariae. *Diplostomum* spp. are normally found within the lens of the eye (Figure 21.24). *Sanguinicola* spp. may be identified by the

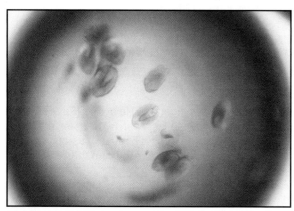

Figure 21.24 Photomicrograph of *Diplostomum* sp. in the lens of a fish. (Wet mount preparation.)

presence of eyespots in the metacercarial stage and by the presence of triangular eggs within the blood and tissues and adult flukes in the fish. Identification to species can be complex and time-consuming.

Treatment and control: Metacercariae close to the surface of the skin may be removed surgically. Praziquantel has been shown to be effective in reducing numbers of some digeneans in fish. If the fish is already parasitized, it is unlikely that the infection will spread to other fish within the aquarium unless an alternate host is available.

Introduction of infected wild molluscs can lead to infections in fish. Lymnaeid snails are hosts for *Sanguinicola* spp. and should therefore be avoided. The best approach in preventing infection is avoidance or removal of the mollusc host and the infective stage.

Cestodes

Cestodes, or tapeworms, are found in most fish species and occur in both freshwater and marine habitats. They rarely cause disease in captive fish but some are known pathogens that may be cause for concern.

Cestodes can be divided into the Cestodaria (infecting mainly elasmobranchs) and the Eucestoda (infecting teleosts). The latter have an attachment organ (scolex) and visible external segmentation with concomitant internal segmentation, and lack a gut. The scolex can be simple or may bear hooks, spines, grooves or suckers. The body segments (proglottids) contain the reproductive organs; cestodes are hermaphroditic.

Most cestodes are whitish or yellowish in colour and range from a few millimetres to around 20 cm long in fish. They are usually found in the gastrointestinal tract or visceral cavity, though some forms may encyst in various tissues.

Freshwater cestode species of concern include *Bothriocephalus acheilognathi* and *Khawia sinesis* in carp and *Ligula* sp. in cyprinids.

Life cycle: Aquatic cestode life cycles are complex and require at least two hosts (Figure 21.25). Fish can

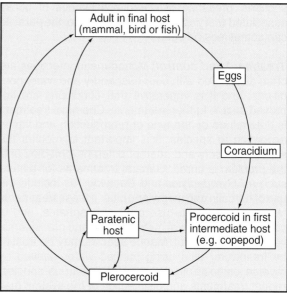

Figure 21.25 Simplified life cycle of cestode parasites.

be the second intermediate, the paratenic or the final host, depending on species; the first intermediate host is usually a copepod.

Pathology: Fish infected with cestodes generally show no clinical signs, though there may be visible distension of the abdomen due to the size of the parasite. Large numbers of cestodes in the gastrointestinal tract may lead to general malaise and reduction in growth due to occlusion of the gut and destruction of the gut epithelium at the site of parasite attachment (Figure 21.26). Migration of cestodes through the fish can cause localized damage to tissues.

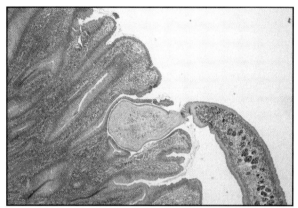

Figure 21.26 Histological section through the intestine of a carp infected with a cestode. (H&E stain.)

Diagnosis: Diagnosis is by finding and identifying the parasites within the fish. Identification to genus on external features is often possible, though speciation may require histological sectioning to determine the arrangement of the reproductive organs.

Treatment and control: There are no known treatments for cestode larval stages. To avoid introduction to naïve fish, no potential alternative hosts (including live food and infected fish) should be added to the system. Adult cestodes may be eradicated using praziquantel or a suitable anthelmintic but it should be noted that killing cestodes with any anthelmintic might cause eggs to be released into the water to continue the cycle. To ensure that no reinfection occurs, treatments should either include eradication of intermediate hosts or be carried out in a separate quarantine tank.

Nematodes

Nematodes, or roundworms, are present in most freshwater and marine wild fish. They do not usually pose a risk in aquaria, due to their inability to complete their complex life cycles. Some can produce live young without the need for an intermediate host and these can be problematic.

Nematodes are elongate with a round cross-section and usually less than 3 cm long. They are usually white or red and are speciated on the basis of the morphology of the head (Figure 21.27) and tail, on the arrangement of the oesophagus and gut, and on size. In most cases, they are host-specific. Adults are generally found within the gastrointestinal tract, and

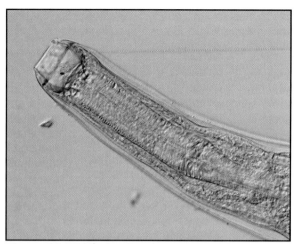

Figure 21.27 Head region of a nematode (*Camallanus* sp.) showing mouthpart detail (Wet mount preparation.)

larval stages may encyst within the visceral cavity, the liver, muscle or other organs. *Anguillicola crassus* is a parasite of the swim-bladder of eels.

Life cycle: Most nematodes have a complex life cycle (Figure 21.28) involving at least two hosts. The sexes are separate. Some nematodes have a direct life cycle; these are usually members of the capillarids and numbers of parasites can build rapidly in aquaria.

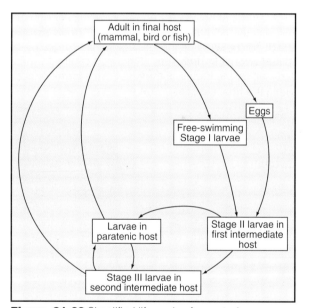

Figure 21.28 Simplified life cycle of nematode parasites.

Pathology: Most marine forms do not cause problems but a number of freshwater forms can be problematic. These include *Capillaria* spp. in the gut of species such as angelfish and cichlids, *Capillostrongyloides* sp. infecting armoured catfish, *Camallanus* spp. ('red worm') infecting live-bearers and *Philometra* sp. under the skin, fins or in the visceral cavity.

Fish infected with large numbers of nematodes may be emaciated, anaemic and lethargic. Often the migration of larval stages through the tissues will cause damage. Damage and subsequent ulceration of the gastrointestinal tract due to the feeding action of parasites may be noted. Excess mucus may be produced as a result of this invasion.

Diagnosis: Presence of roundworms in the fish is indicative of infection. Identification of eggs of some species from fish faeces can provide a non-destructive means of identifying infections. Infections of *Capillaria* spp. may be diagnosed by clear faeces (due to excess mucus production). The presence of red worms protruding through the anal vent is indicative of *Camallanus* spp.

Treatment and control: There are no known chemotherapeutants for encysted larval forms of nematodes; adults may be controlled by the use of anthelmintics. Avoidance or elimination of intermediate hosts may reduce the incidence of nematodes with complex life cycles. For nematodes with direct life cycles, infected fish should be isolated and the system cleaned and sterilized.

Acanthocephalans

Acanthocephalans, or spiny-headed worms, are not usually considered as pathogens in aquaria, though pond-reared or wild-caught fish with access to the intermediate hosts may be infected. Normally, only fish with abnormally high loads of these parasites are debilitated.

Acanthocephalans are generally whitish or orange and usually no more than 2 cm long. Adult stages attach to the wall of the gastrointestinal tract by a spined eversible proboscis (Figure 21.29), with their body within the lumen of the gut. Larval forms encyst within the host tissues.

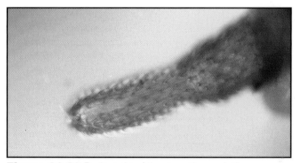

Figure 21.29 Proboscis of the acanthocephalan *Echinorhynchus truttae*, showing numerous spines. (Wet mount preparation, DIC microscopy.)

Typical of the acanthocephalans are representatives of the genera *Echinorhynchus* and *Pomphorhynchus*. Taxonomy of the acanthocephalans is based primarily on the size, number and arrangement of the hooks on the proboscis.

Life cycle: The sexes are separate. Eggs are released into the water via the host faeces. The larval stage (acanthor) infects a first intermediate host (arthropod or other crustacean) and develops into a cystacanth. The first host is ingested by a fish and the parasite either matures into an adult or utilizes the fish as a second intermediate or paratenic host (Figure 21.30).

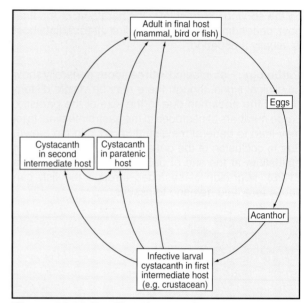

Figure 21.30 Simplified life cycle of acanthocephalan parasites.

Pathology: In heavy infestations, fish may be anorexic due to damage to the intestinal mucosa as a result of attachment by the parasite.

Diagnosis: Presence of the adult worm in the gastrointestinal tract or encysted larval forms in the liver or mesenteries is indicative of infection.

Treatment and control: Low levels of infection can be tolerated by most fish. Avoidance or elimination of intermediate hosts such as arthropods will prevent infections. There are no published methods for treating acanthocephalan infections in fish but piperazine citrate may remove the worms.

Annelids

Fish leeches occur in both marine and freshwater environments. They rarely cause problems in aquaria, though they may be present on wild or pond-reared fish.

Leeches are segmented and contractile, with posterior and anterior suckers used for feeding and attachment to the host. Parasitic leeches are blood feeders and may transmit blood parasites and viruses. Common fish-infecting species can be up to 5 cm in length.

Some species, such as the freshwater *Piscicola*, have a wide host range and are able to survive for long periods off the fish host. In marine systems, infestations by *Myzobdella* and others may occur.

Life cycle: Life cycles are direct and the hermaphroditic adults leave the host to lay cocoons on a suitable substrate. After hatching, the larvae infect a suitable fish host.

Pathology: Typically, fish infested with leeches can be anaemic and ulcerations may occur on the skin due to the feeding action of the parasite.

Treatment and control: Low numbers of leeches may be removed manually. Systems may need to be drained and dried to remove adults and egg stages. Judicious use of organophosphates will eliminate leeches.

Molluscs

Larval stages (glochidia) of some freshwater bivalve molluscs have an obligatory parasitic stage encysted primarily on the gills, and also the skin and fins, of suitable fish hosts. Members of the family Unioidae are primarily implicated in this mode of parasitism. They include members of the genera *Anodonta*, *Lampsilis*, *Martigifera*, *Unio* and *Quadrula*.

Life cycle: Fertilized eggs are passed through the female bivalve and, after a period of development, larval forms (glochidia) are released into the water. They come into contact with a suitable fish host, encyst and develop before leaving the fish host to develop into adults. The time spent on the fish host varies from a few days to several weeks.

Pathology: There may be signs of respiratory distress due to large numbers of glochidia interfering with respiration and a hyperplastic response to the infestation. On release from the fish host, there may be severe damage to gill epithelia, allowing secondary pathogens to invade.

Diagnosis: The presence of white nodules with characteristic bivalved larvae within them is indicative of infection.

Treatment and control: There are no known treatments for glochidial infestations. Avoidance or elimination of bivalve molluscs with a parasitic phase should be attempted in order to break the life cycle. After release of larval forms, prophylactic treatment for secondary opportunistic bacterial and fungal infections may be beneficial.

Crustaceans

Many crustaceans are parasitic and can occur in both marine and freshwater habitats. Due to their direct life cycles, they can be serious pathogens in captive environments. Wild-caught or pond-reared fish with access to natural water may be affected. The parasites are in the orders Copepoda (typified by *Ergasilus*, *Lernaea* and *Caligus*), Branchiura (*Argulus*) and Isopoda (*Gnathia* and typical isopod forms).

Copepods

Parasitic copepods are normally ectoparasitic, infecting skin, fins and gills. They may either be anchored within the host fish or move freely about the surface and can be highly modified for a parasitic life. There are several suborders (based primarily on the morphology of the mouthparts), of which the three main ones of importance in captive fish are the Poecilostomatoida, the Cyclopoida and the Siphonostomatoida.

Poecilostomatoids are typified by the genera *Ergasilus* and *Neoergasilus*, potential pathogens in freshwater systems. Members of the genera can be up to 3 mm in length and are found on the gills and skin. They are similar in appearance to free-living copepods except that the antennae are highly modified into grasping hooks. Only adult female *Ergasilus* spp. are parasitic. After mating, the female attaches to a suitable fish host.

The main cyclopoid of concern is the anchor worm *Lernaea cyprinacea*, a cosmopolitan freshwater species with a low host specificity. Characteristically the female adult is seen attached to the fish host and is usually around 2 cm long (Figure 21.31). The highly modified cephalic process is buried within the fish muscle; the main body of the parasite with egg strings is seen on the outside. Only the female of *L. cyprinacea* is parasitic. Copepodid stages attach to a fish host, the separate sexes mate and the male dies. Females then burrow into the body of the fish and undergo metamorphosis. Temperature plays an important role in transmission of the parasite, as it will not reproduce below 15°C.

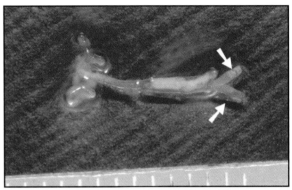

Figure 21.31 *Lernaea cyprinacea*. The holdfast, or 'anchor', is normally buried under the skin of the host. The distal portion, showing two egg strings (arrowed), is normally the only part of the parasite that is visible externally. Scale in millimetres. (Wet mount preparation.)

Most of the parasitic copepods are siphonostomatoids. Of greatest importance are the dorsoventrally flattened caligiforms that live on the surface of the fish. Marine species include *Caligus elongatus* (with a wide host range), *Pseudocaligus brevipedis* (parasitic on marine flatfish) and several species of *Lepeophtheirus*. The suborder also includes the lernaeopodids, which are usually found firmly attached to the gills. They feed mainly on epithelial cells and mucus of the fish. Both the male and female stages of caligiform copepods are parasitic. Chalimus stages are firmly attached to the fish by means of a chalimus filament at the anterior end of the parasite, which is unable to move around the host. Lernaeopodids have a simpler life cycle, without the chalimus stage, and the males are often dwarf and hyperparasitic on the females (i.e. relying on them wholly for sustenance).

Life cycle: Life cycles of parasitic copepods are normally direct and the sexes are separate. Eggs released into the water hatch into free-swimming naupliar stages. There can be up to six moults prior to the parasitic copepodid stage and up to a further five moults during this phase and up to four chalimus stages, in which the parasite is firmly attached to the host. There may be one or two pre-adult stages before the parasite becomes an adult.

Pathology: In most copepod infections, death can be associated with osmoregulatory failure due to the feeding actions of the parasite. *Ergasilus* spp. in the gills can cause destruction of the secondary lamellae, with concurrent necrosis, reduction in growth rates and mortality. *Lernaea* infections, even in low numbers, can cause serious damage. Fish can be lethargic and are susceptible to secondary infections through the site of parasite attachment, which is usually inflamed and haemorrhagic. Caligids can cause localized petechial haemorrhages at the site of feeding, again exposing the fish to the risk of secondary infections.

Diagnosis: Infected fish frequently show agitated behaviour, including increased flashing (rubbing). The parasites can often be seen in skin or gill scrapes, or on close examination of the skin or gills. Anchor worms are clearly visible attached to the body surface, and *Ergasilus* spp. can be seen attached to the gills.

Treatment and control: In all cases, infected fish should be quarantined to avoid cross-infection. Complete draining and disinfection of the system may be needed in order to break the life cycle of *Ergasilus* spp. Generally, copepod infections are treated with organophosphates and it may be necessary to carry out more than one treatment. Adult *L. cyprinacea* may be removed manually by grasping them at the point where they enter the body, but the wounds may need prophylactic treatment and careful monitoring for a few days. Free-swimming stages can be removed by treating the system with organophosphates. All stages are sensitive to drying.

Branchiurans
The most important branchiuran genus is the fish louse *Argulus* (Figure 21.32), normally parasitic in freshwater fish. *Argulus* spp. are dorsoventrally flattened and oval and have eyespots on the carapace. Most are less than 1 cm in length and live on the skin surface, feeding on blood. They can be differentiated from parasitic copepods by the presence of two suckers on the ventral surface of the body and a proboscis-like mouth. *Argulus* spp. are not normally found in aquaria, though wild-caught or pond-reared fish with access to natural waters may be infected. There are over 100 different species and perhaps the most important in freshwater systems is *A. foliaceus*. Also potentially problematic is *A. japonicus*, which is parasitic on ornamental koi and goldfish.

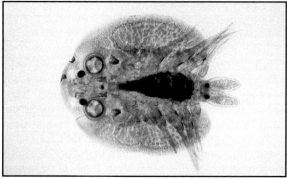

Figure 21.32 The branchiuran *Argulus foliaceus* isolated from the skin of a carp. (Wet mount preparation.)

Life cycle: Life cycles are direct. Both sexes are parasitic. After mating, the female deposits the eggs on a suitable substrate, such as aquatic plants, then returns to the fish host. The eggs hatch, develop, infect the fish and metamorphose into adults.

Pathology: Infected fish may show increased flashing, agitation and excess mucus production. Low numbers of parasites are usually tolerated by the fish. Sites of feeding by the parasite are often inflamed with local haemorrhaging. *Argulus* spp. may act as transport hosts for the virus causing spring viraemia of carp (SVC) and some nematodes that will be transmitted during the feeding process.

Diagnosis: *Argulus* spp. can be readily identified on the surface of the fish. When fish are removed from the water, the parasites may leave the host and can be seen swimming in the water.

Treatment and control: Adult *Argulus* spp. can be removed physically from the fish but this may not eliminate the parasite completely from the environment. Treatment with organophosphates, formalin or potassium permanganate will eradicate adult forms; juveniles can be killed by immersion in a 2% salt bath. The life cycle can be broken either by draining and drying out the system or by providing special egg-laying surfaces, removing them every few days and allowing them to dry.

The effective use of chitin inhibitors (e.g. diflubenzuron) has been documented and there are anecdotal reports of successful treatment using lufenuron. These chemicals inhibit the formation of larval chitin structures, thereby inhibiting the development of parasitic larvae and providing environmental control.

Isopods
Most parasitic isopods are found in marine systems and on almost any fish host. They are an infrequent problem in aquaria. The group is subdivided into two suborders: the Flabellifera, with a typical isopod shape, and the less common Gnathiidae (Figure 21.33), of which the most important are *Gnathia* spp. Flabellifera can be up to 6 cm in length and are generally ectoparasitic; they may be found on the skin surface or

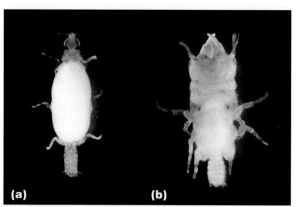

Figure 21.33 Two examples of a gnathid isopod: (a) a juvenile stage (praniza), which is parasitic; (b) a large adult, which is not normally parasitic.

in the mouth. Gnathids are much smaller (usually less than 1 cm) and for the most part only the larval or praniza stage is parasitic (on the skin or gills); adult stages are non-feeding and live in mud tubes.

Life cycle: Life cycles are simple. The non-parasitic adults produce larvae, which infect fish and live on the skin or gills.

Pathology: Because they are large, single individuals of the Flabellifera can cause problems due to their feeding action and potential occlusion of the host's mouth, which can lead to a reduction in growth. Infections with *Gnathia* spp. can kill small fish and may cause local haemorrhaging in areas of feeding.

Diagnosis: Isopods are easily seen when attached to the fish host.

Treatment and control: Individual isopods may be removed manually from the fish host. Removal of suitable habitats for adult gnathids will break the life cycle and reduce numbers. It is possible that isopods are susceptible to organophosphate treatments.

Further reading and references

Brown AF, Chubb JC and Veltkamp CJ (1986) A key to the species of Acanthocephala parasitic in British freshwater fishes. *Journal of Fish Biology* **28**, 327–334

Feist SW (1997) Pathogenicity of renal myxosporeans of fish. *Bulletin of the European Association of Fish Pathologists* **17**(6), 209–214

Kabata Z (1979) *Parasitic Copepoda of British Fishes.* Ray Society, London, 468 pp.

Kabata Z (1988) Copepoda and Branchiura. In: *Guide to the Parasites of Fishes of Canada. Part II: Crustacea* (eds Margolis L and Kabata Z). Canadian Special Publications, Fisheries and Aquatic Science, No. 101. Department of Fisheries and Oceans, Ottawa, pp. 3–127

Khalil L, Jones A and Bray RA (1994) *Keys to the Cestode Parasites of Vertebrates.* CAB International, Wallingford, 751 pp.

Kirk RS and Lewis JW (1994) Sanguinicoliasis in cyprinid fish in the UK. In: *Parasitic Diseases of Fish* (eds Pike AW and Lewis JW). Samara Publishing, Dyfed, pp. 101–117

Lom J and Arthur JR (1988) A guideline for the preparation of species descriptions in Myxosporea. *Journal of Fish Diseases* **12**, 151–156

Lom J and Dyková I (1992) *Protozoan Parasites of Fishes.* Vol. 26 in *Developments in Aquaculture and Fisheries Science.* Elsevier Science Publishers, Amsterdam

Rafi F (1988) Isopoda. In: *Guide to the Parasites of Fishes of Canada. Part II: Crustacea* (eds Margolis L and Kabata Z). Canadian Special Publications, Fisheries and Aquatic Sciences, No. 101. Department of Fisheries and Oceans, Ottawa, pp. 129–148

Shaw RS and Kent ML (1999) Fish microsporidia. In: *The Microsporidia and Microsporidiosis* (ed. Wittner M, contributing ed. Weiss LM). American Society for Microbiology, Washington DC

Thoney DA and Hargis WJ Jr (1991) Monogenea (Plathyhelminthes) as hazards for fish in confinement. *Annual Review of Fish Diseases* **1**, 133–153

Yokayama H, Ogawa K and Wakabayashi H (1990) Chemotherapy with fumagillin and toltrazuril against kidney enlargement disease of goldfish caused by the myxosporean *Hoferellus carassii. Fish Pathology* **25**, 157–163

Acknowledgements

The authors would like to acknowledge the numerous colleagues who over the years have supplied parasite material, some of which has been used here. In addition, we are grateful for the support from our families during the preparation of this chapter.

22

Bacterial diseases

Gavin Barker

Bacteria are probably the most significant pathogens of cultured fish, causing the highest levels of both morbidity and mortality. The rapid expansion of the aquaculture industry over the past two decades has led to a reasonable understanding of the pathogenesis of bacteria causing disease to farmed fish, but this information remains relatively poor compared with our understanding of bacterial diseases in humans and other animals. The knowledge concerning bacterial diseases of ornamental fish (in particular, tropical ornamental fish) is extremely limited and studies on ecology, epidemiology and management of diseases still remain to be carried out.

Causal factors

Bacterial diseases of fish are the result of many factors working together, ranging from environmental conditions, stress and susceptibility of the host through to virulence of the pathogen. Many bacterial pathogens are ubiquitous in the aquatic environment and are virulent over a wide range of environmental temperatures, affecting both coldwater and tropical species. They are nearly all capable of existing and multiplying in the aquatic environment outside the fish host. A few obligate fish pathogens do occur, but even these are capable of survival in the aquatic environment for considerable periods.

Stress

Over recent years it has become increasingly obvious that the host's physiology is very closely linked to the establishment of disease. It is likely that many potential bacterial pathogens coexist with fish either in the environment or even within carrier fish, without causing clinical disease until 'stress' occurs. Any deleterious alteration in the fish's environment can trigger a series of characteristic physiological changes (namely, a stress response) within the fish.

Invariably, fish respond to all forms of environmental stress by activation of the hypothalamic–pituitary–interrenal axis, with a resultant elevation in blood cortisol levels. In a fish-farming environment, stress can be continuous and can have a negative impact on the fish by suppressing growth rate, interfering with reproductive processes and increasing susceptibility to disease.

Bacterial virulence

In order for disease to occur, bacteria have to adhere to or penetrate fish tissues. Bacteria must then over-come various components of the fish immune system and obtain macronutrients and essential micronutrients to grow and proliferate.

All these characteristics are various aspects of an organism's virulence. Some bacteria, such as *Aeromonas salmonicida*, are extremely virulent; they are classified as primary pathogens and can potentially cause disease when the host is only marginally stressed. Other bacterial pathogens, such as *A. hydrophila*, are less virulent and are considered secondary pathogens, causing clinical disease only when fish are subjected to far greater levels of stress.

Disease prevention

During the rapid expansion of the salmonid fish-farming industry in the 1980s, bacterial diseases had a dramatic effect on production and resulted in considerable widespread use of antibiotics. The situation today is very different, with bacterial diseases being managed through a combination of improved husbandry and the use of increasingly effective vaccines.

The salmonid industry is well serviced with appropriate and effective vaccines supplied by a number of specialist manufacturers. Vaccines are also available for other sectors of the fish-farming industry and are continually being developed to service the needs of new, emerging aquaculture species. In contrast, only a few vaccines have been developed for the ornamental industry and these are still undergoing clinical trials. This reflects the paucity of knowledge surrounding ornamental fish and bacterial diseases as well as the fragmented nature of the market and the diversity of fish species within it.

Without vaccines being currently available, preventive methods rely almost entirely on husbandry and hygiene. Effectively this means good water quality, acceptable stocking densities, quick removal of moribund or dead fish and scrupulous disinfection procedures. It is likely that vaccines will become more widely used in the ornamental fish industry and that a range of other techniques to promote fish health will become available. Undoubtedly, these will include nutritional approaches such as micronutrients, immunostimulants, prebiotics and probiotics. In the longer term it is likely that more disease-resistant fish will be bred through the use of genetic markers and accelerated breeding programmes where appropriate.

Clinical signs

Frequently, one of the first clinical signs of bacterial disease is loss of appetite. Other signs include:

- Lethargy
- Change in colour (faded pigment or darkened pigment)
- Eye damage (corneal opacity, exophthalmos or hyphaema)
- Gill damage
- Fin rot
- Swollen abdomen
- External abscesses and ulcers.

Internal lesions often associated with bacterial infection include:

- Fluid in the abdominal cavity
- Swollen intestines
- Liver and spleen abnormalities (pale or swollen)
- White nodules on internal organs
- Haemorrhages on internal organs
- Muscle and skeletal deformities.

In a few cases, some clinical signs are pathognomonic, but generally a number of non-specific signs are observed. For accurate disease diagnosis some form of histopathological or bacteriological sampling, followed by isolation and identification of bacteria, is usually required.

Diagnosis and interpretation of results

In an ideal world, laboratory reports would clearly identify a single organism as the causative agent of a particular disease, treatment would be straightforward and a positive clinical outcome would be achieved. However, there are a number of problems concerning identification and treatment that must be considered.

Sampling

Under laboratory conditions, it is relatively easy to take bacteriological samples using swabs or loops under aseptic conditions. In contrast, this is rarely achievable in the field and it is easy to contaminate loops or swabs by inadvertently sampling adjacent tissues, especially in small fish. This will probably result in the culture of secondary as opposed to primary pathogens.

Under laboratory conditions, it is also practical to inoculate directly a range of selective and non-selective agar to assist in the recovery of suspected pathogens. In veterinary practice, it is often expensive and impractical to maintain a wide range of bacteriological media and often impossible to purchase small quantities of ready-made specialized media. Therefore, samples are frequently taken using swabs, placed in transport media and sent by post to specialist laboratories for diagnosis. This is a tried and tested technique in medical and other veterinary fields but is far from ideal in the case of fish pathogenic bacteria.

Some of these bacteria are fastidious, with specific nutritional and environmental requirements, and are unlikely to be recovered from transport media after several days in the post. Others will survive but are unlikely to be recovered, due to overgrowth by less fastidious bacteria capable of growth at the higher temperatures often associated with transport. In particular, organisms such as *Aeromonas hydrophila* and *Pseudomonas fluorescens* often seem to be dominant when transport swabs are used.

Identification

Many of the techniques used to identify pathogenic bacteria of fish, e.g. commercial biochemical test strips such as API are 'adapted' from their normal use in identifying bacteria associated with human disease. In experienced hands, these 'adaptations' can still provide accurate and reproducible results but the sensitivity required to split a genus clearly into separate species can be lost. One such example is aeromonads, where laboratory results can confuse *Aeromonas hydrophila*, *A. sobria* and *A. caviae*. In less experienced hands, when bacteria are unreactive, a spurious result can be achieved, generating a false identification and an illogical diagnosis, which is then passed to the veterinary practitioner and is of no value at all.

Interpretation

For some of the reasons outlined above, it is possible that results obtained from a laboratory will frequently highlight secondary pathogens such as *A. hydrophila* and other aeromonads or pseudomonads. In some cases, such as ulcer disease in coldwater ornamental fish, this may still be of great value, because unless attempts are made to inhibit these abundant secondary pathogens it is likely that existing ulcers will never heal. In these cases, the most important laboratory result is not so much the name of the bacteria present, but the antibiotic susceptibility tests that identify compounds that could inhibit the growth and proliferation of the organisms.

Antibiotic susceptibility tests

In human medicine there are national and international standards regulating the way in which antibiotic susceptibility tests are carried out in the laboratory. In principle, the disc diffusion assay is a simple technique providing reproducible results.

Without standardization (as in fish bacteriology), there are numerous procedures that can be conducted in a variety of different ways which, taken together, can significantly affect the inhibition zone sizes and the interpretation of the results. These differences include selection of media, inoculation density, inoculation method, antibiotic discs (drug concentration, diameter, thickness), incubation time and temperature, and measurement of inhibition zones (ruler, callipers, including/excluding microcolonies). In addition, in human medicine there are published tables linking inhibition zone sizes with minimum inhibitory concentration (MIC) values, which, coupled with pharmacokinetic data, give a good indication of clinical efficacy. Needless to say, no such data or tables exist for fish bacteriology.

Clinical outcome

Despite all the problems listed above, a positive clinical outcome can still be achieved, but there are many unknown factors to be overcome and it is best to be realistic about the difficulties of treating bacterial fish diseases.

Bacterial pathogens

Figure 22.1 lists the bacterial pathogens that are most commonly associated with diseases of ornamental fish. In the sections below, bacteria are listed according to their prevalence.

Motile aeromonads

Characteristics

Motile aeromonads are ubiquitous mesophilic organisms, frequently found in soil, freshwater lakes and streams, brackish waters, sea water (less often) and sewage and are part of the normal gut flora of humans. They are most commonly associated with aquatic animals, where they are considered part of the normal flora and as both primary and secondary pathogens.

Classification of the motile aeromonads remains confused. Typically, three species are recognized: *Aeromonas hydrophila*, *A. sobria* and *A. caviae*. Due to the problems associated with using biochemical identification kits designed for medical use, it is likely

Species	Staining characteristics	Physical characteristics	Freshwater or marine	Clinical feature
Motile aeromonads	Gram –ve	Rod 0.8–1.0 × 1.0–3.5 μm Motile	Both but mainly freshwater	Possibly primary pathogens. Definitely secondary pathogens. Acute systemic diseases and haemorrhagic skin lesions, frequently ulcerating. Chronic disease also occurs
Aeromonas salmonicida subsp. *achromogenes*	Gram –ve	Rod 0.3–1.0 × 1.0–3.5 μm Non-motile	Both but mainly freshwater	Haemorrhagic skin ulcers, often without general septicaemia
Cytophaga–Flavobacterium–Flexibacter group	Gram –ve	Rod 1.5–8.0 × 0.5–0.8 μm Non-motile, or motile by gliding	Both	Mainly gill diseases but also lesions on skin, fin and muscle. Extensive mouth erosions and general bacteraemia also occur
Edwardsiella species	Gram –ve	Rod 1.0 × 2–3 μm Motile	Both but mainly freshwater	Sepicaemia with dermal lesions that may ulcerate. Foul-smelling gas produced in lesions with necrotic tissue
Mycobacterium species	Gram +ve Acid-fast	Rod 1.5–2.0 × 0.25–0.35 μm Non-motile	Both	Chronic systemic disease with granulomas both externally and internally
Nocardia species	Gram +ve Weakly acid-fast	Rod 0.5–1.2 μm diameter mycelia fragmenting into rods and cocci	Both	Chronic disease causing nodular or diffuse granulomas internally
Photobacterium damselae subsp. *piscicida* (formerly *Pasteurella piscicida*)	Gram –ve	Cocco-bacilli 0.3–1.0 × 1.0–2.0 μm Non-motile	Both but mainly marine	Acute systemic disease. Granulomatous pseudo-tubercles formed in kidney and spleen with widespread internal necrosis
Pseudomonas species	Gram –ve	Rod 0.5–1.0 × 1.5–5.0 μm Motile	Both but mainly freshwater	Acute systemic diseases and haemorrhagic skin lesions that may ulcerate. Often associated with fin or tail rot
Streptococcus species	Gram +ve	Coccus 0.5–1 μm diameter Non-motile	Both	Acute systemic disease. Lesions (on dorsum and operculum and around the mouth) extend to form ulcers
Vibrio species	Gram –ve	Rod 0.3–0.3 × 1.4–2.6 μm	Marine and brackish	Acute systemic disease with haemorrhagic skin lesions leading to ulcers on the skin surface or mouth. Often produces anaemia
Chlamydia-like organisms	Gram –ve	Intracellular coccus or coccobacillus 0.2–1.2 μm	Both	Benign white or yellow nodules up to 1 mm in the gills and skin. Rarely causes dyspnoea and mortality

Figure 22.1 Important bacterial pathogens of ornamental fish.

that any of the three species could be diagnosed. The most probable organism to be involved is *A. hydrophila*, which will usually be recovered from all lesions and ulcers and which, by the time veterinary advice is sought, may also be isolated from many internal organs.

A. hydrophila survives well in transport media and will grow on all general-purpose bacteriological media, including many low-nutrient and selective media designed to inhibit it. For these reasons alone, its presence is frequently diagnosed, especially in diseases of freshwater fish.

Motile aeromonads are capable of growing at an extremely wide range of temperatures, from 5 to 37°C, but there is some evidence to suggest that they are unlikely to be pathogenic to fish at temperatures below 8°C.

Motile aeromonad septicaemia can be acute or chronic in fish and external lesions can ulcerate, with necrotic tissue present throughout the dermis, epidermis and muscle. Internal lesions include oedema, haemorrhaging and diffuse necrosis.

Treatment and control

Whether *A. hydrophila* is considered a primary or secondary pathogen, existing clinical conditions will not improve unless the organism is inhibited. Ideally, it is best to control all underlying factors that may have caused stress to the fish population and predisposed them to infection. In practice, it is often difficult to determine these factors and what primary pathogens, if any, are present.

Dead or moribund fish should be removed immediately and, where possible, stocking densities reduced. Filtration should be improved and organic loading (nutrient input) reduced significantly. Antibiotic therapy is often required but this may not always be successful, as resistance to antibiotic compounds is widespread among motile aeromonads and some isolates can be resistant to a wide range of antibiotics (Figure 22.2). Motile aeromonad infections can cause widespread and devastating losses among ornamental fish; therefore, on welfare grounds alone, antibiotic therapy should be attempted.

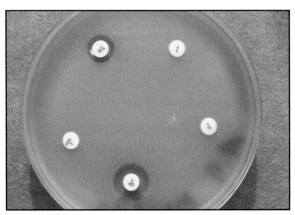

Figure 22.2 The problem of bacterial resistance to antibiotics is illustrated by this *Aeromonas hydrophila* isolated from a koi, which is resistant to all five antibiotics tested.

Pseudomonads

Characteristics

Pseudomonads are ubiquitous in water but they are also found in soil and often associated with spoiled foods. Most pseudomonads are saprophytic but can be opportunistic pathogens of tropical fish.

The classification of pseudomonads remains confused. At present, there are probably four species that are considered pathogenic to fish or eels: *Pseudomonas fluorescens*, *P. anguilliseptica*, *P. chloraphis* and *P. pseudoalcaligenes*. It is almost certain that nearly all septicaemia caused by pseudomonads seen in ornamental fish will be associated with *P. fluorescens*. This organism causes a haemorrhagic septicaemia that can be acute or chronic and that is clinically similar to motile aeromonad septicaemia.

Pseudomonad septicaemia can often occur through the results of poor husbandry, such as low dissolved oxygen, overcrowding, elevated ammonia levels, high water temperatures or poor nutrition.

P. fluorescens is capable of causing infection over a wide temperature range but is more commonly recovered at water temperatures ranging from 15 to 25°C. The organism survives well in transport media, is easy to culture (Figure 22.3) and is thus frequently diagnosed.

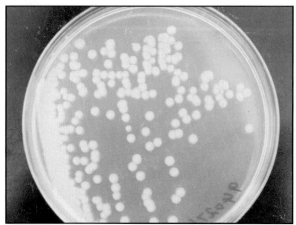

Figure 22.3 The characteristic green pigment that is produced by *Pseudomonas fluorescens* is fluorescent under ultraviolet light.

Treatment and control

It is important that all factors that may cause stress are addressed in order to reduce infection with *P. fluorescens*. Although the organism can be a devastating pathogen, it is only weakly virulent and a reduction in stress will allow fish to recover. Antibiotic therapy may be required but, due to problems of widespread antibiotic resistance, success may be limited.

Aeromonas salmonicida subsp. *achromogenes*

Characteristics

Aeromonas salmonicida is a true primary pathogen of fish. It is an obligate pathogen and has limited ability to survive outside the host. It is the cause of furunculosis in salmonid fish and outbreaks of the disease, related to stress, can pose a real threat, with extremely high mortality rates.

Originally, some isolates of *A. salmonicida* (Figure 22.4) were referred to as 'atypical' isolates because they were recovered from non-salmonid fish. However, classifying isolates based on the host from which they were recovered has subsequently led to significant classification problems. Atypical strains are heterogeneous in nature, with varying biochemical characteristics and growth conditions, but in the main are differentiated from typical isolates by their lack or very slow production of pigment on bacteriological media – hence the name *achromogenes*.

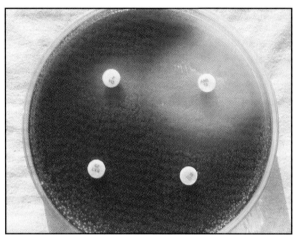

Figure 22.4 The characteristic brown pigment produced by typical *Aeromonas salmonicida* isolated from a salmonid. Atypical strains are more commonly isolated from ornamental fish and do not produce pigment.

The best-known diseases associated with atypical *A. salmonicida* are carp erythrodermatitis and goldfish ulcer disease. It is most probably the cause of ulcer disease seen in koi; it is the cause of ulcer disease of flounder; and has been associated with diseases of many other marine and freshwater fish.

Atypical *A. salmonicida* infection in ornamental fish is usually seen as skin ulcers without septicaemia. Initially some scales become infected, and then inflamed and raised. The scales are shed, resulting in necrosis of the epidermis, dermis and then the muscle. Secondary pathogens invade the wounds in abundance and it is often organisms such as *A. hydrophila* and *Pseudomonas fluorescens* that are recovered, masking the presence of atypical *A. salmonicida*.

Isolation of atypical *A. salmonicida* can be improved by carefully sampling tissues on the very edge of ulcers with small sterile plastic loops and directly inoculating a general-purpose agar containing the dye coo-massie brilliant blue. The growth of dark blue colonies on this agar (Figure 22.5) is a good indication of *A. salmonicida achromogenes*.

Treatment and control

At present, most treatments rely on the use of antimicrobial therapy. Frequently, this is best administered by injection for large valuable ornamental fish. In addition,

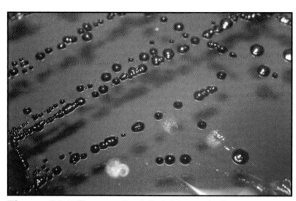

Figure 22.5 The growth of dark blue colonies on coomassie brilliant blue agar is characteristic of *Aeromonas salmonicida achromogenes*. (Courtesy of M. Algoet. © W.H. Wildgoose)

success has been achieved through debridement, disinfection and topical dressing of individual wounds and ulcers. Since ulcers very quickly become colonized by secondary pathogens it is also important to improve environmental conditions if possible, and to remove infected individuals to isolation or recovery tanks.

Atypical *Aeromonas salmonicida* may not survive well in the environment but it may remain dormant within the host. Carrier fish are a very real problem and caution should be exercised for a long time after an outbreak of the disease. It is likely that effective vaccines will eventually be developed to protect coldwater ornamental fish against atypical *A. salmonicida*. Before significant progress can be made, further studies are required to determine which isolates are virulent and problematical, and which ones can be ignored.

Vibrios

Characteristics

Vibrios are ubiquitous organisms in the marine and estuarine environment, particularly when there is a high organic load. Some species are considered harmless, some as opportunistic pathogens to fish in a compromised state and others seem to be highly virulent primary pathogens.

For many years vibriosis referred only to diseases of fish in cold water caused by *Vibrio anguillarum* but it is now widely accepted that vibrios are an emerging group of pathogens causing widespread mortalities among tropical marine fish. Others implicated in fish disease are *V. salmonicida*, *V. ordalii*, *V. alginolyticus*, *V. parahaemolyticus*, *V. vulnificus* and *V. damsela*.

Vibriosis is very similar to motile aeromonad septicaemia; it is usually associated with a haemorrhagic septicaemia and produces extensive haemorrhaging and skin lesions. Internal lesions include anaemia and necrosis of the liver, spleen and kidney.

Vibrios will nearly always be isolated from any ulcer or lesions of marine fish. The two species most likely to be encountered with ornamental fish are *V. anguillarum* and *V. ordalii* but without the help of a specialized laboratory it is unlikely that the species will be identified. As with aeromonad infections, identification of the species is less important than its antibiotic susceptibility.

Treatment and control

Treatment relies on improving husbandry and reducing stress. Where practical, wounds can be debrided and disinfected or antimicrobial therapy can be applied topically. However, oral medication with antibiotics in sea water is always problematical and in many cases, coupled with antibiotic resistance problems, treatment can prove ineffective. No vibriosis vaccines are produced for the ornamental market.

Mycobacteria

Characteristics

Infections of fish by mycobacteria are generally referred to as mycobacteriosis or fish tuberculosis. Mycobacteriosis has been observed in over 150 marine and freshwater fish species. There are more than 50 recognized species of mycobacteria but only two are commonly involved with fish diseases: *Mycobacterium marinum* and *M. fortuitum*. *M. chelonae* is also considered a rare fish pathogen.

Most mycobacteria are free-living in soil and water but are recognized as pathogens of a wide range of animals, including humans. Both *M. marinum* and *M. fortuitum* cause localized non-healing ulcers and lymph node infections in humans and can occur after exposure to infected fish (Chapter 34).

Mycobacteriosis in fish may manifest itself as localized lesions in the skin but usually no external clinical signs are observed. A range of non-specific clinical signs, such as reduced appetite, emaciation, lethargy, colour change, body deformation and lack of coordination, may be present. Internally, grey/white granulomas are seen in many organs, especially the kidney (Figure 22.6), liver and spleen.

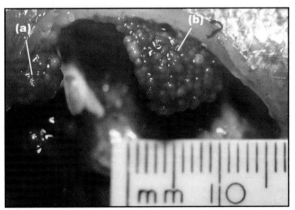

Figure 22.6 Mycobacterial granulomas in (a) anterior and (b) posterior kidney of a goldfish that was sampled from an aquarium experiencing chronic mortalities. Despite the extensive lesions, only a few acid-fast bacteria were found on histological examination. (© W.H. Wildgoose)

Identification of mycobacteria is often carried out using stained histology samples confirming the presence of Gram-positive pleomorphic rods that are acid-alcohol fast. Theoretically, mycobacteria can be cultured on general-purpose bacteriological agar but this requires a large inoculum. Usually, culture requires specialist media such as Löwenstein–Jensen agar and

even then it is not always successful. The use of immunohistochemistry and PCR techniques is currently being investigated as an aid to confirmation of mycobacterial infection.

Treatment and control

Various measures can be taken to prevent or reduce the risk of infection with mycobacteria. The most important is to quarantine new fish for a period of up to 2 months. Overcrowding should be prevented and the use of raw and 'natural' feeds avoided where possible.

Once established, mycobacteriosis is a difficult infection to eradicate. Realistically, the only practical step that can be taken is elimination of infected fish and disinfection. Many drugs have been suggested for treating this disease but few rigorous trials have been published. Various authors have suggested rifampicin, erythromycin, streptomycin, kanamycin, doxycycline and minocycline (van Duijn, 1981) but a successful clinical outcome may be limited. The use of environmental disinfectants has also been suggested as an aid to controlling the disease.

Cytophaga–Flavobacterium–Flexibacter group

Characteristics

Gram-negative yellow-pigmented bacteria have been associated with diseases in a wide range of fish species, both marine and freshwater, and under warm and cold conditions. Genera that are frequently encountered include *Cytophaga*, *Flavobacterium*, *Flexibacter*, *Myxobacterium*, *Myxococcus* and *Sporocytophaga*. These genera are often difficult to identify, since they can be fastidious in their growth requirements and biochemically unreactive. This has led to confusion among taxonomists and a long process of classifying and reclassifying the organisms, with the result that the nomenclature changes frequently.

Many of these bacteria cause gill diseases and usually produce hyperplasia of the gill epithelium. This often results in fish gathering at water inlets and 'gasping' at the water surface. Fortunately, not all of the group are significant pathogens of ornamental fish.

One of the most frequently encountered is *Flavobacterium columnare*, the causative agent of columnaris disease, sometimes referred to as 'saddleback' or 'cotton-wool disease'. It can affect freshwater fish at both high and low temperatures. The gill is usually the area of infection, although lesions also occur on the skin and musculature. On the body these lesions start at the base of the dorsal or pelvic fins and at first appear as patches of discoloration that have the characteristic appearance of a saddle.

Flexibacter maritimus causes an ulcerative syndrome in marine fish at high and low temperatures. The disease has been called 'eroded mouth syndrome' or 'black patch necrosis', depending on fish species infected. As these names suggest, the common sites of infection include the mouth, gill and tail. In larger fish the lesions appear on the head, body and fins. Large numbers of long, slender bacterial rods colonize the infected tissue and produce a pale yellow appearance.

'Fin rot' is a term used to describe a characteristic necrosis of the fins caused by various bacteria within this group of organisms. Although the bacterium formerly known as *Cytophaga psychrophila* causes fin rot, 'peduncle disease' and 'coldwater disease' in salmonids, the problem in ornamental fish is more complicated and may involve several different species of bacteria, including *Flavobacterium columnare* and *Flexibacter maritimus*.

Both *Flavobacterium columnare* and *Flexibacter maritimus* can be identified through their characteristic slow, gliding movement, which can be seen in wet preparations. Here, *Flavobacterium columnare* cells are often seen to gather into characteristic column-like groups (Figure 22.7). Specialized low-nutrient medium is required to culture both these organisms.

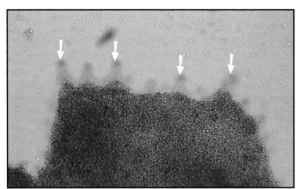

Figure 22.7 Wet preparation revealing colonies of *Flavobacterium columnare* in columns (arrowed), amorphous masses of bacteria attached to pieces of necrotic tissue (× 100 original magnification). (Reproduced with the permission of *In Practice*.)

Flavobacterium branchiophilum is a filamentous, non-gliding bacterium and is considered the causative agent of 'bacterial gill disease'. Typically, this is a disease of salmonids but other freshwater fish are likely to be affected by this organism or other bacteria belonging to the *Cytophaga–Flexibacter–Flavobacter* genera. The clinical signs of the disease and culture of *Flavobacterium branchiophilum* are similar to those described for *Flavobacterium columnare* and *Flexibacter maritimus*.

Treatment and control
All bacteria in the *Cytophaga–Flavobacterium–Flexibacter* group can spread rapidly through water. Attention to hygiene is essential and water quality should be improved by increasing dissolved oxygen levels, reducing suspended solids and ammonia and, where possible, reducing stocking density.

In cases of *Flavobacterium columnare*, a controlled reduction in water temperature is often beneficial and surface bactericides added to water as a dip can be effective in treating external lesions. Sulphonamides have been used to treat systemic infections effectively. *Flexibacter maritimus* can be more difficult to control, though oxytetracycline has proved effective in some cases.

For *Flavobacterium branchiophilum* and other freshwater gill disease problems, dipping fish in 1–5% sodium chloride (salt) solution for 1–2 minutes can be effective. It can also be stressful and result in significant mortalities but it is worth considering before resorting to compounds such as quaternary ammonium compounds, chloramine-T or antibiotics.

Streptococci

Characteristics
Streptococci are found in a wide variety of human, animal and plant habitats. They are also significant pathogens of fish, causing systemic diseases in both fresh and sea water.

Clinical signs differ depending on the species of bacteria and fish involved. Externally, darkening of the body colour, loss of coordination, exophthalmos, ulceration and haemorrhages at the base of fins and operculum are observed. Internally, an enlarged spleen and pale necrotic liver are seen, together with infection of the eye and brain. Disease is usually associated with high temperatures (about 30°C) but increasingly bacteria are recovered at relatively low temperatures.

Classification of streptococci (or streptococci-like bacteria) that are pathogenic for fish is always being reviewed and isolates are frequently being reclassified as *Vagococcus*, *Lactococcus* or *Enterococcus*. Streptococci are maintained well in transport media and the Gram-positive organism can be isolated and cultured relatively easily.

Treatment and control
It is thought that streptococci are present in water and mud and may be present in carrier fish. During an outbreak, environmental improvements such as reductions in feeding, handling and stocking density may be useful. In warmwater outbreaks, reducing water temperatures and dipping freshwater fish in 1–5% sodium chloride (salt) solution for 1–2 minutes may be beneficial. If the disease occurs in alkaline waters, lowering the pH may also be effective. Antibiotics such as erythromycin have been used to treat streptococcal diseases in fish.

Edwardsiellae

Characteristics
Unlike most other genera, the classification of *Edwardsiella* is not confused. Two species – *E. ictaluri* and *E. tarda* – are recognized pathogens of fish.

E. ictaluri is the causal agent of enteric septicaemia of catfish and is responsible for 'hole-in-the-head' disease in young catfish. It is not exclusively a disease of catfish and outbreaks of disease have occurred in non-ictalurid species. Two forms of disease are caused by the pathogen: an acute gastrointestinal septicaemia, and a chronic form producing a 'hole-in-the-head' lesion followed by septicaemia and death. Erratic swimming behaviour or listlessness is seen, with white ulcerations (1–10 mm in diameter) over the entire body. Internal clinical signs are typical of an acute septicaemia.

E. tarda is arguably not so pathogenic as *E. ictaluri* but does affect a wider range of fish species. *E. tarda* infections are characterized by small lesions located over the body, which develop into abscesses, and by a reddening of the fins and body surfaces. The abscesses contain many neutrophils and necrotic material, which becomes liquefactive and foul smelling. In later stages the infection spreads to internal organs and muscle, where suppurative abscesses develop.

Edwardsiellae are easy to sample, well maintained in transport media and simple to culture and identify. An accurate and rapid diagnosis should be possible.

Treatment and control

Edwardsiellae are able to survive in pond water and mud. There is some confusion as to whether a true carrier state exists, but it is probable that recently introduced fish could be infective. Vaccine development has not proved to be straightforward and is unlikely to be available for the ornamental sector for some time. During a disease outbreak, a reduction in feeding rates and a lowering of water temperature can be helpful.

E. tarda is sensitive to a wide range of antibiotics and is relatively easy to control. *E. ictaluri* can also be treated with orally administered antibiotics but is susceptible to only a narrow range of antimicrobials.

Photobacterium damsela subsp. *piscicida* (formerly *Pasteurella piscicida*)

Characteristics

Pasteurellosis, a disease caused by *Photobacterium damselae* subsp. *piscicida*, was traditionally associated with sea bass, sea bream and yellowtail. It is now thought to affect a wider range of fish species but is more likely to occur in public aquaria than in domestic situations. The organism has limited survival in the environment and is probably transmitted through carrier fish.

Both acute and chronic forms of pasteurellosis occur. Externally there may be few clinical signs, such as darkening of the skin, but the disease can be dramatic with large numbers of mortalities. The acute form results in little gross pathology, but the liver, kidney and spleen are colonized by bacteria that cause tissue necrosis. In chronic lesions prominent white granules may be visible in the spleen and kidney, giving rise to the name 'pseudotuberculosis' or 'bacterial tuberculoidosis'. The organism is not difficult to grow but can often be misdiagnosed, especially where it is rarely encountered.

Treatment and control

A range of antibiotics can be administered orally and usually with good effect but antibiotic resistance is becoming more widespread. The disease may be prevented by improved husbandry and water quality and by avoiding overcrowding. Frequently, the disease occurs when temperatures rise to over 25°C coupled with a reduction in salinity. If possible, this combination of events should be avoided or rectified quickly.

Nocardiae

Characteristics

Nocardiae are widely distributed in soil. Two species have been implicated in fish diseases: *Nocardia kampachi* is associated with disease in cultured yellowtail only; but *N. asteroides* has been implicated in disease of a number of fish species, especially tropical ornamental fish.

Clinical signs attributed to nocardiosis are very similar to those described for mycobacteria and this has often led to confusion. *N. asteroides* causes a chronic disease with typical clinical signs such as emaciation, lethargy and skin discoloration. Only a small percentage of a given population is affected and mortalities are few.

In theory, nocardiae are easy to culture and identify. In practice, they are rarely seen and misdiagnosis or confusion with mycobacteria undoubtedly occurs.

Treatment and control

Prevention and treatment methods for nocardiae are very similar to those advocated for mycobacteria. In a clean environment the bacterium can survive for only a limited period outside the host but survival increases considerably as the quality of the environment deteriorates. As with mycobacteria, treatment with antibiotics is possible and could be attempted for rare or valuable fish. This involves a combination of antibiotics administered for at least a 3-week period. Where possible, the removal of moribund fish and scrupulous disinfection of the environment are recommended.

Chlamydia

Characteristics

A *Chlamydia*-like organism is thought to be the cause of epitheliocystis, an uncommon disease that affects both freshwater and marine fish. The intracellular organism produces small white or yellow nodules on the gill, and less commonly on the skin, that measure up to 1 mm. In small numbers, the disease is an incidental finding but severe infection may cause dyspnoea and mortality, particularly in juvenile fish. The disease can be identified on wet mount preparations but is confirmed by histological examination (Figure 22.8) and

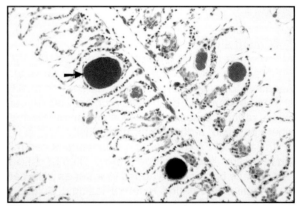

Figure 22.8 Histological section of a gill with epitheliocystis. A large granular basophilic inclusion is seen in an infected epidermal cell (arrowed) (H&E stain, × 400 original magnification). (Courtesy of P. Southgate)

electron microscopy. Infected epidermal cells become enormously enlarged (up to 400 μm) due to a large granular basophilic inclusion that occupies most of the cell. Histologically the disease resembles lymphocystis, a viral infection of the dermal fibroblasts.

Treatment and control

There is no known treatment. At present, the life cycle and mode of transmission is unknown; therefore, quarantine and disinfection may be the only means of limiting the spread of the disease. Until the organism can be successfully isolated and because of the low mortality, it is unlikely that a vaccine will be developed.

Further reading and reference

Austin B and Austin DA (eds) (1993) *Bacterial Fish Pathogens: Disease in Farmed and Wild Fish.* Ellis Horwood, Chichester

Inglis V, Roberts RJ and Bromage NR (eds) (1993) *Bacterial Diseases of Fish.* Blackwell Scientific Publications, Oxford

Puttinaowarat S, Thompson KD and Adams A (2000) Mycobacteriosis: detection and identification of aquatic *Mycobacterium* species. *Fish Veterinary Journal* **5**, 6–21

van Duijn C (1981) Tuberculosis in fishes. *Journal of Small Animal Practice* **22**, 391–411

Acknowledgement

The author is very grateful to Debbie Page for her assistance during the preparation of this chapter.

23

Fungal diseases and harmful algae

Andrew Holliman

The biological feature that characterizes fungi, above all else, is their osmotrophic (absorptive) mode of nutrition. They can neither ingest their food nor manufacture it in the way that plants do. In addition, the majority of fungi are composed of characteristic branching filaments (hyphae) that grow by apical (tip) extension. The mass of hyphae is called the mycelium. Upon reaching a certain stage of maturity, the mycelium forms reproductive cells called spores, which may be produced directly by asexual methods or indirectly through sexual reproduction. Spores are released and dispersed by a variety of mechanisms and are typically resistant to heat, drying and a variety of chemical disinfectants.

The organisms traditionally studied by mycologists, although mostly falling within the kingdom Fungi, are now known to include representatives phylogenetically lying within the kingdoms Protozoa and Chromista, and others whose taxonomic position is unresolved. These latter include at least two genera containing important fish pathogens, as described below. The most economically important fungal pathogen of fish, *Saprolegnia parasitica*, belongs to the oomycetous fungi, or water moulds, whose phylogenetic roots lie with the chromophyte algae in the kingdom Chromista rather than the main evolutionary line of fungi.

Healthy skin is usually covered with a layer of mucus and this generally serves as an effective barrier to fungal invasion. This protection is typically thought to have three components (though it is unknown whether all fish species respond in this way to fungal pathogens):

- Physical removal of attached spores as the external mucus is continually renewed
- Substances within the mucus that inhibit mycelial growth
- Cellular response within the mucus directed at the growing mycelium (Willoughby, 1989).

Fungal diseases of fish are usually secondary, being precipitated by factors such as poor environmental conditions, poor nutrition, physical injury and bacterial or parasitic diseases. These serve to weaken a fish's natural defences by either disrupting the natural integrity of the skin or acting as stressors and thereby reducing the specific and non-specific immune defences.

Fungal infections are typically superficial, being confined to the skin, with deeper involvement only in more severe or more chronic cases. Occasionally (but rarely) systemic disease may occur, with multi-organ involvement. Fish eggs are also susceptible to infection.

Saprolegniasis

Infection with fungi of the family *Saprolegniaceae* represents probably the most important mycotic disease of fish worldwide. Important genera in terms of pathogenicity include *Saprolegnia*, *Achlya* and *Aphanomyces*. In the UK and Europe, *Saprolegnia* is the predominant species in fresh water. When aquarists refer to 'fungus disease' in their fish they are usually referring to saprolegniasis. Virtually all species of freshwater fish are susceptible, and it is being increasingly recognized as important in estuarine species. Marine fish species are not affected, as even half-strength seawater is lethal to *Saprolegnia* spores. This disease has a worldwide distribution and commonly occurs at temperatures between 3°C and 33°C.

Whilst there is evidence that *Saprolegnia* can act as a primary pathogen, it is typically a secondary invader and a number of factors may increase susceptibility.

- Epidermal integrity: large wounds are always potential sites for *Saprolegnia* colonization and these may result from netting, handling, skin parasites, overcrowding etc.
- Stress: increased plasma corticosteroid levels appear to increase susceptibility, associated with immunosuppression, and factors as described above may all act as stressors
- Sexual maturation: mature male fish, in particular, appear to have a reduction in the natural resistance of skin to fungal invasion; this is dramatically illustrated in spawning salmonids
- Infection may be seen following a fall in water temperature, presumably related to a reduction in immune function.

Characteristics

Members of the *Saprolegniaceae* belong to the oomycetous fungi (water moulds). The vegetative mycelium is made up of a series of thick, branched, aseptate filaments. The life cycle is complex. Primary zoospores released from zoosporangia settle and round-up to produce thin-walled cysts. A secondary zoospore is released and this is the main motile stage, remaining motile for hours or even days. It also encysts, forming a secondary cyst, and this is thought to be the main infective stage, locating and attaching to suitable food substrates. Oomycete spores are often present in high concentration in many types of waters, with some seasonal variation, and levels can increase dramatically following colonization of fish skin.

Fish tissues *per se* are suitable growth substrates for many oomycetes, and dead fish may be colonized by a range of species of *Saprolegniaceae*, including *Saprolegnia*, *Achlya* and *Aphanomyces*. Basically, they act as saprophytes, living on dead material. Similarly, severely damaged necrotic tissue will almost certainly yield many different oomycete species.

Only the parasitic species are able to colonize live fish efficiently. For instance, spores of the common pathogenic species, *S. parasitica*, are successfully able to colonize fish epidermis but the exact basis for fish pathogenicity has not yet been clearly defined. Fish-lesion isolates from wide geographical origins are all characterized by their distinctive cyst coat morphology and germ tube growth.

Many *Saprolegnia* isolates taken from fish are asexual and cannot be identified to species level. Speciation is based on the morphology of the sexual organs but it is generally accepted that asexual isolates taken from moribund fish or fish eggs belong to the species *S. parasitica* whilst the common saprophytic isolates belong to either the species *S. diclina* or occasionally *S. ferax*.

There is significant variation within the group identified as *S. parasitica*. It has been suggested that isolates of *S. parasitica* from salmonid fish fall into their own distinct subgroup, defined as Type 1, whilst isolates from coarse fish fall into a Type 2 subgroup. The exact nature of isolates from aquarium fish is unclear (Willoughby, 1978).

Clinical signs

Saprolegnia invades epidermal tissues, generally beginning on the head or fins, and may spread over the entire body surface (Figure 23.1). It presents as white or grey cotton wool-like patches, radiating out in a

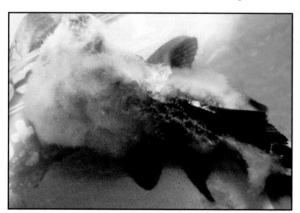

Figure 23.1 A fancy goldfish with *Saprolegnia* infection. The disease produces a dense mass of cotton wool-like growth when viewed under water. (By permission of *In Practice*.)

circular or crescent-shaped pattern. Removal of an infected fish from water causes the mat to collapse and appear as a slimy mass (Figure 23.2). The entrapment of suspended solids or other debris within the mass of mycelia may alter both its colour and appearance (Figure 23.3). Dead and dying fish eggs may be infected by *Saprolegnia*, followed by direct-contact spread to adjacent viable eggs.

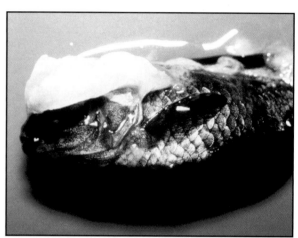

Figure 23.2 The same fish as in Figure 23.1, having been removed from the water. The delicate fungal structure has collapsed into a slimy mass. (By permission of *Koi Health Quarterly*.)

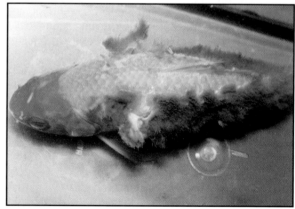

Figure 23.3 Algae frequently become entrapped in the fungal mass and give the lesion a green coloration, as seen in this goldfish. The epidermis has been lost from the dorsum and is continuing to detach further down the sides of the fish. (© W.H. Wildgoose.)

Pathology

Damage to the skin is often sufficient to kill a fish, the degree of severity being related to the surface area affected. Death results from osmoregulatory failure and loss of electrolytes and serum protein. Any involvement of the gills is invariably fatal. Loss of epithelial integrity occurs because of epithelial cell necrosis, resulting in eventual penetration of the dermis by fungal hyphae. The secretion of proteolytic enzymes aids the growth and spread of the fungus. Deep muscular penetration is uncommon, though it may occur in small fish and even involve vital organs. Host inflammatory responses are weakly developed. There is no evidence of toxin production with systemic effects.

Diagnosis

- White mycelial patches on fish skin are likely to be due to a member of the *Saprolegniaceae*
- Examination of the fungus mounted in water on a glass slide may allow confirmation of the identity of the fungus (Figure 23.4). Staining with lactophenol cotton blue or methylene blue will aid the visualization of branched aseptate hyphae
- Much more information can be obtained if small pieces of fungus, plus underlying fish tissue, are placed in 20 ml of sterilized water in a Petri dish. Since fish fungal pathogens are facultative necrotrophs, they will continue to grow on dead tissue. After 48 hours at 10°C, they will produce a luxuriant clear mycelium bearing sporangia at the tips of fertile hyphae (Figure 23.5), each zoosporangium bearing mature zoospores, enabling generic identification. Ideally, culture should only be attempted from a live fish. After death, the fish will be subject to saprophytic colonization by a variety of aquatic fungi (Willoughby, 1994).

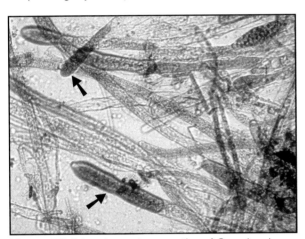

Figure 23.4 A wet mount preparation of *Saprolegnia* revealing a tangled network of aseptate hyphae and zoosporangia (arrowed). The latter are not always present in samples from lesions. × 100 original magnification. (Courtesy of Peter Scott.)

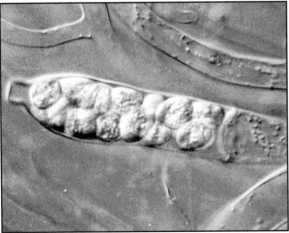

Figure 23.5 A club-shaped zoosporangium of *S. parasitica* containing primary zoospores. SEM mount, × 1000 original magnification. (Courtesy of Gordon Beakes.)

Treatment

Recovery from the disease is directly related to the area of skin affected, therefore prompt diagnosis and treatment are vital. Fungal infections are difficult to treat but various chemicals can be used:

- Zinc-free malachite green is considered the most effective chemical for controlling saprolegniasis. There are reports of toxicity to tetras, scaleless fish and some marine species
- Formalin has been used but is much less effective
- Salt, potassium permanganate, methylene blue and copper sulphate have also been used to some effect
- A new therapeutic bath or flush treatment containing bronopol (Pyceze®, Novartis) is currently obtaining registration in the UK and internationally. It has been shown to be effective in salmonids but has not been fully investigated for use in ornamental species.

Control

Control and prevention can be aided by:

- Identifying and correcting the predisposing factors (including malnutrition, physical injury, bacterial or parasitic infection) that may lead to saprolegniasis. The reduction of stress appears to be the single most important factor in resisting infection and it is essential to address this aspect and not rely solely on medication
- Removal and treatment of affected fish
- Removal of all dead fish and dead fish eggs
- Avoidance of overfeeding.

Branchiomycosis

The exact taxonomic classification of *Branchiomyces* spp. is uncertain but they are placed within the order *Saprolegniales*. This disease is associated with *Branchiomyces sanguinis* and *B. demigrans* infection and is commonly called 'gill rot'. Cyprinid fish appear particularly susceptible. It is typically recognized as a disease of carp in farm ponds. Tench, sticklebacks and eel are also susceptible.

The disease is most often reported from Europe, Japan and the United States but only rarely from the UK. Infection commonly occurs in association with abundant organic matter at high water temperatures (20–25°C) in high stocking density situations.

Clinical signs

Affected fish become weak, show respiratory distress with gasping at the surface, often lose equilibrium and die. Gill tissue appears eroded, necrotic and pale and takes on a marbled appearance. Necrotic tissue may slough, leaving denuded areas.

Pathology

Fungal spores attach to the gills, germinate and produce hyphae. Hyphal growth is intravascular, resulting in infarctive necrosis due to vascular obstruction and thrombosis. Maturing spores may be seen within the aseptate branching hyphae and mature spores are released from necrotic gill tissue. Hyperplasia and fusion of gill lamellae are accompanying features.

Diagnosis

This is often based on:

- Previous history of disease in an endemic area
- Clinical signs and characteristic gross appearance of gills
- Hyphae and spores that may be seen in gill squash preparations
- Distinctive intravascular hyphae that are easily recognized in gill section (almost diagnostic)
- Relative ease of culture on agar media, such as Sabouraud's.

Treatment

- Formalin is reported to be effective, using an initial treatment of 15 ml/l followed by an application of 25 ml/l. Repeated treatments are necessary to control infection
- Malachite green at 0.1 mg/l for extended periods may be effective.

Control

- Avoidance is best achieved by not feeding raw-fish products and not introducing infected fish from an endemic zone
- Control may be achieved by preventing the accumulation of decomposing organic matter (e.g. by reducing stocking densities, improving water quality, decreasing feed and destroying and removing infected fish)
- Elimination from earth ponds requires emptying, drying and the use of quicklime or copper sulphate, the latter at the rate of 0.2–0.3 g/m^2
- Infection often reappears unless adhering strictly to the above procedures.

Ichthyophonus

Ichthyophonus hoferi is an obligate parasite with a relatively simple life cycle. The exact phylogenetic position of the parasite is still unclear; it shows affinities with both fungi and protozoa. It is thought to be a member of a lower protistan group. Many marine and freshwater species, including aquarium species, can become infected. The organism is primarily of marine origin but can be transferred to freshwater fish when carnivorus species are fed on tissues from infected marine fish. The disease has a worldwide incidence.

Clinical signs

These are not pathognomonic and include erratic swimming movements and loss of equilibrium. Fish appear emaciated and listless and may darken, initially along the lateral line. Many organs, including skin, may be infected. Affected skin areas appear granular and roughened. Scoliosis is occasionally seen.

Pathology

The parasite can be found in a wide variety of organs, including the brain, appearing as whitish-grey or occasionally orange foci. Affected organs may be noticeably swollen and nodular. Muscle may be extensively affected and appear necrotic.

Histologically the lesion consists of a granulomatous reaction around variably sized spherical bodies – the 'resting' spores (Figure 23.6). Larger spores have varying numbers of nuclei and typically thick, multi-layered cell walls that stain strongly PAS-positive. The characteristic parasite germination (i.e. the formation of branched germination tubes or 'hyphae'), seen after death of the host, is a useful diagnostic feature.

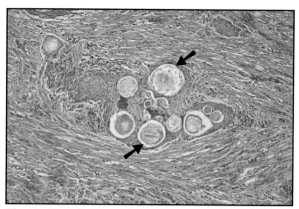

Figure 23.6 Cross-section of a granulomatous lesion in the heart caused by *Ichthyophonus hoferi* infection. There is a chronic inflammatory response surrounding some spores (arrowed). H&E stain, × 100 original magnification. (Courtesy of David Bruno.)

Infection is thought to be via the gut by ingestion of 'resting' spores, followed by germination, gut penetration and systemic invasion into the circulatory and lymphatic systems. In target organs, nuclear proliferation of the invasive stage results in the formation of the typical multinucleate, spherical bodies.

Diagnosis

This usually relies on a combination of clinical history, gross pathology and microscopic examination of organ squashes. The latter may reveal the presence of spherical bodies with thick cell walls typical of the 'resting' spore, varying in diameter from 10 to 250 μm. Massive replication of the parasite occurs after host death and demonstration of the characteristic germination tubes provides a definitive diagnosis.

Treatment

There is no effective treatment.

Control

- The 'resting' spores of *Ichthyophonus* are resistant to a variety of physical treatments. Spores may survive for months, even years, and can grow at a wide range of temperatures and pH

- Feeding of raw fish or raw-fish products is to be discouraged
- Infected fish should be removed and destroyed and any dead fish removed daily
- Complete disinfection with chlorine or other strong disinfectants is recommended where practical
- In earth ponds, drying and exposure to ultraviolet light for months, or sometimes years, may be the only effective solution.

Dermocystidium

This organism is closely related to *Ichthyophonus* and is thought to belong to the same lower protistan group. A number of species have been described, including *Dermocystidium koi* from koi and *D. salmonis* from salmonid species. Infection in a wide range of other fish species has been described. There is very little information on the true incidence but it is presumed to occur worldwide. It has been only rarely described in aquarium species.

Clinical signs

The organism may infect the skin (e.g. *D. koi*) or gills (e.g. *D. salmonis*) but may occasionally be found in visceral organs.

In the skin, *D. koi* produces smooth raised lesions up to 10 mm in diameter; they are typically noticed when 5–8 mm in size (Figure 23.7). The surrounding skin shows little inflammatory reaction and fish remain in good health. As the lesion grows, the overlying skin becomes thinner and white filamentous 'hyphae' (Figure 23.8) can be seen within the swelling. This eventually ruptures, causing the release of hundreds of spores measuring 6–15 μm in diameter (Figure 23.9) from the broken ends of the 'hyphae'. The skin heals with minimal damage (Wildgoose, 1995). Lesions are most commonly seen between May and July in the UK, when water temperatures are about 17–22°C.

D. salmonis is a more significant pathogen, resulting in extensive gill pathology and high mortality (Olson and Holt, 1995).

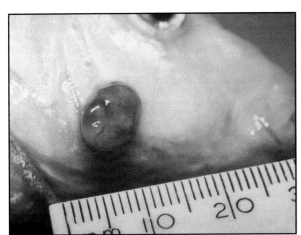

Figure 23.7 A raised lesion on the operculum of a koi due to infection with *Dermocystidium koi*. Scale in millimetres. (By permission of *The Veterinary Record*.)

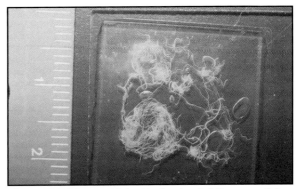

Figure 23.8 Strong thick white 'hyphae' of *Dermocystidium koi* plucked from a mature lesion on a koi. Scale in centimetres. (By permission of *The Veterinary Record*.)

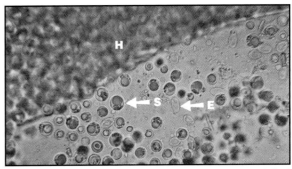

Figure 23.9 Spores (S) released from the 'hyphae' (H) of *Dermocystidium koi*. The characteristic spherical spores contain a large central vacuole or refractile body, with the cytoplasm and nucleus restricted to the narrow periphery. They are similar in size to an erythrocyte (E). Wet mount preparation, × 400 original magnification. (By permission of *The Veterinary Record*.)

Pathology

Histological examination of a koi (Dyková and Lom, 1992) revealed a loose network of individual 'hyphae' in the dermis and hypodermis (Figure 23.10). Large agglomerations of spores were present within the mature 'hyphae'. Each spore contained a large, refractile central inclusion and peripheral nucleus. The presence of spore-filled 'hyphae' is characteristic of *D. koi* and not seen in most other *Dermocystidium* species.

The spore-filled cysts of *D. salmonis* are located within the gill epithelium.

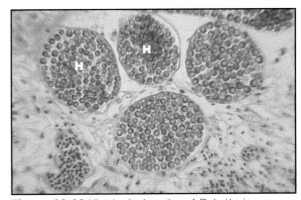

Figure 23.10 Histological section of *D. koi* lesion showing 'hyphae' (H). The thin-walled hyaline capsules are filled with spores but show little inflammatory reaction in the surrounding tissue. PAS stain, × 400 original magnification. (By permission of *The Veterinary Record*.)

Diagnosis

- Typical skin swellings containing white tangled mass of 'hyphae' in *D. koi*
- Characteristic spores present within 'hyphae' seen microscopically in *D. koi*
- Typical histopathological appearance as described above.

Treatment

- No specific treatment is available
- Self-cure is probably the norm but surgical excision and debridement may improve the rate of recovery (Wildgoose, 1995).

Control

Culling of infected fish to prevent further spread should be considered.

Other fungal diseases

Other fungal diseases have been described in many species, including aquarium fish. Such infections are often systemic and granulomatous but occasionally superficial and ulcerative. The incidence of such infections is presumed to be both low and sporadic. Definitive diagnosis usually requires histopathological confirmation and specialized mycological support. Implicated fungal genera include *Exophiala*, *Aureobasidium*, *Verticillium*, *Phoma*, *Rhizopus*, *Achlya* and *Aphanomyces*.

Harmful algae

Algae are members of a group of predominantly photosynthetic organisms of the kingdom Protista. They have been defined as eukaryotic (nucleus-bearing) organisms that photosynthesize but lack the specialized reproductive structures of plants. Some algae have a closer evolutionary relationship with the protozoa or fungi than they do with other algae. The prokaryotic (nucleus-lacking) blue-green algae or cyanobacteria are included in this section for convenience.

Algae are ubiquitous and they are most common in aquatic habitats. When nutrients (especially nitrogen and phosphorus) are abundant, algal cell numbers can become great enough to produce obvious patches or 'blooms'.

Several algal species, such as the flagellate *Prymnesium parvum*, produce ichthyotoxins that may be lethal and occasionally result in massive fish kills. Some, especially diatoms, may kill by physically damaging the gills or clogging gill tissue. Others, including cyanobacteria (*Anabaena*, *Aphanizomenon*, *Microcystis*, *Oscillatoria*), flagellates and dinoflagellates, have been linked to fish kills because of oxygen depletion. This may occur following bloom respiration at night or high microbial oxygen demand during bloom die-off. Such events are not uncommon. High pH levels and high ammonia levels during bloom senescence may also be important factors.

Many algae are suspected of being harmful to fish but few have been confirmed. Their identification requires a trained specialist, since noxious algae often resemble non-harmful species. When making a diagnosis, not only is the type of algae important but also the numbers present.

Treatment and control

Where possible, fish should be removed from the affected body of water and placed in unpolluted water. The occurrence of algal blooms in outdoor ponds is often unpredictable and sometimes unavoidable. Chemical treatment of algal growth is possible but bloom collapse must be avoided, since this may cause hypoxia.

Several methods are used to control algal growth in ponds but not all are effective against all types of algae (Chapter 5). Avoiding runoff from surrounding soil (e.g. rockeries) during heavy rain will prevent plant nutrients washing into the pond. Some methods include the use of:

- Proprietary chemical algicides
- Shading to reduce exposure to bright sunlight
- Vegetable filter (e.g. watercress) to compete for the uptake of plant nutrients
- Ultraviolet filter units
- Barley straw (produces anti-algal factors during decomposition when exposed to sunlight and oxygenated water)
- Commercial electronic and magnetic devices.

Further reading and references

Bruno DW and Wood BP (1999) *Saprolegnia* and other *Oomycetes*. In: *Fish Diseases and Disorders, Vol 3: Viral, Bacterial and Fungal Infections*, eds PTK Woo and DW Bruno, pp. 599–659. CABI Publishing, Wallingford, Oxon

Codd GA (1995) Cyanobacterial toxins: occurrence, properties and biological significance. *Water Science Technology* **32(4)**, 149–156

Dyková I and Lom J (1992) New evidence of fungal nature of *Dermocystidium koi* Hoshina and Sahara 1950. *Journal of Applied Ichthyology* **8**, 180–185

McVicar AH (1999) *Ichthyophonus* and related organisms. In: *Fish Diseases and Disorders, Vol 3: Viral, Bacterial and Fungal Infections*, eds PTK Woo and DW Bruno, pp. 661–687. CABI Publishing, Wallingford, Oxon

Olson RE and Holt RA (1995) The gill pathogen *Dermocystidium salmonis* in Oregon salmonids. *Journal of Aquatic Animal Health* **7**, 111–117

Wildgoose WH (1995) *Dermocystidium koi* found in skin lesions in koi carp (*Cyprinus carpio*). *Veterinary Record* **137**, 317–318

Wildgoose WH (1998) Skin disease in ornamental fish: identifying common problems. *In Practice* **20**, 226–243

Willoughby LG (1978) Saprolegniasis of salmonid fish in Windermere: a critical analysis. *Journal of Fish Diseases* **1**, 51–67

Willoughby LG (1989) Continued defence of salmonid fish against *Saprolegnia* fungus after its establishment. *Journal of Fish Diseases* **12**, 63–67

Willoughby LG (1994) *Fungi and Fish Diseases*. Pisces Press, University of Stirling

Acknowledgements

The author is grateful to Gordon Beakes (University of Newcastle), David Bruno (SERAD), the editor of the *Veterinary Record*, Peter Scott and William Wildgoose for the use of their photographs to illustrate this chapter.

24

Viral diseases

David Bucke

The detection and diagnosis of viral diseases in fish is best performed by specialist laboratories with facilities for the isolation of aquatic viruses. Most viruses are detected in tissue cultures and identified by serological and molecular procedures such as an immunofluorescent antibody test, enzyme-linked immunosorbent assay and polymerase chain reaction techniques. Even with this biotechnology, some viruses or suspected viruses can only be diagnosed by electron microscopy. Nevertheless, even though virus detection may not be the work of the practising veterinarian, it is important that there is awareness about the current state of viral diseases of ornamental fish.

Over the past decade, at least nine different rhabdoviruses have been isolated from wild cyprinids and other freshwater fish species. Recently, there have been reports of epizootics caused by other viruses in some commercial ornamental fish farms. Related to those events, and of concern to the UK ornamental fish industry, a number of viral diseases have been diagnosed in koi in parts of the Middle East, Europe and North America. This chapter will describe the important viral diseases that are known to affect ornamental fish.

Spring viraemia of carp

Spring viraemia of carp (SVC) is a well known disease of wild and farmed carp. It affects all varieties of carp, including common, mirror, leather and koi, as well as other cyprinid species, including orfe, goldfish, grass carp, Crucian carp and tench. The disease has also been recorded in some non-cyprinids, including pike and Wels catfish (Plumb, 1999).

The disease is caused by spring viraemia of carp virus, also known as *Rhabdovirus carpio*. The disease, as its name suggests, usually occurs in the spring when the water temperature rises above 7°C, and is most severe between 10° and 15°C. The virus can exist above 23°C but mortalities are rare at high water temperatures. Occasionally, disease may also occur in the autumn when the water temperature falls. On continental European carp farms, yearling fish are the group most affected. After overwintering, these carp are in poor physiological and immunological condition and are highly susceptible to the disease. In the UK, it affects fish of all ages, causing mortalities of between 10% and 100%. Since 1988, between 10 and 40 cases have been confirmed each year in the UK but most of these have occurred in sport fisheries rather than premises with ornamental fish. Fish that survive the disease may become carriers.

Clinical signs and pathology
Clinical signs are varied and include lethargic swimming with loss of balance and affected fish swimming at the surface, close to the edge of ponds. There is often darkening and haemorrhages in the skin (Figure 24.1). Exophthalmos, abdominal swelling and trailing faecal casts may also be present. On occasions, fish appear emaciated and swim erratically.

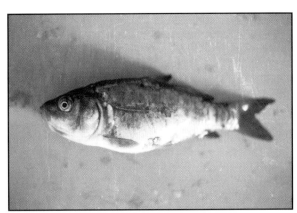

Figure 24.1 A juvenile common carp infected with spring viraemia of carp virus. There are extensive haemorrhages in the skin and slight abdominal enlargement. (Courtesy of Peter Dixon.)

Postmortem examination may reveal pale or bleeding gills together with petechiation of the skin, abdominal wall, intestines and other viscera. Inflammation of the swim-bladder may be present but this sign is not pathognomonic, because the myxozoan parasite *Sphaerospora renicola* can produce similar pathology. Classical signs of viraemia also include petechiation of the musculature, which is seen on incision of the tissue (Schlotfeldt and Alderman, 1995).

Treatment and control
There is currently no effective treatment for SVC but the use of antibacterial medications may reduce the extent of secondary bacterial disease. The greatest risk of infection is from the introduction of infected fish into ponds; for this reason, the disease is notifiable in

the UK under the Fish Diseases Act 1937 (Modified 1983). It is also listed in Category 3 of European fish health legislation and is notifiable to the Office International des Epizooties (OIE, 1997). Therefore, suspicions of SVC must be reported to a government fisheries laboratory where the appropriate tests will be performed. Following a positive identification, various statutory measures will be taken to control and eradicate the infection. This may include a movement restriction order with periodic testing performed every 2 years until no infection can be isolated. Alternatively, a slaughter and disinfection programme may be used in commercial premises where this action is an economic necessity.

Herpesvirus diseases

Two diseases in ornamental carp are caused by herpesviruses. The first is the benign disease known as 'carp pox' or *Papillosum cyprini* and is one of the oldest known fish diseases. The other disease is caused by a more pathogenic type of herpesvirus, which has been implicated as the cause of recent epizootics in koi in Europe and North America.

Carp pox

For many years, this disease was only regarded to have a viral aetiology because of observations by electron microscopy. It is now accepted that cyprinid herpesvirus I is the causative agent of the disease (Plumb, 1999). Although it commonly infects carp, it has also been found in other coldwater species (e.g. orfe, rudd) and some tropical aquarium fish.

Clinical signs and pathology

The signs of epidermal hyperplasia are usually seen in fish after their second year and often observed during the winter months in the UK. The smooth raised lesions resemble drops of milky white candle wax (Figure 24.2) and affect all areas of the body surface and fins. The lesions are usually benign, rarely causing clinical problems. Although they may regress, they often reappear and may persist for

several years. Histological examination of the lesions reveals typical hyperplasia of epithelial cells with few mucus cells. In more advanced cases, the hyperplasia progresses to form papillomatous growths characterized by hyperplastic epithelial cells supported by connective tissue. Other organs are not affected.

Treatment and control

There is no effective treatment for this disease and surgical removal is unlikely to provide an effective or lasting result. Occasionally, the lesions may slough spontaneously when the water temperature is raised to above 20°C. The disease may be unsightly in appearance and reduce the commercial value of the fish; therefore affected fish may need to be culled if these are important considerations.

Pathogenic herpesvirus disease

A separate herpesvirus similar to cyprinid herpesvirus I has been isolated from diseased goldfish and koi (Jung and Miyazaki, 1995; Groff *et al.*, 1998; Chang *et al.*, 1999; Hedrick *et al.*, 2000). The virus that affects koi, called koi herpesvirus, appears to be highly infectious, causing an acute gill disease and producing up to 100% mortality. The disease appears to be more severe at water temperatures between 18° and 25°C and is thus more common in the summer months in the UK. There have been suspicions of the disease for several years but there have been only a few confirmed cases of this herpesvirus in koi in the UK.

Clinical signs and pathology

Affected fish often become lethargic and swim close to the surface. They may gather at the water inlets and show respiratory distress. The body surface and gills may be covered in excess mucus and occasionally the gills are pale and mottled. These lesions are the main clinical finding and may vary from very subtle changes to severe necrosis of the gill tissues (Figures 24.3 and 24.4). Standard tissue samples from the gill, heart, spleen and kidney should be taken for light microscopy, electron microscopy and virus isolation.

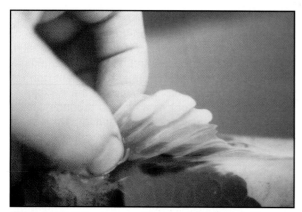

Figure 24.2 Carp pox on the dorsal fin of a koi. The smooth milky-white lesions of epidermal hyperplasia resemble drops of candle wax. (Reproduced with the permission of *In Practice*.)

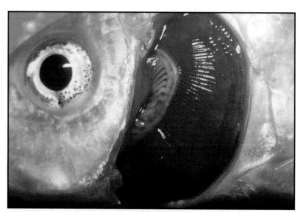

Figure 24.3 Gill of a koi with pathogenic koi herpesvirus infection. Only mild pathological changes are visible with excess mucus and secondary bacterial infection. (© W.H. Wildgoose.)

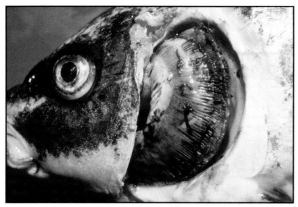

Figure 24.4 Gill of a koi with pathogenic koi herpesvirus infection. Extensive tissue necrosis and secondary disease are also present. (© W.H. Wildgoose.)

Histological examination often reveals advanced gill necrosis, but pathological changes may also be present in other organs. Infected epithelial cells are usually found in gill tissue, where the cells may be enlarged and contain nuclei with distinctly marginated chromatin (Figure 24.5). It may be possible to identify faint intranuclear inclusions in these cells under oil immersion; viral inclusions may be seen using electron microscopy.

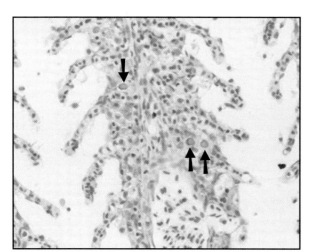

Figure 24.5 Histological changes in the gill of a koi with pathogenic herpesvirus infection. Some epithelial cells exhibit enlarged nuclei with marginated chromatin (arrowed). Giemsa stain, ×400 original magnification. (Courtesy of Keith Way.)

Treatment and control
There is no effective treatment for this disease but improving the water quality and the use of antibacterial drugs to minimize secondary infections may help some fish to survive. There is only limited scientific information about this disease and diagnostic laboratory tests are still under development. Therefore, it is advisable to purchase koi and other cyprinids only from reputable dealers. If the disease is confirmed on a site, slaughter and disinfection of the facility and equipment are recommended before introducing new fish.

Lymphocystis

Lymphocystis is a well known benign disease that predominantly affects flatfish and percoid-like fish (Anders, 1989). In captivity, the disease is usually seen in marine angelfish, butterflyfish, clownfish and freshwater cichlids. It is caused by an iridovirus, which invades the dermal fibroblasts and causes the cells to enlarge by up to 100,000 times their normal size.

Clinical signs and pathology
The hypertrophied cells are just visible to the naked eye and can measure up to 1 mm in diameter. They often occur in clusters and have a raspberry-like appearance. They are usually white or pink and occur mainly on the body and fins (Figure 24.6). Their presence may disfigure some ornamental fish but the disease rarely affects their health and causes only low mortality. Histological examination enables confirmation of the disease (Figure 24.7).

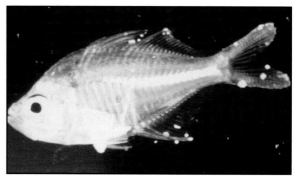

Figure 24.6 Artificially coloured glassfish with lymphocystis disease. The white nodules on the fins represent clusters of hypertrophied cells. (Courtesy of Peter Burgess.)

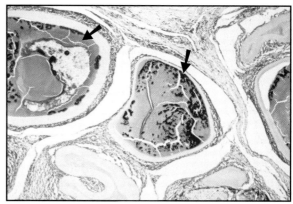

Figure 24.7 Histological section of lymphocystis lesion in a butterflyfish. Grossly hypertrophied cells (arrowed) have a thick hyaline capsule and an enlarged nucleus. H&E stain, ×20 original magnification.

Treatment and control
There is no effective treatment. Since the disease is infectious, eradication of affected fish is recommended, but isolation of infected fish together with improved nutrition and environmental conditions will often cause the lesions to regress spontaneously. Although

there may be complete recovery in some fish, many will relapse when stressed by poor water conditions or transportation.

Other viral diseases

A number of other viruses have been isolated from ornamental fish. For a virus to be considered the causal agent of a disease, specific experimental evidence is required to establish an aetiological relationship. These conditions are commonly known as Rivers' postulates. To fulfil the first of these postulates, the virus must be found in all cases of the disease in question. Secondly, the agent must be isolated, grown and propagated in another system, such as tissue culture. The third postulate to be fulfilled is to infect test animals and reproduce in them the essential clinical features of the original disease. After having reproduced the disease, the virus must be further isolated and identified as the same at the start of the experimental infection (Wolf, 1970).

In many cases, there is not always hard evidence that these viruses are associated with significant clinical diseases. Examples of these include the following:

- Iridoviruses have been isolated from goldfish, guppies and doctorfish (Plumb, 1999). In one case, freshwater angelfish with abdominal distension, exophthalmos and pale gills experienced mortalities in excess of 70% (Rodger *et al.*, 1997)
- Ramirez's dwarf cichlid virus may cause up to 80% mortality in some species of South American cichlid. Although the virus has been found in lesions using electron microscopy, it has not yet been isolated (Leibovitz and Riis, 1980)
- Birnaviruses, similar to infectious pancreatic necrosis virus, have been isolated from zebra danio (Ahne, 1982)
- Viral erythrocytic necrosis virus has been described from electron micrographs of many marine fish species, including blennies (Eiras and Santos, 1992)
- A coronavirus was recently isolated in Japan from koi experiencing high mortalities due to a non-bacterial ulcer disease called 'ana-aki-byo' (Miyazaki *et al.*, 2000)
- A reovirus was isolated from a marine angelfish with head and lateral line erosion syndrome, though this has not been proved to be the cause (Varner and Lewis, 1991).

Occasionally, viruses or virus-like particles have been reported to be the cause of some fish tumours, including epidermal papillomas (Anders and Yoshimizu, 1994; Grizzle and Goodwin, 1998). On the rare occasion when viral isolation from tumours has been successful, the viruses have mostly been identified as herpesviruses similar to that described for carp pox (Plumb, 1999). Lip fibromas in freshwater angelfish are thought to be associated with retrovirus-like particles but the lesions are sometimes referred to as odontogenic hamartomas, due to the presence of teeth in the tissue (Francis-Floyd *et al.*, 1993).

It is inevitable that the exploitation of new fish species for aquaculture will reveal further viral-related diseases. Veterinarians should therefore be aware that many ornamental fish are closely related to food-fish species and that they may carry or be susceptible to the same viral diseases.

Further reading

Ahne W (1982) Isolation of infectious pancreatic necrosis virus from zebra danio, *Brachydanio rerio*. *Bulletin of the European Association of Fish Pathologists* **2**, 8

Anders K (1989) Lymphocystis disease of fishes. In: *Viruses of Lower Vertebrates* (ed. W Ahne). Springer, Berlin, pp. 141–160

Anders K and Yoshimizu M (1994) Role of viruses in the induction of skin tumours and tumour-like proliferations of fish. *Diseases of Aquatic Organisms* **19**, 215–232

Chang PH, Lee SH, Chiang HC and Jong MH (1999) Epizootic of Herpes-like virus in goldfish, *Carassius auratus* in Taiwan. *Fish Pathology* **34**, 209–210

Eiras JC and Santos PJ (1992) Presumptive viral erythrocytic necrosis (VEN) in fishes off the Portuguese coast. *Bulletin of the European Fisheries Society* **12**, 45–47

Francis-Floyd R, Bolon B, Fraser W and Reed P (1993) Lip fibromas associated with retrovirus-like particles in angel fish. *Journal of the American Veterinary Medical Association* **202**, 427–429

Grizzle JM and Goodwin AE (1998) Neoplasms and related lesions. In: *Fish Diseases and Disorders, Vol. 2, Non-infectious Disorders* (ed. JF Leatherland and PTK Woo). CABI Publishing, Wallingford, pp. 37–104

Groff JM, LaPatra SE, Munn RJ and Ziukl JG (1998) A viral epizootic in cultured populations of juvenile goldfish due to a putative herpesvirus etiology. *Journal of Veterinary Diagnostic Investigation* **10**, 375–378

Hedrick RP, Gilad O, Yun S, Spangenberg JV, Marty GD, Nordhausen RW, Kebus MJ, Bercovier H and Eldar A (2000) An herpesvirus associated with mass mortality of juvenile and adult koi *Cyprinus carpio*. *Journal of Aquatic Animal Health* **12**, 44–57

Jung SJ and Miyazaki T (1995) Herpesviral haematopoietic necrosis of goldfish, *Carassius auratus* (L.). *Journal of Fish Diseases* **18**, 211–220

Leibovitz L and Riis RC (1980) A viral disease of aquarium fish. *Journal of the American Veterinary Medical Association* **177**, 414–416

Miyazaki T, Okamoto H, Kageyama T and Kobayashi T (2000) Viremia-associated ana-aki-byo, a new viral disease in color carp, *Cyprinus carpio* in Japan. *Diseases of Aquatic Organisms* **39**, 183–192.

OIE (1997) *OIE Diagnostic Manual for Aquatic Animal Diseases*, 2nd edn. Office International des Epizooties, Paris, pp. 63–73

Plumb JA (1999) *Health Maintenance and Principal Microbial Diseases of Cultured Fishes*. Iowa State University Press, Ames, Iowa

Rodger HD, Kobs M, Macartney A and Frerichs GN (1997) Systemic iridovirus infection in freshwater angelfish, *Pterophyllum scalare* (Lichtenstein). *Journal of Fish Diseases* **20**, 69–72

Schlotfeldt H-J and Alderman DJ (1995) *What Should I Do? A Practical Guide for the Freshwater Fish Farmer*. European Association of Fish Pathologists, Weymouth, 60 pp

Varner PW and Lewis DH (1991) Characterization of a virus associated with head and lateral line erosion syndrome in marine angelfish. *Journal of Aquatic Animal Health* **3**, 198–205

Wolf K (1970) Guidelines for virological examination of fishes. In: *A Symposium on Diseases of Fishes and Shellfishes* (ed. SF Snieszko). Special Publication No. 5, American Fisheries Society, Washington DC, pp 327–340

Acknowledgement

The author would like to thank Keith Way of the CEFAS Fisheries Laboratory, Weymouth, for his helpful comments on this chapter.

25

Environmental disorders

Todd R. Cecil

Deviant environmental factors are often the trigger to a cascade of events leading to unhealthy fish. In many cases, these result from poor husbandry and can be divided into water quality disorders and exogenous factors. Many of these disorders can be avoided with planning and routine monitoring of the pond or aquarium.

This chapter will discuss environmental disorders that result in disease. The cause of such a disorder, its effect on the fish and action required to correct the disorder will be highlighted. Chapter 1 gives a more detailed discussion of the aquatic environment and parameters highlighted here.

Water quality disorders

The most commonly reported environmental problems revolve around water quality. Parameters that should be monitored routinely include temperature, pH, ammonia, nitrite and nitrate. Other aspects that may require testing include dissolved oxygen, hardness, alkalinity, salinity and carbon dioxide.

Temperature

Temperature fluctuations are usually well tolerated by freshwater pond and aquarium fish but only if the changes are gradual. Fish are poikilothermic and rely on environmental temperatures to optimize enzyme activity such as digestion and respiration, and functioning of the immune system. Rapid or prolonged hyperthermia or hypothermia can precede stress and compromise the immune system.

Meaningful temperature readings can only be taken on site, at the pond or tank. Fish keepers should use a thermometer capable of recording daily high and low temperatures.

Clinical signs associated with temperature extremes vary depending on the species of fish, temperature range and elapsed time of change. Saltwater tropical fish are very sensitive to changes in temperature. Freshwater fish, particularly temperate species, are more resistant and can often tolerate variations of 8–10°C in a 24-hour period.

Treatment involves returning the fish to its preferred optimum temperature zone. Too rapid a reversal of temperature can cause temperature shock and subsequent death.

Hypothermia

For tropical fish, suboptimal water temperatures may arise through malfunction of the aquarium heater or thermostat. Pond fish may experience hypothermia during severe winter weather, particularly in shallow ponds. This may be exacerbated by excessive movement of the whole water column, resulting from the water pump or outlet to the filter being positioned at the bottom of the pond. This breaks up any stratification of water temperatures in deep ponds and creates a chilling effect.

Effect

- Inactive (torpid)
- Lying on bottom (often listing to side)
- Lethargic
- Anorexic.

Action: Water temperatures can be raised by installing suitable electric water heaters and providing insulation.

Hyperthermia

All bodies of water exposed to direct sunlight, whether an aquarium close to the window or an outdoor pond without shade, are subjected to potentially severe temperature fluctuations. Lethal high temperature changes can quickly result from the malfunction of aquarium heaters and thermostats.

Effect

- Restlessness
- Sudden death.

The increased body temperature stimulates metabolism, in turn accelerating oxygen demands by the tissues. Indirect effects of increased water temperatures include increased toxicity of ammonia and a reduced oxygen solubility that may lead to hypoxia.

Action: Cold or frozen water bottles or sealed bags of ice can be submerged in the water to reduce water temperatures. Temperature corrections should be limited to 1°C per hour and no more than several degrees per day. Providing shade (such as window blinds, or floating mats in ponds) can prevent water from overheating. Small electric chillers are available and can be installed for use with indoor aquaria. In order to limit oxygen demand by the body, hyperthermic patients should not be fed.

pH

The pH of a recirculating system is influenced by many factors, such as dissolved gases, particulate matter, organic load, buffering capacity and temperature. Although some fish can tolerate wide variances, most have adapted to a limited pH range; in general, fish have adapted to environmental pH conditions ranging from 5.8 to 8.5.

Low pH

If the pH drops below the optimal range, acidosis occurs. This can happen rapidly in systems with a low buffering capacity.

Effect

- Lethargy and general signs of stress
- Skin irritation with excess mucus production, colour change, rubbing and attempting to jump out
- Gill irritation with excess mucus production and hypertrophy/hyperplasia; in extreme cases, fish gasp at the surface, due to reduced gaseous exchange
- Blood acidosis causing sudden death below pH 4
- Increased toxicity of heavy metals and some medications (e.g. chloramine-T, copper sulphate, formalin, malachite green).

Action: Treatment involves increasing the pH and improving the buffering capacity of the system. In freshwater ponds and aquaria, the addition of a proprietary buffering compound or sodium bicarbonate (baking soda) can be used, the latter at a rate of 3 mg/l. In large ponds, it may be necessary to use lime. A pH test 1 hour later should indicate an improvement. For long-term control, limestone or crushed oyster shell can be used.

High pH

If the pH rises above a tolerable range, alkalosis can follow. This is common during an algal bloom (Figure 25.1) and in heavily planted ponds and aquaria, or untreated concrete ponds where calcium compounds leach into the water.

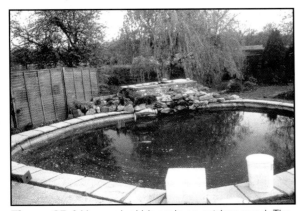

Figure 25.1 Heavy algal bloom in an outdoor pond. The effects of photosynthesis produced pH 10.5 at midday, resulting in corneal oedema, skin lesions and mortality. (© W.H. Wildgoose.)

Effect

- Damage to fins, skin and gills, causing fish to gasp at the surface or attempt to jump out
- Eye damage (corneal oedema, cataract)
- Blood alkalosis, causing death above pH 10
- Increased toxicity from ammonia, iron and some medications (e.g. potassium permanganate)
- Reduced effect of some medications (e.g. organophosphates).

Action: In freshwater ponds and aquaria, the addition of a proprietary buffering compound can be used to decrease the pH. Alternatively, use white vinegar (dilute acetic acid) titrated slowly into the water, ensuring even distribution, and carefully monitor the pH. Concrete ponds can be treated with non-toxic sealant or scrubbed with hydrochloric (muriatic) acid to prevent leaching of calcium salts. Submerged plants should be removed and algal growth controlled with the judicious use of an algicide or installation of an ultraviolet unit.

Nitrogenous compounds

Nitrogen compounds (ammonia, nitrite and nitrate) can rapidly rise to toxic levels in aquaria and ponds.

Ammonia

This is the primary nitrogenous waste product of fish metabolism and the by-product of bacterial degradation of organic material in the water column. Elevations in ammonia levels are common in aquaria and ponds, particularly in new systems or after vigorous cleaning of filters. 'New tank/pond syndrome' occurs when the nitrifying biological filter has not matured and ammonia production exceeds the capacity of the filtration system. Ammonia is more toxic in warm water, at high pH levels and with decreasing salinity. Toxic levels vary between species but for freshwater aquarium fish the lethal level is 0.2–0.5 mg un-ionized ammonia per litre.

Effect

- Behaviour change (listlessness, excitability)
- Anorexia
- Hyperplasia and hypertrophy of gill filaments
- Osmoregulatory disturbance
- Impaired transport of oxygen in haemoglobin
- Increased susceptibility to disease
- Retarded growth
- Death.

Action: Treatment requires frequent water changes (carefully matching temperature and pH). If the problem persists, then the adequacy of the filter system must be investigated. Excess detritus in the filter unit (Figure 25.2) must be removed and the addition of a proprietary solution of filter bacteria or some medium from a mature filter system can help to establish or repopulate the biological filter.

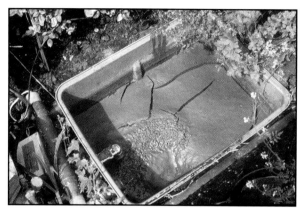

Figure 25.2 Excess detritus in a single chamber filter unit used on a garden pond. The brown sediment was only noticed after the water was drained out. This thick sediment blocked the filter medium, preventing any biological activity and causing poor water quality. (Courtesy of W.H. Wildgoose.)

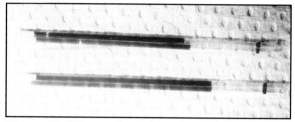

Figure 25.3 The capillary tube at the top is from a catfish suffering from methaemoglobinaemia. The distinctive brown coloration is clearly visible when compared with the other tube, which contains blood from a normal fish. (Courtesy of Lester Khoo, VMD.)

The clay resin, zeolite (clinoptilolite), binds ammonia and can be used in the tank or pond. Zeolite is reusable and can be recharged by soaking in a strong salt solution. However, this competitive binding of salt and ammonia makes it unsuitable for use in marine systems or if salt is present in freshwater systems.

A gradual lowering of the pH will reduce any ammonia toxicity, as will the addition of a low dose of salt to freshwater systems. Reduction in the feeding rate and removal of uneaten food are also helpful.

Prevention through good husbandry and regular monitoring of water quality is the best policy. It is important to limit overcrowding and overfeeding. Control of plant and algal growth by the judicious use of an algicide or installation of an ultraviolet unit is helpful.

Nitrite

Nitrite is produced by the bacterial oxidation of ammonia. It is toxic to fish but less so than ammonia. New tanks commonly experience high levels, due to the slow multiplication and insufficient numbers of *Nitrobacter* and the other microorganisms that convert nitrite into nitrate.

When nitrite levels increase in the water system, nitrite is actively transported across the gill epithelium, where it oxidizes haemoglobin (Hb) to methaemoglobin (MetHb). The structural change of haemoglobin due to oxidation decreases the affinity of haemoglobin for oxygen, leading to hypoxia, cyanosis and death. Confirmation of a diagnosis is dependent on a colorimetric measurement of MetHb in the blood. Increased nitrite levels in the blood stream cause 'brown blood disease', or methaemoglobinaemia (Figure 25.3). Toxicity varies according to species but levels between 10 and 20 mg/l are lethal.

Effect

- Listlessness
- Dyspnoea and gasping at the surface
- Dark brown gills
- Death.

Action: Treatment success depends on the severity and duration of toxicity. Chloride ions competitively inhibit nitrite absorption over the gill epithelium; therefore, adding salt to the water often alleviates clinical signs. After measuring the level of nitrite, 3 mg of non-iodized salt (sea salt) per litre can be added for every 1 mg of nitrite per litre detected by the test method. Obtaining an exact measurement of nitrite with standard colorimetric chemical test kits can be difficult and this dosage should be considered a minimum starting point. Partial water changes every 2–3 days can be used to remove nitrite from the system. Clinical signs will often resolve 24 hours after lowering nitrite levels. Increasing aeration will ensure maximum dissolved oxygen levels and minimize environmental hypoxia. Adding a proprietary solution of filter bacteria or some medium from a mature filter system will help to establish or repopulate the biological filter.

Nitrate

This is the final product of the nitrification process of ammonia. In the absence of regular partial water changes, nitrate can accumulate in aquaria and other closed circulation systems. In some areas, high levels of nitrate are found in the domestic water supply but these can be removed using proprietary ion exchange resins (e.g. Nitragon®) or reverse-osmosis units. If nitrate is allowed to accumulate, further conversion of ammonia through the nitrogen cycle by nitrifying bacteria could be hindered. As the nitrate levels increase, the bacterial oxidation of nitrite to nitrate decreases; consequently, nitrite levels start to increase.

Nitrate is considered the least toxic of the nitrogenous compounds but eggs and fry are more sensitive to it than adult fish. Currently, the effect of low-grade, long-term exposure of fish is unknown but water levels should be maintained below 50–100 mg/l. High levels may encourage algal blooms and result in associated water quality problems. Routine testing and water changes are recommended for control. In outdoor ponds, a vegetable filter (e.g. watercress) can be used to extract nitrates from the water.

Salinity

The salt concentration of water is termed salinity and is expressed in parts per thousand (ppt) or grams per litre (g/l). In general, freshwater has a salinity lower than

0.5 ppt and sea water in marine aquaria varies from 33 to 37 ppt. Each species of fish can tolerate various salinities but will thrive best within a narrow range.

In freshwater systems, increasing the salt concentration can be therapeutic. Mild elevations in salinity reduce stress on fish by balancing internal electrolyte equilibrium with the external environment. However, sudden or extreme changes in salinity will cause osmoregulatory disturbance and can lead to renal compromise. Saltwater fish are often given short, timed freshwater dips as a treatment for ectoparasites but prolonged exposure to low salinities can lead to overhydration and cardiac failure. It should be noted that zeolite will release any ammonia that has been absorbed when salt is used in freshwater systems and that nitrate becomes more toxic with increased salinity.

Dissolved gases

Oxygen

All fish require oxygen for many life processes and hypoxaemia is a frequent complication in pond and aquarium management. Dissolved oxygen concentrations are maintained through diffusion at water/air interfaces. The surface area of such interfaces can be increased using air-stones, fountains, waterfalls, venturis and other aeration devices.

Oxygen can also enter the water as a product of photosynthesis of plants and algae. Oxygen concentrations are usually highest after long periods of direct sunlight or artificial illumination. Animals, plants and algae all become consumers of oxygen after prolonged periods of darkness and the oxygen concentration decreases. Fish that had appeared normal the previous evening but are found gasping at the surface in the morning could be suffering from hypoxaemia. Algal blooms will often cause environmental hypoxia due to respiration during the hours of darkness, producing low levels of dissolved oxygen just before daybreak.

Hypoxaemia occurs when fish are unable to extract adequate amounts of oxygen from the water to sustain proper metabolic functions. Underlying causes can be environmental or physiological in origin (Figure 25.4).

Although the biological requirement varies with fish species, size, age and health, most species require a minimum of 4 mg of dissolved oxygen per litre and some have a higher requirement. Prolonged exposure to environmental hypoxia causes stress and will lead to secondary disease. Environmental hypoxia can develop quickly and soon reaches lethal levels. Larger fish have a higher total oxygen demand and usually die first.

Effect

- Lethargy (may be preceded by aggression)
- Anorexia
- Dyspnoea, gasping at surface and water inlets (Figure 25.5)
- Increased respiratory rates
- Sudden death.

Environmental Factors

Excess consumption from a high biological demand:
    Overstocking with fish
    High consumption by bacteria in the biological filter or
      decomposing detritus
    Heavy growth of algae and other submerged plants

Poor gas exchange:
    Oil or dust on the surface
    Excessive growth of leafy surface-growing plants
    Mechanical failure of air pumps or fountains
    Poor water movement
    Stagnation within the water column

Reduced holding capacity or availability:
    High water temperatures
    High salinity
    Use of oxygen-binding medications (e.g. formalin)

Physiological Factors

Poor absorption:
    Gill disease: any pathogen or disease process that causes
      thickening of the gill epithelium (hyperplasia or hypertrophy)
      or reduced surface by tissue necrosis reduces the fish's
      ability to extract oxygen from the water

Internal disease:
    Anaemia (e.g. haemoparasites)
    Methaemoglobinaemia (e.g. nitrite toxicity)
    Poisoning (e.g. malachite green)

Figure 25.4 Environmental and physiological causes of hypoxaemia.

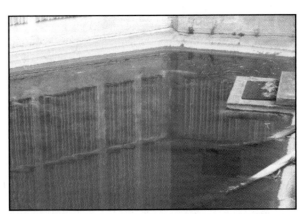

Figure 25.5 Fish crowding around a water inlet in a pond with poor aeration. The decomposition of dead algae (brown sediment) in the pond further depletes dissolved oxygen levels. (© W.H. Wildgoose.)

The diagnosis of hypoxaemia is difficult and often symptomatic. Observing the response to additional aeration and oxygenation often provides supporting evidence.

Action: Additional aeration such as air-stones, fountains or a venturi should be installed and kept running 24 hours per day.

Control of algal growth by the judicious use of an algicide or installation of an ultraviolet unit is helpful but dead algae must be removed from the system, since their decomposition will consume more oxygen. Filamentous algae and other submerged plants should be removed manually, particularly

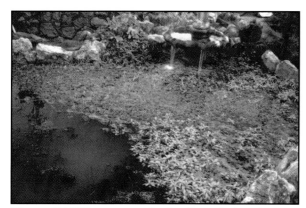

Figure 25.6 The overgrowth of surface plants reduces the surface area for gas exchange. This causes environmental hypoxia and prevents the growth of aquatic algae. (© W.H. Wildgoose.)

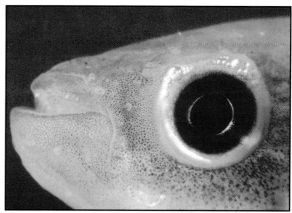

Figure 25.7 'Gas bubble disease' affecting the eye of a mummichog. Gas bubbles are visible in the dorsal periorbital tissue. (© National Aquarium in Baltimore.)

if there is heavy growth. Leafy surface-growing plants should also be removed if they cover a large surface area (Figure 25.6). Decomposing material should be removed from the system, including detritus in the filtration unit.

In an emergency, injection of hydrogen peroxide into the water column (using a squirt bottle) will bring temporary improvement. A 3% solution of hydrogen peroxide can be used at a rate of 0.5 ml/l. Care must be taken to avoid spraying fish, as hydrogen peroxide can be harmful to live tissue. Potassium permanganate liberates oxygen and has been used at the rate of 2 mg/l as an emergency source of oxygen; it is toxic in water with a high pH and must be used with great care.

Medications that contain formalin should be avoided, since they will absorb oxygen from the water.

Gas supersaturation

'Gas bubble disease', caused by supersaturation of water, is a relatively rare independent finding. When gases are forced into liquids under pressure, supersaturation can result. Venturi injectors, faulty pumps and waterfalls are the most common cause of gas bubble disease in aquatic systems. This condition can also be caused by rapid changes in air pressure during air transportation, or when fresh borehole water is used in some large facilities.

Disease occurs when fish absorb the gases from supersaturated water which then form gas emboli in the circulation and tissues. Although most cases of gas bubble disease involve supersaturation with nitrogen, occasionally excessive amounts of oxygen are produced by heavy algal blooms in hot sunny weather and may result in a similar clinical condition.

Effect

- Gas bubbles seen in the eyes (Figure 25.7), on the fins and gills and under the skin
- Behavioural abnormalities (e.g. circling)
- Excess positive buoyancy in small fish
- Death.

Diagnosis can be made based on clinical signs and presence of excess gas bubbles on submerged surfaces. A simple test is to place a hand or small object in the aquarium or pond and observe for the formation of small gas bubbles on the object's surface. Acute disease often results in death, whereas chronic disease results in lower mortality.

Action: Treatment requires elimination of excess gas from the water by performing a water change and allowing the gas to equilibrate with air. The underlying cause must be identified and corrected. Commercial degassing systems are available for use on fresh borehole water supplies.

Carbon dioxide

Elevated levels of carbon dioxide can lead to disease in fish. High levels of bicarbonate, used as a buffering compound or added to raise pH, complicate the fish's ability to eliminate bicarbonate ions and absorb oxygen through the gills. The disease process can be exaggerated by acidosis, preventing the dissociation of gaseous carbon dioxide in the blood to form carbonates. Affected fish show signs of respiratory distress even in the presence of adequate dissolved oxygen levels. Vigorous aeration will reduce dissolved levels of carbon dioxide and allow the gas to equilibrate with air.

In some species, high calcium carbonate levels in the blood have been associated with nephrocalcinosis of the renal tubules. At present, there is no treatment for nephrocalcinosis.

Hydrogen sulphide

Hydrogen sulphide is produced under anaerobic conditions by certain bacteria at the bottom of ponds and aquaria. In the absence of oxygen, these bacteria proliferate and utilize sulphur for respiration. The end-product of this pathway is hydrogen sulphide. This problem occurs more frequently in marine than freshwater systems.

Levels greater than 0.5 mg/l may cause acute mortality. A chronic low-grade problem is suspected when other water parameters are within normal ranges and there are no signs of infectious disease. Stirring of the gravel or bottom sediment often liberates trapped pockets of gas, with the pathognomonic smell of rotten eggs, though levels detectable by smell are not necessarily toxic. High temperature and low pH will increase toxicity.

Effect

- Lethargy
- Anorexia
- Dyspnoea, with gasping at the surface
- Sudden death in acute toxicity.

Vigorous aeration of the water will help to remove the toxic gas from solution. Frequent partial water changes may also be necessary. Removal of any decomposing detritus will remove the source of the hydrogen sulphide.

Hardness and alkalinity

The sum of the concentrations of divalent cations, especially calcium and magnesium, is defined as water hardness. Hardness is expressed as mg/l equivalents of $CaCO_3$. In general, the total (or general) hardness of fresh water and sea water is less than 200 and 6500 mg/l as $CaCO_3$, respectively. Freshwater fish species usually tolerate a wide range of hardness, but if water is too 'soft', susceptibility to poor water quality conditions becomes greater. Increased water hardness decreases toxicity of ammonia and dissolved metals such as copper and zinc, and reduces stress on fish. Rarely is hardness a problem in marine environments, due to the high concentrations of calcium and magnesium in sea water.

Alkalinity is a measure of the capacity of water to neutralize strong acid and is derived from the presence of bicarbonate (HCO_3^-) and carbonate (CO_3^{2-}) in water. It is usually expressed as milligrams per litre as calcium carbonate or occasionally as milliequivalents per litre (mEq/l). Other buffering compounds such as phosphates, borates and organic bases can also contribute to alkalinity. Water of low alkalinity (<10 mg/l as $CaCO_3$) is rarely suitable for rearing fish. This can result in wide pH fluctuations, leading to acidosis or alkalosis. Higher alkalinity protects fish from potentially lethal exposure to heavy metals such as zinc, aluminium and copper, by forming carbonate precipitates and bicarbonate complexes. The buffering capacity of a system with high alkalinity also protects against the acid production of the nitrification process.

Exogenous factors

Algal overgrowth

Algal blooms or 'floating scum' can wreak havoc in an established system. Controlled algal growth can add many benefits to an aquatic system. Algae can augment dissolved oxygen levels by photosynthesis, are utilized as a food source by many fish and remove nitrogenous compounds from the water column. Overgrowth of algae can foul filter systems, consume oxygen during non-photosynthetic periods, cause dramatic pH fluctuations and add undesirable compounds to the water. Many blue-green algae (e.g. *Microcystis*) produce hepato- and neurotoxins capable of devastating aquatic systems. Clinical signs in fish are often non-specific, such as lethargy and anorexia. Fatalities can be acute or chronic. Water changes and control of algal populations are the only means of treatment.

Chlorine and chloramine

Chlorine and chloramines are often added to drinking water by relevant authorities to ensure potability. The reaction of chlorine with organic material, particularly ammonia, can precipitate the formation of chloramines. Toxicity is a common problem when steps are not taken to remove these compounds from the water before introducing them to the fish tank or pond. The threshold for detecting chlorine by smell is 40 mg/l but levels of 0.1 mg/l can be lethal. Chronic low-grade exposure will lead to gill hyperplasia.

Effect

- Dyspnoea, with gasping at the surface
- Sudden death.

Commercial test kits are available for detecting chlorine and chloramine concentrations in water samples, but tentative diagnosis can be made with a complete history and clinical signs. Any detectable levels can cause chronic damage to skin and gills.

Action: Aeration of water for 24 hours in an open-topped container will allow chlorine to dissipate. Several proprietary dechlorinating solutions are available for use with fish; they bind to chlorine and chloramine and remove them from the water column. Granulated sodium thiosulphate can be dissolved in water to eliminate chlorine. Dechlorination can be accomplished by adding sodium thiosulphate to produce a final concentration of 3.5 mg/l of water. Where it is impractical to store large volumes of water for dechlorination, such as when adding to large ponds, domestic tap water can be passed through selective water purification filters. Water should be retested for chlorine and chloramine content before being added to the aquatic system.

Electrical shock

Fish subjected to strong electrical charges, whether from faulty wiring or lightning strike, are often found swimming erratically or dead. Electrocution can cause disorientation or abnormal posture due to fractured vertebrae (Figure 25.8). Fish may also be found in lateral recumbency on the bottom of the pond or aquarium. Spinal damage is usually permanent in those fish that survive.

All electrical outlets must be grounded and equipped with a ground fault interrupter or residual current device (RCD). Stray electrical current may originate from submersible heaters and pumps, underwater lighting sources and other electrical devices. Equipment and wiring should be inspected at regular intervals for signs of physical damage and where necessary should be either repaired or replaced. Dexamethasone at 1–2 mg/kg can be given by injection and may be of help to shocked patients.

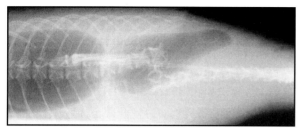

Figure 25.8 Dorsoventral radiograph of a koi following lightning strike. The fish exhibited a stiff swimming motion and inability to fully flex the caudal peduncle, due to the severe fracture and dislocation of the vertebral column. (Courtesy of Alex Barlow.)

UV exposure/sunburn

Fish exposed to strong sunlight or ultraviolet radiation without shade can develop sunburn. Outdoor ponds are areas of greatest risk. Light-coloured and non-pigmented fish are most at risk of severe exposure. Conditions that force fish up to the surface (e.g. low dissolved oxygen, gill disease) increase surface swimming and exposure. Poorly constructed shallow ponds make it difficult for fish to escape exposure. Shade plants growing inside and beside the pond, overhanging shade constructions or floating mats may provide some relief. Sunburn produces areas of erythema and petechiation on the dorsal surfaces of the fish (Figure 25.9).

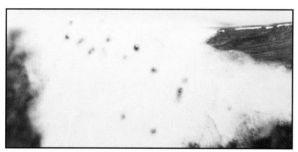

Figure 25.9 Sunburn on the dorsum of a koi in a shallow outdoor pond. The generalized inflammation and petechiation affected only the white areas on the dorsal surfaces. (© W.H. Wildgoose.)

Treatment is aimed at minimizing exposure. Topical ointments are discouraged, as the potential for fouling gills and water quality is significant. Severe sunburn may cause skin necrosis and lead to secondary bacterial infections, requiring systemic antibacterial treatment.

Flooding and runoff

Both situations are preventable by proper selection and planning of the pond site.

Flooding is often the result of a forgotten hose or severe weather conditions. The concerns with flooding are escape of the fish and pollution problems. If advanced warning of severe rainfall is given, then partially draining the pond may help to combat flooding. In some circumstances, dropping the water level by one third of the volume should not harm the fish and, if flooding is averted, will allow for an unplanned water change.

Pollution from the influx of contaminants by flooding may also occur with runoff from the raised areas surrounding the pond fish. Runoff is the result of a poorly located and constructed pond, where watershed terrain has not been taken into account.

Both situations can add suspended solids, organic debris, chemicals or other toxins to the pond. Organophosphates and fertilizers used in the surrounding soil can achieve high concentrations in runoff and may be lethal to fish and the delicate ecosystem in which they live. Similar events may follow in large ponds fed by natural streams that drain from the surrounding countryside. The construction of drainage ditches and raised pond walls can easily redirect running water away from ponds.

Less obvious toxic contaminants may come from the leaves, fruits, seeds or sap from overhanging vegetation. Rainwater may cause wood preservatives to leach from treated structures assembled over the pond.

Physical damage

Self-trauma

Fish with skin irritation due to ectoparasites can excoriate themselves on rough surfaces. Exposed wire or other sharp items can cause punctures or lacerations that may be prone to secondary infection.

Fighting

Overcrowding precipitates aggression in some species and fighting may result in external injury. Less dominant fish frequently suffer injured tail fins and opercular wounds during fighting. Depressed or wounded fish should be isolated for observation and treated. Topical, oral or parenteral antibiotics should be administered as required.

Escape

Some fish attempt to jump out of ponds and tanks, commonly landing on hard surfaces. In addition to desiccation, impact injuries such as fractured fin spines, torn rays and damaged skin may occur. Fish exposed to air can develop corneal opacity and severe skin damage as result of 'flopping' around. Fish should be returned to the water as soon as possible. The addition of salt to freshwater and injection of dexamethasone may alleviate shock and stress. Improved aeration and controlled heating may assist recovery. Fish have been known to survive and recover even after several hours out of water.

Further reading

Andrews C, Exell A and Carrington N (1988) *The Manual of Fish Health.* Salamander Books, London

Bassleer G (1996) *Diseases in Marine Aquarium Fish: Causes, Symptoms, Treatment.* Bassleer Biofish, Westmeerbeek, Belgium

Blasiola GC (1992) Diseases in ornamental marine fishes. In: *Aquariology: the Science of Fish Health Management*, eds JB Gratzek and JR Matthews, pp. 275–300. Tetra Press, Morris Plains, New Jersey

Branson EJ and Southgate PJ (1992) Environmental aspects. In: *Manual of Ornamental Fish*, ed. RL Butcher, pp. 50–53. British Small Animal Veterinary Association, Cheltenham

Cecil TR (1999) Husbandry and husbandry-related diseases of ornamental fish. In: *The Veterinary Clinics of North America: Exotic Animal Practice, Husbandry and Nutrition*, ed. JR Jenkins, pp. 1–18. WB Saunders, Philadelphia, Pennsylvania

Johnson EL (1997) *Koi Health and Disease*. Reade Printers, Athens, Georgia

Moe MA (1992) *The Marine Aquarium Handbook: Beginner to Breeder*. Green Turtle Publications, Plantation, Florida

Moe MA (1992) *The Marine Aquarium Reference: Systems and Invertebrates*. Green Turtle Publications, Plantation, Florida

Noga EJ (1996) *Fish Disease: Diagnosis and Treatment*. Mosby-Year Book Inc, St Louis, Missouri

Post G (1987) *Textbook of Fish Health*. TFH Publications, Neptune City, New Jersey

Stoskopf MK (1993) Environmental requirements and disease of carp, koi, and goldfish. In: *Fish Medicine*, ed. MK Stoskopf, pp. 455–463. WB Saunders, Philadelphia, Pennsylvania

Acknowledgements

The author is grateful to Lester Khoo, The National Aquarium in Baltimore and William Wildgoose for the use of their photographs to illustrate this chapter.

26

Toxins

Peter J. Southgate and Edward J. Branson

The intimate interrelationship between fish and their environment renders them very susceptible to changes in that environment. There is a vast range of elements and compounds that are potentially toxic and many interacting factors that influence their toxicity. The susceptibility of fish to toxins varies greatly with the species involved and may also vary with size, age and general condition and in particular with the health of the gills. Changes in water quality due to the metabolic activities of the fish and the natural breakdown products of nitrogenous waste are discussed in Chapter 1. This chapter is concerned with the effects of exogenous toxic substances introduced into the water.

Clinical signs

Although the range of toxic compounds is large, the gross clinical signs commonly associated with poisoning are limited.

Death
Acute poisoning frequently results in a complete kill with the fish exhibiting little gross abnormality or pre-mortem signs. This is in contrast to primary infectious diseases, which rarely cause such high levels of acute mortality. The event often resembles acute oxygen deficiency, from which it must be distinguished. The situation is often complicated by the fact that the toxin itself may be creating an oxygen deficiency – either directly, due to its reducing activity, or indirectly (for example, by causing an algal die-off).

Respiratory distress
Sublethal levels of many poisons cause direct damage to the gills, resulting in pathology, which reduces the capability of the fish to exchange gases across the gill epithelium. This produces clinical signs of respiratory distress such as gasping at the surface or crowding at water inlets. Some poisons (e.g. malachite green, cyanide) affect respiration at the cellular level, which also results in clinical signs of respiratory distress. Whereas oxygenating the water may alleviate respiratory distress due to toxins that damage the gills, it is unlikely to help in situations where cellular respiration is blocked. The effect of these toxins will be exacerbated if there is any underlying gill pathology due to established water quality problems or gill parasitism, which further complicates investigation and action.

Behavioural changes
Some toxins, such as organophosphorous insecticides, may affect the nervous system, resulting in a variety of 'nervous' signs. On detecting the presence of a toxin in the water, fish may attempt to take avoiding action, which may result in erratic swimming behaviour and jumping.

Osmotic imbalance
Subacute exposure to a toxin may result in impairment of the ability to maintain osmotic control, which may manifest as abdominal swelling, exophthalmos and raised scales.

Other clinical signs
A variety of other signs may be seen, including skin lesions such as hyperplasia or ulceration, and colour changes.

Chronic effects
The long-term effects of exposure to sublethal levels of some toxins, especially metals, can result in poor growth, loss of reproductive capability, deformity, immunosuppression and neoplasia.

Water sources

The quality of the water supply to fish-holding facilities can vary considerably and depends on geographical location, the nature of the water supply and water treatment processes. Natural supplies of water, such as rainwater, boreholes and springs, can be of good and consistent quality but there are potential hazards from each of these supplies and the suitability of the supply should be assessed before use.

Rainwater
Dissolved gases such as sulphur dioxide, carbon dioxide and hydrogen sulphide produce a low pH (acid rain). In addition to the damaging effect of the low pH, particularly on gill tissue, some of these gases can be toxic in themselves (e.g. hydrogen sulphide). There may also be dissolved and suspended organic and inorganic material from atmospheric pollution, which may give rise to a reduction in water quality.

Boreholes and springs

Low pH, particularly in areas prone to acid rain or runoff from acidic soils (e.g. forestry land), may be a problem. There may be the additional effect of the acidified water dissolving metals from the environment. These sources are vulnerable to pollution incidents (e.g. from oil spills and agricultural or industrial discharge) that may enter the watercourse over a protracted period and have a relatively insidious effect.

Rivers, streams and sea water

Used infrequently for ornamental fish, these carry similar risks to boreholes or springs. Rivers and streams are likely to have less consistent water quality and may carry an increased risk from pollution, in addition to the danger of the transmission of disease organisms. The quality of sea water can be influenced by tidal movement and pollution at the point of extraction.

Domestic water supply

Most fish keepers use a domestic water supply and in general this is of consistent good quality. There are regional variations in quality and it is always preferable to obtain a basic water quality analysis and assess its suitability for the fish species to be stocked. The water supply can be affected by the domestic pipework and pre-treatment by the water authority.

- Dissolved metals may be a problem in domestic systems, particularly older ones. Preliminary analysis will determine whether this is likely to be significant
- Chlorine and chloramine are added to the domestic water supply to ensure that it is suitable for human consumption. They can cause acute mortalities and it is essential that any water is allowed to stand for at least 24 hours, preferably with aeration, to allow dissolved chlorine to dissipate. Commercial water conditioners or activated carbon filtration can be used to remove both chlorine and chloramine.

Toxic agents

The majority of toxic substances can be grouped into five broad categories:

- Toxic metals
- Toxic organic compounds
- Biocides
- Toxic gases
- Toxic therapeutic agents.

Many variables influence the toxicity of a compound and there is also marked variability of susceptibility between fish species. The toxic levels for some specific elements and compounds are given in Figure 26.1 but these should be treated as only a rough guide. More detailed information can be obtained from a number of sources, including those listed in the further reading section.

Compound	Level (mg/l)
Metals	
Aluminium	0.3
Copper	3.0
Cadmium	0.1
Iron	0.1
Lead	1.0
Zinc	1.0
Gases	
Chlorine	0.003
Hydrogen sulphide	0.006
Biocides	
Organochlorines (e.g. lindane, toxaphene)	< 0.1
Organophosphates (e.g. dichlorvos, trichlorfon)	0.1–10
Pyrethrum	< 0.1
Rotenone	< 0.1
2,4-D	1–10
Glyphosate	1–10

Figure 26.1 Levels generally considered toxic to fish (based on LC50 data after 48 or 96 hour exposure). The toxicity of most substances will vary according to one or more water quality factors (e.g. alkalinity, hardness, pH, temperature).

Toxic metals

Many metals have been implicated in causing fish kills and having toxic effects. Those most frequently cited as potentially harmful are aluminium, copper, cadmium, iron, zinc and lead. The source is often the water supply.

- Domestic water supplies are a potential source of lead, iron and zinc, particularly in older systems. Newer domestic systems may be a source of copper toxicity. It is important to flush thoroughly any water that has been static in such a system before any is used for fish
- Other sources of metal poisoning include therapeutic agents and biocides deliberately introduced into the system
- The use of unsuitable or contaminated equipment and decorative items within the tank or pond may also present problems
- Water abstracted from springs and boreholes may pass through metal-bearing rocks and contain toxic levels of dissolved metals, particularly if the water is low in pH following acid rainfall or acid snowmelt
- Contamination with industrial effluent may be a source of toxic metals and other potentially toxic substances.

Factors influencing toxicity

The toxicity of a metal will be greatly influenced by other water quality parameters, including pH, temperature, hardness and the presence of organic material and suspended solids, all of which must be taken into account when assessing a situation for evidence of metal toxicity.

pH

In general, a low pH results in higher solubility and therefore a more toxic effect. There are exceptions to this:

- Iron and aluminium are toxic at low pH (aluminium toxicity is greatest at about pH 5 and is a frequent cause of gill pathology in acid conditions)
- In water above pH 7, iron will be precipitated as a colloid on the gills and block gaseous exchange
- Aluminium becomes toxic above pH 8 but the character and toxicity of any aluminium present depend on a complex interaction with pH and other water quality factors. Therefore, the presence of elevated levels of aluminium should always be viewed as potentially toxic.

Temperature

- Increasing temperature tends to increase metal toxicity
- Dissolved oxygen decreases and the metabolic rate increases with rising temperatures, which may further exacerbate the toxic effect of metals.

Alkalinity

Copper toxicity decreases with an increase in alkalinity. It is important to assess alkalinity when contemplating dosing systems with copper-based medications.

Hardness

- In general, metals tend to be more toxic in soft water
- Higher levels of metals will be tolerated in hard water.

Other factors

- The presence of organic material and suspended solids tends to reduce the toxic effect of a metal by adsorbing some of the element
- In contrast, additional metals and other chemicals in the water may have an additive or synergistic effect.

Clinical signs and pathological effects

The toxic effects of metals can vary from the immediate and sudden death of an entire stock to a slow chronic pathology resulting in poor growth rate, deformities and low-grade mortalities. Sublethal effects include respiratory distress and osmotic imbalance.

Species and age have a bearing on the effect of exposure. Young fish are more susceptible to the lethal effects of acute exposure and are more likely to show developmental abnormalities caused by exposure to sublethal levels. Raised levels of mortalities in eggs are found in cases of metal toxicity, and developmental abnormalities are more likely in fish hatched from surviving eggs.

The principal organs affected by metal toxicity are the gills, the kidney and the liver.

Gills

The gill reacts in only a limited number of ways to the presence of a toxic insult. Therefore the clinical signs and pathology are very similar for a wide range of toxins and water quality problems.

In acute metal toxicity, gill damage may be the only pathology detected. Histological examination usually reveals necrotic and hypertrophic changes of the gill epithelium, with some increase in mucus activity. The latter may be detected grossly, as may a similar increase in skin mucus.

Subacute to chronic exposure results in proliferative changes (hyperplasia) of the gill epithelium. These hyperplastic changes reduce the respiratory capabilities of the fish and give rise to the respiratory distress seen particularly at times of limited oxygen availability. They also impede the excretion of carbon dioxide and ammonia. Examination of fresh gill preparations may suggest the presence of gill hyperplasia but this can only be confirmed by histopathological assessment.

With continuing or frequent exposure there may be a combination of acute and chronic effects. A fish with chronic damage to the gills will be more susceptible to the acute effects of a toxin or other water quality problem. The damaged gills are very prone to secondary bacterial and fungal infections and this underlying gill pathology must be considered if any treatment for secondary infections is to be given, since some medications can themselves be damaging to the gills or reduce available oxygen.

The pseudobranch is sensitive to toxic insult and reacts in a manner similar to the gill. Pseudobranch pathology may be seen with heavy metal toxicity and may be affected by biocides and organic toxins. This tissue is valuable in histopathological examination in cases of suspected poisoning and should be sampled in addition to the gill.

Kidney

Absorption of a toxic metal is likely to cause necrosis of the haematopoietic and excretory tissues of the kidney. Hydropic swelling and necrosis of the renal tubules are frequently described. In surviving fish, this results in fibrosis and loss of tubular tissue with a subsequent reduction in excretory ability and produces clinical signs of osmotic imbalance.

Liver

Toxic metals can directly damage the liver, giving rise to a patchy necrosis and perivascular fibrosis in surviving fish. Patchy liver necrosis may also be a consequence of anoxia or hypoxia resulting from gill damage or low dissolved oxygen.

Toxic organic compounds

The range of organic compounds that are potentially poisonous to fish is wide but the risk of exposure for ornamental fish is relatively small. It is mainly restricted to accidental introduction by domestic use or in the construction and decoration of the pond or aquarium.

Ponds that are fed from springs or boreholes are at risk from pollution incidents such as oil spills, sewage and industrial or agricultural discharge.

The toxic effect varies with the nature of the pollutant and the speed at which the pollutant enters the water supply.

- Silage and sewage discharges may have a rapidly toxic effect, mainly due to their deoxygenating nature and the possible presence of toxic components such as hydrogen sulphide
- Phenols, benzene, oils and grease from industrial and refining processes can make their way into the water table from discharges and oil spills and may have an acutely lethal effect. Oil fractions can coat the skin and gills and cause asphyxiation as well as causing direct pathology to the gills, pseudobranch and internal tissues. They may also be much more insidious, resulting in a variety of sublethal and often subtle chronic effects such as glomerulonephritis, osmotic imbalance, skin lesions, anaemia, poor growth and reduced reproductive capability
- Polychlorinated biphenyls (PCBs), mainly from electrical industries, are very persistent contaminants in the environment and have been implicated in suppression of reproductive capability and immunosuppression
- Many organic toxins have been implicated as carcinogens.

Due to the insidious, variable and subtle nature of poisoning from organic compounds, diagnosis can be difficult, protracted and expensive unless a specific pollutant is suspected.

Household compounds

Domestic aquaria and ponds supplied by the domestic water supply are at much less risk of contamination. The major risk here is from human activity in the vicinity of the fish.

- Many household compounds (e.g. ammonia-based cleaning agents, detergents, disinfectants, polishes) are extremely toxic to fish and should never be used where there is a risk of contamination
- Substances used to clean and disinfect aquaria and equipment must be thoroughly flushed from the system
- Nicotine is a highly soluble and toxic compound. Fish should not be housed in smoky atmospheres, particularly where air pumps draw smoke-laden air into the system.

Styrene

Many ponds are constructed from glass-reinforced plastic (GRP). It is essential that the GRP is properly 'cured' (at appropriately high temperature and duration) before it is used for holding fish. Styrene and other hydrocarbons leaching from improperly cured GRP are acutely toxic to fish and are a risk in ponds that are homemade or repaired or not supplied by a reputable manufacturer. Acetone, used to dissolve benzocaine anaesthetic, can dissolve styrene from temporary holding units (e.g. polystyrene boxes).

Wood preservatives

Wood is often used in the construction and decoration of ponds and aquaria. Great care must be taken in the selection and use of wood preservatives near aquatic facilities. The majority of preservatives become non-toxic when properly dried and cured but some, such as creosote, remain toxic. It is preferable to use only preservatives that are recommended for aquatic environments.

Barley straw

Barley straw is occasionally used in garden ponds for its anti-algae effect. Various algal growth-inhibiting factors are produced when barley straw is allowed to rot in water. For aerobic decomposition to occur the straw must be situated near the surface, where it is exposed to sunlight and fresh oxygenated water. It should also be removed after 6 months. Toxic effects in fish have been noted if the straw is not used correctly and is allowed to decompose anaerobically at the bottom of the pond. A foul smell is often detected when the straw is removed in these cases.

Biocides

This group includes pesticides, herbicides and molluscicides. The majority of these compounds are directly toxic and their use should be avoided, unless they are formulated for use in a fish-holding facility and used correctly.

Pesticides

The major risk to pond fish is often from garden or agricultural runoff and potentially from aerial sprays. Indoor aquaria are at risk from the household use of domestic insecticidal aerosol sprays. Veterinary aerosols used to control flea infestations are also very toxic to fish. The effect can be lethal or sublethal, with many of the compounds having a cumulative effect in the fish. Pesticides that pose a hazard to fish include the organochlorines (OCs), organophosphates (OPs) and 'natural' pesticides such as pyrethrum and its synthetic derivatives.

OCs are fat-soluble and may accumulate in fat depots, from which they can be slowly released – their pathological effect can be delayed for some time. Toxic effects of OCs include damage to the central nervous system and necrosis of liver and kidney tissue.

OPs are used extensively in agriculture and horticulture, in the home and in the treatment of crustacean parasites of fish. They act as cholinesterase inhibitors and can be acutely toxic, causing paralysis and death. They may also have a cumulative effect of reducing brain and tissue cholinesterase, which has been implicated in poor growth and deformities.

Pyrethrum and rotenone are natural insecticides of plant origin, and synthetic pyrethroids have a wide application as pesticides. All are toxic to fish and rotenone has long been used as a piscicide to eliminate unwanted fish populations.

Herbicides, algicides and molluscicides

The use of herbicides to control weeds around ponds may pose a hazard. Some products are designed for the control of aquatic weeds but great care must be exercised. Their toxicity may vary with water conditions; for example, glyphosate is more toxic at higher temperatures and at higher pH. Some compounds contain surfactants, which are directly toxic to gill tissue.

Copper formulations such as copper sulphate are used as algicides and molluscicides and great care must be taken in their use. Their toxicity is due mainly to the copper component and varies with water conditions, as discussed earlier. A secondary effect due to the use of herbicides and algicides is the dramatic oxygen depletion resulting from the decomposition of dead weeds and algae.

Toxic gases

Chlorine

The main toxic effect of chlorine (found in domestic water supplies) is destruction of the gill epithelium and respiratory failure. Sublethal exposure results in chronic gill epithelial changes, which restrict the respiratory capabilities of the fish.

Hydrogen sulphide

Hydrogen sulphide can be acutely toxic and can be introduced into water supplies from effluent discharges. The principal source is from the anaerobic decomposition of organic matter within pond and aquarium systems. Disturbing decomposing organic matter on the bottom of a pond or filter unit can result in the release of hydrogen sulphide, leading to acute mortalities. Anaerobic decomposition can also occur within aquaria, and occasionally within decorative items such as shells. Marine aquaria may be more prone to hydrogen sulphide poisoning, due to the larger amounts of sulphate present. Pump breakdown or electrical failures can rapidly lead to anaerobic conditions within filters, again leading to hydrogen sulphide poisoning.

Toxic therapeutic agents

All therapeutic agents are biocidal and potentially toxic to fish, particularly in unfavourable water conditions or if the fish is compromised in any way (e.g. by intercurrent disease).

Many bath treatments are potentially harmful to gill tissue in particular, and any established gill pathology or parasitism may render the fish more vulnerable to the toxic effects of the treatment. It is important to make a basic assessment of fish health and gill condition prior to treatment. Water quality should also be assessed, because it may also affect toxicity. A test treatment on a few fish is always advisable. All treatments must be evenly distributed in the water, avoiding 'hot spots' with high concentrations.

Several bath treatments, including formaldehyde, reduce dissolved oxygen levels and it is important to oxygenate or aerate the water during medication. Paraformaldehyde, seen as white crystals in formaldehyde solutions, is highly toxic and must be removed by filtration if necessary.

It is possible for stock solutions to become more concentrated at the bottom of their containers. To avoid accidental overdose, thorough mixing must take place before use.

Several compounds used as therapeutic agents may cause internal pathology and may result in cumulative effects with repeated use:

- Malachite green is hepatotoxic and very persistent within fish tissues: it has also been implicated in causing developmental abnormalities when used to treat fish eggs
- Sulphonamides are reported to crystallize in the kidney, resulting in renal failure – particularly in marine species
- Gentamicin is nephrotoxic in some species, even at therapeutic doses
- Oxytetracycline can be hepatotoxic following intraperitoneal injection and has also been shown to be immunosuppressive.

Investigating cases

Unless there are strong indications of the agent involved, the limited presenting signs are unlikely to suggest a specific toxin in the majority of cases. An indiscriminate fish kill, possibly with the death of invertebrates and plants and a sudden deterioration in water quality, will be strongly indicative of an acute toxic episode but must be distinguished from an acute primary oxygen deficiency, which may present with a similar clinical history. It must be appreciated that many toxic agents will cause an acute oxygen deficiency.

Many of the sublethal signs are identical to those seen with other water quality problems or infectious disease. It is imperative to carry out adequate investigations into possible water quality problems and pathogenic infections. In addition, underlying disease, parasitism or water quality problems may render fish more vulnerable to a toxic episode or exacerbate the effects of a toxin.

Acute cases with total fish kills may be easier to identify than a more chronic exposure to a toxin, which will have a far more insidious effect.

If a toxic agent is strongly indicated, it may be extremely difficult to determine the exact nature of the agent involved without embarking on a range of complex and expensive laboratory investigations. It is vital to collect as much circumstantial evidence as possible and obtain a comprehensive history of the episode (Figure 26.2).

A full risk assessment should be carried out to determine the possible source of a toxin. Water supplies should be investigated, including records of recent water changes and installation of new equipment. General water quality analysis should

Immediate investigation
• Assess environment for sources
• Check clinical history for clues associated with water changes or medications
• Examine surviving fish for behaviour changes and clinical signs
• Investigate other possible causes or contributory factors such as poor water quality, low oxygen levels or ectoparasitic infestations
• Notify water authority if pollution or poisoning is suspected
• Notify insurers if a claim is likely.
Sampling for analysis
• Notify laboratory of any samples being taken and confirm their suitability
• Collect water samples (at least 1 litre); where possible, obtain comparative samples from 'unaffected' site
• Remove dead fish; freeze carcasses in case of insurance claim or for further investigations
• Obtain samples for histopathology and toxicology from moribund or very recent dead fish (at least 200 g of tissue is required for toxicological analysis); where possible, obtain comparative samples from 'unaffected' fish, preferably from unaffected site
• Consider which analytical tests are to be carried out and whether to request general screen (e.g. for organic compounds) if no specific toxin suspected. Potential cost must be fully appreciated.
Care of survivors
• Remove source of toxin if known
• Consider moving affected fish to 'unaffected' site if possible
• Flush fresh water through the system or carry out water changes, using conditioned water where possible
• Oxygenate or aerate water
• Withhold feeding until some sign of recovery
• Establish preventive procedures to avoid recurrence
• Closely monitor situation for prolonged effect or secondary disease.

Figure 26.2 Action in cases involving a possible toxic agent.

be carried out to ensure that the problem does not originate from an acute deterioration in water quality. Standard measurement of ammonia, nitrite, nitrate and pH should be performed.

A full postmortem and pathological examination should be performed to establish the contribution of pathogens and parasites to the problem. Histopathological analysis may provide a strong indication of a toxic event. Water and tissue analysis for the presence of toxins may also be valuable, but it will be necessary to try to narrow down the range of suspected toxins.

Water samples

Water samples should be taken as soon as practical after poisoning is suspected, though it is quite possible – indeed probable – that the offending toxin has been flushed from the system or dissipated by the time the sample is taken. If a serious pollution episode is indicated, the appropriate water authority should be notified. If there is a possibility of litigation or if malicious poisoning is suspected, duplicate samples of the water should be obtained and these should be sealed and signed in the presence of an independent witness. The following points should be considered:

• Containers must be chemically clean. At the very least they should be rinsed several times in distilled water (including the cap) and then rinsed at least five times in the water to be analysed
• Containers should be of inert plastic with plastic tops when sampling for heavy metals. Glass bottles should be used for samples to be tested for most other substances
• At least 1 litre of water should be collected and the container filled to the top, excluding all air
• The sample should be kept cool and immediately forwarded to the laboratory on ice. Refrigeration is acceptable for short-term storage. Freezing of samples should be avoided if at all possible.

Tissue sampling

Where possible, whole fish should be submitted on ice to the laboratory, with appropriate protection against contamination. If tissues are removed and submitted, care must be taken not to contaminate the samples (e.g. by using metal instruments). Containers must not contaminate the samples.

The most useful tissues for toxicological analysis are gill, liver, kidney and muscle/skin. Samples should be as large as possible: often the minimum is 200 g of liver, kidney or muscle tissue. Brain tissue should be collected when testing for cyanide or organophosphates.

Samples should be deep frozen if there is any delay before analysis. It is also worthwhile retaining some frozen specimens in case further analysis is required.

Malicious poisoning

Cases of deliberate poisoning are not unknown and cyanide is the most frequently employed compound. Tissue analysis for cyanide is essential if malicious poisoning is suspected.

Further reading

Leatherhead JF and Woo PTK (1998) *Fish Diseases and Disorders. Volume 2: Non-infectious Disorders.* CABI Publishing, Wallingford
Mayer FL and Ellersieck MR (1986) *Manual of Acute Toxicity: Interpretation and database for 410 chemicals and 66 species of freshwater animals.* Resource Publication 160. Department of the Interior, Fish and Wildlife Service, Washington DC
Treves-Brown K (2000) *Applied Fish Pharmacology.* Kluwer Academic Publishers, Dordrecht, The Netherlands
Weber LJ (ed.) (1982) *Aquatic Toxicology.* Raven Press, New York

27

Neoplasia and developmental anomalies

John C. Harshbarger

A neoplasm, or tumour, is a clone of mutated cells characterized by some degree of proliferation, autonomy and anaplasia. Solid tumours can vary from benign small intact populations of slowly growing cells with minimal cytological and pattern atypia, to cancerous masses of rapidly dividing, poorly differentiated cells that invade and destroy adjacent normal tissue and may spread or metastasize to distant locations via the blood. Leukaemias arise in circulating blood cells rather than forming a mass.

Mutations that transform cells neoplastically include aneuploidy, activation of growth genes (proto-oncogenes) into oncogenes (tumour genes) and inactivation of suppressor genes (regulator genes). Mutagens are chemical or physical agents that induce or increase genetic mutation by causing changes in DNA. Ornamental fish can be exposed to various mutagens, which include:

- Electrophilic chemicals that bind to DNA
- Viruses or virus templates that are inserted into the DNA
- Ionizing radiation or ultraviolet (UV) light that breaks DNA.

Veterinarians in practice will often encounter neoplasms in ornamental fish. At least 220 species of captive fish with tumours are known from the literature combined with unpublished cases archived by the Registry of Tumors in Lower Animals (RTLA). These tumours originated from cells in every organ or tissue system.

This chapter presents an overview of common fish tumours to enable clinicians to reach a provisional diagnosis. As neoplasia is a disease of cells and because non-neoplastic lesions can have a superficial resemblance to neoplasms, the definitive diagnosis of a tumour requires histopathological examination to confirm the gross impression.

Skin

The most conspicuous tumours occur on the skin and can originate from various cells including epidermal cells, dermal fibrocytes, peripheral nerve sheath cells, pigment cells, endothelial cells lining blood vessels and subcutaneous fat cells.

Papillomas

Epidermal tumours occur anywhere on the body surface but particularly on the head and mouth, where the propensity for abrasion and trauma increases exposure to oncogenic agents, and the ensuing reparative hyperplasia promotes tumour growth. They present as three papillary patterns: exophytic, endophytic and flat.

Epidermal papillomas with an exophytic pattern result from the outward buckling of the thickening epidermis (Figure 27.1). A fibrovascular core continuous with the dermis nourishes the outgrowing fronds or epidermal papillae. Exophytic papillomas have a verrucal surface as seen with oral tumours long known in the European eel.

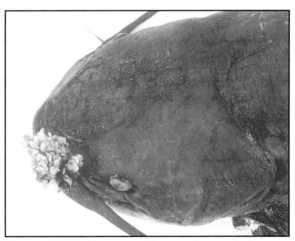

Figure 27.1 Epidermal papilloma on the snout of a brown bullhead. Nodules on the surface of the lesion are manifestations of exophytic papillary growth of neoplastic epidermis. (Courtesy of G.G. Combs, RTLA 328.)

Epidermal papillomas with an endophytic pattern result when pegs of neoplastic epidermis grow down and interdigitate with dermal fibrovascular papillae. Grossly, endophytic papillomas are convex or nodular protrusions with a smooth surface (Figure 27.2). Endophytic epidermal papillomas can often undergo squamous metaplasia, form layered swirls or 'pearls', breach the basement membrane and invade adjacent normal tissues. These are known as squamous cell carcinomas. This occurs less commonly in exophytic papillomas and is rarely seen in flat papillomas. Occasionally endophytic papillomas occur on the anus (Figure 27.3).

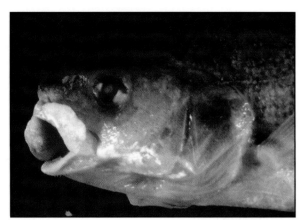

Figure 27.2 Epidermal papilloma of the labia oris in a white croaker. The smooth raised lesions are manifestations of the distension of the surface by endophytic growth of neoplastic epidermal pegs. (Courtesy of K.P. Lindstrom.)

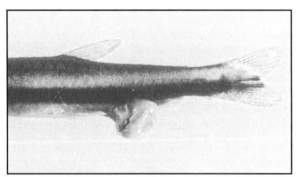

Figure 27.3 Epidermal papilloma of the anus in a black-stripe pencilfish. A smooth doughnut-shaped mass of papillary neoplastic anal epithelium encircles the anus. (Courtesy of S.H. Weitzman, RTLA 432.)

Epidermal papillomas with the flat pattern form when the epidermis thickens but epidermal pegs remain short. Flat papillomas expand laterally as sheets, in part because tumour growth does not exceed 1–2 mm in thickness without vascularization.

In many species there is evidence of a viral aetiology for flat papillomas and some may be transmissible. An example of this is carp pox (Figure 27.4), which is a misnomer since it is neither pox-like

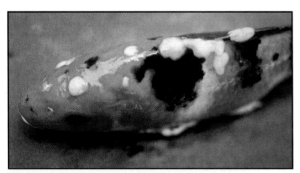

Figure 27.4 A koi affected with multiple flat-type epidermal papillomas, sometimes called carp pox. The skin is thickened by a laterally expanding milky-white epidermal proliferation of cells infected with herpesvirus. (Courtesy of W.H. Wildgoose.)

nor caused by a poxvirus but is caused by *Herpesvirus cyprini*. This herpesvirus is temperature sensitive; therefore as the seasonal water temperature rises above 20°C, papilloma cells containing virus particles begin to lyse, an inflammatory response ensues and the tumours slough. The virus DNA persists in the genome of a number of cell types, probably including epidermal cells. During the next cold season, epidermal cells infected with herpesvirus proliferate again.

Sloughing is often equated with regression and it is argued that carp pox is a hyperplastic proliferation of normal cells rather than neoplasia. However, sloughing of carp papilloma cells results from virus-induced necrotic cell death rather than apoptosis or physiological cell death that occurs in regression. Two additional observations support the view that this is a neoplasm rather than hyperplasia:

- Carp with flat papillomas have been known to grow large squamous cell carcinomas in extended low temperature-controlled situations
- Seasonal lysing of tumour cells is also a feature of the epizootic metastasizing renal adenocarcinoma of the northern leopard frog (*Rana pipiens*) which is also caused by a herpesvirus and which is unarguably a cancer. As in carp tumours, frog renal carcinoma tumour cells containing assembled virus particles lyse in rising summer temperatures while the cancer cells that only contain viral DNA in their genome remain viable.

The exophytic and endophytic patterns do not have any aetiological or physiological significance but merely a fortuitous opportunistic difference. However, the flat type is significant because it indicates a possible viral aetiology.

Pigment cell tumours

Pigment cell tumours predominantly develop on the skin as abnormal pigmented areas or masses. Among different fish species there is a vast array of colours and patterns imparted by a subepidermal layer of specialized pigment cells. Tumours of the specialized pigment-producing cell types usually exhibit the colour of the cell of origin. Thus, in general, melanomas (Figures 27.5 and 27.6) are black, iridophoromas are silver, erythrophoromas (Figure 27.7) are red and xanthophoromas are orange. Pigment cells can be multicoloured because, as shown *in vivo*, neoplastic goldfish pigment cells from the same tumour are capable of differentiating into several pigment phenotypes (Matsumoto *et al.*, 1989). To reflect this variable potential, multicoloured pigment cell tumours *in vivo* are called chromatoblastomas.

Several routes to melanoma formation are illustrated in platy × swordtail hybrids. Certain crosses selectively eliminate the suppressor genes that regulate an activated pigment oncogene carried by the platy, and melanomas arise spontaneously in the offspring. In some other hybrids, melanomas do not arise spontaneously but do so after exposure

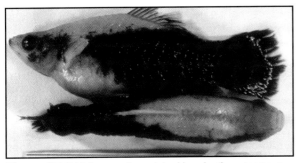

Figure 27.5 Melanoma in a platy. Neoplastic cutaneous melanophores spreading via the dermis are encircling the platy and extend from the head to the tip of the tail. Tumour cells have destroyed and replaced most of the elements of the normal skin and their bulk has significantly expanded the surface outline. (Courtesy of I.S. Gorman, RTLA 230.)

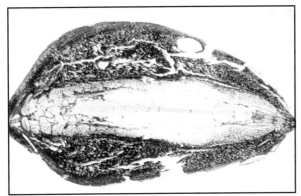

Figure 27.6 Histological cross-section of the melanoma in Figure 27.5. Tumour cells have aggressively invaded the underlying skeletal muscle to the midline. (H&E, × 4 original magnification.) (Courtesy of I.S. Gorman, RTLA 230.)

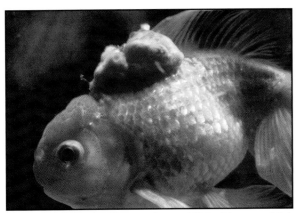

Figure 27.7 Erythrophoroma in a goldfish. A large reddish lobulated neoplasm between the head and the dorsal fin consisted of erythrophores producing carotenoid pigment. (Courtesy of F.M. Hetrick, RTLA 2609.)

to UV light or carcinogenic chemicals, either of which could inactivate suppressor genes through mutations.

Not all coloured lesions can be assumed to be pigment cell tumours. As examples, the metacercariae of some trematode parasites are melanotrophic, some epidermal papillomas concentrate melanophores, and some red lesions are blood-filled vascular tumours in the skin.

Connective tissue

Lipomas originate from fat cells in the subcutaneous layer and elsewhere. They can grow quite large; for example, a 20 kg lipoma was found in a bluefin tuna. Cutaneous lipomas (Figure 27.8) are often ulcerated, exposing fatty yellowish tissue under the skin. The cut surfaces often feel greasy to the touch. Histologically, lipomas are composed of mature fat cells often separated by fibrous septa of varying thickness or containing fibrous areas. Liposarcomas that arise from fetal fat cells have rarely been diagnosed in fish.

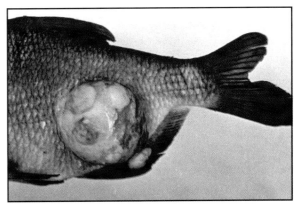

Figure 27.8 Lipoma in a bream. The large spherical ulcerated mass protruding laterally from an area between the anus and the tail exhibits yellowish discoloration from fat stored in the neoplastic lipocytes. (Courtesy of L.E. Mawdesley-Thomas and D. Bucke, RTLA 220.)

Vascular system

Vascular tumours most commonly originate from endothelial cells lining blood vessels and form an array of vascular spaces from the size of capillaries to cavernous cysts. Grossly, they usually appear red because the spaces are engorged with blood and those that are poorly formed by tumour cells are prone to haemorrhage. However, other spaces will be empty because they do not communicate directly with the circulatory system. Non-invasive vascular neoplasms are called haemangiomas and haemangioendotheliomas. Vascular cancers are called angiosarcomas.

Nervous system

Peripheral nerves consist of individual axons which have an endoneural myelin sheath produced by Schwann cells. A fascicle of axons is enclosed by a perineurium, and a nerve trunk made up of fascicles is enclosed in an epineurium. Fibroblasts are present in the perineurium and epineurium. Peripheral nerve sheath tumour cells, common on many species of fish, are frequently multiple and occur anywhere on the body surface as well as internally. They can also develop along the same nerve, as illustrated by Morrison *et al.* (1993) in a rainbow smelt. Tumour diagnosis reflects differences in histology and behaviour of the tumour cells, due in part to the covering from which they

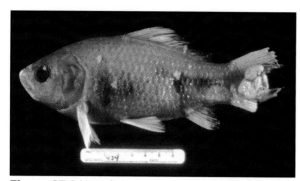

Figure 27.9 Neurofibroma in a goldfish. A large lobular mass on the tail and smaller scattered cutaneous masses originated from neoplastic peripheral nerve sheath. (Courtesy of B.M. Levy, RTLA 454.)

originate. Depending on the components of these tumours, they are diagnosed as schwannomas or neurofibromas (Figure 27.9). When cancerous, they are called malignant peripheral nerve sheath tumours.

Digestive system

Tooth tumours (Figure 27.10) are seen on freshwater angelfish. Fish teeth develop similarly to those of mammals, as an interaction of dental epithelium or dental lamina (ectodermal) with connective tissue (mesodermal). However, rather than becoming permanently anchored to bone, as in mammals, fish teeth are only ankylosed to oral bones and are continually shed and replaced by newly developing teeth. Among various fish species, teeth can develop on most bones of the oral cavity. Thus, tooth tumours are not restricted to the dental plate just behind the lips, but these are the most common. Poorly differentiated ameloblastomas and ameloblastic odontomas cannot be distinguished grossly from lip papillomas without histology, but well differentiated odontomas can sometimes be distinguished by misdirected abortive teeth present on the surface.

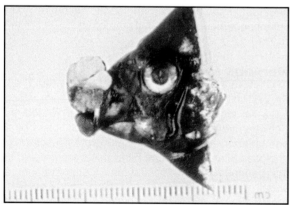

Figure 27.10 Compound odontomas in a freshwater angelfish. Large oral growths of papillary dental epithelium are inducing many well formed teeth in association with a thickened matrix of loose connective tissue containing numerous bony spicules. (Courtesy of G.C. Blasiola Jr, RTLA 2189.)

Liver cancer in fish is epidemiologically related to exposure to chemical carcinogens in the environment (Harshbarger and Clark, 1990). This relationship is confirmed by experimental studies and biochemical data. No alternative aetiology has been found. This suggests that the finding of hepatocellular carcinoma or cholangiocarcinoma in ornamental fish is an indication of carcinogenic contamination of the food or water. Many liver cancers occur below the surface of the organ but when on the surface they often present as flush or slightly raised discolorations that can only be confirmed by histological examination.

Urinary system

Urinary bladder tumours are most commonly found in oscars that present with a swollen abdomen, protruding anus, lethargy or emaciation. Internally, a large retroperitoneal mass (Figure 27.11) in the caudal abdomen often displaces other organs in a cranial direction. The mass appears cystic with brown or yellow fluid. Histologically the tumours are papillary cystadenomas of the urinary bladder epithelium.

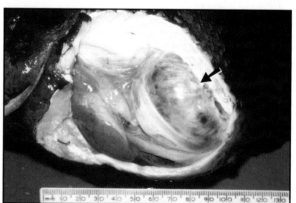

Figure 27.11 Urinary bladder papillary cystadenoma in an oscar. This anorexic oscar had a swollen abdomen with a large retroperitoneal mass (arrowed) containing reddish-brown fluid in a large central cyst formed by neoplastic bladder epithelium. Scale in millimetres. (Courtesy of W.H. Wildgoose, RTLA 7299.)

Reproductive system

Gonadal tumours are common in carp hybrids (including ornamental carp). These are large, often circumscribed masses attached to mesenteries in the body cavity (Figure 27.12). Histologically they present a mix of gonadal tissues that vary between different tumours as well as among different locations within the same tumour. Consequently, they have been diagnosed as a fibroma, granulosa-cell tumour, gonadoblastoma and teratoma. Regardless of the diagnosis, they could result from the difficulty of certain hybrid combinations to produce a gonad and they therefore represent dysmorphogenesis instead of neoplasia. With that in mind it seems prudent to refer to them generically as either gonadal

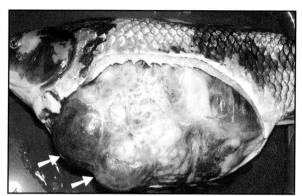

Figure 27.12 A gonadoblastoma in a carp. A huge lobular mass (arrowed) in the body cavity is partly enveloped by mesenteric membranes. The pluripotent neoplastic cells were differentiating into various germinal and stromal gonadal elements in different locations throughout the mass. (Courtesy of W.H. Wildgoose, RTLA 6228.)

tumours or as a gonadoblastoma, to indicate variable potential for differentiation. The successful surgical removal of one case has been reported by Lewbart *et al.* (1998).

Other neoplasms

Many other spontaneous neoplasms can be seen externally. For example:

- Olfactory neuroepithelioma protrudes from the nares
- Retinoblastoma can be associated with exophthalmos, though protrusion of the globe can also result from parasitic or bacterial infections
- Fibroma and osteoma of scales or skeletal bone are hard or gritty in texture
- Thymic lymphoma (Figure 27.13) deflects the operculum, as does thyroid hyperplasia (goitre).

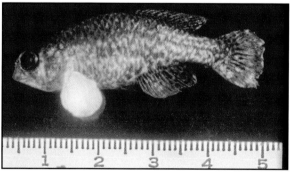

Figure 27.13 A thymic lymphoma in a black-fin pearlfish. The white mass protruding from the opercular cavity is packed with proliferating neoplastic lymphocytes. Scale in centimetres. (Courtesy of G.C. Blasiola Jr, RTLA 1646.)

Internally, nephroblastomas are well recognized kidney tumours and mesotheliomas can arise from serous peritoneal membranes. Tumours of the pancreas, including acinar cell adenocarcinoma, have been recorded in goldfish presenting with abdominal distension. Ependymoblastomas that originate from the nerve cord invade and destroy the skeletal muscle, and may protrude through the side of the fish. These arise spontaneously in 0.35% of cultured coho salmon fingerlings.

Developmental anomalies

Thousands of developmental anomalies have been reported in fish, ranging from simple overgrowths of tissue to hamartomas that include two germ layers and teratomas that include a mixture of cells from all three germ layers. Tumour-like teratoid anomalies in the form of Siamese twinning (Figure 27.14) have been seen many times in fish. They have been well studied in the guppy (Hisaoka, 1961), where lesions range from near-perfect Siamese twins to double and triple monsters, often recognized by a partial fin. Teratoid anomalies are frequently attached ventrally but have been noted in the body wall, the intestinal wall and elsewhere. The lesions consist of a collage of normal tissues but neoplasms, teratomas or teratocarcinomas can arise within the teratoid anomaly. The rate of growth of Siamese embryos can be disproportionate, due to an inhibitory effect by the dominant embryo. Postulated origins of these abnormalities include:

- Development of two embryos in one ovum, possibly triggered by double fertilization
- Latent activation of a nest of pluripotent cells resulting in the secondary development of independent embryonic tissue.

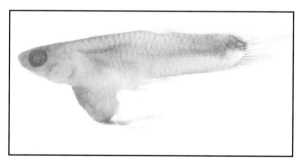

Figure 27.14 Teratoma in a guppy. The scale-covered ventral abdominal growth with attached fins contains various normal tissues, including brain, suggestive of abortive Siamese twin formation. Neoplasms arising in such malformations are called teratomas or teratocarcinomas. (Courtesy of R. Wenk, RTLA 75.)

Polycystic kidney is a developmental anomaly most often seen in goldfish and causes significant abdominal distension. The body cavity is filled with a multilocular, thin-walled, fluid-filled mass (Figure 27.15). The cysts are Bowman's capsules that failed to develop a connection to the nephrogenic tubules. Glomeruli continue filtering urine into these

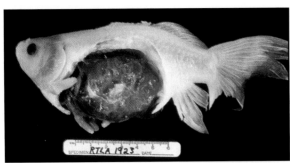

Figure 27.15 Polycystic kidney in a goldfish. The multilocular fluid-filled thin-walled mass of grossly dilated Bowman's capsules occupies much of the body cavity. This is a non-neoplastic developmental anomaly that is due to the failed development of a connection to nephrons for drainage. (Courtesy of TJ Dodgeshun, RTLA 1923.)

non-draining capsules (Schlumberger, 1950). A grossly similar lesion referred to as 'kidney enlargement disease' is caused by infection with the myxosporean, *Hoferellus* spp. (see Chapter 21).

Further reading and references

Ferguson HW (1989) *Systematic Pathology of Fish: A Text and Atlas of Comparative Tissue Responses in Diseases of Teleosts.* Iowa State University Press, Ames, Iowa

Harshbarger JC and Clarke JB (1990) Epizootiology of neoplasms in bony fish of North America. *The Science of the Total Environment* **94**, 1–32

Hisaoka KK (1961) Congenital teratoma in the guppy, *Lebistes reticulates. Journal of Morphology* **109**, 93–113

Hoover KL (ed.) (1984) *Uses of Small Fish Species in Carcinogenicity Testing.* National Cancer Institute Monograph 65. US Government Printing Office, Washington DC

Lewbart GA, Spodnick G, Barlow N, Love NE, Geoly F and Bakal RS (1998) Surgical removal of an undifferentiated abdominal sarcoma from a koi carp (*Cyprinus carpio*). *Veterinary Record* **143**, 556–558

Matsumoto J, Wada K and Akiyama T (1989) Neural crest cell differentiation and carcinogenesis: capability of goldfish erythrophoroma cells for multiple differentiation and clonal polymorphism in their melanogenic variants. *Journal of Investigative Dermatology* **92**, 255S–260S

Mawdesley-Thomas LE (ed.) (1972) *Diseases of Fish. Symposia of the Zoological Society of London, Number 30.* Academic Press, London

Morrison CM, Harshbarger JC and McGladdery SE (1993) Schwannomas in rainbow smelt. *Journal of Aquatic Animal Health* **5**, 317–323

Reichenbach-Klinke H and Elkan E (1965) *The Principal Diseases of Lower Vertebrates.* Academic Press, London

Roberts RJ (ed.) (2001) *Fish Pathology*, 3rd edn. WB Saunders, London

Schlumberger HG (1955) Polycystic kidney (mesonephros) in the goldfish. *Archives of Pathology* **50**, 400–410

The Registry of Tumors in Lower Animals (RTLA) is supported by National Cancer Institute contract NO1-CB-77021 for the study of tumours and related diseases in cold-blooded vertebrates and invertebrates. Specimens are received from donors worldwide and their cooperation is greatly appreciated. Further information about the RTLA can be found on its website at **http://fact.gwumc.edu/tumour**

Acknowledgements

The invaluable assistance of Marilyn S. Slatick, Phyllis M. Spero, Kathy L. Price and Norman M. Wolcott in the registration and histotechnology of the specimens, abstracting the literature and querying the specimens and literature bases is gratefully acknowledged.

28

Nutritional disorders

Roy P.E. Yanong

There is such a diversity of ornamental fish species that nutritional requirements may vary considerably, though some generalities can be made. Familiarity with basic life history, anatomy and physiology is helpful, especially when working with less common species. For example, the size and shape of the mouth, the presence and type of teeth and the type of digestive tract are important clues to diet. Good references are essential and provide invaluable information about the feeding habits of many species. The three major groupings include herbivore, carnivore and omnivore.

Fish require significantly fewer calories by mass than warm-blooded counterparts. There are several major reasons for this:

- Fish are poikilothermic ('cold-blooded') and therefore do not expend energy to maintain their body temperature
- Most teleost fish have a swim-bladder that allows them to be neutrally buoyant in water, further reducing energy requirements
- Fish can excrete products of protein metabolism directly as ammonia, without using energy for biochemical conversions.

Nutritional requirements

Proteins

Protein is one of the most expensive parts of any diet; therefore optimizing protein availability is critical. Excess protein, or protein that is not well assimilated, will result in increased waste and ammonia production, as well as being diverted from use as an energy source. Most fish require from 25% to 50% protein in the diet but exact requirements are determined by temperature, size, age, genetics, feeding rate, protein source, availability of natural sources and the ratio of protein to energy. For example, younger fish require significantly more food in proportion to their bodyweight than older fish.

Fishmeals are preferred protein sources, but not all fishmeals are equal in quality. Essential amino acids for fish are listed in Figure 28.1. Feeds with protein sources derived primarily from plants are deficient in methionine and lysine and must be supplemented by the manufacturer.

Essential amino acids	Dietary vitamins	Minerals
Arginine	Water-soluble	Major
Histidine	Thiamine	Calcium
Isoleucine	Riboflavin	Phosphorus
Leucine	Pyridoxine	Magnesium
Lysine	Pantothenic acid	Sodium
Methionine	Biotin	Potassium
Phenylalanine	Niacin	Chlorine
Threonine	Folic acid	Sulphur
Tryptophan	Cyanocobalamin	Trace
Valine	Ascorbic acid	Iron
	Choline	Iodine
	Inositol	Manganese
	Fat-soluble	Copper
	A, D, E and K	Cobalt
		Zinc
		Molybdenum
		Aluminium
		Nickel
		Vanadium
		Tin
		Silicon
		Chromium
		Selenium
		Fluorine

Figure 28.1 Nutrient requirements for ornamental fish.

Carbohydrates

Carbohydrates are an inexpensive form of energy. Generally assimilated well by omnivores and herbivores, carbohydrates are poorly utilized by some carnivores. Some fish have been raised successfully on diets free of carbohydrate.

Lipids

Lipids serve many important functions. They are integral to cell membrane structure, they are hormonal precursors and they are a very important source of energy. Certain species have requirements for specific fatty acids, in particular omega 3, omega 6, or a combination of the two. Omega 3 fatty acids appear to be more important in fish that spend more time in cooler waters: the membrane phospholipids of these fish contain a greater proportion of unsaturated fatty acids, since they allow membranes to remain more fluid at these temperatures. The ratio of protein to energy/lipid in the diet will determine whether a fish wastes valuable protein sources (too much protein) or stops eating before receiving an adequate supply of essential amino acids (too much lipid).

Vitamins

Specific vitamin requirements vary depending on the anatomy and physiology of individual species. Some species (e.g. some cichlids, common carp) have gut microflora that can manufacture certain vitamins. The vitamins listed in Figure 28.1 are considered necessary components of any diet.

Some processing methods may destroy vitamins. Stabilized forms of vitamin C have become more common because non-stabilized forms degrade rapidly. Vitamin deficiency syndromes have been documented primarily in food fish and many of these are believed to occur in ornamental fish as well.

Minerals

Figure 28.1 lists the major and trace minerals that are assumed to be required. Fish have the ability to take up many dissolved minerals through their gills; marine fish, in particular, drink water and ingest minerals in this manner. Some groups of fish, such as Cyprinidae (e.g. koi, goldfish, barbs and danios) and Scaridae (marine parrotfish), lack a true acid stomach. This limits their ability to utilize mineral forms requiring gastric acid dissolution for uptake.

Nutrient interactions in certain species can be complex. For example, phytate or phytic acid, which comprises the majority of phosphorus in soybean meal and other feeds of plant origin, forms complexes that reduce the absorption of iron, zinc, copper, manganese, calcium and magnesium. High concentrations of dietary calcium and phytates in a diet will significantly reduce zinc absorption, resulting in clinical signs of zinc deficiency. Toxicity of some heavy metals, especially lead and cadmium, can induce vertebral abnormalities in certain species of fish.

Diet and colour

One of the most important features of many ornamental fish is their coloration. Diet is a key to good coloration, though other factors such as age, sex and social hierarchy may play a role.

In the wild, natural foods such as shrimp and algae (e.g. *Spirulina*) have colour-enhancing elements. In captivity, prepared feeds must be supplemented.

- Carotenoids such as astaxanthin and beta-carotene promote yellow, orange and red pigmentation
- Carotenoids bound to protein promote blue and green pigmentation.

Commercially prepared colour-enhancing additives are available and are now included in many commercial diets.

Live foods

Live foods used in the hobby (Figure 28.2) are readily obtainable from commercial producers or from other hobbyists and, with proper precautions and caveats, can be a welcome addition to the diet of many tropical fish.

Fish
Earthworms
Brine shrimp (*Artemia*)
Water fleas (*Daphnia* and *Moina* spp.)
Micro-worms (*Panagrellus silusiae*)
Grindal worms (*Enchytraeus buchholtzi*)
Infusoria (ciliated protozoans such as *Paramecium*)
Vinegar eels (*Turbatrix aceti*)
Wingless fruit flies (*Drosophila melanogaster*)
Rotifers (*Brachionus* spp.)

Figure 28.2 Live foods for ornamental fish.

The benefits imparted by live foods include natural colour enhancement, increased nutritional value in the diet and the eliciting of natural feeding responses. In fact, larval or fry stages of many commonly bred species, as well as adult stages of some more exotic freshwater and marine fish species, may not accept commercially prepared feeds. Many live food cultures can be supplemented by feeding them with products that will increase their nutritional value – such as essential fatty acids or *Spirulina*.

However, live foods can act as carriers of pathogenic organisms, including parasites, fungi, bacteria and viruses. Live foods that come from controlled indoor artificial cultures are preferred over wild-caught foods, but even well controlled cultures may potentially have some detrimental effects. For example, *Tubifex* worms may be one of the least desirable of the live foods, since they can harbour harmful bacteria (such as *Streptococcus*) and intermediate stages of some parasites, including the nematode *Eustrongylides*.

Feeder fish fed to piscivorous species can also be problematic and should always be examined to ensure that they are healthy, even if obtained from a domestic producer. Symptoms of bacterial disease and the presence of internal or external parasites should be identified before feeder fish are fed to piscivores. Apart from the obvious external parasites (e.g. *Ichthyophthirius, Epistylis*, or monogenean trematodes), internal parasites (e.g. microsporidia, *Capillaria, Eustrongylides*) may be transmitted to the predatory species. Feeder fish with known parasites should be either rejected or treated before being fed. It should be noted that freshwater feeder fish fed to marine carnivores may be lacking in certain nutrients, such as essential fatty acids.

Other foods

As an alternative to live foods and to minimize the risk of introducing disease, it is often safer to use frozen or freeze-dried foods. These should be gamma-irradiated to kill all pathogenic organisms, some of which may survive freezing.

Feeding regimen

The frequency of and amount of feeding are complicated by a number of factors, including the species, age and size of the fish, the availability of natural foods, the water temperature and the type and quality of the diet.

- More active species will require more food
- Cyprinids (e.g. barbs, danios, goldfish, koi) lack a true stomach and therefore may benefit from multiple feedings
- Younger fish may require feeding rates as high as 6–10% bodyweight daily and even more for very early life stages
- For mature fish, most maintenance diets are fed at rates of between 1% and 3% bodyweight
- As temperature increases, feed requirement also increases
- The higher the quality of the diet, the more likely it is that essential nutrients will be physiologically available in sufficient amounts in small servings.

Because most hobbyists do not weigh their fish and fish food, a guideline for many of the common tropical fish at typical temperatures (approximately 25°C) is as follows.

- Feed as much as the fish will eat in 1–5 minutes, once or twice a day
- Decrease feeding if uneaten food remains
- Assess the condition of the fish continually and adjust the regimen accordingly.

Fish undergoing starvation typically have sunken bellies and loss of muscle mass dorsally on the body and on top of the head, in addition to other signs described below.

Nutritional disease

Many commercial diets appear adequate: older juveniles and adults of common species that are fed these diets do not exhibit obvious gross abnormalities, and overt nutritional disease is a rarely diagnosed problem. However, nutritional disease is a relative term. One diet may be adequate for baseline maintenance of adult fish, but may be inadequate or inappropriate for juvenile growth or for brood stock conditioning.

Some changes may be subtle, such as reduced colour. Suboptimal nutrition leads to insidious problems such as slow or reduced growth, greater susceptibility to infectious disease, reduced lifespan, reduced fecundity or chronic illnesses. A number of nutritional deficiencies have been linked with specific syndromes in food fish but such dramatic manifestations are more the exception than the rule.

Excessive or inadequate feeding rates

Where dietary components are appropriate, the most likely problem is either excessive or inadequate feeding.

- Fish fed more than their daily requirement will develop obesity and excess fat stores. Uneaten food will contribute to water quality degradation
- Starvation resulting from inadequate quantity of food can be caused by several factors, including:
  - Underestimation of requirement of a fish or group of fish

  - Interspecific or intraspecific competition, with dominant or more aggressive fish obtaining most of the food (common in community tanks)
  - Temperature increases, resulting in increased metabolic rate and increase in requirement.

Inappropriate diet

A totally inappropriate diet includes both micronutrient and macronutrient imbalances, as opposed to deficiency or excess in only one or a few micronutrients. Examples include:

- Feeding vegetable matter alone to carnivorous species such as red-tailed catfish or pike cichlids
- Feeding only sausages or hot dogs to oscars
- Feeding strictly animal matter to herbivores such as pacu.

In addition to significant micronutrient deficiencies, macronutrient imbalances often lead to starvation or excess fat deposition with resulting disease development such as hepatic lipidosis or fatty liver.

Poor quality or contaminated diet

Most of the popular commercial diets do not cause grossly obvious nutritional disease but less rigorously controlled diets may be lacking in one or more micronutrients or macronutrients. Likewise, components in old or improperly stored diets frequently become degraded: vitamins quickly degenerate and lipids oxidize and become rancid, increasing vitamin E requirements.

Diets stored under warm moist conditions favour the growth of fungi, whose products may be cytotoxic, carcinogenic or neurotoxic. Algal toxins and bacterial toxins (such as botulinum toxin) can also cause disease in fish. In addition to specific toxin production, live or prepared food contaminated with parasites, fungal spores, pathogenic bacteria (e.g. *Mycobacterium*) or viruses may produce acute or chronic systemic infection in fish fed these diets.

Therapeutic agents and organic chemicals (e.g. polychlorinated biphenyls, pesticides, other hydrocarbons) may be present as contaminants. Clinical signs or the presence of a known toxic contaminant may warrant further analysis but toxicity data are not available for most ornamental fish species.

Specific micronutrient deficiency or excess

Micronutrient (and macronutrient) requirements have been experimentally determined for several economically important food fish species, for which nutritionally complete diets are available. By contrast, the complete nutritional requirements of most ornamental tropical fish are not fully understood. Most of the specific micronutrient deficiency or excess syndromes have been extrapolated from studies of food fish, especially salmonids and catfish (Figure 28.3), though work has been done on other food fish species and some ornamental species.

Pathology	Vitamin deficiency	Mineral deficiency	Amino acid deficiency	Other
Ocular disease	Vitamin A, Riboflavin, Vitamin C, Choline, Niacin	Zinc, Copper, Magnesium	Methionine, Tryptophan	
Vertebral deformity	Vitamin C	Phosphorus, Calcium, Magnesium, Manganese	Tryptophan	*Toxicity:* Lead, Cadmium
Opercular deformity	Vitamin A, Vitamin C			
Anaemia	Vitamin B$_{12}$ (cyanocobalamin), Inositol, Vitamin C, Folic acid, Riboflavin, Pantothenic acid, Biotin, Niacin, Vitamin E, Vitamin K	Iron		*Toxicity:* Zinc
Fatty liver degeneration	Choline		Methionine	*Essential fatty acid deficiency Excess dietary fat Toxicity:* Oxidized fat
Muscular disease	Vitamin B$_1$ (thiamine), Biotin, Vitamin D	Selenium and Vitamin E		
Clubbed gills	Pantothenic acid			
Neurological disease or convulsions	Vitamin B$_1$ (thiamine), Vitamin B$_6$ (pyridoxine), Niacin, Riboflavin	Magnesium		
Hyperthyroidism/goitre		Iodine		
Skin/fin haemorrhages	Multiple deficiencies			

Figure 28.3 Specific pathologies and possible nutritional aetiologies.

In all species, it is important to remember that external factors, as well as concurrent dietary factors, may increase or decrease micronutrient or macronutrient requirements or availability. For example, the percentage of polyunsaturated fatty acids in the diet of carp will affect the vitamin E requirement, and methionine deficiency will increase choline requirement in channel catfish. Foods soaked in water for some time before consumption will leach important nutrients such as water-soluble vitamins. This is particularly relevant to flaked foods, where contact with the water for only 30 seconds may result in the loss of up to 90% of various vitamins (Pannevis and Earle, 1994).

The gut microflora of some species are capable of vitamin synthesis. For example, vitamin B$_{12}$ is synthesized in the intestinal tract of Nile tilapia by resident bacteria. Similarly, folic acid is synthesized in common carp. Therefore, vitamin deficiency of B$_{12}$ or folic acid may not occur in these and possibly similar species unless there is concurrent dietary deficiency and antibiotic usage.

Investigating nutritional disease

It is often difficult to identify the presence of a nutritional disease, as many of the associated symptoms, such as reduced growth, are non-specific and chronic.

Nutritional disease should be considered if there is a history of poor growth, poor survival, low fecundity, chronic illnesses or presence of any of the more specific signs previously mentioned. Histopathology of affected fish may provide supportive information but is not definitive.

If a nutritional pathology has not developed beyond the point of recovery, a change in diet or nutritional supplementation may be all that is needed to bring about improvement in condition and further investigation may be unnecessary. A more detailed investigation into the cause of a suspected nutritional disease can be difficult, time consuming and costly. Important considerations are as follows.

- Species – the species involved and their particular nutritional requirements, if known
- Clinical history – the time of onset of the problem, general condition of fish, specific symptoms and concurrent disease (both historically and as determined during routine clinical work-up)
- Nutritional history. Because nutritional disease may take many weeks or months to manifest itself, details of feeding should be obtained over an extended period of time and include such information as freshness and storage conditions of the food
- Histopathology. Although not definitive, histopathology of affected fish can support a diagnosis of nutritional disease
- Diet analysis. Based on the clinical and pathological findings, one or more specific nutritional imbalances may be identified as an underlying causal factor. Diet analysis may then provide corroborating evidence.

Problems associated with feed analysis

- Nutritional disease often progresses slowly. A diet fed in the past that may have had specific imbalances may differ significantly from the present diet. For this reason, clients may need to retain frozen samples of previous batches of feed, for later analysis. Approximately 200 g is required for detailed nutritional analysis

- For meaningful analysis, large quantities of feed are needed. Unless large volumes of food are consumed, this is frequently impossible
- A specific dietary imbalance may not be clearly indicated by clinical or pathological findings
- Information and data on the nutritional requirements of many species is very limited. Unless there is extreme excess or deficiency, interpretation of diet analysis is usually difficult.

Further reading and references

Gratzek JB and Matthews JR (1992) *Aquariology: the Science of Fish Management*. Tetra Press, Morris Plains, NJ

Lovell T (1989) *Nutrition and Feeding of Fish*. Van Nostrand Reinhold, New York

Macartney A (1996) Ornamental fish nutrition and feeding. In: *Manual of Companion Animal Nutrition and Feeding*, ed. NC Kelly and JM Wills, pp. 244–251. BSAVA Publications, Cheltenham

National Research Council (1993) *Nutrient Requirements of Fish*. National Academy Press, Washington DC, 114 pp.

Pannevis MC (1993) Nutrition of ornamental fish. In: *The Waltham Book of Companion Animal Nutrition*, ed. IH Burger, pp. 85–96. Pergamon Press, Oxford

Pannevis MC and Earle KE (1994) Nutrition of ornamental fish: water soluble vitamin leaching and growth of *Paracheirodon innesi*. *Journal of Nutrition* **124**, S2633–S2635

Southgate PJ and Branson EJ (1992) Nutritional diseases. In: *Manual of Ornamental Fish*, ed. RL Butcher, pp. 121–127. BSAVA Publications, Cheltenham.

Wilson RP (1991) *Handbook of Nutrient Requirements of Finfish*. CRC Press Inc, Boca Raton, FL

Yanong RPE (1999) Nutrition of ornamental fish. *Veterinary Clinics of North America: Exotic Animal Practice* **2**, 19–42

29

Reproductive and genetic disorders

Roy P.E. Yanong

Breeding disorders are of great importance to fish health because of their persistence in the breeding line and their long-term consequences. The artificial circumstances and selective breeding in ornamental fish culture units increase the chance of a genetic disorder becoming established, though this may take several generations in which to become manifest. Identifying the underlying cause and developing a solution requires an understanding of genetic principles and complex environmental interactions. This chapter will discuss various aspects of ornamental fish reproduction and associated genetic disorders.

General considerations

Broodstock selection

Broodstock should exhibit overall good health, excellent conformation and colour. Those selecting or examining broodstock should be aware of sexual dimorphism, if present. A history of lineage is useful and a health record may enable identification of potential disease carriers. Young rather than old adults are preferred but younger stock are typically not as fecund (fertile) as more experienced breeders. Old broodstock are more susceptible to age-related diseases, including mycobacteriosis. Broodstock should be examined for external and internal parasites and treated accordingly.

Broodstock conditioning

Factors for optimal broodstock conditioning depend on the species but important factors include water quality, good nutrition, proper habitat and low pathogen levels. In particular, correct nutrition is vital for egg development in the female. Depending upon the ultimate goal, conditioning may require separation of males and females prior to spawning.

Spawning

Identifying the factors that trigger spawning is critical. These include changes in water quality (e.g. pH, hardness, conductivity, total dissolved solids, dissolved oxygen), water currents, rainfall, presence of spawning substrates (e.g. plants, rocks) or presence of other species. Optimal male to female ratios vary from one species to another and involve pairs, harems or groups. Some species for which these triggers have not been determined or cannot be provided are spawned using hormone injections such as carp pituitary extract (CPE), human chorionic gonadotropin (HCG) or gonadotropin-releasing hormone (GnRH). Eggs must be mature prior to injection, otherwise failure is inevitable. In many species this can be verified by ovarian biopsy in which a round-tipped catheter is passed through the genital pore and some eggs are gently aspirated and examined for maturity and condition.

Egg hatching

Optimal water quality is critical to a good hatch rate and ideal conditions will depend upon the species. Inappropriate levels of sodium, calcium or other ions and the presence of toxins or pathogens will reduce the hatch rate.

Fry survival and growth

Larvae and fry are sensitive to poor water quality and excess current, light and turbulence. In addition, they are much more susceptible to pathogens due to their poorly developed immune system.

If infectious disease develops in the breeding room or hatchery, then appropriate precautions must be taken to prevent further spread of the pathogen. This includes proper sanitation and disinfection, especially of fry holding and growing units.

Breeding strategies

It is important to be familiar with standard breeding requirements for the species in question and to recognize habitat, space and social interactions that may affect breeding success and fish health. Because of the diversity of species in the hobby, only a few of the more common strategies are discussed here and they are based on Loiselle (1992).

Live-bearers

Guppies, mollies, platies, swordtails and variatus (all members of the Poeciliidae) are the most familiar of the live-bearing fishes, which give birth to live young. Internal fertilization is achieved through the use of a gonopodium, a specialized intromittent organ formed by a modification of the third, fourth and fifth anal fin rays in the males: this is one of several sexually dimorphic traits. Spermatozeugmata or sperm packets are introduced into the female and in some species are used to fertilize multiple batches of eggs. Although this may hinder breeding programmes, there is evidence that the sperm of the last male to have entered a female will have precedence over any existing sperm. Pregnant females typically develop a dark 'gravid' spot over and near their vent. Most of the common live-bearers gestate 50–100 young for 4–6 weeks (mollies may require up to 10 weeks). Hybridization occurs readily between congeneric species.

Type 1 egg scatterers

Most species in the hobby are egg layers. Type 1 egg scatterers include many of the Cyprinidae (barbs, danios, koi, goldfish, rasboras), Characidae (tetras) and Corydoras catfish. After conditioning, the sexes are distinguished by body shape, with females showing more abdominal swelling than males. Additional sexual dimorphic traits such as colour differences (e.g. black ruby barb) or presence of nuptial tubercles on the pectoral fins and opercula are present in males of some species and varieties (e.g. goldfish) but most do not have these features. After approximately 1–2 days, fry emerge from their eggs and are nourished by the yolk sac for several days prior to feeding and reaching the free-swimming stage.

Type 2 egg scatterers (without diapause)

Many species of killifish that do not undergo diapause (a period of arrested development) and rainbowfish are Type 2 egg scatterers. These species have offspring that are mobile soon after hatching and can often take food shortly thereafter. The males are generally much more colourful than their female counterparts and may have more prominent fins. Rainbowfish fry require approximately 1–3 weeks to hatch.

Type 2 egg scatterers (with diapause)

This group includes the majority of the annual killifish (Cyprinodontidae). Because these fish have evolved from life in temporary pools of water, many species are spawned in a peat moss substrate (mimicking evaporating water holes) and generally have accelerated life cycles. Peat containing eggs is collected, the majority of the water is squeezed out and, depending upon the species, stored in plastic containers for 6 weeks to 9 months (the diapause). Later, eggs are placed in water and, typically, fry hatch out within 6 hours.

Bubble-nest builders

The majority of the common members of this group are labyrinth fish and include gouramis, paradise fish and Siamese fighting fish. These fish have an accessory respiratory organ (the labyrinth organ) that allows them to utilize atmospheric oxygen. In general, males have more developed coloration and fins: for example, the dorsal fin in male gouramis is longer and more pointed. Conditioned, gravid females are easily recognized by their swollen abdomen. Males in this group build a bubble nest prior to spawning. After fertilizing the eggs, the males place them in the nest and guard them ferociously, even against the female.

Cichlids

The Cichlidae family includes a large diversity of species, requiring different water quality (e.g. soft acidic 'blackwater' for South American dwarf cichlids

and West African species, discus and angelfish; hard water with high pH and total dissolved solids for Rift Lake cichlids), diet, habitat and social groupings for successful breeding. Cichlid reproductive strategies can be grouped in a number of different ways. Monogamous species (including discus and angelfish) form a temporary pair bond; polygamous species have multiple spawning partners during one reproductive cycle. Some species are substrate spawners, laying eggs on a specific type of substrate, while others are mouth brooders, caring for the developing eggs and fry in their mouths.

Reproductive problems

When faced with a breeding-related problem, it is important to obtain a clinical history, knowledge of the species' requirements and a good understanding of overall management. General problems with broodstock may be due to inappropriate species requirements, poor stock selection or aspects relating to genetics, nutrition, water quality, filtration systems, social grouping, habitat or infectious disease control.

Attention to good husbandry may minimize health problems and is adequate for maintenance, but conditioning of broodstock requires increased vigilance. The fish must be of the correct age and size, their nutritional plane must be increased and water quality needs may differ from those for maintenance. Waterborne toxins, such as heavy metals, may reduce fecundity. Some broodstock will only condition seasonally and may require altered light/dark cycles or water temperatures.

Spawning failure

Once conditioned, spawning failure is often due to a lack of proper stimuli. Young breeders or other fish may cannibalize eggs. In addition, subclinical parasitic or bacterial infections may interfere with spawning.

The most important trigger factors often relate to water quality, but others described earlier may also be required. For example, although neon tetras can be raised in relatively hard water with high pH, they require very soft water of very low conductivity and low pH in order to spawn. Hormone-induced spawning failures may be due to improper administration, the use of incorrect, contaminated or degraded product, stress during handling, incorrectly timed stripping of gametes or immaturity of oocytes and spermatocytes.

Egg binding

The term 'egg binding' is frequently used incorrectly by hobbyists to describe any fish that has an enlarged abdomen. Female fish that are exhibiting typical breeding behaviour and are conditioned correctly but do not express their eggs during a 'normal' period, and subsequently have pathological resorption, could be correctly described as egg bound. In some cases, failure to resorb the eggs results in mortalities that may be associated with the condition but further research is required.

Hatchability

The most common cause of poor hatch rates is improper or poor water quality and includes the presence of nitrogenous wastes, low dissolved oxygen, improper levels of minerals (including sodium and calcium) and the presence of toxins. Hatchability is also affected by lack of movement of eggs (required for certain species), poor sanitation and resulting infectious disease, improperly conditioned broodstock due to a poor diet or immature gametes, and poor sperm quality.

Although various chemicals, including iodine and formalin, are commonly used to combat fungal infections in eggs, some eggs are susceptible to fungal infections because they are infertile. Consequently, infertile spawn will become infected much more easily than fertile spawn.

Larvae and fry

Post-hatch larvae and yolk-sac fry are perhaps the most sensitive life stage. In many species, the yolk sac provides nutrition for the first few days of life. Poor water quality, the presence of pathogens and physical disturbance must be minimized.

Nutritional considerations are one of the most common causes of deformity or poor development, because growth is at a peak in the fry and juvenile stages. When fry begin to feed, live foods are often used for the first few weeks of life. These should be of the right size and type, but fish should be weaned on to more complete artificial diets as soon as possible. If hatching brine shrimp nauplii, egg cases must be removed before feeding to the fish in order to avoid bowel impaction. Other live foods, such as microworms (*Panegrellus* spp.) and daphnia (*Moina* spp.) have been used successfully by producers. However, the potential for introducing disease via live food into the fry system is always a possibility and should be considered in the event of an infectious disease outbreak.

Other contributors to disease in these early stages are poor water quality (including presence of nitrogenous and other toxins), high fry stocking densities and poor diet or subclinical disease in broodstock. Angelfish broodstock with intestinal *Spironucleus* infections tend to have poor hatches and weaker fry. Fry are also much more sensitive to chemical treatments, including the presence of a low level of salt. It has been demonstrated that mortalities in danio and tetra fry cultures increased with the use of sodium chloride (1–3 ppt).

Genetics review

No discussion of heritable diseases would be complete without a brief review of genetics.

- A **gene** can be described as a specific **locus** or region of a chromosome that codes for or contributes to the formation of a certain characteristic or trait, typically through formation of a protein
- **Regulatory genes** determine when and where certain genes will be activated; **structural genes** are those that code for specific proteins
- **Autosomal chromosomes** (those not including the sex chromosomes) are present in homologous pairs and contain large numbers of genes, with one set of each group coming from each parent

- Genes that are located on sex chromosomes are referred to as **sex-linked**. Depending upon the species of fish, the number and type of chromosomes that determine sex may vary
- The genetic make-up of a fish is referred to as its **genotype**. Each gene on each chromosome contributes to this 'genetic blueprint'
- Many genes have more than one form or **allele**. Depending upon the form contributed by each parent, a fish may have two of the same allele or two different alleles. The resultant interaction of the two alleles, whether they are the same or different, is referred to as the **phenotype** (i.e. the actual physical manifestation of these genes).

Genetic characteristics

Characteristics can be split into two major groups: qualitative and quantitative.

- Qualitative traits can usually be divided into non-overlapping categories and include colour or scale pattern
- Quantitative traits are continuous and not as easily categorized; they include weight, length and growth rate.

Qualitative inheritance

Simple qualitative traits or phenotypes are usually the result of the interactions of one or two sets of genes and may express themselves as **dominant** (complete or incomplete), **recessive** or **additive**.

- Dominant genes manifest themselves more strongly than their recessive counterparts
- Incomplete dominance results in greater expression of the dominant gene in the heterozygous (one dominant gene, one recessive gene present) state than the recessive gene, but not complete dominance. The recessive gene is expressed to a lesser degree
- In additive gene action, each allele contributes equally to the phenotype
- **Epistasis** is the ability of one gene to suppress or change the qualitative phenotype produced by a second gene.

An example of incomplete dominance is seen in the colour of Mozambique tilapia. Genotype *GG*– exhibits a black phenotype; *Gg*– exhibits a bronze phenotype; and *gg*– exhibits a gold phenotype. Because the gene exhibits incomplete dominance, *Gg* phenotypes are not black.

Quantitative inheritance

Quantitative traits are genetically more complex and are often the result of three or more different interacting loci. Factors contributing to phenotypic variation include effects of genetic variance, differences in environmental factors and the interactions between genetic variance and environment.

- **Additive genetic variance**: the sum total effect of all an individual's alleles on its phenotype
- **Dominance genetic variance**: the interaction at each locus between pairs of genes (cannot be inherited)

- **Epistatic genetic variance**: the interaction between non-homologous alleles (effect of one set of genes on another).

Heritability is the proportion of a quantitative phenotype contributed by the additive genetic variance. This factor is important for selective breeding programmes based on quantitative phenotypes. Environmental factors including nutrition must be controlled in order for true heritability to be determined.

Environmental effects on phenotype

Environmental conditions can alter phenotype (Norton, 1992). For example, silver and black lace strains of freshwater angelfish raised in continuous light fail to develop stripes. Other strains of angelfish will develop different patterns and coloration depending upon whether or not they have been provided with continuous, or 14 hours or 4 hours of light.

Nutrition can also affect phenotype. Genetic half-black angelfish can look like silver angelfish if they have not been provided with adequate amounts of food.

Substrate can influence coloration. Swordtails raised in tanks with dark bottoms will develop deeper red coloration than those raised in tanks with light-coloured bottoms.

Genetics and disease

Genetic diseases are not as well studied as diseases with environmental or infectious aetiologies. Ferguson and Danzmann (1998) reviewed genetic disorders at great length and Tave (1995) discussed genetics and selective breeding programmes from a production standpoint.

Genetic disease is a relative term. Some heritable traits may be favoured by some consumers but the same traits may be considered abhorrent or unacceptable by others. One example in ornamental fish is the Southeast Asian variant, the balloon molly. These fish are shorter, stouter and much deeper bodied dorsoventrally than their wild-type ancestors. Though not true breeding, the balloon molly trait is heritable to a degree.

Because inbreeding causes increases in percentage of homozygous recessive traits, highly inbred variants of ornamental fish often demonstrate reductions in fecundity, fry survival, growth rate and/or overall health.

While many recessive deleterious genes probably exist in low frequencies in natural populations, spontaneous gene mutations can occur at either regulatory or structural gene loci. Gene mutations that adversely alter early developmental processes can result in early embryonic, larval or fry mortalities. This can manifest as poor hatchability or reduced fry survival. Mutations that alter later processes can result in 'weaker' older fish. Different chemicals have been shown to be teratogenic (e.g. malachite green) in some animals and may also affect fish.

It is important to rule out other aetiologies before suggesting a genetic origin. Some traits, especially gross deformities, are often not genetically determined but are caused by nutritional, infectious, toxin or other environmental factors. If a specific mutation or deformity is believed to be inherited and of significant concern, appropriate progeny testing should be carried out to rule out a simple Mendelian inheritance. Progeny testing is the method of choice for determining the genotype of an individual fish through analysis of specific traits of offspring resulting from planned crosses.

It is important to appreciate that some undesirable traits may have specific environmental triggers. For example, the lack of a specific micro- or macronutrient may act as a trigger and so the appearance of that trait may be prevented by providing adequate nutrition.

Genetics of fancy goldfish

Over the centuries, the Chinese have modified the wild-type *Carassius auratus* into numerous fancy variations of goldfish such as the fantail, pearl scale, bubble-eye and oranda. Smartt and Bundell (1996) provided a good introduction to goldfish genetics and breeding and highlighted areas where knowledge is still lacking. While some of the genetics of these variants have been worked out, overall goldfish breeding still requires a significant amount of culling even in strains that breed true. This is one reason why these morphs are called varieties and not breeds.

Certain variations, such as long fins, are best produced by crossing one fish with the desired trait with a different variety of fish. Environmental conditions for the growth and development of juvenile fish also have a significant effect on phenotypes, such as body shape and head growth. Further complicating genetics in both goldfish and koi is the fact that they exhibit polyploidy (i.e. have roughly twice the normal number of chromosomes and genes).

Telescope eyes is a recessive trait in domesticated goldfish (Matsui and Axelrod, 1991). However, when fish with telescope eyes are crossed with the goldfish predecessor, Crucian carp, to form the F_1 generation, the presence of another suppressor gene that inhibits telescope eyes skews the ratio of normal eyes to telescope eyes 15:1 in the resulting $F_1 \times F_1$, (F_2).

Tail fin inheritance also appears to have some logic (Matsui and Axelrod, 1991). A long-tailed variety crossed with a short-tailed variety will have offspring with tails of intermediate length (F_1). $F_1 \times F_1$ results in tails of short, long and intermediate length in the offspring. However, besides length, fin quality is important and so attention to detail and quality in the broodstock is paramount.

Depending upon the specific trait desired, efficient culling may occur within a few weeks of hatching. The presence of single, twin or tri-tails can be determined with the use of a microscope. Other features, such as scale type, colour in metallic varieties and globe-eye characteristics, can be selected after 3–6 months. Still other traits, such as head growth in orandas and lionheads and narial bouquets (fleshy protuberances on the nostrils) in pompons, may require as much as a year or more prior to selection. Final colour selection in certain varieties may require 2 years.

Pattern inheritance is not yet well understood. Colour development and inheritance are complex and readers are referred to Smartt and Bundell (1996) for a more detailed discussion of colour in goldfish. Briefly, major genetic determinants of colour in goldfish include:

- Presence/absence of melanin and variation in chemical composition of melanin
- Presence/absence of xanthine and variation in chemical composition of xanthine
- Surface distribution of pigment
- Vertical distribution of pigment (located in dermis, adipose tissue or other layers).

Scale transparency (caused by presence of guanine) will also determine overall appearance. Fish with normal amounts of guanine have metallic-looking scales, while those without guanine have transparent scales. Neither type of scale appears to be genetically dominant.

In addition to genetic determinants, nutritional and environmental components are important, as evidenced by the effectiveness of carotenoids and other colour-enhancing feed additives. Development of colour in goldfish also depends upon the time of action of a demelanization mutant gene. Juvenile fish typically produce more melanin early in life, with loss of melanin during subsequent growth. This timing may be delayed, with fish losing melanin production much later in life.

While many of these variants are considered attractive to some consumers, to others they are merely more diseased variants, prone to specific ailments such as buoyancy control problems because of their sanctioned deformities. Some of these buoyancy disorders appear to be caused by the resultant physical features of these fancy varieties. For example, a more rounded body shape combined with a deformed swimbladder that is more centralized within the body of the fish will displace the fish's centre of gravity. In some of the varieties examined radiographically, the swimbladder lacked the typical prominent posterior chamber usually found in cyprinids.

Scale pattern in koi

Scale pattern in common carp is a good example of inheritance with both positive and negative repercussions on variety and fecundity, respectively. Scale pattern inheritance is determined by epistatic interaction between two genes, *S* and *N* (Tave 1995). The four major scale patterns are:

- *SSnn* or *Ssnn*: wild-type scaled pattern with scales over the entire body
- *SSNn* or *SsNn*: line pattern, with scales along the dorsal, mid-body and ventral aspect
- *ssnn*: mirror or doitsu type; some scales are highly metallic and reflective, while others have a missing reflective layer
- *ssNn*: leather type, with scales that are greatly reduced in size and koi appear to be scaleless

Matings resulting in *NN* genotypes affect overall fecundity, since *SSNN*, *SsNN* or *ssNN* genotypes result in early death.

Black angelfish

Norton (1992) gave an excellent overview of genetics of several ornamental fish species, including *Xiphophorus* spp. and freshwater angelfish. One example discussed is the inheritance of black lace pattern and black coloration in angelfish involving the dark gene (*D*) and the wild-type pattern/colour (ı). The gene for dark demonstrates incomplete dominance. *DD* angelfish are black, *D*+ angelfish are black lace (like wild type, but somewhat darker) and ++ angelfish are wild-type silver. However, because *DD* angelfish have a higher mortality rate, the actual number of black angelfish produced from this type of cross will be less.

Spontaneous melanomas in *Xiphophorus* hybrids

Spontaneous melanoma formation has been studied by researchers for decades in the Xiphophorine spotted dorsal Gordon–Kosswig platy–swordtail model. Although these hybrids are not commonly observed in the hobby, the model is famous enough to warrant a brief explanation of the genetics involved.

The model was developed using an inbred (*Sd/Sd*; *Diff/Diff*) strain of female platy with: (i) a sex-linked receptor tyrosine kinase gene (*Xmrk*) that is associated with the spotted dorsal gene (*Sd*); and (ii) the autosomal regulatory gene (*Diff*) that regulates macromelanophore pigment cell differentiation and acts as a tumour suppressor (Figure 29.1a). The loss of species-specific alleles in pigmented backcross hybrids causes tumour formation. The notation '–' signifies absence of the particular gene in question.

The F_1 female hybrids (*Sd/-*; *Diff/-*) have an extended pigmented dorsal pattern. Crossing these with a male swordtail (-/-; -/-) (no spotted dorsal pattern; Figure 29.1a) produces the genotypes shown in Figure 29.1b.

FEMALE platy (*Xiphophorus maculatus*) *Sd/Sd*; *Diff/Diff* (spotted dorsal pattern)	**MALE swordtail** (*Xiphophorus helleri*) –/–; –/– (no spotted dorsal pattern)

(a)

–/–; *Diff/-* (no pattern)	*Sd/–*; *Diff/–* (benign melanoma)
–/–; –/– (no pattern)	*Sd/–*; –/– (malignant melanoma)

(b)

Figure 29.1 Genetics of the xiphophorine spotted dorsal Gordon–Kosswig platy–swordtail model. (a) Genotypes of inbred strain of female platy and male swordtail. (b) Genotypes produced by crossing F_1 female hybrids with male swordtail.

Saddleback in tilapia

The saddleback syndrome of tilapia is a disease controlled by a single autosomal gene with incomplete dominant gene action (Tave, 1995).

- The homozygous dominant genotype *SS* results in death

- The heterozygous genotype *Ss* results in an abnormal dorsal fin in affected fish (saddleback)
- The recessive genotype *ss* results in a normal phenotype.

Preventing inbreeding depression

Inbreeding in fish can result in the increased frequency of deleterious genes, especially with small populations and minimal genetic diversity. A minimum breeding population of 25 males and 25 females is recommended to reduce inbreeding depression (Tave, 1995). Thus, approximately 100–200 fish should be maintained to help to optimize genetic diversity. If a higher than natural incidence of a particular deleterious gene or set of genes is present in this population, increased genetic diversity is recommended by introducing additional fish and increasing numbers. Close attention to the selection of broodstock and resulting progeny will assist the breeder in maintaining high quality, healthy stock.

References and further reading

Ferguson MM and Danzmann RG (1998) Genetic Disorders. In: *Fish Diseases and Disorders*, Vol. 2, *Non-Infectious Disorders* (ed. JF Leatherland and PTK Woo) pp. 19–36. CAB International Publishing, Wallingford

Loiselle PV (1992) Breeding aquarium fish. In: *Aquariology: The Science of Fish Health Management* (ed. J Gratzek and JR Matthews) pp. 135–156. Tetra Press, Morris Plains, New Jersey

Matsui Y and Axelrod HR (1991) *Goldfish Guide*, 3rd edn. TFH Publications Inc., Neptune City, New Jersey

Nairn RS, Kazianis S, McEntire BB, Coletta LD, Walter RB and Morizot DC (1996) A CDKN2-like polymorphism in *Xiphophorus* LG V is associated with UV-B-induced melanoma formation in platyfish–swordtail hybrids. *Proceedings of the National Academy of Science* **93**, 13042–13047

Norton J (1992) Fish genetics. In: *Aquariology: The Science of Fish Health Management* (ed. J Gratzek and JR Matthews) pp. 95–134. Tetra Press, Morris Plains, New Jersey

Smartt J and Bundell JH (1996) *Goldfish Breeding and Genetics*. TFH Publications Inc., Neptune City, New Jersey, 256 pp.

Tave D (1995) *Selective Breeding Programmes for Medium-Sized Fish Farms*. FAO Fisheries Technical Paper 352. Food and Agriculture Organization of the United Nations, Rome, 122 pp.

Yanong RPE (1996) Reproductive management of freshwater ornamental fish. In: *Seminars in Avian and Exotic Pet Medicine* **5**, 222–235 (October). WB Saunders Co., Philadelphia

30

Therapeutics

William H. Wildgoose and Gregory A. Lewbart

The aim of therapy is to treat the patient. This involves not only curing the fish and removing the pathogens but also eliminating the predisposing stress factors. Occasionally the morbidity, mortality or the extent of a disease may preclude the need for treatment and in those cases the welfare of the fish must be considered. Experience is often the only means by which to judge situations where fish should be humanely killed. However, many cases can be treated successfully without much effort.

With fish disease, one problem often results in a multitude of secondary infections and it is quite common to identify several separate infections or environmental factors that have contributed to the disease problem. As a result, all factors must be treated and it is therefore essential to prioritize these to achieve both short-term and long-term improvement:

- Where possible, establish a diagnosis
- An environmental crisis will require moving fish to uncontaminated water or performing substantial frequent water changes
- The treatment of infectious diseases is less urgent but protozoan infections such as 'white spot' and *Ichthyobodo* can be severe and must be treated immediately
- Bacterial, fungal and other parasitic infections are less acute problems
- Non-infectious lesions such as skin tumours can be removed if necessary, but many may be left untreated without compromising the health of the fish.

Hobbyists frequently attempt treatment themselves using a variety of proprietary medicines available without prescription. They may also have access to some prescription-only drugs that were obtained illegally. The misuse of antibacterial drugs has been shown to increase the incidence of resistant strains of pathogenic bacteria in fish (Trust and Whitby, 1976; Dixon and Issvoran, 1992). Owners will often use a variety of medications before requesting veterinary assistance and cases that fail to respond may finally be presented for investigation. In some cases, over-use or unsuitable combinations of these medications are responsible for aggravating health problems. These cases can prove challenging but many can be resolved successfully by following a logical approach.

Although many treatment regimens have been derived from the food fish industry, there are significant differences in the approach to the treatment of farmed fish and ornamental fish in a pond or public aquarium (Figure 30.1). The economics of treating farmed fish is an important factor, whereas the emotional value of pet fish often permits treatment far in excess of their financial value. As a result, many ornamental fish are treated on an individual basis and by injection. Apart from the treatment of broodstock, the large numbers of fish on farms are usually treated by in-feed medication. In addition, many farmed fish live in water that is constantly being refreshed (from a river, or the surrounding sea) while pet fish live in an enclosed body of water that is either static or being recirculated. This has great significance when using waterborne treatments, since ornamental fish remain exposed to the chemicals for much longer or until the chemical becomes inactive. Therefore, depending on circumstances, it is best to provide 'first aid' to pet fish by improving the environment before using specific medications.

	Ornamental fish	Farmed fish
Age	All ages (often 'old')	Young (< 3 years old)
Diet	Variable	Specific, formulated
Species	Often mixed	All same species
Size	Variable	Uniform for age

Figure 30.1 Differences between ornamental and farmed fish.

Environmental improvement

In general, improving the environment and management will help to avoid many fish health problems. When fish are ill, environmental improvement is the first priority, often speeding recovery and even avoiding the need for medication. Fish can recover from illness without medication if their environmental conditions are good. Practical methods of improving the environment include the following.

- Maintain stable water conditions – increase aeration and avoid water changes that are greater than 50% per day
- Instal a biological filter and improve its function by cleaning out detritus regularly

- Remove stressors – reduce stocking levels where possible, avoid handling and remove aggressive or predatory fish
- Avoid the use of unnecessary prophylactic medications
- Perform regular water changes in aquaria – change 20% every 2 weeks.

First aid advice

Some clients may be unwilling or unable to bring fish to a clinic or afford visit fees. In these cases simple telephone advice will be required and this may include some of the following.

- Test water quality, particularly ammonia, nitrite, nitrate and pH. These should be within acceptable limits for the type and species kept (see Chapters 5, 6 and 7)
- Change 30% of the tank or pond water in order to dilute poor environmental conditions (draining down the water level by the required amount before refilling is more effective than letting water trickle in and allowing the excess to drain out through the overflow)
- Add salt at the rate of 2 g/l water to reduce physiological stress in freshwater fish. This is particularly valuable if osmoregulation is compromised from skin ulceration or gill disease
- To avoid further waste excretion, stop feeding until a cause has been established. This will also improve acceptability of medicated foods
- Improve aeration with a venturi, air-stones, fountains or waterfall
- Do not add medications indiscriminately since they may cause further stress or reduce dissolved oxygen content: use activated carbon or charcoal to remove medications.

Specific medication

Despite improving water conditions, it is often necessary to use therapeutic agents to improve the health of the fish. Particular diseases, such as infection with ectoparasites and bacteria, require specific compounds to eliminate the pathogen. Prior to their use, the practical aspects, route of administration, and the choice of drug need to be considered.

Practical considerations

The pathogen

'In-contacts': Many fish pathogens are infectious or potentially infectious, therefore all in-contact fish should be treated *en masse*.

Difficulty of treatment: Not all bacteria can be treated easily (e.g. mycobacteria) and some ectoparasites (e.g. fish lice, anchor worms, leeches) are only susceptible to organophosphates or similar compounds.

Drug resistance: Bacterial resistance to antibacterial drugs is now an important factor. Culture and antibacterial drug sensitivity tests may take up to 2 weeks to complete but it is often essential to start treatment as soon as possible in order to limit the progress of an infection. Some ectoparasites (e.g. fish lice) are also thought to show resistance to organophosphate compounds.

Life cycle of parasites: Some parasites (e.g. fish lice) lay eggs in the environment, and some adults may have free-swimming periods off the fish. Therefore, treatment with medicated dips alone will not eliminate the parasite and the whole environment must be treated. Similarly, only the free-swimming stage of the 'white spot' parasite is susceptible to treatment and therefore repeated treatment is required.

The patient

Body size: Small fish and fry may be too small to inject safely. In-water or in-feed treatment should be used.

Severe illness: Some fish may be too ill to inject or handle without causing serious stress. In-water treatment may be more appropriate.

Anorexia: Anorerxia and unpalatable drugs (e.g. nitrofurans) may limit the use of in-feed medications.

Shoaling behaviour: Some fish, particularly in isolation facilities, recover more quickly in the presence of other fish, even if they are of different species.

The environment

Filters: Bacterial filtration systems may be adversely affected, particularly where in-water treatments are used. This is an important factor, since high stocking densities are very dependent on good, stable water quality.

Discharge consents: If substantial quantities of chemicals are used, a discharge consent may be required by the local water authority or environment protection agency, particularly if discharge is to a natural waterway with food-fish farms downstream.

Pond size: Some ponds or facilities may be too large to enable capture of the fish without draining or using a seine-net. Large ponds or natural lakes can make it difficult to treat and achieve an even distribution of medication throughout the water.

Organic matter: Inactivation of the drug by organic matter in the environment can reduce the efficacy of some in-water medications (e.g. potassium permanganate).

Non-target organisms: Harmful effects on non-target organisms (e.g. copepods) in natural waters may affect the availability of food items for raising fry.

Routes of administration

Aim to treat the fish, not the water. Use the least stressful method of treatment to achieve effective therapeutic levels of medication. Administration methods include:

- In-water
- In-feed
- Gavage
- Injection
- Topical application.

In-water medication

This route is most suitable for the treatment of external parasite and fungal infections, though some chemicals may be absorbed through the skin, gills or bowel (by 'drinking'). Bacterial filtration systems will be damaged by some drugs (e.g. antibacterial drugs) unless treatment is carried out in an isolation facility with careful monitoring of water quality. Ozone and ultraviolet systems should be switched off and activated carbon removed before in-water administration, since they may reduce the efficacy of the medication.

In-water medication may involve short timed dips in strong chemical solutions or a permanent bath involving low-dose medication of the tank or pond.

Antibacterial drugs

In-water administration of antibacterial drugs is problematic, since some drugs (e.g. oxytetracycline, quinolones) are chelated by hard water and drug uptake is uncertain. However, this may be the most practical method of treating fry and very small fish and sometimes appears to be effective. Although most carrier compounds are inert, their effect on fish is often unknown and therefore only pure drugs (100% active ingredient) should be used, if available. Some chemicals alter the pH of the water when in solution and this may affect their uptake. To minimize the development of drug-resistant strains of bacteria, treatment using antibacterial drugs by in-water medication should be restricted to high-strength short dips.

Short dips

Short dips are stressful, since they involve netting fish and holding them in a small facility with a strong concentration of chemical, often with poor water quality. To minimize stress due to changes in water chemistry, water used for the dip treatment should be taken from the aquarium or pond of origin. Antibacterial dips also obviate any harmful effect on the biological filter. Some concentrated dips (e.g. organophosphates) may be harmful to the operator.

Permanent baths

Permanent baths are less stressful to the fish but the effects of long-term exposure to some chemicals are unknown. Many fish keepers do not know the exact volume of their own ponds and in such cases miscalculation and overdosing can cause problems, requiring large volumes of water to be changed immediately. Where possible, baths should be filled

using an accurate water meter (Figure 30.2), since it is the total volume of water (in the pond and filter) that must be treated, not just the water in the pond. Formulae for calculating the size of tanks and ponds are given in Figure 30.3. The cost of in-water treatment of large volumes of water may be prohibitive.

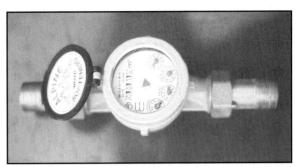

Figure 30.2 A water meter is useful for measuring the total volume of water in large ponds and filtration systems. When performing partial water changes and to maintain the salinity at the same level, the correct amount of salt can be added according to the volume changed.

(a) Rectangular shape
Volume = length × breadth × depth

(b) Circular shape
Volume = 3.14 × radius² × depth

(c) Irregular shape
The volume of irregular shaped ponds can be estimated by using pegs and twine to map out a grid of 1 m squares and measuring the depth of each square. By averaging the partial squares at the edge of the pond and totalling the volumes it is possible to calculate an approximate water volume.

NB: The volume of water in external filters must also be included but allowance must be made for space-occupying media.

Figure 30.3 Calculating the volume of tanks and ponds (1 cubic metre = 1,000 litres).

Absorption, timing and weather

- The rate at which different drugs are absorbed is often unknown. As a general rule, non-polar compounds cross biological membranes faster than polar compounds
- Medications should be added early in the day so that fish can be observed during the following 6 hours for any sign of adverse reaction
- In outdoor ponds, avoid using chloramine-T in sunny weather since chemical breakdown is faster. Avoid using products containing formalin in hot weather since the chemical reduces dissolved oxygen levels.

Distribution

Chemicals should be distributed evenly. In small ponds, the diluted chemical can be applied evenly across the surface by using a watering-can with a rose sprinkler. This can be difficult to achieve in large ponds or lakes, where a boat with an outboard motor can be used to disperse the chemical throughout the water column. The chemical is slowly added to the water behind the propeller as the boat makes several traverses across the pond. Alternatively, large air-stones can be used to create water currents, with chemicals being added slowly to the water over a period. Air-stones and bubble diffusers create an upward flow of water in static ponds, resulting in the movement of large volumes of water.

In-feed medication

Oral medication is the least stressful method of treatment and can be very effective if the fish are still eating. Several antibacterial drugs and a few anthelmintics are administered by this route. Small quantities of pure antibacterial drugs suitable for mixing with fish food can be ordered from specialist wholesalers (e.g. Alpharma Animal Health Ltd in the UK).

Some fish are fastidious eaters and may prove difficult to treat orally due to the poor palatability of some drugs. Withholding food for 24 hours prior to oral medication or feeding a small amount of unmedicated food will stimulate a feeding frenzy among others and improve acceptance of the medicated diet.

Calculating the inclusion rate accurately for an oral medication should be based on either the total bodyweight or the daily food intake (Figure 30.4). Where the total bodyweight is not known, it is best to make up a standard concentration feed mixture with a set amount of drug added, assuming a 1% feeding rate. This should be fed daily, *ad libitum*, removing any food that is uneaten after 5 minutes. It is often easier to make up the whole course of medicated food at the beginning and keep the prepared food in a sealed container in the refrigerator.

Dose rate

This is normally expressed in milligrams per kilogram of bodyweight per day. It is important to check the percentage content of the drug, since the dosage given usually relates to the amount of active ingredient (AI) required. This must be calculated for. Due to the high percentage content, the quantities of drug involved will be small and scientific scales may be required in order to measure the dose accurately. In some cases, the supplier may be able to provide measuring spoons (e.g. 2.5 ml or 5 ml) with approximate weight equivalents for the drug. Note that not all powders have the same weight per unit volume.

Bodyweight

Without weighing each fish individually, the total bodyweight is rarely known. It is occasionally possible to estimate weight from charts relating weight to length (as in Chapter 5), but in most cases an approximation is made by visual assessment.

> **TIP:** Fish bodyweight can be deceptive. In order to gain experience in estimating bodyweight, it is advisable to weigh routinely all fish that are anaesthetized for examination, sampling and treatment.

Feeding rate

Although this will vary according to water temperature as in outdoor ponds, feeding rates of 0.5% to 1.0% can be used as a guideline. In many cases, the owner will know how much food will be eaten over any treatment period.

Calculation based on known bodyweight

1. The daily dose rate (D)
   = D mg of active ingredient per kg bodyweight per day
2. Calculate the dose of commercial product according to the percentage of active ingredient (AI)
   = D mg ÷ AI% = X mg product/kg bodyweight/day
3. Calculate the amount of commercial product required for the known bodyweight (BW)
   = X mg × BW kg = Y mg product/day
4. Calculate the total amount required for the number of days (N) of treatment
   = Y mg × N days = Z mg product
5. The total amount of commercial product is mixed with the total amount of food to be fed (usually 1% bodyweight/day) during the treatment period

Example: to treat 10 kg fish with Aquatrim®*
40% (sulphadiazine + trimethoprim) for 10 days

1. see Figure 30.8
   = 30 mg/kg bodyweight/day
2. 30 mg ÷ AI%
   = 30 mg ÷ 40%
   = 75 mg Aquatrim®
3. 75 mg × BW (kg)
   = 75 mg x 10 kg
   = 750 mg Aquatrim®/day
4. 750 x N days
   = 7500 mg Aquatrim®
   = 7.5 grams Aquatrim®
5. 7.5 grams mixed with 1% x bodyweight (kg) x N days of food
   = 7.5 grams mixed with 1% × 10 kg × 10 days of food
   = 7.5 grams mixed with 1 kg of food

* Aquatrim® (Alpharma Animal Health Ltd, UK)

Calculation based on food intake

1. The daily dose rate (D)
   = D mg of active ingredient per kg bodyweight per day
2. Calculate the dose of commercial product according to the percentage of active ingredient (AI)
   = D mg ÷ AI% = X mg product/kg bodyweight/day
3. Calculate the amount of active ingredient required per kg of food to be fed at 1% of bodyweight per day
   = X mg ÷ 1% = Y mg product/kg food

Example: to prepare a medicated feed with Aquatrim® 40% (sulphadiazine + trimethoprim) for feeding at 1% bodyweight per day

1. see Figure 30.8
   = 30 mg/kg bodyweight/day
2. 30 mg ÷ AI%
   = 30 mg ÷ 40%
   = 75 mg/kg bodyweight/day
3. 75 mg ÷ 1% feed rate per day
   = 7500 mg
   = 7.5 grams Aquatrim®/kg food

Figure 30.4 Calculation of rates for oral medication.

Interval

Licensed products always stipulate the treatment interval. However, due to the nature of disease in ornamental fish and the management of their health problems, it is often necessary to extend the duration of medication. All oral preparations should be fed daily for 10–14 days but this may need to be extended to 21 days in some cases.

Methods of in-feed medication

Pre-medicated feed: Commercial fish flake or pellet food medicated with antibacterial drugs can be manufactured by some feed companies. In the UK, a few products can be incorporated into fish food by Sinclair Animal & Household Care Ltd. on receipt of a medicated feedingstuffs (MFS) prescription and are fed at the rate of 1% bodyweight per day. These medicated pellets are a sinking variety, since the heating process used to manufacture a floating pellet would degrade the antibacterial drug. Consequently, some fish may take a few days to accept this type of pellet. In the USA, similar products are available from Zeigler Brothers Inc.

Surface-coating of pellet food: The oral drug is thoroughly mixed with a small volume of vegetable oil (2–3% per volume of pellets). This slurry is then used to coat the foodstuff by thorough mixing. Alternatively, the drug can be mixed with the dry pellets then oil added as a binding agent. Fish oil is occasionally used to surface-coat food and increase palatability for salmonids but the bioavailability has been shown to be less with fish oil than with vegetable oil.

Gelatin-treated food: A solution is prepared using 5 g of gelatin dissolved in 500 ml of boiling water and allowed to cool to room temperature. The required amount of drug is mixed into an appropriate volume of the gelatin solution (about 2–3% volume of food), then applied to the food and allowed to set. If pellet food is used, the pellets should be gently coated with the mixture to avoid disintegration.

Flake food is mixed into the gelatin solution to form a thick slurry that is allowed to set in a block before being cut into pieces of appropriate size for daily feeding. However, it has been shown that gelatin-treated feed is less palatable to some species than oil-treated feed.

Soaking pellet food: Water-soluble drugs are dissolved in a small volume of water and mixed into food pellets. These are then allowed to dry in air or in a warm oven. Unless the food is eaten quickly, the drug will leach out into the water.

Ice-cube method: A slurry is made by mixing food with the required quantity of drug and a small amount of water. The mixture is frozen in an ice-cube tray and an appropriate number of cubes are given to the fish per day.

Medicated food items: Large food items can be injected with the required daily dose of medication before being fed to individual fish. Small live foods such as brine shrimp larvae and bloodworms can be bathed in solutions of antibiotics for up to several hours before being rinsed in clean water and fed immediately to the fish. Some drugs may be toxic to these invertebrates at high dose rates.

Gavage

This involves stomach-tubing the fish and force-feeding using a syringe with a soft plastic or metal tube attached (Figure 30.5). A suspension containing a known amount of an oral formulation (e.g. crushed tablets) is then administered into the stomach or gastro-intestinal tract. This method can be used to administer unpalatable drugs (e.g. nitrofurans, erythromycin) to small numbers of fish but the procedure is stressful to conscious fish and sedated patients can regurgitate the medication, which may then damage the delicate gill tissues. The pharyngeal teeth in some species (e.g. carp) can make this method of treatment impractical or difficult to perform. In addition, there is a risk of perforating the oesophagus when metal tubes are used.

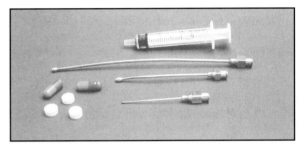

Figure 30.5 Metal tubes for attachment to a syringe and administering medicine by gavage. Rubber and plastic catheters may also be used.

Injection

This route enables a precise dose of drug to be given and is very useful if fish are anorexic. Antibacterials are more effectively and commonly given by injection. Sites for injection (Figure 30.6) vary according to personal preference.

Intramuscular: Intramuscular injections are often given into the flank above the lateral line and lateral to the dorsal fin. Some practitioners prefer to inject into the midline, between the muscle fillets just anterior or posterior to the dorsal fin.

Intraperitoneal: Intraperitoneal (or intracoelomic) injections are preferred in some species and are given into the ventral midline between the vent and pelvic fins, using a short needle or butterfly catheter. It is recommended that the fish be starved for 24 hours prior to injection to reduce the risk of puncturing an organ.

This route may be hazardous in koi and other carp, due to the extensive peritoneal adhesions normally found in these fish. This could result in drugs being injected into a solid organ (e.g. liver or spleen) or into the bowel and then expelled through the vent without being absorbed.

Injection procedures

- Preparation of the injection site is rarely necessary. The use of skin disinfectants may remove much of the protective cuticle and cause damage to the underlying epidermis: alcohol is particularly harmful

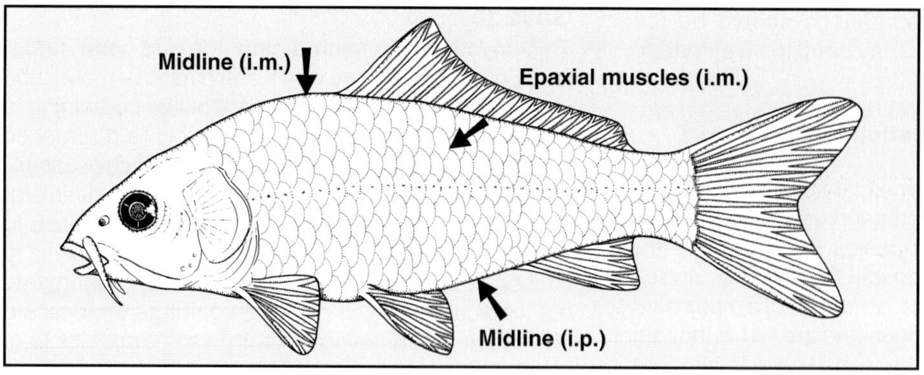

Figure 30.6 Commonly used sites for intramuscular (i.m.) and intraperitoneal (i.p.) injections in ornamental fish.

- The needle should be carefully angled at about 45 degrees between the scales so as not to damage or remove them when injecting
- It is often difficult to assess bodyweight and it may be necessary to sedate the fish with an anaesthetic agent and weigh it out of the water in order to calculate the correct dose.

TIP: In large fish, use long needles (0.7 × 40 mm) for intramuscular injections. This reduces the risk of the drug being expressed through the injection hole by the fish. In these cases, the use of colourless injectable drugs reduces the risk of professional embarrassment.

Topical preparations

These are often applied after debridement of skin wounds under general anaesthesia. They include skin disinfectants, such as povidone–iodine, and topical antibacterial drugs. Adhesion and retention of the medication at the site often requires the use of a waterproofing compound (e.g. Orabase® or Orahesive®, ConvaTec) before returning fish to the water.

Tincture of iodine and oxytetracycline aerosols have been used by hobbyists but are not recommended, due to their harmful effects on the epidermis.

Mercurochrome is the trade name for products containing the red dye, merbromin. This old-fashioned antiseptic was used for topical treatment of skin lesions but it is rarely used now due to its mercury content and concerns about its absorption through the skin.

Friars' balsam is a volatile liquid of natural plant extracts and is commonly used as an inhalant in humans. It has mild antiseptic properties when applied topically, as it has been in the course of treatment of skin ulcers.

Choice of drug

Several factors determine the final choice of the drug used to treat fish. The first consideration is that it should be effective against the microorganism or disease process. The health status of the fish may require the use of a less effective but safer compound in situations where the stress involved in treatment may be unacceptable.

The antibiotic sensitivity of a bacterial infection may require one drug rather than another to be used. As an example, bacteria that cause body ulcers in koi are commonly resistant to oxolinic acid and oxytetracycline.

There are no known effective treatments for some diseases, such as those due to microsporidia, mycobacterial and viral infection.

A variety of commonly used therapeutic agents are listed in Figures 30.7 to 30.10, and should enable an appropriate choice to be made. Despite the diversity of medications, only a few products are licensed for use in fish by the relevant authorities in the UK and USA, and these are listed in Figure 30.11.

The few drugs licensed for use in fish have strict dosages and withdrawal times in food-fish for consumer safety. The dosages for ornamental fish are usually empirical and are often derived from studies on food-fish. Therefore, when using unfamiliar drugs in uncommon species, it is essential to test the product on one or a few fish to avoid potential adverse effects due to unusual water conditions and species susceptibility.

Many commercial products are available to the hobbyist over the counter and without a prescription. In the case of external fungal and parasitic infection, and unless financial restrictions apply, it is often best to use a commercial product first rather than mix one's own preparation, so that an appropriate dosage is applied in what may be a very small volume of water. These products are often tried and tested from years of use in the hobby and most are based on standard ingredients such as formalin and dyes. Many are available in easy-dose bottles with measuring reservoir heads, which reduces the risk of accidental overdosing. The manufacturer will often have information about the effects on many different species and is usually responsible for the quality, safety and efficacy of the product.

Not all non-prescription products are effective, particularly against systemic bacterial disease. Equally, some manufacturers make unrealistic claims (e.g. 'will treat dropsy and virus infections'). Others are reluctant to divulge information on the active ingredients, even though this is routine for ethical drug companies. Proprietary products available without prescription are listed in Figures 30.12 and 30.13.

Individual facilities and environmental circumstances make it impossible to guarantee the safe use of any chemical. While every effort has been made to ensure that the information given here is accurate, no liability can be accepted for fish loss associated with the use of products and dosages listed. The details are presented for information only and do not constitute a claim of safety or efficacy.

Agent	Dosage and route	Interval	Parasite	Comments	Warnings
Acetic acid, glacial	2 ml/l × 30–40 s bath		Trematode, crustacean ectoparasites	Safe for goldfish	May be toxic to small tropical fish
Chloramine-T	Prolonged bath 	pH	Soft water	Hard water
---	---	---
6.0	2.5 mg/l	7.0 mg/l
6.5	5.0 mg/l	10.0 mg/l
7.0	10.0 mg/l	15.0 mg/l
7.5	18.0 mg/l	18.0 mg/l
8.0	20.0 mg/l	20.0 mg/l		Repeat after 48 h if necessary	Protozoal and some monogenean infections		Avoid contact with metal Avoid use in bright sunlight More toxic in soft water and low pH
Chloroquine diphosphate	10 mg/l permanent bath × 1	Monitor for 21 days, repeat as required	*Amyloodinium*	Removed by activated carbon	
Copper sulphate	100 mg/l × 1–5 min bath Maintain free copper ion levels at 0.15–0.2 mg/l as permanent bath until therapeutic effect (use 3 g copper sulphate, 2 g citric acid in 750 ml for stock solution of 1 mg/ml)	Copper levels must be measured daily using standard test kits and maintained by adding stock solutions or performing water changes	Marine fish ectoparasites		Very toxic to invertebrates, elasmobranchs and many plants
Diflubenzuron (Dimilin®)	0.01 mg/l permanent bath	6 days × 3 treatments	Crustacean ectoparasites	Inhibits chitin synthesis Sold to control terrestrial insects	Drug persists in environment
Fenbendazole	2 mg/l permanent bath 50 mg/kg orally, in feed	7 days × 3 treatments 24 h × 2 days, repeat in 14 days	Non-encysted intestinal nematodes		
Formalin	All doses based on full strength formalin (= 37% formaldehyde) 0.125–0.25 ml/l up to 60 min bath 0.015–0.025 ml/l permanent bath	 Repeat at 24 h × 2–3 days 48 h × 6 days	Ectoparasites		Do not use if contains toxic white precipitates (paraformaldehyde) Some fish very sensitive Increased toxicity in soft water, at high temperature and at low pH Requires increased aeration during treatment (binds to oxygen) Toxic to plants Do not use with potassium permanganate Harmful to humans, may cause skin sensitization
Fresh water	3–15 minute bath	Repeat at 7 days as required	Ectoparasites on marine fish	Aerate well	Harmful to small fish; remove fish if distressed
Fumagillin (Fumidil B®)	1–15 mg/kg in feed	24 h × 3–8 weeks	Systemic protozoal infections		
Hydrogen peroxide (3%)	17.5 ml/l × 4–10 min bath		Ectoparasites		Harmful to small fish; remove if distressed
Ivermectin	0.1–0.2 mg/kg i.m.		*Lernaea*		May cause neurological signs or death in some species
Leteux–Meyer mixture (formalin + malachite green)	Use stock solution (malachite green 3.3 g/l formalin) 0.015 ml/l permanent bath	48 h × 3 treatments	Protozoal ectoparasites	For *Ichthyophthirius*, change 50% on alternate days	As for formalin and malachite green
Levamisole	1–2 mg/l × 24 h bath		Internal nematodes		May cause anorexia at higher doses
Lufenuron (Program®)	0.088 mg/l × 1		Crustacean ectoparasites	Used by koi hobbyists Very insoluble: use suspension formulation for cats	Very persistent in the environment

Figure 30.7 Antiparasitic agents used in ornamental fish. (See text on page 242.) (continues)   ►

Agent	Dosage and route	Interval	Parasite	Comments	Warnings
Malachite green	50–60 mg/l × 10–30 s bath 0.1 mg/l permanent bath 100 mg/l topical to skin lesions	3 days × 3 treatments	Protozoal infection in freshwater fish	Can be removed by activated carbon	Mutagenic, respiratory poison, toxic to some species (e.g. tetras) and fry More toxic at high temperatures, low pH Toxic to plants Stains many objects
Mebendazole	1 mg/l × 24 h bath		Monogenean trematodes		
Mebendazole + closantel	(Use mebendazole 75 mg/ml + closantel 50 mg/ml e.g. Supaverm®) 1 ml/400 l × 1			Monogenean trematodes	May be harmful to some species
Metronidazole	25 mg/l permanent bath 100 mg/kg in feed	48 h × 3 treatments 24 h × 3 days	Internal flagellates (e.g. *Hexamita*, *Spironucleus*)	Poorly soluble in water	
Piperazine	10 mg/kg in feed	24 h × 3 days	Non-encysted intestinal nematodes		
Potassium permanganate	100 mg/l × 5–10 min bath 2 mg/l permanent bath		Freshwater protozoal and crustacean ectoparasites	Inactivated by organic matter	Toxic at high pH Toxic to some species Do not use with formalin
Praziquantel	2–10 mg/l up to 4 h bath 5–12 g/kg feed 50 mg/kg by gavage × 1	5 days × 3 treatments 24h × 3 days	Monogenean trematode ectoparasites, cestodes	Aerate water well	Harmful to some marine fish
Salt (sodium chloride)	1–5 g/l permanent bath 30–35 g/l × 4–5 min bath		Freshwater protozoal ectoparasites	Use non-iodinized salts Remove fish if exhibit distress	Some anti-caking agents may be harmful Some species may be sensitive
Toltrazuril	30 mg/l × 60 min	48 h × 3 treatments	Myxozoans		
Trichlorphon	0.5 mg/l permanent bath 0.5–1.0 mg/l permanent bath	10 days × 3 treatments (7 days × 4 treatments for anchor worm and monogeneans) (3 days × 2 treatments for marine monogenean trematodes)	Crustacean ectoparasites		Organophosphate; neurotoxic May be harmful to some species Harmful to humans

Figure 30.7 continued Antiparasitic agents used in ornamental fish. (See text on page 242.)

Agent	Dosage and route			Interval	Comments	Warnings
Acriflavine	500 mg/l × 30 min bath 5–10 mg/l prolonged bath			24 h	Resistance by some bacteria	May cause skin hypersensitivity
Amikacin	5 mg/kg i.m.			72 h × 9 days		
Amoxycillin	40–80 mg/kg in feed 12.5 mg/kg i.m. × 1			24 h × 10 days	Rarely indicated in ornamental fish since few Gram-positive pathogens Use long-acting formulation	
Aztreonam (Azactam®)	100 mg/kg i.m., i.p.			48 h	Used by koi hobbyists in US	
Chloramine-T	Prolonged bath 	pH	Soft water	Hard water
6.0	2.5 mg/l	7.0 mg/l
6.5	5.0 mg/l	10.0 mg/l
7.0	10.0 mg/l	15.0 mg/l
7.5	18.0 mg/l	18.0 mg/l
8.0	20.0 mg/l	20.0 mg/l				Repeat after 48 h if necessary	Treatment of bacterial gill disease, fin rot	Avoid contact with metal Avoid use in bright sunlight More toxic in soft water and low pH

Figure 30.8 Antibacterial agents used in fish. (See text on page 242.) (continues) ▶

Agent	Dosage and route	Interval	Comments	Warnings
Enrofloxacin	2.5–5.0 mg/l × 5 h bath 5–10 mg/kg orally 5–10 mg/kg i.m., i.p.	24 h × 5–7 days 24 h × 10–14 days 48 h × 15 days	Change 50% water between treatments Chelated by hard water	
Erythromycin	100 mg/kg orally, in feed 10–20 mg/kg i.m.	24 h × 10 days 24 h × 1–3	Variable palatability	
Florfenicol	40–50 mg/kg orally, i.m., i.p. 10 mg/kg in feed	12–24 h 24 h × 10 days		
Furazolidone	1–10 mg/l prolonged bath (> 24 h) 50–100 mg/kg in feed	 24 h × 10–15 days	Absorbed from water Inactivated by bright light	Carcinogenic Toxic to scaleless fish

Gentamicin	2.5 mg/kg i.m.	72 h		Nephrotoxic; substantial risk in
				  species for which dosages
				  have not been determined

Kanamycin	50–100 mg/l × 5 h bath 50 mg/kg in feed 20 mg/kg i.p.	72 h × 3 24 h 3 days × 14 days	Change 50% water between treatments	Nephrotoxic to some species

Methylene blue	2 mg/l prolonged bath	48 h, up to
		  3 treatments
				Harmful to biological filters
				Toxic to some scaleless
				  species and plants
				Stains many objects

Neomycin	66 mg/l prolonged bath	3 days, up to 3 treatments		Harmful to biological filters
Nifurpirinol (Furanace®)	1–2 mg/l × 5 min to 6 h bath 0.1 mg/l prolonged bath 4–10 mg/kg in feed	 24 h × 3–5 days 12 h × 5 days	Absorbed from water Inactivated by bright light Variable palatability	Carcinogenic Toxic to scaleless fish
Nitrofurazone	100 mg/l × 30 min bath 2–5 mg/l prolonged bath	 24 h × 5–10 days	Absorbed from water Inactivated by bright light	Carcinogenic Toxic to scaleless fish
Oxolinic acid	25 mg/l × 15 min bath 1 mg/l prolonged bath × 24 h 10 mg/kg in feed 30 mg/kg in feed	12 h × 3 days 24 h × 10 days 24 h × 10 days	Chelated by hard water For marine fish	

Oxytetracycline	
	
	10–100 mg/l × 1 h bath
	
	400 mg/l × 1 h bath
	10–100 mg/l tank water
	
	55–83 mg/kg in feed
	25 mg/kg i.m., i.p.
		
		Treat again on
		  day 3 after 50%
		  water change
		24h × 10 days
		24 h × 5–7 days
			Chelated by hard water
			Less than 1% bioavailability in
			  goldfish and carp
			Freshwater fish
			Higher dose in hard water
			For marine fish
			Higher dose in hard water
				Immunosuppressive
				
				Light-sensitive drug, avoid
				  bright light during treatment
				
				Long-acting formulations may
				  cause sterile fluid-filled cavity
				  at injection site

Potassium permanganate	5 mg/l × 30–60 min bath 2 mg/l permanent bath		Readily inactivated by organic matter	Toxic in water with high pH Do not mix with formalin Stains many objects
Povidone–iodine	Topical application to wounds			
Sarafloxacin	10 mg/kg in feed	24 h × 5 days		
Sulphadimethoxine and ormetoprim (Romet®)	50 mg/kg in feed	24 h × 5 days	Also available as medicated feed in USA	
Sulphadiazine and trimethoprim (Aquatrim®)	20 mg/l × 5–12 h bath 30 mg/kg in feed 30 mg/kg i.m., i.p.	24 h × 5–7 days 24 h × 7–10 days 2 days × 10 days	Change 50% water between treatments	
Sulphadoxine and trimethoprim	75 mg/kg i.m.	4 days × 8–12 days		Overdose may cause crystalluria

Figure 30.8 continued Antibacterial agents used in fish. (See text on page 242.)

Agent	Dosage and route	Infection	Comments	Warning
Bronopol (Pyceze®, Novartis)	20–50 mg/l × 30–60 min bath	Mycotic infections in fish and eggs (use higher dose for eggs)		
Formalin	All doses based on full strength formalin (= 37% formaldehyde) 1–2 ml/l bath, up to 15 min 0.23 ml/l bath, up to 60 min	Mycotic infections on eggs (do not treat within 24 h of hatching)		Do not use if contains toxic white precipitates (paraformaldehyde) Some fish very sensitive Increased toxicity in soft water, at high temperature and low pH Increase aeration during treatment (binds to oxygen) Toxic to plants Do not use with potassium permanganate Harmful to humans, may cause skin sensitization
Itraconazole	1–10 mg/kg daily in feed for 1–7 days	Systemic mycoses		
Malachite green	1–2 mg/l × 30–60 min bath 0.1 mg/l permanent bath 1% topical to skin lesions	Mycotic infections in freshwater fish	Can be removed by activated carbon	Mutagenic, respiratory poison, toxic to some species (e.g. tetras) and fry More toxic at high temperatures, low pH Toxic to plants Stains many objects

Figure 30.9 Antifungal agents used in ornamental fish. (See text on page 242.)

Agent	Dosage	Comments
Acetazolamide	2–10 mg/kg	Treatment of 'gas bubble disease' and some swim-bladder disorders
Activated carbon	Use to effect, replace every 2–4 weeks	Removes medications and other organic compounds by adsorption
Ammonium chloride	10–100 mg/l (depending on intended stocking density)	To maintain biological filter in absence of fish
Atropine	0.1 mg/kg i.m., i.p., IV	Treatment of toxicity due to organophosphate and chlorinated hydrocarbons
Butorphanol	0.05–0.5 mg/kg i.m.	Postoperative analgesia; dilute with sterile water
Carp Pituitary Extract	1.0–12.0 mg/kg i.m.	Inducement of maturation of eggs and inducement of spawning Often used in conjunction with human chorionic gonadotropin Dose and frequency of administration are species dependent
Dexamethasone	1–2 mg/kg i.m., i.p.	Treatment of shock, trauma, stress
Doxapram	5 mg/kg i.p., IV	Respiratory stimulant
Fresh water	0.4–1.0 litre for medium and large sharks by gavage, every 2–3 days	Gavage for sharks to stimulate appetite (by rehydration?)
Hydrogen peroxide 3%	0.5 ml/l	In emergency, to increase dissolved oxygen levels (note that this is only a temporary treatment)
Peat	Use to effect	Reducing pH, softening water
Potassium permanganate	5 mg/l × 5 min	To disinfect plants
Sodium bicarbonate	Use to effect	Raising pH, increasing alkalinity
Sodium chloride	1–3 mg/l	Treatment of nitrite toxicity Reduction of osmotic and physiological stress in freshwater fish
Sodium thiosulphate	10 mg/l 100 mg/l	Use in municipal water when performing water changes Treat chlorine toxicity
Zeolite (clinoptilolite)	Use to effect (recharge in water with 40 mg/l salt at pH 12)	Removal of ammonia from water by exchanging sodium ions for ammonia

Figure 30.10 Miscellaneous agents used with ornamental fish. (See text on page 242.)

Agent	% Purity	Proprietary name	Manufacturer or distributor
Antibacterial agents			
Amoxycillin	80 100	Aquacil Vetremox	Novartis, UK Alpharma, UK
Florfenicol	50	Florocol	Schering-Plough, UK
Ormetoprim with sulphadimethoxine	30	Romet 30	Hoffman-La Roche, USA
Oxolinic acid	100	Aqualinic	Alpharma, UK
Oxytetracycline	100 22	Aquatet TM 100F	Alpharma, UK Pfizer, USA
Sarafloxacin	100	Sarafin	Alpharma, UK
Sulphadiazine with trimethoprim	50	Sulfatrim	Novartis, UK
Sulphamerazine		Sulphamerazine in Fish Grade	American Cyanamid Co., USA
Antiparasitic agents			
Azamethiphos	50	Salmosan	Novartis, UK
Cypermethrin	1.0	Excis	Novartis, UK
Emamectin	0.2	Slice	Schering-Plough, UK
Formalin		Formalin-F Paracide-F	Natchez Animal Supply Co., USA Argent, USA
Hydrogen peroxide	50 35 & 50	Salartect 500 Paramove	Brenntag, UK Solvay Interox, UK
Teflubenzuron	100	Calicide	Trouw, UK
Antifungal agent			
Bronopol	50	Pyceze	Novartis, UK
Anaesthetic agent			
Tricaine methane sulphonate	100 100	MS-222 Finquel	Thomson & Joseph, UK Argent, USA

Figure 30.11 Proprietary medications licensed for use in fish in the UK and USA. (See text on page 242.)

Medication	Manufacturer	Active ingredients	Indications[a]	Species	Warnings
Acriflavine	PPI, UK	Acriflavine	External bacterial, protozoal and fungal infection	Pond fish	
Acriflavine	UK Pond Products, UK	Acriflavine	External bacterial, fungal and protozoal infections	Pond fish	
Aquarium Care Fin-Rot	NT Labs, UK	Acriflavine, aminoacridine hydrochloride, formaldehyde	Flukes and external bacterial infections	Freshwater aquarium fish	
Aquarium Care Fungus	NT Labs, UK	Malachite green	Fungal and ectoparasitic infections	Aquarium fish	
Aquarium Care White Spot	NT Labs, UK	Acetic acid	Protozoal (*Ichthyophthirius, Costia, Chilodonella, Oodinium*) infections	Freshwater aquarium fish	
Aquarium Doctor: BSB (Broad Spectrum Bactericide)	TAP, UK	Acriflavine hydrochloride, malachite green	External bacterial and fungal infections	Freshwater and marine aquaria fish (safe to invertebrates)	
Aquarium Doctor: FC11 (Fungus cure)	TAP, UK	Acriflavine, EDTA, silver, copper, organic salts	External bacterial infections	Freshwater and marine aquarium fish	
Aquarium Doctor: MM2 (Marine Multicure)	TAP, UK	Copper sulphate, malachite green, polyvinylpyrrolidone, organic sulphur	External bacterial, protozoal (*Oodinium*) and fungal infections	Marine fish	Harmful to marine invertebrates
Aquarium Doctor: WSP (White Spot & Parasite Cure)	TAP, UK	Formaldehyde, malachite green, methylene blue, para rosaniline, sodium chloride	Protozoal infections and flukes	Freshwater and marine aquaria fish	Harmful to mormyrids (elephant-noses); use half the dose if marine invertebrates present
Ark-Klens	Vetark, UK	Benzalkonium chloride	External bacterial infections, bacterial gill disease	Pond fish	Use in treatment tank, not in pond

Figure 30.12 Some proprietary medications available without prescription in the UK. (See text on page 242.) (continues) ▶
[a] Derived from manufacturers' literature.

Medication	Manufacturer	Active ingredients	Indications[a]	Species	Warnings
Bacterial Terminator	Sinclair, UK	Allantoin, formaldehyde, magnesium sulphate, sodium chloride	External bacterial and fungal infections	Freshwater aquarium fish	
Bacta-pure	UK Pond Products, UK	Acriflavine, aminoacridine, formaldehyde	Flukes and external bacterial infections	Pond fish	
Bactocide	NT Labs, UK	Acriflavine, aminoacridine hydrochloride, formaldehyde	External infections with bacteria, flukes, *Oodinium*	Freshwater and marine aquarium fish (safe to invertebrates)	
Baktopur	Sera, Germany	Acriflavine, 1,3-butylglycol, methylene blue	External bacterial infections	Freshwater aquarium fish	Harmful to filters
Baktopur direct	Sera, Germany	Nifurpirinol	Internal and external bacterial infections	Freshwater and marine aquarium fish	Harmful to marine invertebrates
Chloramine-T	Vetark, UK	Chloramine-T	External bacterial, protozoal (*Ichthyobodo*, *Ichthyophthirius*) and fluke infections	Pond fish	Use at higher dosage in high pH and hard water
Costapur	Sera, Germany	Malachite green	Protozoal infections (*Ichthyophthirius*, *Costia*, *Chilodonella*)	Freshwater and marine aquarium fish	Harmful to marine invertebrates
Cryptopur	Sera, Germany	1,3-dihydroxybenzol, phenol	Protozoal infections (*Cryptocaryon* and other parasites)	Marine aquarium fish	
Cyprinopur	Sera, Germany	1,3-dihydroxybenzol, ethanol, phenol	Treatment of open wounds and ulcers	Pond fish	
Diseasolve for Ponds	NT Labs, UK	Acriflavine, methylene blue	External bacterial and parasitic infections	Ornamental pond fish	
Diseasolve Aquarium Antiseptic	NT Labs, UK	Acriflavine, methylene blue (methylthioninium chloride)	External bacterial and protozoal infections	Aquarium fish	
Ectopur	Sera, Germany	Sodium borate, sodium chloride, sodium perborate	Ectoparasitic and fungal infections	Freshwater and marine aquarium fish	
Fin Rot Terminator	Sinclair, UK	Silver proteinate	External bacterial infections	Freshwater aquarium fish	Harmful to marine fish; best at 10–30°C
Formalachite	PPI, UK	Formaldehyde, malachite green	Protozoal (*Ichthyophthirius*, *Costia*, *Trichodina*) and fluke infections	Pond fish	
Formaldehyde 30% solution	UK Pond Products, UK	Formaldehyde	Ectoparasitic infections	Pond fish	
Formalin	PPI, UK	Formaldehyde	Protozoal (*Ichthyophthirius*, *Costia*, *Trichodina*) and fluke infections	Pond fish	
Fungal Terminator	Sinclair, UK	2-phenoxyethanol	Fungal infections	Freshwater aquarium fish	Harmful in salt; best at 16–27°C
Gill-Pure	UK Pond Products, UK	Benzalkonium chloride	External bacterial and parasitic infections	Pond fish	Harmful to filters; use half dosage in soft water
Ichcide	NT Labs, UK	Formaldehyde, malachite green	Fungal and protozoal (*Ichthyophthirius*, *Chilodonella*) infections	Freshwater aquarium fish	
Koi Anti Fungus and Bacteria	Interpet, UK	Acriflavine, malachite green, methylene blue	External bacterial and fungal disease	Pond fish	Harmful to orfe, rudd and other sensitive species
Koi Anti Parasite FS	Interpet, UK	Formaldehyde, malachite green, methylene blue	Flukes and protozoal infections	Pond fish	
Koi Care Acriflavin	NT Labs, UK	Acriflavine	External bacterial infections	Pond fish	
Koi Care Formaldehyde 30% Solution	NT Labs, UK	Formaldehyde	Protozoal (*Ichthyophthirius*, *Trichodina*, *Costia*) and fluke infections	Pond fish	
Koi Care F-M-G	NT Labs, UK	Formaldehyde, malachite green	Fungal and parasitic infections	Koi and goldfish	Harmful to orfe, rudd, tench and sterlets
Koi Care Gill-Wash	NT Labs, UK	Benzalkonium chloride	Bacterial gill infections	Pond fish	Harmful to filters; use half the dose in soft water

Figure 30.12 continued Some proprietary medications available without prescription in the UK. (See text on page 242.) (continues)

[a] Derived from manufacturers' literature.

Medication	Manufacturer	Active ingredients	Indications[a]	Species	Warnings
Koi Care Koi Calm	NT Labs, UK	Clove oil	Use as a calmative		
Koi Care Malachite Green Solution	NT Labs, UK	Malachite green	Fungal and external parasitic infections	Pond fish	
Koi Care Ulcer-Swab	NT Labs, UK	Benzalkonium chloride, povidone	Cleanser and disinfectant for skin wounds	Koi and other pond fish	Topical use only
Koi Care Wound Seal	NT Labs, UK	Zinc cream	Use to seal wounds and assist healing	Koi and other pond fish	Topical use only
Malachite	PPI, UK	Malachite green	Fungal, parasitic and some bacterial infections	Pond fish	Harmful
Malachite Green 2% solution	UK Pond Products, UK	Malachite green	Fungal and some parasitic infections	Pond fish	
Methylene Blue (No.10)	Interpet, UK	Methylene blue	Fungal and protozoal infections	Freshwater and marine aquarium fish	Harmful to plants and filters
Methylene Blue	Sinclair, UK	Methylthioninium chloride	Fungal, fluke and protozoal infections	Freshwater aquarium fish	Harmful to filters, marine fish and plants; best at 10–30°C
Miracle Cure	Aquajardin, UK	Oil of cloves and associated anti-bactericides	External bacterial infections	Coldwater ornamental fish	For topical treatment only; harmful to tropical or marine fish; avoid contact with gills and eyes
Mycopur	Sera, Germany	Acriflavine, copper chloride, copper sulphate	Flukes and fungal infections	Freshwater aquarium fish	Harmful to filters
Nishi-Care Anti-Fin Rot	Nishikoi, UK	Acriflavine, aminoacridine hydrochloride, formaldehyde	External bacterial infections	Pond fish	
Nishi-Care Anti-Fungus	Nishikoi, UK	Malachite green	Fungal infections	Pond fish	Use above 6°C
Nishi-Care Anti-White Spot	Nishikoi, UK	Formaldehyde, malachite green	Protozoal infections	Pond fish	Use above 6°C
Omnisan	Sera, Germany	Malachite green	Fungal and ectoparasitic infections	Pond fish	
Oodinopur A	Sera, Germany	Copper chloride, copper sulphate	Protozoal (*Oodinium*) infections	Freshwater and marine aquarium fish	Harmful to marine invertebrates
Paracide	NT Labs, UK	Citric acid, cupric sulphate, formaldehyde	Protozoal (*Oodinium, Cryptocaryon*) infections	Freshwater and marine aquarium fish	Harmful to invertebrates
Para-Pure	UK Pond Products, UK	Formaldehyde, malachite green	Protozoal and fungal infections	Pond fish	May be applied topically for *Argulus, Lernaea*
Pond Care Bacterad	NT Labs, UK	Acriflavine, aminoacridine hydrochloride, formaldehyde	External bacterial and fluke infections	Pond fish	
Pond Care Clear Gills	NT Labs, UK	Benzalkonium chloride	Decongestant bath for gill disease	Pond fish	Harmful to filters
Pond Care Erad-Ick	NT Labs, UK	Formaldehyde, malachite green	Protozoal (*Ichthyophthirius, Chilodonella, Costia*) infections	Pond fish	
Pond Care Fin-Rot	NT Labs, UK	Acriflavine, aminoacridine hydrochloride, formaldehyde	External bacterial and fluke infections	Pond fish	
Pond Care Fungus	NT Labs, UK	Malachite green	Fungal and ectoparasitic infections	Pond fish	
Pond Care White Spot	NT Labs, UK	Formaldehyde, malachite green	Protozoal (*Ichthyophthirius, Chilodonella, Costia, Oodinium*) infections	Pond fish	
Pond Doctor Anti-Bacteria	TAP, UK	Acriflavine, malachite green, sulphur compounds	External and internal bacterial infections	Pond fish	
Pond Doctor Anti-Fungus	TAP, UK	Formaldehyde, metanil yellow, methyl violet, silver nitrate	External bacterial and fungal infections	Pond fish	Switch off UV for 1 day
Pond Doctor Anti-Parasite	TAP, UK	Formaldehyde, malachite green	Flukes and protozoan (*Ichthyophthirius, Costia, Trichodina*) infections	Pond fish	Switch off UV for 1 day
Pond Doctor Anti-Ulcer	TAP, UK	Iodine and sulphur compounds	External bacterial infections	Pond fish	
Pond Pride No. 3: Parasite Control	Sinclair, UK	Acriflavine neutral, malachite green, quinine sulphate	Protozoal infections	Pond fish	
Pond Pride No. 4: Fungus Control	Sinclair, UK	Formaldehyde, malachite green	Fungal infections	Pond fish	

Figure 30.12 continued Some proprietary medications available without prescription in the UK. (See text on page 242.) (continues)
[a] Derived from manufacturers' literature.

Medication	Manufacturer	Active ingredients	Indications[a]	Species	Warnings
Pond Pride No. 5: Fin and Tail Rot Control	Sinclair, UK	Silver proteinate	External bacterial infections	Pond fish	
Pond Pride No. 8: Open Wound Treatment	Sinclair, UK	Allantoin, formaldehyde, magnesium sulphate, sodium chloride	External bacterial infections	Pond fish	
Pond Professional: Acriflavine Gold	TAP, UK	Acriflavine, ethanol	External bacterial, protozoal and fungal infections	Pond fish	
Pond Professional: Aquabath	TAP, UK	Glutaraldehyde compounds, quaternary ammonium salts	External bacterial and ectoparasitic infections; also as disinfectant for nets and equipment	Pond fish	Harmful to filters
Pond Professional: Aquagel	TAP, UK	Calamine, silicone, zinc oxide	For treatment of wounds	Pond fish	Topical application only
Pond Professional: Aquaswab	TAP, UK	Ethanol, iodine compounds	For treatment of external wounds	Pond fish	Topical application only
Pond Professional: Formalin Gold	TAP, UK	Formaldehyde 40%, methanol	Flukes and protozoal infections	Pond fish	
Pond Professional: Malachite Gold	TAP, UK	Malachite green medical	Flukes and protozoal infections	Pond fish	
Pond Professional: MS10	TAP, UK	Formaldehyde, potassium permanganate, tin oxide	Flukes and ectoparasitic (*Trichodina, Argulus,* leeches) infections	Pond fish	Harmful to orfe and rudd
Potassium	PPI, UK	Potassium salts	Anchor worm, protozoal (*Ichthyophthirius, Trichodina*) and fungal infections	Pond fish	
Propolis	NT Labs, UK	Bee propolis	Sealing wounds and ulcers	Pond fish	For topical application or use in feed
Protoban	Vetark, UK	Formaldehyde, malachite green	External bacterial, protozoal (*Costia, Trichodina, Chilodonella*) and fluke infections	Pond fish	
Tamodine	Vetark, UK	Povidone–iodine	Topical application to skin ulcers and wounds	All fish species	Topical use only
Tamodine-E	Vetark, UK	Iodophor	Disinfection	All fish species	Toxic to fish, do not use as treatment
TetraFin GoldMed: Goldfish disease treatment	Tetra, UK	Formaldehyde, malachite green oxalate	Flukes, external bacterial, protozoan and fungal infections	Aquarium goldfish	
TetraMedica ContraSpot	Tetra, UK	Formaldehyde, malachite green chloride	Flukes and protozoal infections	Freshwater aquarium fish	
TetraMedica FungiStop	Tetra, UK	Collidon, metanil yellow, silver colloid	Fungal infections on fish and eggs	Freshwater aquarium fish	Not recommended for marine aquaria
TetraMedica General Tonic	Tetra, UK	Acriflavine, aminoacridine, ethacridine lactate, methylene blue	External bacterial infections	Freshwater aquarium fish	
TetraPond Medifin	Tetra, UK	Formaldehyde, malachite green oxalate	Flukes, external bacterial, fungal and protozoal infections	Pond fish	
Ultimate Solution: Paracure	TAP, UK	EDTA, malachite green, tin chloride	Ectoparasitic infections	Freshwater and marine aquarium fish	Harmful to orfe, rudd, piranha, silver dollars, sharks, rays, crustaceans, cartilaginous fish and marine surgeon fish
Velvet Terminator	Sinclair, UK	Cupric sulphate	*Oodinium* infection	Freshwater aquarium fish	Use half dose for light scaled fish (e.g. sharks, loaches); use at 20–30°C
White Spot Terminator (WS3)	Sinclair, UK	Acriflavine, malachite green, quinine sulphate	Protozoal infections	Freshwater aquarium fish	Harmful to marine fish; best at 25–30°C

Figure 30.12 continued Some proprietary medications available without prescription in the UK. (See text on page 242.)
[a] Derived from manufacturers' literature.

Medication	Manufacturer	Active ingredients	Indications[a]
Ampicillex	Aquatronics, USA	Ampicillin trihydrate	Bacterial infections
Bettamax	Aquatronics, USA	Nitrofurazone, methylene blue, vitamins, sodium chloride, sulphamethazine, sulphadiazine, sulphamerazine	Bacterial infections
BGDX	Argent, USA	p-Toluene sulphonylchloride (chloramine-T)	Bacterial gill disease
Clear-ich	Aquatronics, USA	Quinine monohydrochloride, gentian violet, sodium chloride, diatomaceous earth	*Ichthyophthirius* infections
Clout	Aquarium, USA	4-p-Dimethylamino-o-phenylbenzylidene-2,5-cyclohexadien-1-xylidenedimethyl ammonium chloride; dimethyl (2,2,2-trichloro-1-hydroxy-ethyl) phosphonate; 2-methyl-5-nitro-1-hydroxyethylmidazole; inert ingredients	Most external parasites
Fluke Tabs	Aquarium, USA	Trichlorfon, mebendazole	Tapeworms, copepods, flukes, lice, *Capillaria*
Formalite I	Aquatronics, USA	Formaldehyde, malachite green, copper sulphate	External parasitic infections
Formalite II	Aquatronics, USA	Formaldehyde, copper, nickel sulphate	External parasites
Fungi Cure	Aquarium, USA	Victoria green, green band, neutroflavins	Fungal infections
Fungus Guard	Jungle, USA	Sodium chloride, potassium chloride, triethylene glycol, EDTA, methylene blue, polyvinylpyrrolidone, nitromersol acriflavine	Fungal infections
Furazone Green	Various manufacturers	Methylene blue, nitrofurazone, furazolidone	External bacterial and fungal infections
General Cure	Aquarium, USA	Metronidazole, copper sulphate, trichlorfon	
Ick Guard	Jungle, USA	Triethylene glycol, Victoria green, nitromersol, acriflavine in aqueous solution	*Ichthyophthirius*
Ick Guard II	Jungle, USA	Formalin, carmisine red, triethylene glycol, Victoria green, sodium hydroxide, nitromersol, acriflavine	*Ichthyophthirius* in scaleless fishes
Kanamycin	Aquatrol, USA	Kanamycin sulphate	Bacterial infections
Maracyn I	Mardel, USA	Erythromycin	Bacterial infections
Maracyn II	Mardel, USA	Minocycline	Bacterial infections
Metrozol	Aquatrol, USA	Metronidazole	'Hole-in-the-head' disease, external protozoal infections
Nitrofurazone	Aquatrol, USA	Nitrofurazone	Bacterial infections
Paracide Green	Argent, USA	p-P-benzylidene-N-N-dimethylalanine, formalin	External parasites (including *Ichthyophthirius*) and fungi
Paragon I	Aquatronics, USA	Dibromohydroxymercurifluorescein (merbromin), aniline green (malachite green)	External parasitic infections
Paragon II	Aquatronics, USA	Metronidazole, neomycin sulphate, furazolidone, naladixic acid, sodium chloride	Wide-spectrum for bacterial and parasitic diseases
Prefuran (Furanace)	Argent, USA	Nifurpirinol	Most bacterial infections, *Saprolegnia*, *Ichthyophthirius*, 'hole-in-the-head' disease
Zeemax	Jungle, USA	Sodium chloride, nitrofurazone, nitromersol, triethylene glycol, potassium permanganate, acriflavine	Wide-spectrum for bacterial and parasitic diseases; safe for species sensitive to organophosphates

Figure 30.13 Some proprietary medications available without prescription in the USA. (See text on page 242.)
[a] Derived from manufacturers' literature.

Alpharma Animal Health Ltd Unit 15, Sandleheath Industrial Estate, Fordingbridge, Hampshire SP6 1PA, UK Tel: +44 (0) 1425 656081	**Brenntag (UK) Ltd** Ham Lane, Kings Winford, West Midlands DY6 7JU, UK Tel: +44 (0) 1384 400 222	**Novartis Animal Health** New Cambridge House, Litlington, Nr Royston, Hertfordshire SG8 0SS, UK Tel: +44 (0) 1763 850500	**TAP** (Technical Aquatic Products Ltd) Blackfriar's Road, West End Trading Estate, Nailsea, Avon BS48 4DJ, UK Tel: +44 (0) 1275 810522
Aquajardin c/o Jardinerie Garden Centre, Bath Road, Haresfield, Nr Stonehouse, Gloucester GL10 3DP, UK Tel: +44 (0) 1452 724341	**Hoffman-La Roche** Roche Animal Health and Nutrition, 340 Kingsland Street, Nutley, NJ 07110, USA Tel: +1 973 235 5000	**NT Laboratories Ltd** Unit B, Manor Farm, Wateringbury, Kent ME18 5PP, UK Tel: +44 (0) 1622 817692	**Tetra** Lambert Court, Chestnut Avenue, Eastleigh, Hampshire SO53 3ZQ, UK Tel: +44 (0) 2380 620500
American Cyanamid Co. One Cyanamid Plaza, Wayne, NJ 07470, USA Tel: +1 201 831 2000	**IZVG** (International Zoo Veterinary Group) Keighley Business Centre, South Street, Keighley, West Yorkshire BD21 1AG, UK Tel: +44 (0) 1535 692000	**Pfizer Animal Health** 812 Springdale Drive, Exton, PA 19341, USA Tel: +1 800 366 5210	**Thomson & Joseph Ltd** T&J House, 119 Plumstead Road, Norwich, Norfolk NR1 4JT, UK Tel: +44 (0) 1603 439511
Aquarium Pharmaceuticals Inc. PO Box 218, Chalfont, PA 18914, USA Tel: +1 800 847 0659	**Interpet Ltd** Vincent Lane, Dorking, Surrey RH4 3YX, UK Tel: +44 (0) 1306 881033	**PPI** (Pet Products International Ltd) Pedigree House, Gamston, Nottingham NG2 6NQ, UK Tel: +44 (0) 115 9811088	**Trouw Aquaculture** Wincham, Northwich, Cheshire CW9 6DF, UK Tel: +44 (0) 1606 561090
Aquatrol Inc. 237 North Euclid Way, Anaheim, CA 92801-6776, USA Tel: +1 714 533 3881	**Jungle Laboratories Corporation** 120 Industrial Drive, Cibolo, Texas 78108-3500, USA Tel: +1 210 658 3505	**Schering-Plough Animal Health** Breakspear Road South, Harefield, Uxbridge, Middlesex UB9 6LS, UK Tel: +44 (0) 1895 626277	**UK Pond Products** 19–20 Riverside, Power Station Road, Rugeley, Staffordshire WS15 2YR, UK Tel: +44 (0) 1889 579055
Aquatronics PO Box 2457, Oxnard, CA 93033, USA Tel: +1 805 486 2614	**Mardel Laboratories Inc.** 1656 West 240th Street, Harbor City, CA 90710-1311, USA Tel: +1 310 326 1249	**Sera GmBH** c/o Aquazoo, 1058 Whitgift Centre, Croydon, Surrey CR0 1UW, UK Tel: +44 (0) 20 8781 0556	**Vetark Professional** PO Box 60, Winchester, Hampshire SO23 9XN, UK Tel: +44 (0) 1962 880376
Argent 8702 152nd Avenue, N.E. Redmond, WA 98052, USA Tel: +1 206 885 3777	**Natchez Animal Supply Co.** 201 John R. Junkin Drive, Natchez, MS 39120, USA Tel: +1 800 647 6760	**Sinclair Animal and Household Care Ltd** Ropery Road, Gainsborough, Lincolnshire DN21 2QB, UK Tel: +44 (0) 1427 810231	**Zeigler Brothers Inc.** 400 Gardners Station Road, Gardners, PA 17324, USA Tel: +1 800 841 6800
AVL (Aquaculture Vaccines Ltd) 24–26 Gold Street, Saffron Walden, Essex CB10 1EJ, UK Tel: +44 (0) 1799 528167	**Nishikoi Aquaculture Ltd** White Hall, Wethersfield, Essex CM7 4EP, UK Tel: +44 (0) 1371 851424	**Solvay Interox Ltd** PO Box 7, Warrington, Cheshire WA4 6HB, UK Tel: +44 (0) 1925 651277	

Figure 30.14 Suppliers and manufacturers of proprietary products used in fish. (Information correct at time of going to press.)

Pharmacokinetics

The characteristics of absorption, distribution, localization in the tissues, biotransformation and excretion of a drug are collectively known as the pharmacokinetics. There is limited information available regarding the fate of many compounds used in aquaculture and reference to textbooks for full details of the drugs is advised (e.g. Stoskopf, 1999; Treves-Brown, 2000). Those details that are available relate mainly to farmed fish rather than ornamental fish and most apply to in-feed medications.

Many factors affect the action of drugs administered to fish and require consideration if treatment is to be effective. They include the following.

Species: Variations in bioavailability, metabolism and drug clearance suggest that what happens to a drug inside in caged seawater salmon may not necessarily apply to koi in a freshwater pond. For example, the bioavailability of oxytetracycline given orally in carp and goldfish is less than 1% whereas it is up to 15% in salmonids.

Temperature: Fish are ectotherms and temperature has a profound effect on the body rate and drug metabolism. Low water temperatures result in a slow uptake of drug and subsequent therapeutic effect.

Gastric emptying time: This is reduced at higher temperatures. Coldwater fish are more active in warmer water, and their metabolic functions accelerate. They eat more and food passes through their gut more rapidly. This may affect drugs that are absorbed from the stomach and not from the intestine, resulting in a reduced uptake of a drug. Digestion of some agents in the stomach will reduce the efficacy of any oral medication but this will be minimal in species without a stomach (e.g. carp and goldfish).

Binding agents: Bioavailability may be affected by the oil vehicle on surface-coated foods. Drug absorption is greater in cases where vegetable oils are used rather than fish oil, which is used to increase palatability.

Concurrent treatment: The administration of other drugs (e.g. immuno-modulating agents such as glucans) may affect the uptake of oral antibacterial drugs.

Environmental factors: Temperature, salinity, stocking density and competition for feed may influence the effect of a drug inside the fish.

Drug characteristics: Particle size and homogeneity (uniformity) may affect the way that a drug is absorbed.

Duration and frequency: It may take a few days for some drugs to reach therapeutic levels in the tissues of the fish, and alternate-day feeding of some less palatable drugs may be just as effective, if not more so, than daily feeding (e.g. potentiated sulphonamides).

Dose rate: Careful calculations of dose are required to avoid both underdosing and overdosing.

Calculations and client instructions

In many cases, it is advisable to calculate the dosage of medication required for the client. This should be done carefully, using an electronic calculator and paying particular attention to the position of any decimal point – it is easy to miscalculate the dosage by a factor of ten. Equally, great care must be taken to note if dosages are given in milligrams or grams, since this may produce a more serious error. Every step of the arithmetic calculation should be written out in full and a copy retained in case of an accident. The figures should be checked at least twice.

It is also important that clear unambiguous instructions regarding treatment are given to the client. It is useful to prepare standard instruction sheets for different products, ensuring that a sufficient amount of detail relating to the drug dosage is added.

Non-chemical control methods

Several non-chemical methods of control have been used in fish medicine with varying degrees of success.

Cleaner fish

Some species of fish will actively remove some ectoparasites from fish. These include goldsinney wrasse, the neon goby and cleaner shrimps (Figure 30.15). Sticklebacks can be used to remove *Argulus* from ponds. Species that rely entirely on ectoparasites as a food source should be avoided since there may be insufficient numbers to maintain their survival.

Environmental manipulation

Moving fish infected with 'white spot' to new aquaria daily for 7 days has been shown to prevent reinfection and eliminate the parasite. Levels of *Argulus* have been controlled in lakes by using removable boards (submerged just below the surface) on which the parasite lays its eggs; prior to hatching, the boards are removed regularly and the eggs scraped off.

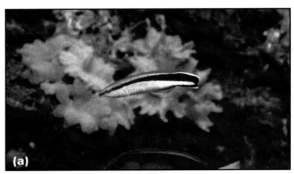

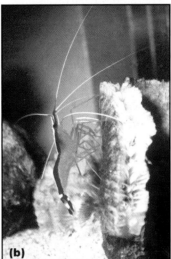

Figure 30.15 In marine systems, 'cleaners' such as (a) neon goby and (b) cleaner shrimps can be used to control some ectoparasite diseases. (Courtesy of Shotgate Koi and Aquaworld, © W.H. Wildgoose.)

Temperature control

Maintaining fish infected with 'white spot' at temperatures over 30°C will eradicate the parasite, since the free-swimming stages are killed at this temperature. Similarly, using temperatures over 25°C for 1 week and over 32°C for 5 days is sufficient to eliminate *Chilodonella* and *Ichthyobodo*, respectively.

Ultraviolet (UV)

Under laboratory conditions, certain wavelengths and intensities of UV light have been shown to control 'white spot' theronts but in practice the scale of equipment required is rarely practical.

Mechanical filtration

Fine nylon socks and large paper cartridge filter units can remove suspended materials (including free-swimming parasites) as small as 5 μm. These systems are commonly used in public aquaria or retail premises.

Leech trap

It is possible to reduce the number of leeches in a pond by placing a piece of raw meat or liver in a plastic container with several small holes. This should be submerged and, if necessary, weighted down with pebbles or stones. Leeches will be attracted to the meat and can then be removed from the trap regularly.

Intermediate host control

Some parasites require an intermediate host, such as a snail, to complete their life cycle. Molluscs can be controlled by stocking snail-eating fish such as black carp, by removal of aquatic weed on which the snails feed, or by using various chemical molluscicides.

Manual removal of parasites

Leeches and adult anchor worms can be removed under anaesthesia when parasite numbers are low but fish lice often leave the host when netting the fish. In all of these cases, eggs are deposited in the environment and in-water chemical control is often required.

Herbal remedies

Water extracts of onion and garlic have been used to a limited degree to control sea lice in salmon. Other extracts such as lilac leaves (*Syringa vulgaris*) and pine needles (*Pinus* spp.) are reported to have some antiprotozoal effect when placed in water. Quinine, an extract from *Cinchona* bark, has also been used to treat protozoan and monogenean infestations.

Supportive treatment

In addition to the use of specific therapeutic products, supportive measures can greatly assist the recovery of the patient. These include:

- Isolation facilities
- Immuno-stimulants
- Appropriate nutrition.

Isolation facilities

A separate aquarium can easily be assembled for small fish but may be unsuitable for large pond fish. In the latter case, a temporary facility can be made using a child's paddling pool or a large rigid box lined with heavy-duty polyethylene. It is preferable to have a larger permanent structure that can also be used to quarantine new arrivals.

Various factors may determine the scale of an isolation facility but some essential features are listed in Figure 30.16. If a unit of suitable size is not available, treating fish in the main pond is preferable to a small isolation facility. An example of a basic facility for aquarium fish is shown in Figure 30.17.

By isolating the diseased fish, the loading of pathogens in the main tank or pond is reduced and the spread of infection to healthy fish is minimized. The use of an isolation facility avoids the harmful effects that some medications may have on a biological filter, resulting in deterioration of water quality. Accidental overdosing of chemicals can be catastrophic in the main tank or pond but this can be limited in an isolation facility. Should overdosing occur, immediate removal of the fish will minimize the effects of toxicity.

Immuno-stimulants

Vitamin C is known to improve the immune response in catfish and there may be a similar effect from other vitamins. Levamisole may help to improve the

- Water capacity as large as possible for the species involved
- Water taken from tank or pond of origin
- Biological filtration constructed using a suitable aquarium filter filled with medium taken from main tank or pond
- Water quality tested daily
- Thermostatically controlled water heaters to maintain water temperatures at 20°C (68°F) for coldwater fish
- Facility insulated with expanded polystyrene or bubble-wrap
- Thermometer
- Air-stones to aerate the water
- Shelter (pieces of large-diameter pipes or similar) to provide simple refuge
- Small companion fish if treating single fish accustomed to shoaling behaviour
- Feeding reduced to minimum (unless medicated feed being given)
- Separate set of equipment (nets, bucket) and disinfectants to avoid transfer of infection
- Facility covered with fine-meshed nylon net or other barrier to prevent fish from jumping out
- Subdued lighting to reduce stress
- Salt (2 g/l, increase to 3 g/l after 3 days if necessary) – may be beneficial to freshwater fish by raising their tolerance to ammonia and nitrite, and reducing physiological stresses in gills and skin wounds.

Figure 30.16 Features of an isolation facility.

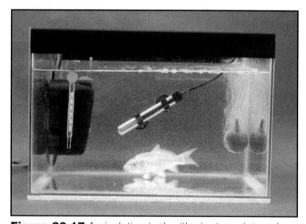

Figure 30.17 An isolation tank with air-stone, internal box filter, thermometer and thermostatically controlled heater. These facilities should be of a suitable size and maintain fish in good water conditions during the course of treatment. The facility can also be used to quarantine new arrivals for at least 4 weeks.

immune response in fish as in mammals. A combination of peptidoglycan, beta glucans and mannan oligo-saccharides, yeast and bacterial extracts (Vetregard®, Alpharma) added to food is known to be effective in ornamental fish (Türnau *et al.*, 2000). Immuno-stimulants are fed for 2 weeks, stopped for 6 weeks, then repeated indefinitely, but constant feeding with an immuno-stimulant may have a reduced benefit. A seaweed extract (Ergosan F1®, AVL) has been added to some brands of food for ornamental fish in the UK and is claimed to 'stimulate' the immune system in fish.

Agent	Dosage	Comments
ACE-High (Vetark, UK)	1 g/kg food	Ascorbic acid, biotin, calcium, cholecalciferol, choline, cobalt, copper, folic acid, iodine, iron, manganese, nicotinic acid, pantothenic acid, phosphorus, pyridoxine, riboflavin, selenium, sodium chloride, thiamine, vitamin A, zinc
Aquaminivits (IZVG, UK)	1 tablet/4 kg bodyweight per week in food	Ascorbic acid, biotin, cholecalciferol, choline, cyanocobalamine, folic acid, inositol, iodine, iron, pantothenic acid, thiamine, alpha-tocopherol, vitamin A
Aquavits (IZVG, UK)	1 tablet/20 kg bodyweight per week in food	Ascorbic acid, biotin, cholecalciferol, choline, cyanocobalamine, folic acid, inositol, iodine, iron, pantothenic acid, thiamine, alpha-tocopherol, vitamin A
Calcium iodate	250 mg/kg food	Treatment of goitre
Potassium iodide	1 mg/kg food/24 h 10 mg/kg bodyweight weekly	Treatment of goitre
Thiamine	25–35 mg/kg food	Supplement for frozen fish fed to carnivorous species (e.g. sharks)
Vitamin E	100 units/kg food	Supplement for frozen fish fed to carnivorous species (e.g. sharks)

Figure 30.18 Nutritional supplements for ornamental fish.

Appropriate nutrition

A well balanced diet is essential to host defence mechanisms and good quality commercial foods or fresh food with vitamin supplements should be used. Supplements suitable for fish are listed in Figure 30.18.

Control and prevention

Following the old adage that prevention is better than cure, several management tools can be applied.

Selection of stock

Buy only healthy fish. Inspect new fish thoroughly and examine a sample of skin mucus and gill tissue.

Quarantine

Quarantine of new arrivals may be of limited benefit, since it may not reveal carrier fish (e.g. aeromonads, mycobacteria, viruses). Treatment with commercial medications on arrival may reduce ectoparasite burdens. A minimum quarantine period of 4 weeks is a safe recommendation.

Water quality

Water quality testing must be performed regularly to prevent environmental stress through poor water conditions.

Batch screening

An 'all-in-all-out' policy to reduce the spread of disease from one batch to the next should be practised in commercial systems. Regular health screening should be performed on a representative sample of fish in each batch. This should include examination of skin and gill samples under light microscopy. Routine postmortem examination should also be performed on all mortalities.

Hygiene

Disinfection and general hygiene of tanks, ponds and nets are part of good husbandry. Several effective disinfectants are available for use in fish facilities (Figure 30.19) but it is important to note that they must be used at the correct strength and for the recommended time. The physical removal of organic debris and waste greatly enhances the effectiveness of all disinfectants. Ozone and UV irradiation can reduce the pathogen burden in the water.

Agent	Use to disinfect	Advantages	Disadvantages
Alcohols	Equipment	Effective against many micro-organisms, including viruses and mycobacteria Inexpensive	Irritant fumes Flammable
Chloramine-T	Equipment; net dips; foot baths	Effective against many bacteria, viruses and fungi Bio-degradable Non-corrosive	Inactivated by high levels of inorganic debris Dry powder corrosive Expensive
Chlorhexidine	Equipment; foot baths	Effective against many bacteria, fungi and viruses Relatively non-corrosive	Not effective against some Gram-negative bacteria (including *Pseudomonas*), mycobacteria or hydrophilic viruses Inactivated by organic matter Expensive
Iodophores	Equipment; foot baths; eggs	Effective against wide range of bacteria, fungi and viruses (including spring viraemia of carp) Changes colour when inactive	Very toxic to fish Some bacterial resistance Stains some materials Inactivated by organic debris, sunlight and heat Expensive

Figure 30.19 Disinfectants for use in aquatic environments. Many products are harmful to fish and therefore should only be used strictly according to the manufacturer's instructions. (continues) ▶

Agent	Use to disinfect	Advantages	Disadvantages
Lime	All types ponds and tanks	Effective against most microorganisms when maintained above pH11 Not inactivated by organic debris Inexpensive	Very caustic Harmful to humans and fish
Ozone	Water	Effective against bacteria and some viruses	Toxic to fish (residual ozone must be removed before water re-used, e.g. with protein skimmer) Harmful to humans Expensive equipment
Peroxygen compounds	Equipment; net dips; foot baths	Effective against wide range of bacteria, fungi and viruses	Inactivated by high level of organic matter Toxic to fish Corrosive to some metals Expensive
Quaternary amines (e.g. benzalkonium chloride)	Equipment; net dips; foot baths	Effective against most bacteria and some fungi Detergent action which removes mucus Non-corrosive	Not effective against viruses, some fungi or some bacteria Inactivated by high levels of inorganic debris Expensive
Sodium hydroxide	All types ponds and tanks; equipment; foot baths	Effective against most microorganisms when maintained above pH11 Not inactivated by organic debris Inexpensive	Very caustic Harmful to humans and fish
Sodium hypochlorite	Equipment; net dips	Effective against most microorganisms Inexpensive	Toxic to fish Inactivated by organic debris and heat Destroys nets rapidly
Ultraviolet irradiation	Water	Effective against some bacteria, fungi and protozoan parasites Controls algae Not harmful to fish	Not effective against all pathogens UV tube replacement every 6 months Efficacy of units depends on narrow water void (< 6 mm) and rate of water flow Expensive equipment

Figure 30.19 continued Disinfectants for use in aquatic environments. Many products are harmful to fish and therefore should only be used strictly according to the manufacturer's instructions.

Diet

To ensure fresh vitamin content, good quality food should always be used. Extra vitamins (see Figure 30.18) added to the diet may be useful to some fish on selective fresh food diets. Mouldy foods may cause fatal systemic aspergillomycosis or result in aflatoxicosis, which can produce hepatoma in trout.

Prophylaxis

Routine prophylactic medication is practised by some hobbyists but is of questionable benefit in the absence of specific problems. It may be used in a quarantine facility to control some ectoparasitic problems (e.g. leeches, fish lice) where management of large ponds may be impractical. Resistance to antibacterial drugs and organophosphate compounds is now a serious problem and the prophylactic use of these chemicals should be discouraged.

Vaccines: Various commercial vaccines are available to protect farmed fish against certain bacterial diseases. Some of these may be of use in ornamental fish keeping where specific bacterial infections are a problem (e.g. *Aeromonas salmonicida, A. hydrophila, Vibrio*). The vaccines are administered by injection, immersion or orally. A commercial vaccine against *A. salmonicida* has been used successfully to protect wolf-fish in a public aquarium (Gibson, 1999) and another (Furogen b, Novartis) is authorized for use in koi in North America. Further advice may be obtained from the suppliers of fish vaccines (Alpharma, AVL and Novartis).

Aquatic invertebrates

Little is known about diseases of many tropical reef invertebrates and even less is known about suitable medications for these animals. The health of most aquatic invertebrates is highly dependent on their environmental conditions and water quality, much of which is described in Chapter 32. Poor water conditions predispose invertebrates to disease and this may involve bacteria, parasites, fungi or viral infections.

Medications similar to those used to treat fish have been found to be effective against diseases of invertebrates, but some products are toxic and some are toxic at different dose rates in different species. Many dose rates have been derived from species farmed for food, such as prawns and shellfish.

Where possible, invertebrates should be removed from the main display tank and treated in isolation. Only a few animals should be treated at any one time, using the lowest dose, and they should be closely monitored for any signs of adverse reaction during the course of treatment. Details of suitable medications can be found in Figure 30.20.

Agent	Dosage	Indications
Chloramine-T	5.5–100 mg/l for 2 days	Protozoal and fungal infections in prawns
Erythromycin	0.65–1.5 mg/l	Bacterial necrosis in crustaceans
Formalin (37% formaldehyde)	0.025 ml/l	Ectoparasites (use with malachite green)
Furazolidone	2–10 mg/l	Bacterial infections
Malachite green	0.1 mg/l	Ectoparasites (use with formalin)
Methylene blue	8–10 mg/l	Protozoal and fungal infections in crustaceans
Neomycin	10–100 mg/l for 2 days	Bacterial infections in prawns
Nifurpirinol	1 mg/l	Bacterial infections in prawns
Nystatin	100,000 units/l	Fungal infections in prawns
Oxytetracycline	60–250 mg/l 450 mg/kg feed 75 mg/kg orally or by injection into abdominal sinus	Bacterial infection in prawns *Vibrio* infection in prawn larvae Gaffkaemia in lobsters

Figure 30.20 Antimicrobial agents suitable for use in aquatic invertebrates.

Failure to respond

Not all affected fish will necessarily survive or recover and there are several reasons why treatment may fail despite thorough investigation and correct diagnosis. For example:

- In many cases, the severity of the disease in individuals is often greater than is initially appreciated, due to additional stress factors and the extent of tissue damage at a cellular level
- The original disease may be superseded by an equally debilitating secondary bacterial or fungal infection
- Incorrect diagnosis, inappropriate medication and resistance of the organism to treatment may affect the outcome
- Inactivation of the drug by chelation in hard water, UV irradiation in filter systems or high organic load in water may reduce the effect of in-water medications
- Various aspects relating to the pharmacokinetics of a drug and the inadequate intake of medicated food will limit the effectiveness of oral medications.

Adverse reactions

Many drugs used in fish health can be toxic to the fish, even when used at the recommended dose. For example, organophosphate, benzalkonium chloride and chloramine-T are more toxic in soft water than in hard water. Chloramine-T, formalin and malachite green are more toxic at low pH, whereas potassium permanganate is more toxic at high pH. Formalin

reduces the oxygen content of the water, and malachite green is a respiratory toxin; therefore both must be used with extreme care when treating fish with gill disease or anaemia.

Impurities and contamination of chemicals are equally hazardous and may not always be detectable. Paraformaldehyde, a white precipitate found in aged stocks of formalin, is very toxic to fish. Some impurities in chloramine-T can produce toxic compounds when in contact with metal surfaces.

In addition to direct adverse reactions, chemical reactions can take place between medications and other substances. For example, potassium permanganate and formalin are extremely toxic when mixed. Therefore, with a few exceptions, only one chemical at a time should be used in a pond or aquarium.

In general, antibacterial drugs are less hazardous than other medications. Despite this, accidental overdosing and variations in species sensitivity to antibacterial drugs may result in adverse reactions or death.

Injections often produce local bruising and haemorrhage but some drugs (e.g. long-acting oxytetracycline) can produce large swellings of sterile serosanguineous fluid when administered by intramuscular injection. Oxytetracycline has also been linked to suppression of the immune system in carp. Gentamicin may be nephrotoxic and sulphonamides can produce crystalluria and renal failure (Figure 30.21).

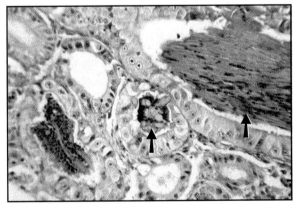

Figure 30.21 Histological section revealing crystals in the renal tubules (arrowed) of a goldfish following an overdose of potentiated sulphonamide that was given by injection. H&E stain, ×400 original magnification. © W.H. Wildgoose.

Human health and safety

This is a seriously neglected aspect of fish therapeutics. Many chemicals used to treat fish are hazardous to human health and it is essential to read the material safety data sheets. Not all dangerous chemicals produce an immediate effect or require long-term exposure. The health hazards may include carcinogenic, mutagenic or teratogenic effects (e.g. malachite green). The data sheet for a brand of trichlorfon states that artificial respiration and even tracheotomy may be required to save the life of humans who become affected by this organophosphate.

In addition to the inhalation hazard from chemical powders and dust, some antibacterial drugs (e.g. amoxycillin) may cause a hypersensitivity reaction to some handlers. While chloramine-T may be irritant to the skin, acriflavine and formaldehyde can produce sensitization by contact with skin. Appropriate protective clothing, such as disposable gloves and face masks, should be worn when handling these substances.

Legislation

Many aspects of fish health are controlled by legislation and these are discussed in Chapter 33. Most of the legislation applies to farmed food-fish but some is equally relevant to ornamental fish. The laws concerning the use of medicines relate primarily to consumer safety and drug residues. Different countries have their own legislation but areas that apply to fish medicines often include:

- Supply of drugs and prescription only medicines
- Restrictions on the use of medicines in particular species
- Incorporation of medicines into fish foods and the need for a medicated feedingstuffs (MFS) prescription
- Health and safety aspects of handling and disposal of medicines
- Environmental safety legislation (this may involve accidental contamination of waterways).

Consent forms

Few medicinal products are authorized for use in ornamental fish and consequently it is often necessary to use medicines outwith the data sheet recommendations. Veterinarians intending to use any such medicine are advised to obtain the written consent of the owner, who should be made fully aware of the possibility of side-effects and of the precautions related to administration of the medication. Consent forms should be drafted carefully and suitable examples may be obtained from various veterinary organizations or found in Bishop (2000).

Conclusion

Due to the diversity of environments in which ornamental fish live, it is not possible to provide a definitive guide to treatment in this book. However, we hope that we have provided enough information for the general practitioner to be able to approach fish therapeutics more confidently and follow a logical course of action. Improving the environment and husbandry is a vital part of therapy in fish. The use of any drug alone, without consideration of underlying management factors, is unlikely to resolve a health problem. Consequently, it is important to adopt a comprehensive approach to achieve a successful outcome.

Further reading and references

Andrews C, Exell A and Carrington N (1988) *The Interpet Manual of Fish Health*. Salamander Books, London

Bishop Y (ed.) (2000) *The Veterinary Formulary, 5th edn*. The Pharmaceutical Press, London

Brown L (ed.) (1993) *Aquaculture for Veterinarians: Fish Husbandry and Medicine*. Pergamon Press, Oxford

Burka JF, Hammell KL, Johnson GR, Rainnie DJ and Speare DJ (1997) Drugs in salmonid aquaculture – a review. *Journal of Veterinary Pharmacology and Therapeutics* **20**, 333–349

Carpenter JW, Mashima TY and Rupiper DJ (2001) *Exotic Animal Formulary*, 2nd edn. WB Saunders Co., Philadelphia

Dixon BA and Issvoran GS (1992) The activity of ceftiofur sodium for *Aeromonas* spp. isolated from ornamental fish. *Journal of Wildlife Diseases* **28** (3), 453–456

Gibson DR (1999) Health care in a large public aquarium: some case studies. *Fish Veterinary Journal* **3**, 40–42

Herwig N (1979) *Handbook of Drugs and Chemicals Used in the Treatment of Fish Diseases*. Charles C Thomas, Springfield, Illinois

Noga EJ (1996) *Fish Disease: Diagnosis and Treatment*. Mosby, St Louis, Missouri

Stoffengregen DA, Browser PR and Babish JG (1996) Antibacterial chemotherapeutants for finfish aquaculture: a synopsis of laboratory and field efficacy and safety studies. *Journal of Aquatic Animal Health* **8**, 181–207

Stoskopf MK (1999) Fish pharmacotherapeutics. In: *Zoo and Wild Animal Medicine, 4th edn*, ed. ME Fowler. pp. 182–189 WB Saunders, Philadelphia

Treves-Brown K (2000) *Applied Fish Pharmacology*. Kluwer Academic Publishers, Dordrecht, Netherlands

Trust TJ and Whitby JL (1976) Antibiotic resistance of bacteria in water containing ornamental fishes. *Antimicrobial Agents and Chemotherapy* **10** (4), 598–603

Türnau D, Schmidt H, Kürzinger H and Böhm KH (2000) Potency testing of β-glucan immuno-stimulating effect in food for ornamental fish. *Bulletin of the European Fish Pathologists Association* **20**(3), 143–147

Whitaker BR (1999) Preventative medicine programs for fish. In: *Zoo and Wild Animal Medicine, 4th edn*, ed. ME Fowler. pp. 163–181 WB Saunders, Philadelphia

Acknowledgements

The authors are grateful for the help and cooperation given by the manufacturers of the proprietary medications and to Keith Treves-Brown for his constructive comments on an early draft.

31

Surgery

Craig A. Harms and William H. Wildgoose

Fish can make excellent subjects for surgery if suitable measures are taken to cater for the patient's aquatic lifestyle. The decision to proceed to surgery in clinical cases can be motivated by rarity of the species involved, economic value of the patient or the owner's emotional attachment to the fish.

Anatomy

Knowledge of the patient's anatomy is critical to any surgical procedure, since there is some striking structural diversity between fish of different species. For example, within teleost fish, body form ranges from the familiar fusiform trout to the more unusual forms such as sea horses and flatfish. Internal fish anatomy is discussed in Chapter 16.

Anaesthesia

Establishing a safe and effective out-of-water anaesthesia protocol is the first step towards a successful surgical procedure. For short-duration procedures such as skin scrapings and gill biopsies that last less than 5 minutes, inexact addition of anaesthetics 'to effect' have traditionally been used. While this approach works for minor procedures, such imprecision is not advised for longer surgery, and continuous delivery of known concentrations of anaesthetic solutions is required. Anaesthetic delivery systems and protocols are discussed in Chapter 11.

Fish eyes do not adapt quickly to the bright light of the surgical theatre and anaesthetized fish should be shielded from glare.

Instrumentation

Surgical instruments commonly used in small animal practice are suitable for use on large fish but ocular or microsurgical equipment is usually required for small fish (Figure 31.1). Head loupe magnification with centre-mounted illumination is helpful for visualizing structures that are small or deep in the coelomic cavity. Access to the internal organs is greatly improved with the use of Gelpi retractors or self-retaining ocular retractors (Figure 31.2). Bipolar electrocautery can be used for haemostasis but must be used with caution in small fish to avoid excessive damage to surrounding tissues.

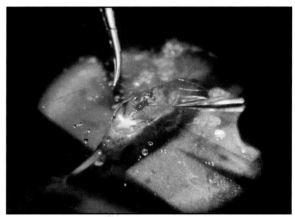

Figure 31.1 An operating microscope and microsurgical instruments are used to close a ventral midline incision in a gourami weighing 8 g. The fish is positioned in a V-shaped foam tray and covered with a clear plastic surgical drape.

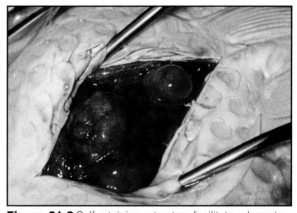

Figure 31.2 Self-retaining retractors facilitate adequate exposure to internal organs. Here, a ventral midline approach is used to remove an undifferentiated sarcoma from a koi. (Courtesy of Greg Lewbart.)

Presurgical investigation

Radiography and ultrasonography are recommended for presurgical evaluation. This helps to identify the best approach and delineate the surgical field, since even superficial lesions may have deep attachments to bone or internal organs. Fish are well suited for ultrasonographic examination, and two-colour Doppler imaging can be used to identify the location of major blood flow to a mass before surgical intervention.

Consent forms

As with all surgical procedures in any animal it is prudent to ask owners to sign a consent form, which may form part of a combined consent for anaesthesia and surgery. It is essential that the surgical risks involved be discussed according to the patient's health status. Written confirmation of the owner's informed consent can then be obtained. The animal's owner or authorized agent should be over 18 years of age. Signed consent forms should be kept for 2 years.

Preoperative preparation

- The fish can be positioned in a foam block with a V-shaped notch, cut to fit the individual patient
- The skin and natural mucus are major barriers to infection, therefore preparation of the surgical site should be minimal. A simple swipe along the intended incision site with a cotton swab soaked in sterile saline, or at most dilute povidone–iodine or chlorhexidine solution, to reduce gross contamination is often sufficient
- A clear plastic surgical drape has many advantages for fish surgery. The plastic helps to retain moisture around the fish, does not allow moisture to leak through and compromise the surgical field, and provides a working surface that stray suture material can contact without contamination. A rim of petroleum jelly can be used to adhere the drape to the fish, if desired
- Skin should be kept moist throughout the surgical procedure, taking care to avoid irrigating the incision site. Pre-soaking the surgical foam support and the use of a clear plastic surgical drape will help to prevent desiccation of the skin and fins
- Removing scales just along the incision line facilitates a smooth entry in those fish with substantial scales, but is not necessary for fine-scaled fish. In fish with bony scales, it may be necessary to cut between scales or make a small initial incision and extend it by cutting from the inside with a scalpel blade.

Techniques

In contrast to mammals, an abundance of freely mobile skin is rarely found in fish; therefore skin defects are difficult to close and must often be managed by second intention healing. Consequently, the osmotic requirements of the fish should be considered and salt should be added to freshwater systems at the rate of 1–3 g/l to reduce the osmotic gradient between the tissues and the environment. The body wall is often inelastic, unless the coelomic cavity is distended by fully developed gonads or a mass, and retraction is often required to maintain coelomic visualization.

Wound closure

A good suturing technique and the natural responses involved in wound healing (see Chapter 15) ensure a watertight seal at the surgical site.

Suture material

The choice of suture material is a personal decision and many types have been used successfully in fish.

Synthetic absorbable material may not be readily absorbed in fish and those that are normally absorbed rapidly in mammalian tissues (e.g. polyglactin) can exhibit long-term retention in fish. Anecdotally, polyglactin 910 and polydioxanone used during intracoelomic surgery or in the muscle layer of an abdominal closure have been recovered intact over a year later. In other instances, polydioxanone skin sutures in wild fish implanted with transmitters for population studies have disappeared in a matter of months, possibly through a process of foreign body expulsion rather than hydrolysis or absorption.

It is best to use a monofilament material to minimize the risk of bacterial infection – particularly for skin closure, where bacterial ingress through the capillary effect of braided suture materials may occur.

Other factors to consider are tissue reactivity and healing time. Polyglactin elicits a strong inflammatory reaction in the skin, compared with strong to intermediate reactions for chromic catgut (which exhibits short retention time in skin) and lesser reactions for polyglyconate and monofilament nylon. The healing time is reduced with suture materials that provoke fewer inflammatory reactions.

Suture technique

Needles with a cutting tip improve skin penetration. Skin closures using simple interrupted, simple continuous and continuous Ford interlocking patterns have all been used with satisfactory results. A single- or double-layer closure can be used, depending on the thickness of the body wall. There is rarely any dead space to eliminate, since the subcutaneous layer is minimal and the dermis is tightly adhered to the underlying muscle. Skin sutures should be removed when the incision is healed (usually in 3–4 weeks in uncomplicated cases).

Tissue adhesive

The use of cyanoacrylate tissue adhesive is recommended by some authors for skin closure and to promote a watertight seal. However, its use in fish is problematic, both alone and in combination with sutures. Although application of tissue adhesive can reduce the surgical time, cyanoacrylate causes severe dermatitis in some species of fish. When used alone it is associated with a higher incidence of wound breakdown due to mucus production, which elevates the tissue adhesive layer away from the skin. When tissue adhesives are used in addition to sutures, the sutures retain the adhesive with mucus trapped beneath, creating extra drag on the sutures. Mucus production and rapid epidermal cell migration are normal responses to injury and quickly provide a watertight seal.

Surgical staples

Surgical staples have been used successfully in fish and theoretically reduce skin closure time when compared with suturing. In some species, however, the tissue handling characteristics of the skin are unfavourable for consistent staple placement.

Postoperative care

As in other species, antimicrobial use should not be considered a substitute for poor technique, even though strictly sterile procedures are rarely achievable in fish surgery. The efficacy of prophylactic perioperative antibiotic therapy in fish has not been systematically evaluated. The need for antibiotic medication depends on the nature of the procedure, the location where it is performed (i.e. in the field or clinic), the conditions to which the fish is returned and the degree of postoperative monitoring.

- A single intramuscular dose of enrofloxacin given at the rate of 5 mg/kg or oxytetracycline at 10 mg/kg may be administered immediately prior to surgery
- Antibiotics can be continued if the surgery involves bowel penetration or repair of contaminated wounds
- A single application of povidone–iodine ointment to the closed incision has reduced the incidence of fungal infections, even though retention time of the ointment is limited
- The use of postoperative analgesia in fish has not been fully evaluated but butorphanol at 0.1–0.4 mg/kg, given as a single intramuscular injection just before recovery from anaesthesia, has produced no evident adverse effects and may provide beneficial effects
- Addition of salt to freshwater systems, at the rate of 1–3 g/l, may ease electrolyte imbalances that freshwater fish can experience following anaesthesia and epithelial disruption, as well as inhibit secondary fungal infection of the incision site
- Raising the water temperature to the upper limits of the preferred temperature range for coldwater species will increase the rate of healing. For example (and where practical), koi and goldfish kept in water that is slowly raised to and maintained at 20–25°C will heal more quickly than those kept in outdoor ponds, particularly in winter.

Surgical procedures

Minor procedures that can be performed quickly without continuous delivery of anaesthesia include debridement of skin ulcers, trimming necrotic fin lesions, excision of embedded parasites (e.g. encysted digenetic trematodes), treatment of corneal ulcers and implantation of microchip transponders.

Skin ulcers

The surgical treatment of skin ulcers is commonly performed in pond fish such as koi and goldfish. These ulcerations can occur on all areas of the body, including the head, mouth, eye and fins. They may be the result of physical trauma from fighting, predation, ectoparasites and bad handling but also develop from chronic infection with *Aeromonas* and other bacteria. Various methods of treatment have been described and much depends on personal preference. The following is a common approach:

1. The fish is anaesthetized and removed from the water.
2. The wound is debrided by removing necrotic tissue with dry cotton buds or gauze swabs. Any damaged scales should be plucked out (Figure 31.3a). Exposed areas of bone and cartilage must be cleaned thoroughly and loose edges may require removal with rongeurs.
3. Dilute povidone–iodine is applied topically and the site is dried (Figure 31.3b).
4. A waterproof preparation is applied to the lesion (Figure 31.3c). Two commonly used products are Orahesive® and Orabase® (ConvaTec), which contain equal quantities of gelatin, pectin and methyl cellulose and are used to treat mouth ulcers in humans.

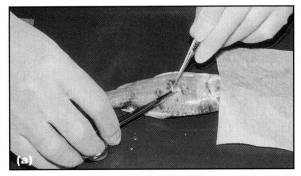
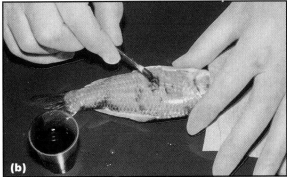
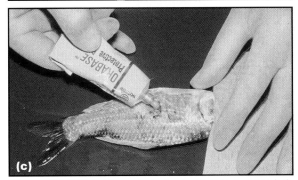

Figure 31.3 Debridement of a body ulcer in a young koi. (a) Loose scales and necrotic tissue are removed using scissors and forceps. A drape covers the eyes and protects them from the glare of the operating lights. (b) Dilute povidone–iodine is applied to the ulcer with cotton buds to ensure thorough disinfection of the site. (c) A waterproof paste is applied to the ulcer to provide temporary sealing of the wound and help to retain some of the skin disinfectant. (© W.H. Wildgoose.)

The debridement is performed only once, since epithelialization will be impeded by further interference unless there is persistent tissue necrosis. An appropriate antibacterial is given by injection and repeated at suitable intervals, or a suitable formulation is given as an in-feed preparation. If any underlying bacterial infection is treated and all necrotic tissue is removed, healing should take 2–4 weeks (Figure 31.4).

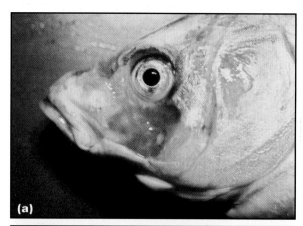

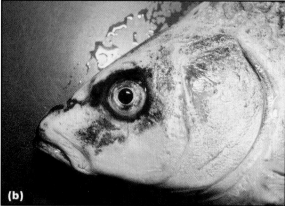

Figure 31.4 Ulceration on the face of an adult koi following injury from a dog bite. (a) This photograph was taken 2 weeks after initial debridement of the wound. Epithelialization has covered most of the wound, which appears less inflamed as a result. (b) The same fish photographed 16 weeks later, showing complete healing of the site. Restoration of normal pigmentation is a slow process and the final coloration may be unpredictable. (© W.H. Wildgoose.)

Masses

The surgical removal of external and internal masses of neoplastic and parasitic origin is a common procedure in clinical practice (Figure 31.5). Dermal masses are difficult to excise completely and are likely to recur if clean margins are not achieved. If excision is attempted, wide and deep margins should be removed despite the impossibility of primary closure. The non-compliant nature of fish skin and underlying muscle necessitates second intention healing following excision of external masses. Skin defects resulting from tumour removal can be treated topically with products such as silver sulphadiazine cream. For example, lip fibromas in freshwater angelfish have been treated successfully by simple excision (Figure 31.6) followed by application of topical antibiotic ointment.

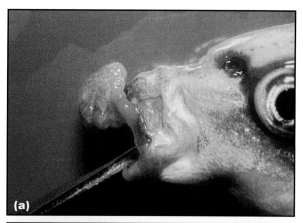

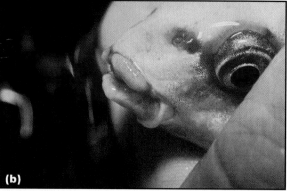

Figure 31.5 (a) A papilloma on the top lip of an adult mirror carp, which interfered with normal feeding and respiration. It was not possible to excise the whole lesion, due to attachment to the underlying cartilage around the mouth. (b) The same fish photographed 4 weeks later. The remaining epidermal hyperplasia on the lip did not cause problems during feeding and resolved over several months. (© W.H. Wildgoose.)

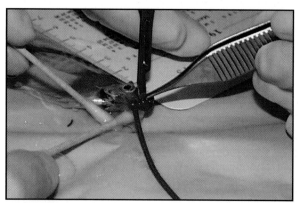

Figure 31.6 Lip fibromas in freshwater angelfish may interfere with normal feeding. Wide excision is not always achievable or necessary, since debulking the lesion can restore normal functional morphology, and recurrence is rare.

Coelomic masses are removed through a standard ventral midline approach. For abdominal exploration and/or mass removal, the following surgical procedure can be applied.

1. The ventral body wall may be swabbed with dilute (1:10) povidone–iodine solution (Figure 31.7a).
2. The scales are removed from the area of the planned incision site with forceps.

3. A ventral midline abdominal incision is made, beginning immediately caudal to the base of the pectoral fins and extending to within 1 cm of the vent (Figure 31.7b).
4. The pelvic girdle (Figure 31.7c) can be separated along the midline using the scalpel blade, or in larger fish by using an osteotome. This can be repaired with steel sutures if necessary or simply by incorporation into the suture line in smaller individuals. Pelvic fin abnormalities following this procedure are rare.
5. Lateral extensions from the midline incision may be necessary for adequate exposure, and to deviate around the vent.
6. Self-retaining retractors improve visualization within the coelomic cavity (Figure 31.7d).
7. Sharp and blunt dissection may be used to free a mass from its attachments. Larger vessels may be divided and ligated, and bipolar cautery can be used to coagulate smaller vascular pedicles.
8. The muscle can be closed in a simple continuous pattern (Figure 31.7e).
9. The skin is closed in a simple interrupted (Figure 31.7f), simple continuous or continuous Ford interlocking pattern.

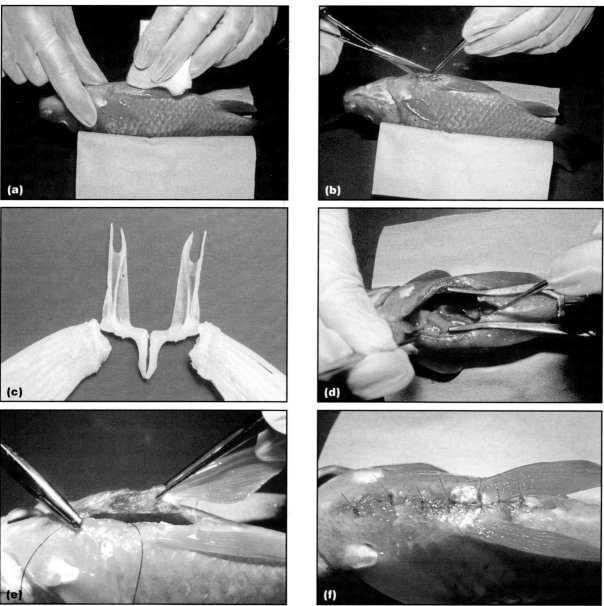

Figure 31.7 (a) Preparation for midline abdominal surgery. Any excess body mucus is removed and dilute povidone–iodine solution is applied. Large scales, where present, are plucked from the incision line with forceps. (b) A ventral midline incision is made with a scalpel and extended caudally to the pelvis. (c) The pelvic girdle of a goldfish. This simple bony structure is embedded in the muscles of the body wall and joined in the midline by a fibrous junction. In old fish, the bones become ossified and fused together. (d) After sectioning the pelvis, the midline incision is extended towards the vent. Retractors improve visualization and access to the internal organs. (e) Closure of the muscle layer with absorbable monofilament suture material using a continuous suture pattern. (f) Closure of the skin with non-absorbable monofilament suture material using a simple interrupted suture pattern. The sutures are removed after 3–4 weeks. (© W.H. Wildgoose.)

Enucleation

Advanced infectious, inflammatory and neoplastic diseases of the eye may require enucleation (Figure 31.8a). Although this is a relatively uncomplicated procedure, damage to the multiple branches of cranial nerves V and VII, which traverse the retrobulbar space, should be avoided.

1. In most cases, the fish will be in lateral recumbency with the affected eye positioned uppermost.

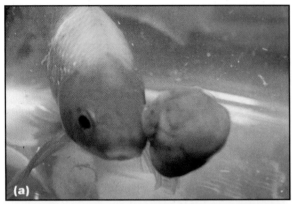

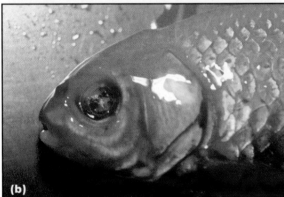

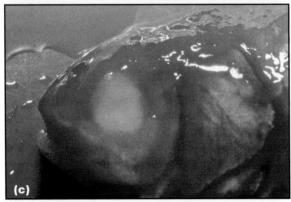

Figure 31.8 (a) An 8-year-old goldfish with a large fibroma involving most of the eye. The tumour had increased in size over a period of 3 months and was removed by enucleation. (b) Heat cauterization was used to control haemorrhage following the enucleation. The empty socket was packed with a waterproof paste and the fish was given systemic antibacterial treatment. (c) The fish was examined 20 months later: the original socket had become a shallow depression, with some resorption of the surrounding facial bone. There was no pigmentation at the surgical site.

2. The eye and periocular tissues may be swabbed with dilute (1:10) povidone–iodine solution.
3. A pair of curved tenotomy scissors is used for blunt dissection of the globe from the circumorbital sulcus.
4. The muscular attachments are transected and the eye removed by transecting the optic nerve and vessels.
5. Haemostasis can be achieved by direct pressure or heat cautery (Figure 31.8b) or with a drop of 2.5% phenylephrine hydrochloride.

The orbit may be left to heal by filling with granulation tissue. Although the empty socket is not cosmetically pleasing, the site will heal quite well. In time, there is often facial remodelling of the bones and the socket becomes less obvious (Figure 31.8c). In some cases, an ocular prosthesis has been implanted (Nadelstein *et al.*, 1997) but long-term retention has been problematic.

Pseudobranchectomy

The teleost respiratory system comprises four paired gill arches situated in two opercular cavities (Chapter 17). Most teleosts also have a pseudobranch located dorsally in the opercular cavity (Figure 31.9). The function of the pseudobranch is uncertain but efferent blood from the pseudobranch passes to the choroid of the eye, suggesting that one function may be oxygenation of the eye.

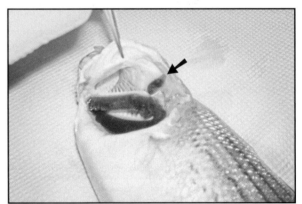

Figure 31.9 The pseudobranch (arrowed) of a striped bass is located in the dorsal opercular cavity. Pseudobranchectomy is one potential treatment for idiopathic gaseous exophthalmos.

Removal of the pseudobranch in conjunction with aspiration of retrobulbar gas has been used as a treatment for idiopathic gaseous exophthalmos in some fish when environmental and medical management have failed. The rationale of this procedure is related to the hypothesized function of the pseudobranch in regulating gas delivery to the eye. Since the pseudobranch is primarily a vascular structure, haemostasis is the primary intraoperative concern during its excision.

Lacerations and skin injury

Lacerations due to bird strike or other trauma are repaired using standard techniques. Lavage of the exposed underlying muscle tissue with a dilute chlorhexidine solution or saline before closure is essential. Skin defects pose an increased osmotic burden on fish, therefore replacement of loose skin flaps is beneficial for maintaining electrolyte balance. In koi, much of their economic value depends on the dorsal coloration and pattern, and therefore a cosmetic restoration is highly desirable.

Swim-bladder disorders

Abnormalities of the swim-bladder are common causes of buoyancy disorders and are readily diagnosed by radiography. Over-inflation, herniation and torsion more frequently affect the caudal portions of the swim-bladder.

Partial pneumocystectomy (swim-bladder reduction) may be performed in cases refractory to environmental manipulation or repeated aspiration. Due to the retroperitoneal position of the swim-bladder, dorsolateral extensions from the ventral midline incision may be necessary for adequate exposure of the organ. The swim-bladder is a fragile structure and may collapse completely if torn; therefore its attachments to the body wall must be carefully dissected.

Removal of the abnormal caudal portion of the swim-bladder may be accomplished by placing an encircling ligature before excision. This leaves the normal cranial portions intact, together with the structures involved in gas exchange, namely the gas gland, the oval and, in physostomes, the pneumatic duct.

Negative buoyancy may result following swim-bladder reduction. Fish can adapt to this condition by behaviour change but a non-abrasive substrate may be necessary to prevent decubital ulcers.

Gonadectomy

There is little indication for routine spays and castrations in fish but ovariectomies have been performed in fish that are egg-bound. Fish reproductive organs are elongated and consequently a long incision is required for their surgical removal. The primary blood supply lies at the cranial pole of the gonad and care must be taken at the caudal pole to avoid damage to the excretory systems. Free eggs released into the coelomic cavity following the breakdown of the ovarian wall at the time of ovulation can be removed by lavage and suction.

Ovarian prolapse

Repair of ovarian prolapse may be performed by applying an encircling ligature and then excising the protruding tissue (Lewbart, 1998). Depending on the fish's spawning condition, manual stripping of eggs may be required to prevent recurrence: a sterile syringe case is inserted through the genital pore to prevent immediate prolapse while eggs are massaged and expressed through the barrel of the syringe case. The use of a purse-string suture may be helpful.

Diagnostic biopsy

Liver and kidney biopsy techniques have been developed and these could be adapted for a diagnostic purpose.

Liver biopsy

The liver is readily accessible in the cranioventral portion of the coelomic cavity. It can be approached via a left caudoventral to craniodorsal incision, dorsal to the pectoral fin. No special haemostasis is required for the liver biopsy site, provided the large vessels are not damaged.

Kidney biopsy

The kidney occupies a retroperitoneal position dorsal to the swim-bladder and ventral to the spinal column. In some species (e.g. trout) it is a fused, long thin organ separated functionally into an anterior haematopoietic organ (anterior kidney) grading caudally into an excretory organ (posterior kidney). In other species (e.g. catfish, koi, goldfish) the two segments can be physically separate.

- Access to the kidney is severely restricted for much of its length by the swim-bladder
- The posterior kidney is approached via a paramedian incision midway between the lateral line and the pelvic fin
- Gonads and mesentery are retracted or partially excised, and the swim-bladder is gently teased away from the kidney by blunt dissection
- The biopsy should be unilateral to avoid compromising contralateral renal function
- Haemorrhage during kidney biopsy can be reduced by application of cyanoacrylate tissue adhesive to the scalpel blade just before incising the kidney. Direct pressure or a drop of 2.5% phenylephrine hydrochloride could also be used
- Nephrocalcinosis is a common sequel of kidney biopsy but does not have a major effect on survival or reproduction.

Percutaneous kidney aspirates: With knowledge of renal anatomy for the particular target species, percutaneous kidney aspirates can be obtained for cytology and culture.

In rainbow trout and other species, the anterior kidney curves ventrally at its cranial limit and lies just beneath the medial surface of the branchial chamber. At this location, it is readily accessible for fine needle aspiration by simply lifting the operculum and visualizing the kidney through the translucent membrane.

In koi, an enlarged segment of the posterior kidney sits in a small saddle created at the isthmus between the two chambers of the swim-bladder and is a useful target for percutaneous kidney biopsy. The needle is inserted perpendicular to the lateral body wall at the level of insertion of the pelvic fin, just dorsal (by 2% of the fish's total length) to the lateral line. The needle is advanced through the muscle layers to the midline of the fish. Gas may be obtained if the swim-bladder is mistakenly penetrated, but a single puncture is not a serious complication. Laceration of the dorsal aorta is a potentially fatal complication of this procedure if the needle is directed too far dorsally.

Because of conformational differences between species, this technique should not be expected to apply to all species and is even problematic in some varieties of koi. Radiographic verification of the landmarks would be warranted in the case of a valuable fish.

Endoscopy

Endoscopic techniques may be used for sex identification and for direct visualization and biopsy of visceral organs (see Chapter 14). Tightly packed coelomic viscera require insufflation to allow instrument manipulation and adequate visualization. Insufflated gas should be removed as completely as possible before closure to avoid excess positive buoyancy problems but residual gas will eventually be absorbed.

Endoscopy may also be useful for the removal of oral and gastric foreign bodies.

Microchip implants

The implantation of microchip transponders in pet animals is now routine in general veterinary practice. These devices register a unique alpha-numerical code when activated by a suitable scanner, and this can be used to identify the individual against details kept on a database. Harmonization of microchip standards across Europe has allowed a more widespread use of these implants but due to the limited range of detection of some scanners it is essential to implant the microchips at the same site in the same class of animal. In the case of fish, guidelines from the British Veterinary Zoological Society advise deep implantation in the midline, anterior to the dorsal fin. Other sites used include the left side at the base of the dorsal fin in fish over 30 cm in length and in the coelomic cavity in smaller fish.

Telemetry implants

Veterinarians may occasionally be consulted by fish researchers for assistance in the implantation of telemetric transmitters. These devices can transmit sonic or radio signals.

Sonic transmitters are used in marine environments, where radio waves are rapidly attenuated; signals are received on a submerged hydrophone. Because there is no antenna, sonic transmitter implantation involves a simple laparotomy, insertion and closure.

Radiotelemetry transmitters often require a length of antenna external to the fish in order to extend the range to a useful distance. The antenna should not exit through the primary incision but should be threaded through a cannula passed at an acute angle through the lateral body wall. Maximizing the distance between internal and external ports reduces any potential contamination of the body cavity. This chronic communication between the coelomic cavity and the external environment is problematic and local inflammation at the antenna exit site may be readily visible in recaptured fish. However, good long-term survival has been observed and useful data on habitat utilization and migration have been collected in fish fitted with internal transmitter/external antenna combinations.

As a rule, the implants should weigh less than 2% of the fish's bodyweight. Transmitter implants should not put pressure on vital organs and should be positioned away from the incision site. Expulsion of the implant can be a problem, possibly dependent on species, transmitter coating, environmental conditions or surgical technique.

Further reading and references

Harms CA and Lewbart GA (2000) Surgery in fish. *Veterinary Clinics of North America: Exotic Animal Practice* **3**, 759–774

Lewbart GA (1998) *Self-Assessment Colour Review of Ornamental Fish*. Manson Publishing, London

Nadelstein B, Bakal R and Lewbart GA (1997) Orbital exenteration and placement of a prosthesis in fish. *Journal of the American Medical Association* **211**, 603–606

Stoskopf MK (1993) Surgery. In: *Fish Medicine*, ed. MK Stoskopf, pp. 91–97. WB Saunders, Philadelphia

Wildgoose WH (2000) Fish surgery: an overview. *Fish Veterinary Journal* **5**, 22–36

32

Aquatic invertebrates

Colin Grist

Keeping invertebrates in aquaria has become increasingly popular, both in domestic tanks and zoological collections. The science of invertebrate husbandry is still in its infancy, with little known about the specific requirements of many species, and disease diagnosis and treatment still poorly understood. However, observations by aquarists over many years have provided much information about the behaviour of invertebrates in captivity. Water quality monitoring and control is now better understood and with other environmental factors also taken into consideration, it is possible to maintain a wide range of species in a healthy condition.

General aspects

Invertebrates should only be maintained in facilities constructed from non-corrosive materials. Many metals are toxic to invertebrates – including copper, which is commonly used to treat marine fish. Some plastics may also contain harmful chemicals that can leach into the aquarium water. Food grade materials and those made specifically for aquarium use are safe.

Heating
Tropical species require thermostat-controlled heating systems that should be powerful enough to provide an even temperature throughout the entire volume of water.

Filtration
Most invertebrates kept in aquaria originate from coral reefs, where environmental conditions are very stable. This stability must be maintained in the captive environment by careful management of the filtration system in conjunction with water quality monitoring and control. Standard filtration units that provide a combination of mechanical, chemical and biological filtration are readily available for aquaria and are discussed in Chapters 6 and 7. There are a wide variety of water testing kits available for monitoring the standard parameters such as ammonia, nitrite, nitrate and pH.

Water movement
Strong water movement is required to improve oxygen distribution and gas exchange. A layer of stagnant water surrounds all submerged solid objects, including living organisms. This is reduced by strong water movement, which prevents impaired respiration and improves other metabolic functions. Water movement can be achieved using several small water pumps and 'wave-making' devices that are commercially available.

Salinity
In marine aquaria, it is best to use a commercial artificial seawater mixture that is added to fresh tap water. Artificial preparations are sterile and also have a better buffering capacity to maintain stable carbonate hardness and pH, which are vital to a large number of organisms.

Relatively few species of freshwater invertebrates, mostly crustaceans and gastropods, are of interest to aquarists. However, the required conditions (e.g. hardness) may be specialized for certain species.

Lighting
Correct light intensity is critical for organisms such as hard (true or stony) corals. Many suitable lighting systems are available but it is important to research the specific requirements for the species in question.

Maintenance
Maintenance of water quality involves regular testing, performing water changes (10–20% weekly) and servicing the filters in order to keep conditions optimum and stable.

The calcium concentration is very important to many invertebrates, especially hard corals and crustaceans. If the correct concentration is difficult to maintain, a calcium reactor should be used. This consists of a closed cylinder filled with aragonite (coral sand) through which aquarium water is slowly circulated. Carbon dioxide is injected into the cylinder and its acidic properties slowly dissolve the alkaline sand, allowing calcium to be delivered to the aquarium.

'Living rock'
The use of 'living rock' in coral reef aquaria is very popular. This natural material is collected and shipped without being allowed to dry, so that any organisms on it remain alive. In addition to providing habitat, the special conditioning powers of such rock on aquarium water are well known. It is possible for the more experienced aquarist to maintain a very stable aquarium using this rock as a means of filtration, sometimes with no equipment other than a foam fractionator.

Disease and medications

There is very little detailed information about specific diseases in many aquatic invertebrate groups. Most research has focused on those that are of economic value, especially food-producing species. Good water quality and correct environmental conditions are of paramount importance in maintaining healthy specimens and failure to provide them inevitably results in secondary disease or poor growth. It is equally essential to avoid incompatible species and an inappropriate diet.

The standard methods of investigation in identifying disease in fish can equally be applied to invertebrates. Water quality tests, wet mount preparations and histopathological examinations are all useful diagnostic techniques.

Several common medicinal products (e.g. copper, acriflavine, organophosphates) used to treat diseases in fish are toxic to invertebrates, but other medications such as formalin, malachite green and many antibacterial agents can be used safely. Most drugs are administered in the water; a list of suitable products can be found in Chapter 30.

Anaesthesia

Anaesthetic procedures for aquatic invertebrates are not well developed but they can be anaesthetized using similar products to those used in fish (see Chapter 11). MS222 and benzocaine can be used safely but dosages vary dramatically between the orders and species. For example, it may take up to an hour to induce anaesthesia in crustaceans using MS222 at 500 mg/l. Therefore in large lobsters and crabs, isobutanol injected at the rate of 0.1 ml/kg into the abdomen produces anaesthesia within 2 minutes. Ethanol at 20 ml/l induces anaesthesia in octopuses and other cephalopods. Recovery from waterborne agents can be hastened by placing the animal in fresh water with bubbling oxygen. Greater detail of these and other agents can be found in Ross and Ross (1999).

Euthanasia

The most effective method of killing many invertebrates is to use an overdose of anaesthetic. When respiratory movements cease, the brain should be destroyed to ensure that no recovery is possible.

Invertebrate groups

Although the underlying requirements of all invertebrates are similar, different groups may have certain specific requirements so that they may be kept successfully in captivity. In general, the conditions for keeping corals are adequate for most coral reef invertebrates but more specific requirements will be covered under the relevant section. The following is a brief overview of common invertebrate families. It is not exhaustive and there are many other groups, such as sponges and sea squirts, that are not within the scope of this chapter.

Corals

Corals can be split into two groups: soft corals and hard corals. Within their tissues they contain photosynthetic algae known as zooxanthellae and rely on these for certain nutrient by-products from the photosynthetic process. It is because of these algae that many corals require high levels of illumination in order to survive themselves. The true or hard corals secrete a calcareous material and lay down structures in a variety of forms unique to each species (Figures 32.1 and 32.2). The combination of this material and the bonding nature of coralline algae creates coral reefs. Soft corals (Figure 32.3) do not secrete such material.

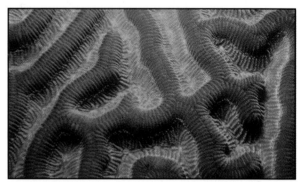

Figure 32.1 Brain corals (*Leptoria* spp.) are typical hard corals that receive most of their nutrition from the symbiotic algae in their tissues. They require intensive lighting and very good water quality. (© W.H. Wildgoose.)

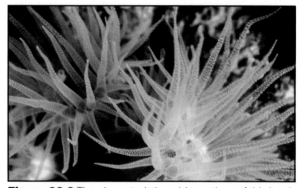

Figure 32.2 The characteristic golden polyps of this hard coral, *Tubastrea* sp., only become extended at night. Unlike many other corals, it does not contain zooxanthellae algae and lives in darkened areas. (© W.H. Wildgoose.)

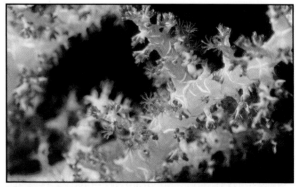

Figure 32.3 The white calcium spicules help to support the water-filled structure of this cauliflower coral, a type of soft coral. It does not contain zooxanthellae but expands and it is most active at night. (© W.H. Wildgoose.)

Hard corals reproduce sexually by releasing masses of small cream-coloured egg packets and sperm into the water column. This event is synchronized with millions of corals spawning at exactly the same time. This has also been observed to a limited extent in aquaria.

Light

In order to maintain corals in a healthy condition in the aquarium, strong lighting with a colour temperature of 10,000°K is recommended. This is possible using fluorescent lamps designed for the purpose, but metal halide illumination penetrates the water more efficiently. The photoperiod should be 12–14 hours per day. If the illumination is insufficient, the zooxanthellae will either die or vacate the corals, causing them to lose their colour and turn white. Since photosynthetic corals are unable to survive without their zooxanthellae, they will also eventually die.

Feeding

Corals rely to a great extent on the nutrients provided by zooxanthellae. However, they can also catch zooplankton with their stinging cells (nematocysts) by extending their tentacles into the water column. Liquidized shrimps and shellfish can be offered once a week by dropping the solution into water currents within the aquarium. Hatched brine shrimp nauplii (*Artemia*) are also excellent food for corals.

Water quality

On a natural reef, the water is warm, very clear, rich in oxygen and low in nutrients. There is also a lot of water movement. These conditions must be replicated in the aquarium if corals are to survive. Good filtration is necessary to ensure water clarity and quality, coupled with strict routine maintenance to avoid excess nutrient levels. Conditions must remain stable and the various water quality parameters that should be strictly maintained include:

- Salinity 33 g/l (SG 1.024)
- pH 8.3
- Temperature 26°C
- Nitrate 20–40 mg/l
- Temporary (carbonate) hardness 6–8 °KH
- Calcium carbonate concentration approximately 400 mg/l.

Note that it is important to check the calcium concentration if the temporary (carbonate) hardness falls below 6 °KH.

New stock

Only healthy animals should be purchased and specimens that show signs of tissue damage should be avoided. A healthy specimen should always have a clean, intact and firm appearance. Corals may sustain damage in transit, either from poor handling or from poor water conditions. Some fleshy corals occasionally have sections of tissue detaching from their calcareous 'skeleton' but this often heals when the coral is placed into good water conditions.

A strong sulphurous smell may develop from dead organisms on the rock, which often appears as a black patch. The smell and black patches may also occur with progressive tissue degeneration that advances up the stem of the coral. This may be caused by pathogenic bacteria or protozoans, and may be accompanied by a brown jelly-like substance, or a white film.

White film on a coral is due to excess mucus production following stress caused by poor handling and shipment. This will resolve when the coral has settled into its new environment.

Many corals offered for sale, particularly the branching types, are 'cuttings' from a larger head, and may appear to have broken edges (Figure 32.4). These heal easily and quickly.

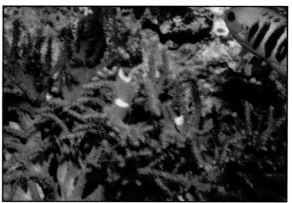

Figure 32.4 Physical injury has caused a few branches to break off from this hard coral (*Acropora* sp.). The areas of exposed white flesh usually heal uneventfully over several weeks if the coral is kept in good water conditions. (© W.H. Wildgoose.)

New corals may be given a short freshwater bath for 2–3 minutes to avoid introducing ectoparasitic diseases into aquarium. To reduce the risk of further stress, it is essential that the water temperature and pH in the bath are the same as the water from which the coral has been taken.

Specific diseases

Much of what is known about coral diseases may only be speculation at present. Diseases affecting corals in the wild are rarely encountered in the aquarium, although 'black band disease' and 'white band disease' are seen with a characteristic indication of tissue recession.

The most significant cause of death in captive corals is known as rapid tissue necrosis (RTN). Clinical signs of RTN include changing colour (often darker and more pinkish) and a strong odour of decomposition that can be detected some distance away from the aquarium. The polyps will be withdrawn. Mucus production is reduced and becomes thicker and stickier prior to actual tissue death, when the necrotic tissue sloughs rapidly (Figure 32.5). The condition appears to be highly infectious and will rapidly spread through a collection. If early signs are noted it is possible to transfer the coral to another tank, where the process

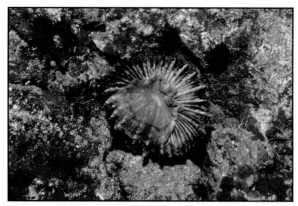

Figure 32.5 The ridged radial skeleton of this hard coral has become exposed due to the effects of rapid tissue necrosis. The fleshy tissue on the surface has become discoloured and is peeling off. (© W.H. Wildgoose.)

may slow down to some degree. The best and most successful solution at present is fragmentation, in which a section of still healthy coral is cut away and allowed to recover in optimum conditions.

Aggression results in corals vying for the best position by extending their tentacles and stinging their neighbours. This causes severe damage and even death; therefore care should be taken to avoid this problem by ensuring adequate spacing.

Predation by butterflyfish, gastropods and nudibranchs that feed on nematocysts can cause significant damage to corals, but this is often species-specific.

Anemones

As with the corals, anemones belong to the phylum Cnidaria. The basic anatomy of corals and anemones is the same, except that an anemone exists as a single polyp, whilst corals are colonial polyps connected by a membrane. Anemones also possess zooxanthellae and require strong illumination.

A unique feature of the anemones is their ability to roam using their single 'foot'. When they are first introduced into the aquarium, they will often spend several days or weeks wandering until they find a position that seems to suit them best. They usually settle quickly if conditions are good.

The most popular species found in aquaria tend to be rock dwellers but some species, like the tube anemones, live partly buried in sand. Some species have a commensal association with anemone fish and survive much better when kept with these fish in the aquarium.

Feeding

Anemones are capable of paralysing fish and other invertebrates with their nematocysts and draw them into their mouth with their tentacles. Anemones should be fed individually by offering them small chunks of fish or prawn, once or twice a week, depending on the species and its size.

Water quality

This should be the same as for corals where reef species are concerned, although some like very strong water movement. Temperate species do not require heating and the use of a chilling system may be necessary.

New stock

Only healthy full-bodied specimens without obvious tissue damage should be selected. They should be introduced gradually by mixing the transport water with that from the aquarium.

Specific diseases

Little is known about the diseases of anemones but lesions similar to RTN in corals have been observed occasionally. Unhealthy anemones either disintegrate rapidly or close up into a tight ball and gradually shrink over a period of time (e.g. several weeks), then die. The cause of this is unknown.

Disc anemones

Also known as mushroom corals, these belong to the Order Corallimorpharia and are often regarded as intermediate between corals and anemones. Their internal morphology is closer to that of hard corals but their general appearance is more like anemones. They are relatively small and make attractive additions to a tropical marine aquarium and several may inhabit one rock. They are generally hardy and in a well kept aquarium will reproduce by sexual reproduction, budding or division.

Feeding

Disc anemones rely greatly on the nourishment provided by their symbiont algae, but supplementary foods must be offered once or twice per week. A liquidized mixture of fish, shrimp and shellfish can be offered by delivering it directly down a small plastic tube or by transmitting it freely throughout the aquarium water. Filtration must always be operating when this type of food is used. Newly hatched *Artemia* nauplii can also be offered.

Water quality

Water conditions are not quite so critical as for corals and other anemones but, nevertheless, it is always good practice to maintain a high standard.

New stock

Specimens with a wrinkled withered appearance should be avoided. Before release into the aquarium, the temperature and pH should be the same as the transport water before release. Sudden shock will often cause polyps to vacate their rock and they may find it difficult to become re-established.

Specific diseases

Disc anemones appear relatively resistant to disease and other ailments.

Colonial anemones

These zoanthids superficially resemble corals, with their short stems and small diameter. They are generally very hardy in the aquarium and are commonly seen living in organically polluted areas in the wild. They propagate asexually by producing daughter buds from the parent polyp, which can grow to full size in around 6 months.

Feeding

The zooxanthellae provide most nourishment but supplementary offerings of zooplankton (e.g. newly hatched *Artemia*) is recommended.

Water quality

Although zoanthids are hardy, they are best kept in conditions similar to those required by corals and survive best in a strong flow of water.

Specific diseases

Colonial anemones are prone to being smothered by filamentous algae. This can be prevented by maintaining good water quality.

Jellyfish

Jellyfish are related to corals and anemones, and also possess nematocysts. Unlike their benthic relatives, jellyfish are able to swim in open water. Modern public aquaria commonly display a variety of jellyfish, particularly the moon jelly, whereas the most common species found in hobbyist tanks is the upside-down jelly, which characteristically spends much of its time lying upside-down on the substrate looking more like an anemone, although it can swim. It is very important for open-water species to have water currents, to prevent them from making contact with solid objects (which may cause them to fragment very easily).

Ctenophores, commonly known as sea-walnuts or comb-jellies, are also commonly kept in public aquaria and are interesting because of their bioluminescence. Their husbandry requirements are similar to those of jellyfish.

Feeding

Newly hatched *Artemia* and rotifers are good for small recently metamorphosed polyps.

Water quality

Water quality is as for corals and with steady, but not aggressive, water movement. Many species, other than upside-down jellies, require chilled water.

Specific diseases

It is possible that the early developmental stages (i.e. ephyrae) are vulnerable to bacterial and protozoan infections. The most common problem in adult medusae is damage caused by parasitic arthropods or from contact with solid objects. Nothing can be done once damage has been sustained.

Molluscs

Considering the vast size of the phylum Mollusca, only a relatively small number of molluscs are of interest to hobbyists. Many enter aquaria via 'living rock' and are incidental.

The larger and more interesting species are important aquarium subjects. Octopuses make fascinating exhibit animals and are occasionally kept by hobbyists. The tiny blue-ringed octopus has often been kept in home aquaria, despite being one of the most venomous animals on Earth. The larger species, such as the common octopus and the giant Pacific octopus, are impressive and popular in big exhibits.

Octopuses require tightly fitting covers to prevent their escape, which is often through the smallest of gaps. Other cephalopods, such as cuttlefish, squid and the distinctive nautilus, are regularly displayed in public aquaria but are very rare in domestic fish tanks. In general, they prefer subdued lighting.

Clams have become popular in both commercial and domestic aquaria. Like hard corals, some clams possess zooxanthellae in the exposed tissues of their mantles (Figure 32.6) and, as such, require the same high level of illumination and water quality.

Other molluscs frequently seen in aquaria include nudibranchs and scallops, such as the flame scallop.

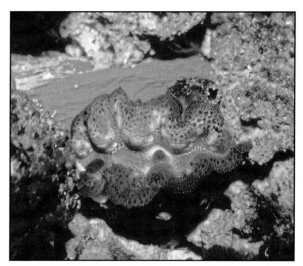

Figure 32.6 Different species of zooxanthellae produce different vibrant colours in the mantle of clams. The large opening on the left side is the inhalant siphon and the everted tube in the centre is the exhalant siphon. (Courtesy of London Aquarium, © W.H. Wildgoose.)

Feeding

The food requirements of molluscs vary according to group. Octopuses and other cephalopods are predators, feeding on crabs and other crustaceans as well as fish. Depending on species, some nudibranchs graze on algae whilst others feed upon corals and anemones. Scallops are filter feeders and should be offered liquidized shrimp, fish and clam meat or live newly hatched *Artemia*. Their own photosynthetic algae provide most of the nutrition required by clams but liquidized foods and *Artemia* nauplii can also be offered.

Water quality

It is essential that water quality is optimum for these animals. Octopuses and clams are sensitive to even the smallest traces of nitrate. Good water movement is important, particularly when liquidized food must be kept in suspension.

Specific diseases

Some molluscs can suffer rapid tissue necrosis similar to that seen in corals. Many cephalopods live in cool water and if subjected to temperatures above their tolerance level will suffer changes to their haemoglobin and quickly die.

Worms

Although some worms are associated with health problems (e.g. platyhelminths, nematodes), others are decorative and often seen in aquaria, such as the sabellid fan worms and feather duster worms, and the serpulid Christmas-tree worms. These are all sessile tubeworms and are usually seen in large congregations. The tubes of sabellids are membranous or made from sand particles, whilst serpulids have calcareous tubes that are usually embedded in coral rock. Their fan-like or feathery crowns (Figure 32.7) are tentacles derived from the gill structures and serve as respiratory organs but are also used for catching food. They are very sensitive to changes in light and the crown can be instantly withdrawn in defence (i.e. a startle response).

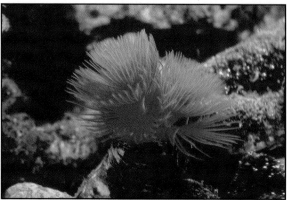

Figure 32.7 This serpulid worm lives in a self-made hard calcareous tube. It has two feathery plumes with which it feeds and breathes. These can be retracted quickly in response to danger and local disturbance. (© W.H. Wildgoose.)

Feeding
Tubeworms are plankton filter feeders, using the feathery crowns to collect their food, which is transported to the mouth via tiny cilia. Suspended food matter, newly hatched *Artemia* and rotifers are ideal foods.

Water quality
Although sabellids are often seen close to waste outfalls in nutrient-rich waters, it is advisable to maintain good water quality with good water flow to aid the delivery of suspended food.

Specific diseases
The occasional shedding of the crown should not be regarded as a problem, because a new one will often regrow over a period of time (e.g. several weeks). The cause is not clearly understood.

Marine crustaceans

There is a wide variety of marine crabs, shrimps and lobsters commonly kept in tropical and coldwater aquaria. Many are secretive or nocturnal and some are voracious predators. The larger lobsters and spiny lobsters are generally too big for domestic aquaria, but there are numerous smaller species that are more suitable. Some have fascinating

lifestyles (such as anemone crabs and shrimps that live within the tentacles of anemones), whilst others have different associations, such as the sponge crabs that allow sponges to grow on their carapace and boxing crabs that carry a small anemone on each claw. Some shrimp species remove parasites and other irritating particles from the skin of fish. The banded coral shrimp is a popular species and, unusually, pairs for life: unpaired individuals will fight aggressively to the death. Although it is commonly regarded as a food item for other organisms, the brine shrimp (*Artemia* spp.) has recently been presented as a pet (Figure 32.8). Hermit crabs (Figure 32.9) are useful additions to the aquarium because they are very effective scavengers, removing uneaten food and cleaning the substrate.

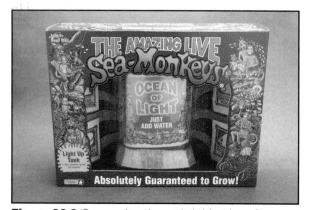

Figure 32.8 'Sea-monkeys' are a hybrid variety of *Artemia salina*, the brine shrimp. They have recently been commercially packaged and sold as pets in gift shops and supermarkets. The complete kit contains a small aquarium, water purifier, *Artemia* eggs and food. (© W.H. Wildgoose.)

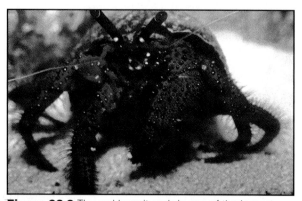

Figure 32.9 The red hermit crab is one of the largest species of hermit crabs. They are active climbers and may cause considerable damage in a small invertebrate aquarium. (Courtesy of the Horniman Museum, © W.H. Wildgoose.)

Feeding
Due to the secretive nature of many species it is important to ensure that enough food is offered and they are fed individually. Some species are algae grazers but for most others, a variety of chopped fish, shrimp, clam and mussel and dry aquarium foods should be offered. Some species are filter feeders and require suspended food matter and *Artemia* nauplii.

Water quality

Crustaceans moult frequently and the period following when they are hardening their new skin is crucial, since they are vulnerable to predation. To ensure rapid hardening, good quality water with the correct alkalinity, hardness and pH is essential.

Specific diseases

Crustaceans are prone to losing limbs but are capable of growing replacements. Regenerated limbs appear during the next moult, though it may take several moults to regain full size.

Many bacterial and viral infections are known to affect crustaceans. 'Shell disease' is commonly observed in captive lobsters and believed to be the result of overcrowding and poor water quality; any of 30 known bacteria may be responsible. Infection may develop in damaged carapaces, possibly caused by aggression. Shell disease appears as erosion, pitting, melanization and necrosis of the exoskeleton and can probably affect many crustacean species. Improving water quality and reducing the stocking density may enable the problem to clear with the next moult.

Sudden deaths in lobster populations have recently been attributed to an infection by a protozoan parasite, *Paramoeba*. This parasite destroys the nervous system, resulting in a condition commonly referred to as 'limp lobster syndrome', followed by death within 24 hours. There is no known cure.

A Gram-positive bacterium, *Aerococcus viridans*, causes 'red-tail disease' or gaffkaemia. It is commonly seen in lobsters but is also known in several species of crabs and prawns. Heavily infected specimens show a slight reddish discoloration through the integument of the ventral abdomen and death is usually rapid. Mortality may be reduced temporarily by lowering the temperature to decrease bacterial reproduction; for example, death occurs within 2 days at 20°C, but infected specimens can survive for up to 250 days at 1°C. Improved water quality and reduced stocking levels are also beneficial and vaccines may be useful.

Freshwater crustaceans

Historically, only crayfish species have been kept in domestic and public freshwater aquaria, but a much wider variety has recently become available. Many are colourful and make interesting aquarium subjects. Atyids are fan and dwarf shrimps that have fan-like 'hands' instead of claws and have become popular because they are effective at controlling algae. They are found naturally in large groups and should not be kept singularly. Long-arm shrimps are distinguishable by their thin, elongated arms. Floating shrimps, also known as glass or ghost shrimps, are small but interesting because of their unusually long swimmerets, which paddle so rapidly that they appear to float in the water column.

Several crab species have become popular, including fiddler crabs and land crabs, such as the colourful Cameroon crab. Fiddler crabs possess one claw that is substantially larger than the other and they live in mud burrows under brackish conditions. Land crabs will enter freshwater but remain on damp ground for much of the time.

Feeding

Details are similar to those for marine crustaceans.

Water quality

Clean and well oxygenated water is required for most species. Alkalinity and hardness are also important for many, particularly as they aid moulting.

Specific diseases

Freshwater crustaceans may be susceptible to bacterial shell disease problems similar to those described for marine species. Crayfish plague has caused the rapid decline of European species due to the introduction of North American signal crayfish, which are regarded as carriers and are resistant to the disease. The plague is caused by the fungus *Aphanomyces astaci*, which infects the soft non-calcified parts of the crayfish's cuticle and spreads systemically, often along the nerve cord. Infected animals die within a few weeks of exposure.

Australian crayfish are known to be susceptible to only one major disease, known as 'porcelain disease' or 'white tail disease', which is caused by a microsporean, *Thelohania* sp. There are no known cures for these diseases but regular examination and removal of unhealthy specimens may help to control the spread of infection.

A small temnocephalan flatworm is often seen on the shells and gills of freshwater crayfish but it is not regarded as a serious problem and can be controlled with saltwater baths.

Echinoderms

Echinoderms are characterized by their radial symmetry and their water vascular system, which they use for motivation, feeding and respiration. Starfish (Figure 32.10), sea urchins, sand dollars and sea cucumbers (Figure 32.11) are all echinoderms. Both tropical and temperate species are common in public aquaria, but temperate species are rare within the hobby. The majority of starfish species have five limbs but species with more exist. Sea cucumbers and urchins have five segments that are joined at the edges to form a cylinder shape or a dome, respectively. A tough outer layer, sometimes with hard knobbly extensions, protects most starfish and sea cucumbers, whilst sea urchins use their spines for protection. Feather stars, basket stars and brittle stars are quite delicate.

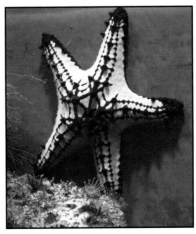

Figure 32.10
The red knobbed starfish is popular among marine hobbyists and can reach up to 30 cm in diameter. However, they are omnivorous and will consume sessile marine invertebrates such as molluscs and corals. (Courtesy of Underwater World, © W.H. Wildgoose.)

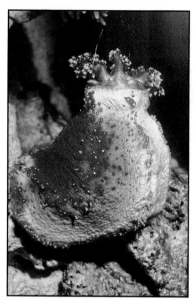

Figure 32.11 The 'sea apple' is one of the most colourful sea cucumbers and a popular species in marine aquaria. The feathery tentacles on the head are used for filter feeding and they can be fed on brine shrimp and rotifers. (Courtesy of Aquaworld, © W.H. Wildgoose.)

Feeding

Some species are algae grazers whilst others are carnivorous. Some urchins will eat corals, and many of the larger starfish are capable of prising open mollusc and bivalve shells to access the flesh within. Sea cucumbers tend to be scavengers and are efficient at removing detritus.

Water quality

Water conditions similar to those required by corals are suitable for most echinoderms. Temperate species may cope with wider parameters and lower temperatures.

Specific diseases

Starfish occasionally lose limbs but are able to regenerate them slowly. A detached limb is capable of regenerating into a full starfish.

Sea urchins are prone to casting off spines, often following shipment, which may be a stress response caused by poor water conditions in transit.

Some starfish species are known to contract the ciliate disease caused by *Orchitophyra stellarum*. This disease infects the gonads of males in particular and can substantially reduce the numbers of males in a population and impair reproductive potential. There is no known cure.

Acknowledgements

The author is grateful for the information and help provided by Kelly Rakow, Brian Nelson and Lance Adams of the New England Aquarium, Charles Delbeek at Waikiki Aquarium, Gary K. Ostrander at Johns Hopkins University Baltimore, Eric H. Borneman and Esther C. Peters.

Further reading

Anderson I (1993) The veterinary approach to marine prawns. In: *Aquaculture for Veterinarians, Fish Husbandry and Medicine* (ed. L Brown) pp. 271–296. Pergamon Press, Oxford

Borneman EH (2000) *Aquarium Corals: Selection, Husbandry and Natural History*. Microcosm, Shelburne, Vermont

Bower SM (1995) Parasitic diseases of shellfish. In: *Fish Diseases and Disorders*, Vol.1, *Protozoan and Metazoan Infections* (ed. PTK Woo) pp. 673–728. CABI Publishing, Wallingford

Boyle PR (1999) Cephalopods. In: *The UFAW Handbook on the Care and Management of Laboratory Animals*, 7th edn, Vol. 2 *Amphibious and Aquatic Vertebrates and Advanced Invertebrates* (ed. T Poole) pp. 115–139. Blackwell Science, Oxford

Debelius H and Baensch HA (1994) *Marine Atlas*. Mergus, Melle, Germany

Delbeek JC and Sprung J (1994) *The Reef Aquarium*, Vol. 1. Ricordea Publishing, Coconut Grove, Florida

Erhardt H and Moosleitner H (1997) *Marine Atlas*, Vol. 2. Mergus, Melle, Germany

Erhardt H and Moosleitner H (1998) *Marine Atlas*, Vol. 3. Mergus, Melle, Germany

Ingle RW (1999) Decapod crustaceans. In: *The UFAW Handbook on the Care and Management of Laboratory Animals*, 7th edn, Vol. 2, *Amphibious and Aquatic Vertebrates and Advanced Invertebrates* (ed. T Poole) pp. 140–172. Blackwell Science, Oxford

McGladdery SE (1999) Shellfish diseases (viral, bacterial and fungal). In: *Fish Diseases and Disorders*, Vol. 3, *Viral, Bacterial and Fungal* (ed. PTK Woo and DW Bruno) pp. 723–842. CABI Publishing, Wallingford

Moe MA (1989) *The Marine Aquarium Reference: Systems and Invertebrates*. Green Turtle Publications, Plantation, Florida

Ross LG and Ross B (1999) Anaesthesia of aquatic invertebrates. In: *Anaesthetic and Sedative Techniques for Aquatic Animals*, 2nd edn. (ed. LG Ross and B Ross) pp. 46–57. Blackwell Science, Oxford

Werner U (1998) *Shrimps, Crayfishes and Crabs in the Freshwater Aquarium*. Verlag ACS, Rodgau, Germany

UK legislation

Peter W. Scott

Much of the law relating to ornamental fish has not truly been challenged or even clarified, and there are serious problem areas, notably the perception of pain and the concept of suffering. This chapter is written from the standpoint of a practising veterinary surgeon, rather than that of a member of the legal profession. For a strict legal interpretation the appropriate references should be read. This chapter covers:

- Veterinary legislation
- Medicines legislation
- Welfare legislation
- Disease control legislation
- Zoo legislation
- Wildlife-related legislation
- Other legislation.

Veterinary legislation

Veterinary Surgeons Act 1966

For the purposes of this Act the definition of 'animals' includes birds and reptiles but not fish. Pressure at the time that the Act went through the House of Lords resulted in fish being removed, despite strenuous efforts to have them included. Treatment of fish, however, is still controlled under the *Medicines Act 1968*.

In the past, the Royal College of Veterinary Surgeons (RCVS) has held that it is the responsibility of a veterinary surgeon to provide emergency first aid for all species and to ensure that the owner can reach more experienced help if necessary. In circumstances where no practice in an area has the necessary expertise, the RCVS makes it clear that practices must take all reasonable steps to obtain assistance so that the public (and the animals) are not denied help. The veterinary surgeon personally should make contact with another colleague who can deal with the case. In general, veterinary surgeons in 'fish' practice are usually more than willing to advise colleagues directly.

Veterinary Surgeons Act 1966 (Schedule 3 Amendment) Order 1988

This amendment changes the type of treatment that can be carried out on animals (as covered by the 1966 Act) by the owner. It therefore makes no reference to fish.

Medicines legislation

Legislation controlling the prescribing and classification of medicines in the UK is currently under review. This particularly affects the treatment of ornamental or exotic fish; the treatment of food fish is at least partially defined and is unlikely to change in any significant manner. When prescribing for ornamental fish, it is strongly recommended that veterinary surgeons use consent forms. These should make it clear that the medicines may be unlicensed for a particular use, and that the use of these medicines is a matter of informed consent.

Medicines Act 1968

This Act, despite the definition of 'animals' in the *Veterinary Surgeons Act 1966*, does include fish. Therefore, prescription only medicines may be prescribed only for animals under the care of a veterinary surgeon. There is no legal definition of the phrase 'animals under his/her care', the expression used in the application of this Act. However, the RCVS interprets the term as follows.

- The veterinarian must have been given responsibility for the health of the animals
- That responsibility must be real and not merely nominal
- The animals must have been seen immediately before prescribing medication or recently and often enough to have personal knowledge of the animals to make a diagnosis
- The veterinarian must keep clinical records of those animals.

The stage at which a tank of fish realistically comes 'under one's care' is open to discussion. Similarly, whether the examination of one cadaver brought to the surgery is sufficient to satisfy this requirement or whether a site visit is required may vary with circumstances. The issues of accepting responsibility for taking animals under one's care when one is totally unfamiliar with their general anatomy, physiology and husbandry may also be debated in the future.

The vast majority of treatments used for ornamental fish are not currently licensed as medicines. Medicinal products are defined as any substance that is administered for a medicinal purpose. Traditionally, most proprietary medications have been sold through pet shops and garden centres, and many of these outlets may also give advice regarding fish health. Therefore veterinary surgeons may be placed in an invidious position regarding the supply and use of unlicensed medicines, since failure to do so may itself cause welfare problems.

A further concern is that many fish outlets sell chemicals that under some circumstances would be considered as 'medicines'. Here, the law has also been rather vague. For example, benzocaine becomes an anaesthetic (and hence a medicine) only when the customer chooses to use it as such. Hopefully, this anomalous situation will be resolved in due course.

Medicines (Restrictions on the Administration of Veterinary Medicinal Products) Regulations 1994 (SI 1994/2987), as amended by SI 1997/2884 (Amelia 8)

These Regulations establish in UK law the prescribing cascade, and the requirements for minimum withdrawal periods and record keeping by veterinary surgeons adopted by the European Community in 1990. These requirements were incorporated in the *Code of Practice for the Prescribing of Medicinal Products by Veterinary Surgeons* introduced by the British Veterinary Association (BVA) in 1991 and subsequently, in the *Guide to Professional Conduct* of the RCVS.

In summary, these state that when no authorized veterinary medicinal product exists for a condition in a particular species, and in order to avoid causing unacceptable suffering, veterinary surgeons exercising their clinical judgement may prescribe for one or a small number of animals under their care in accordance with the following sequence.

(i) A veterinary medicine authorized for use in another species or for a different use in the same species ('off-label use'); or

(ii) a medicine authorized in the UK for human use; or

(iii) a medicine to be made up at the time on a one-off basis by a veterinary surgeon or a properly authorized person.

There are additional requirements for treating food-producing animals.

The limitation of a small number of animals, and the requirement to follow the three stages of the cascade in strict order, do not apply to non-food-producing animals of minor or exotic species. The Veterinary Medicines Directorate suggests that as a working rule 'minor and exotic species' is taken to cover all companion, laboratory and zoo animals (except any whose produce might enter the food chain) other than cats and dogs.

Welfare legislation

Protection of Animals Act 1911 (1912 Scotland)

This Act deals with the subject of unnecessary suffering and it includes fish within its definition of 'animal'. It states that:

1.1   If any person–

a)   shall cruelly beat, kick, ill-treat, over-ride, over-drive, over-load, torture, infuriate, or terrify any animal, or shall cause or procure, or, being the owner, permit any animal to be so used, or shall, by wantonly or unreasonably doing or omitting to do any act, or causing or procuring the commission or omission of any act, cause any unnecessary suffering, or, being the owner, permit any unnecessary suffering to be so caused to any animal; or

b)   shall convey or carry, or cause or procure, or, being the owner, permit to be conveyed or carried, any animal in such manner or position as to cause that animal any unnecessary suffering, ... such person shall be guilty of an offence of cruelty within the meaning of this Act...

Cooper (1987) has discussed the implications of this in detail, and explains that to prove that an offence under Section 1 has been committed, it is necessary to show that an act both causes suffering and that it was unnecessary. It also needs to be unreasonable and, by case law, 'substantial'.

The above is of significance in relation to whether fish suffer or feel pain. Although difficult to argue, there is considerable evidence to support the premise and little to refute it. The Government-commissioned *Report of the Panel of Enquiry into Shooting and Angling (1976–1979)* (Kelly, 1997) recommended that:

where considerations of welfare are involved, all vertebrate animals (i.e. mammals, birds, amphibians and fish) should be regarded as equally capable of suffering to some degree or another, without distinction between 'warm-blooded' and 'cold-blooded' species.

Protection of Animals (Anaesthetics) Acts 1954 and 1964

These Acts specifically exclude fish. Cooper (1983) speculates that this may be because satisfactory methods of anaesthesia for fish were not envisaged at that time. It is likely, however, that suffering resulting from failure to use an anaesthetic where appropriate, would be regarded as an offence under the *Protection of Animals Act 1911*.

Pet Animals Act 1951 and Pet Animals Act 1951 (Amendment) Act 1982

Shops selling ornamental fish are included within the remit of this Act although its terms are relatively loose. The BVA and Local Authority consultative groups have guidelines for inspections under the *Pet Animals Act*, which specify water quality standards for shops (LGA, 1998).

Abandonment of Animals Act 1960

This Act makes it an offence of cruelty under the 1911 Act to abandon an animal without reasonable excuse, in circumstances likely to cause it suffering. Although intended to apply to abandoned pets, this might also apply to the release of captive-bred animals into the wild, such as restocking a river or lake with brown or rainbow trout. In 1991, the RSPCA brought a successful prosecution of an ornamental fish wholesaler under the provisions of this Act (RSPCA v. Durier 1991).

Animals (Scientific Procedures) Act 1986 as amended

Regulated procedures involving pain, suffering, distress or lasting harm in live vertebrate animals and the octopus must be authorized. This includes procedures such as fin clipping and tagging of wild fish. Researchers and premises must also be authorized. The Act applies to zoos and fieldwork but not to procedures that are recognized veterinary, agricultural and animal husbandry practices. Most behavioural observation is not covered by the Act.

Disease control legislation

Diseases of Fish Act 1937

This Act is very important and has various significant areas of interest. It deals with restrictions on the importation of live fish and eggs of fish. All fish importations require a licence under this Act. Contraventions result in seizure and detention of the fish or eggs. It also gives the power to designate infected areas and so can prohibit or regulate the movement of live fish or foodstuffs from that site. This takes the form of a renewable 16-day order. The owner is entitled, on application, to a report of the evidence on which the order was made. The Minister for agriculture can direct the owner regarding removal of dead or dying fish, and their disposal. This is covered in Section 2, Subsection 4, and appears to exclude non-fish farms, though fish dealers are defined under the Act as 'fish farms'.

The Act requires 'any person entitled to take fish from any inland water, or employed for the purpose of having the care of inland waters' to report any suspected notifiable diseases to the Minister: in actuality, to his agents, until recently the Ministry of Agriculture Fisheries and Food (MAFF). The view from the ministry's legal department was that this obligation does not extend to a veterinarian asked to examine or screen fish. However, they would expect the veterinarian to advise the owner of his obligation to report such findings. In 2001 the Department of the Environment, Food and Rural Affairs (DEFRA) was established, incorporating those responsibilities formerly handled by MAFF.

If the Minister believes that any direction is not being complied with, he can direct an inspector to carry out that direction, and then recover the cost from the owner by civil proceedings.

The Minister can authorize the owner to remove fish from an infected area if he believes it to be appropriate. This only applies to fish farms and it *authorizes* removal rather than *requires* removal.

Diseases of Fish Act 1983

This modifies 'infected area' to 'designated area' and extends the controls to prohibiting the taking into or out of the area any live fish, eggs or foodstuff for fish. It changes the 16-day order to 30 days, and this can then be extended to 60 days and further renewed. Although there are no powers of compulsory slaughter, this can be applied to ornamental fish dealers to prevent sale of live fish until the infected fish (normally all of the fish on the premises at the time) are slaughtered and the premises are disinfected satisfactorily.

The Act updates the definition of 'fish farm' to:

> any pond, stew, fish hatchery or other place used for keeping, with a view to their sale or to their transfer to other waters (including any other fish farm) live fish, live eggs of fish, or foodstuffs for fish, and includes any buildings used in connection therewith, and the banks and margins of any water therein.

It also refers to the 'business of fish farming' as meaning 'business of keeping live fish (whether or not for profit) with a view to their sale or to their transfer to other waters'. This widens the definition and essentially brings within the Act ornamental retailers, wholesalers and many hobbyists who breed and sell fish.

The Act also requires registration of the fish farm and requires the submission of records relating to stock movements.

The Minister has the right to add diseases to the list of those covered by the provisions of the *Diseases of Fish Acts 1937 & 1983*.

Import of Live Fish (England and Wales) Act 1980

This Act provides for the licensing of the importation, release or keeping of non-indigenous fish. To date, licences for the importation of ornamental fish have been granted freely although changes being examined in the European Community (EC) may alter this in the future.

New measures set out in the *Prohibition of Keeping or Release of Live Fish (Specified Species) Order 1998* reinforces the above Act. Anyone wishing to keep any of the listed species requires a licence before obtaining the fish. Species covered by this order include some salmonids, catfish (including Wels catfish), sturgeons, sterlets, paddlefish, cyprinids (including grass carp), pumpkinseed and pike-perch.

Zoo legislation

Zoo Licensing Act 1981

This Act, in its definitions, includes all places where animals (including fish), not normally domesticated in the UK, are displayed to the public for more than seven days per year whether a charge is made or not. This could range from a conventional zoo or public aquarium to a restaurant or even a veterinary surgery. The Act does not cover circuses or pet shops, which are covered under separate legislation. In practice, the majority of small commercial situations where fish are used for decoration (i.e. shops and restaurants) are exempted by simply not being asked to register. Some have been specifically exempted where there are a number of tanks and their case merited inspection.

This Act is primarily concerned with public safety, although animal welfare issues have been brought within its influence. *The Secretary of State's Standards of Modern Zoo Practice* (DETR, 2000) are the standards to which zoos and public aquaria must operate. These are based on the 'Five Freedoms' drawn up for livestock by the Farm Animal Welfare Council and apply to fish exhibits.

EC Zoos Directive (1999/22/EC)

Council Directive 1999/22/EC relating to the keeping of wild animals in zoos (and public aquaria) came into force on 29 March 1999. The Directive provides for the licensing and inspection of zoos and for good standards of animal care. It also sets the framework for the participation of zoos in conservation, research and education.

National legislation will need to be brought into line with the Directive by 9 April 2002. Pending implementation, advice is offered to zoos and inspectors on the requirements that will apply once the Directive is translated into domestic legislation.

The Directive will require Member States to ensure that all zoos:

* 'Participate in research from which conservation benefits accrue to the species, and/or training in relevant conservation skills, and/or the exchange of information relating to species conservation and/or, where appropriate, captive breeding, repopulation or reintroduction of species into the wild'
* 'Promote public education and awareness in relation to the conservation of biodiversity, particularly by providing information about the species exhibited and their natural habitats'
* 'Accommodate their animals under conditions which aim to satisfy the biological and conservation requirements of the individual species, *inter alia*, by providing species-specific enrichment of the enclosures; and maintaining a high standard of animal husbandry with a developed programme of preventive and curative veterinary care and nutrition'
* 'Prevent the escape of animals in order to avoid possible ecological threats to indigenous species and preventing intrusion of outside pests and vermin'
* 'Keep up-to-date records of the zoo's collection appropriate to the species recorded.'

Wildlife-related legislation

Wildlife and Countryside Act 1981

This has many powers to regulate the taking of listed species from the wild, their sale and possession, to prohibit injuring and prohibit release of non-native species without a licence.

Convention on International Trade in Endangered Species (CITES)

Sometimes known as the Washington Convention, this originally came into force on 1 July 1975 and was ratified by the UK Government in 1976. At present, 145 coun-tries are now signatories to the Convention. CITES aims through international cooperation to protect certain species of wild fauna and flora (listed in Appendices) against over-exploitation through international trade.

Currently, over 2,700 animals (and 21,000 plants) are listed in the Appendices of CITES. Not all the species are exotic: many species native to the UK are listed in the Appendices. The listings may be amended from time to time.

Appendix I includes:

all species threatened with extinction that are or may be affected by trade. Trade in specimens of these species must be subject to particularly strict regulation in order not to further endanger their survival and must only be authorized in exceptional circumstances.

Appendix II includes:

(a) all species which although not necessarily now threatened with extinction may become so unless trade in specimens of such species is subject to strict regulation in order to avoid utilization incompatible with their survival; and

(b) other species that must be subject to regulation in order that trade in specimens of certain species referred to in sub-paragraph (a) of this paragraph may be brought under effective control.

Appendix III includes:

all species identified by a country as being subject to regulation within its jurisdiction for the purpose of preventing or restricting exploitation, and as needing the co-operation of other Parties in the control of trade.

The European Community in total, and the UK in particular, is one of the largest consumers of wildlife and wildlife products in the world (along with the USA and Japan). Due to the European single market and the absence of internal border controls, CITES provisions are applied uniformly in the European Community through two EC regulations (as amended):

* Council Regulation (EC) 338/97 on the protection of species of wild fauna and flora by regulating trade therein
* Commission Regulation (EC) 939/97 laying down detailed rules concerning the implementation of Council Regulation (EC) 338/97 on the protection of species of wild fauna and flora by regulating trade therein.

These are enforced in the UK by *The Control of Trade in Endangered Species (Enforcement) Regulations 1977* (or COTES Regulations) and the *Endangered Species (Import and Export) Act 1976*. Some of the measures taken by the European Community are more strict than those required by CITES and the Annexes to the EC regulations contain species that are not listed by CITES.

Other legislation

Control of Substances Hazardous to Health Regulations 1999

The COSHH Regulations are to control people's exposure to hazardous substances, which are defined as those that cause harm by ingestion, inhalation, inoculation and direct contact. They apply in a number of areas where ornamental fish are concerned and in particular to the use of chemical treatments, such as formaldehyde, malachite green, benzalkonium chloride and chloramine T. Veterinarians should be aware of the harmful nature of these products and should advise owners or users on appropriate safety measures.

Environmental Protection Act 1990

The safe disposal of clinical waste (which is defined as any waste that contains animal tissue or fluids, pharmaceuticals, syringes and needles) is regulated by the Environmental Protection Act 1990 and subsequent legislation. Consequently, the disposal of cadavers and medicinal products used to treat fish requires the same care as other waste generated by veterinary practice. The disposal of water treated with medicinal products may also require approval or consent from the local water authority.

References and further reading

British Veterinary Association (2000) *Code of Practice on Medicines.* BVA Publications, London

Cooper ME (1983) Anaesthesia: the legal requirements. *Veterinary Practice*, 18 April 1983

Cooper ME (1987) *An Introduction to Animal Law.* Academic Press, London

DETR (2000) *The Secretary of State's Standards of Modern Zoo Practice.* Department of the Environment Transport and the Regions, London

Howarth W (1990) *The Law of Aquaculture: The Law relating to the Farming of Fish and Shellfish in Britain.* Fishing News Books, Oxford

Howarth W (1990) *The Law of the National Rivers Authority.* NRA and Centre for Law in Rural Areas, Aberystwyth

Kelly JS (1979) *Report of the Panel of Enquiry into Shooting and Angling (1976–1979).* Chaired by Lord Medway

LGA (1998) *The Pet Animals Act 1951: Model Standards for Pet Shop Licence Conditions.* Local Government Association, London

RCVS (1990) *Guide to Professional Conduct.* Royal College of Veterinary Surgeons, London

RCVS (1993) *Legislation affecting the Veterinary Profession in the United Kingdom*, 7th edn. Royal College of Veterinary Surgeons, London

Treves-Brown K (2000) *Applied Fish Pharmacology.* Kluwer Academic Publishers, Dordrecht

US legislation

Roy P.E. Yanong

The legal aspects of practising fish medicine in the United States are complicated by different historical factors. Fish had been ignored by most of the US veterinary profession for some time. Fish health specialists with alternative backgrounds emerged to fill the gaps, especially during the formative years of salmonid and channel catfish farming. In aquaculture, many of these experts contributed most, if not all, of the initial body of fish health knowledge.

Over time, veterinarians were given the legal right to practise medicine on all animals. As the veterinary profession became more involved in aquaculture, some tensions were evident. Veterinarians, arriving relatively late on the scene, appeared to be attempting to take over a discipline that already had many well established knowledgeable experts. However, at the same time, the breadth and scope of a veterinary education was not fully appreciated or understood by many outside the profession. Since then, a mutual understanding among the different groups of fish health professionals and an appreciation of the strengths within each group has developed over time. In aquaculture, the role of a veterinarian as a member of a team of experts is just as important as their role in other agricultural commodity groups.

During the major developmental periods of the ornamental fish industry, veterinarians played no role in management of fish health. Exporters, importers, wholesalers and pet stores had to devise fish health management protocols for the collection, shipping and handling of ornamental fish. As the tropical fish industry in Florida increased after the 1930s, farmers also developed their own techniques. When the aquarium hobby was first created, owners had to make significant financial investments. Despite this, fish were still ignored by most veterinarians, who at that time had less knowledge about fish husbandry and health than their potential clientele.

Today, US veterinarians are playing an increasing role in aquaculture, health assessment of wild stocks, management of public aquaria, and in the care of ornamental pet fish.

Veterinary legislation

In the US, as a result of our federal form of government, the right to regulate the veterinary profession was given to each individual state or jurisdiction. Although originally based on a human medicine case, Dent v. W Virginia 1888 recognized that states have policing power to regulate the professions.

Subsequently, each state legislature adopted a 'Practice Act' that empowered a state Board to regulate the veterinary profession. In 1960, the American Association of Veterinary State Boards (AAVSB), comprising all state regulatory boards, was founded. This is the association of governmental agencies whose primary function is to protect the public by regulating veterinarians and the practice of veterinary medicine. Established as a not-for-profit corporation in the mid-1970s, AAVSB membership now includes 56 jurisdictions. Its website address is: *http://www.aavsb.org*

Although veterinary rules and regulations are for the most part uniform across the 50 states and other participating jurisdictions, there are some differences depending upon each state's particular practice act. All states recognize the veterinarian's jurisdiction over animal health, and include fish in their definitions of 'animal'. However, some states explicitly allow non-veterinarians to practise veterinary medicine in fish under certain conditions. For example, in Kansas, 'fisheries biologists employed by the state, the US government, or any person in the production or management of commercial food or game fish while in the performance of such persons' official duties' and rehabilitators in a number of states are allowed to practise veterinary medicine without direct supervision by a veterinarian. In addition, producers and owners are allowed the right to care for their own animals.

Although individual states do have the final authority in the regulation of veterinary medicine, several US Codes (Federal legislation) have played major roles in defining the role of veterinary medicine.

Medicines legislation

The Federal Food, Drug, and Cosmetic Act

This Act, the FFD & CA, empowers the US Food and Drug Administration (FDA) and Centre for Veterinary Medicine (CVM) to regulate all animal drugs. There has been a concerted effort in the past few years by many groups to simplify the FDA's drug approval process through an amendment of the FFD & CA, as outlined in the *Minor Animal Species Health and Welfare Act 2000*, introduced in the House of Representatives as Bill 4780 in June 2000. Better known as 'MUMS' (Minor

Use/Minor Species) Act, this legislation is currently undergoing review and, if passed, will simplify approval of fish chemotherapeutants. In the past, commercial drug sponsors for minor uses and minor species, including fish, have had difficulty meeting all of the FDA's requirements because of the large expenses incurred by drug companies with relatively small returns.

Commercial producers can legally use drugs and chemicals:

- On the FDA's approved list for specific species, specific diseases, and at specific doses and/or concentrations. The approved drugs are manufactured by specific companies
- As registered participants in investigational new animal drugs (INADs) for aquaculture; or
- If the drugs are on the FDA's list of unapproved drugs of low regulatory priority.

Finally, under the extra-label provisions of the *Animal Medicinal Drug Use Clarification Act 1994* (AMDUCA), veterinarians may prescribe other veterinary and human drugs under certain conditions. US veterinarians may also use alternative drugs as accorded by the AMDUCA but they are still legally restricted in several aspects. Ornamental fish have been, and so far continue to be, of low regulatory priority. Consequently, many ornamental fish medications are available over-the-counter to the pet owner, and there is very little regulation over their medicinal claims and contents.

With regard to fish, the following medicines are approved for use:

- Formalin is approved for the control of fungi of the family Saprolegniaceae on all finfish eggs and for control of external protozoa and monogenetic trematodes
- Human chorionic gonadotrophin (HCG) is approved as an aid in spawning
- Tricaine methane sulphonate (e.g. MS222) is approved for hatchery or laboratory use as an anaesthetic
- Oxytetracycline, sulphadimethoxine–ormetoprim, and sulphamerazine are currently legal for use in certain food-fish for certain diseases. A number of other drugs are being examined for use in food fish under INADs.

Except for formalin, there are currently no chemotherapeutants (i.e. for use against infectious diseases: antibacterials or antibiotics, anthelmintics or other antiparasiticides) approved for use in any ornamental fish species.

Unapproved new animal drugs of Low Regulatory Priority are permitted for use by producers according to the FDA (Federal Joint Subcommittee on Aquaculture) provided that:

- The drugs are used for the prescribed indications, including species and life stage
- The drugs are used at prescribed dosages
- The drugs are used according to good management practices

- The product is of an appropriate grade for use in food animals
- An adverse effect on the environment is unlikely.

There are about 18 drugs in this group, but many of these have 'illegal' counterparts that are more safe and effective. Drugs in this category include the following for use as parasiticides:

- Acetic acid (1000–2000 mg/l for 1–10 minutes)
- Calcium oxide (2000 mg/l for 5 seconds)
- Magnesium sulfate (30,000 mg/l magnesium sulfate and 7000 mg/l sodium chloride for 5–10 minutes for external monogenetic trematode and crustacean infestations)
- Sodium chloride (3% for 10–30 minutes).

Hydrogen peroxide (250–500 mg/l) can be used for the control of fungus on all life stages.

Federal Environmental Pesticide Control Act

The *Federal Insecticide, Fungicide, and Rodenticide Act* (FIFRA), originally passed by Congress in 1947, but amended several times subsequently, was significantly changed in 1972 (7 U.S.C. s/s 136 *et seq.*) under a new law titled the *Federal Environmental Pesticide Control Act* (FEPCA). The amended FIFRA mandated that the US Environmental Protection Agency (EPA) regulate all pesticides. These compounds must be registered with the EPA and classified for general or restricted use. The term 'pest' is defined as:

- 'any insect, rodent, nematode, fungus, weed'; or
- 'any other form of terrestrial or aquatic plant or animal life or virus, bacteria, or other micro-organism (except viruses, bacteria, or other micro-organisms on or in living man or other living animals) which the Administrator declares to be a pest under section 136w(c)(1) of this title'.

The act was intended to guarantee efficacy for the target organism, protection to the user and protection to the environment. One major outcome of this Act is that pesticides must be used as directed and only be used in sites described in the label. Additionally, restricted-use pesticides can only be applied by licensed pesticide applicators. Under FIFRA, a federal pesticide label is termed a Section 3 label. In the US, use of Dimilin® (diflubenzuron) is allowable only by licensed pesticide applicators for use in control of only the un-attached form of the anchorworm (*Lernaea cyprinacea*) in commercial ornamental fish and baitfish production ponds and tanks. Under Section 18 of FIFRA, the EPA may temporarily authorize states or federal agencies in emergencies to use a specific pesticide in a non-labelled site. For example, Mississippi catfish farmers can use diuron (dimethyl urea) for blue green algae.

Under FIFRA, states also have the power to issue a 24(c) label. This is a 'special local need' label for use of a pesticide in a non-labelled site issued on an annual basis. For example, in Florida, 24(c) labels have been issued to ornamental fish farmers for the following restricted use pesticides:

- Bayluscide® (niclosamide) (labelled against snails, an intermediate host) for use against digenean trematodes
- Baytex® (fenthion) for use against dragonfly larvae
- Diuron for use against macroalgae.

Bath treatments with chemicals that may find their way into public waterways are technically under the jurisdiction of the EPA. For example, the use of trichlorfon as a bath treatment in outdoor ponds for the treatment of free-swimming stages of crustacean parasites is not legal in most states, even with a private applicator's licence.

Welfare legislation

The Animal Welfare Act

In 1966, the *Laboratory Animal Welfare Act* was passed, with subsequent amendments made in 1970 (when the name was shortened to the *Animal Welfare Act*), 1976 (the *Animal Welfare Act* of 1976), 1985, 1990 and 1991. The Act and its amendments helped to define standards of animal care that became law in the US Code of Federal Regulations (CFR). Title 9, *Animals and Animal Products*, of the CFR empowers the US Department of Agriculture, Animal and Plant Health Inspection Service (USDA-APHIS) with regulating standards of animal care.

Under Title 9 (1994), by definition:

'Animal' means any live or dead dog, cat, nonhuman primate, guinea pig, hamster, rabbit, or any other warm-blooded animal, which is being used, or is intended for use for research, teaching, testing, experimentation, or exhibition purposes, or as a pet.

In the US Code, Title 7, Agriculture, Chapter 54, *Transportation, Sale and Handling of Certain Animals* Sec. 2132, the term animal is defined similarly. In short, fish are not included under these codes.

Wildlife-related legislation

State regulations regarding import, export or sale of ornamental fish

For most of the 50 states, there are no regulations on interstate movement of ornamental fish. Some states do have prohibited species lists and typically these lists include different species of piranha. However, other species may be included, for example members of the Potamotrygonidae (freshwater stingrays), Osteo-

glossidae (bony tongues, arowanas) and Channidae (snakeheads). One or two states have a health certificate requirement for all animals entering the state, but this may change in the near future.

Current information regarding these regulations can be obtained from USDA APHIS Veterinary Services: US State and Territory Animal Import Regulations for Aquatic Species website at *http://www.aphis.usda.gov/guidance/regulations/animal/state/aquatic/*

Federal regulations regarding import, export or transport of wildlife

Current information regarding these regulations can be obtained from the US Code of Federal Regulations website at *http://www.access.gpo.gov/nara/cfr/cfr-table-search.html*

50 Code of Federal Regulations 14 (50 CFR 14)

These rules regulate the importation and exportation of ornamental fish. 'Live farm-raised fish and farm-raised fish eggs' meet the definition of 'bred in captivity'. Ornamental fish shipments that have only live farm-raised fish or eggs are not required to have an import or export licence according to 50 CFR 14.92 (4). However, this does not apply to endangered species (as described in 50 CFR 17, *Endangered Species Regulations*) and CITES-listed fish (as listed in 50 CFR 23), including all sturgeon, paddlefish, lungfish and Asian arowana. For export purposes, koi and goldfish bred in the USA are also exempt but fall under a slightly different category.

Dealers exporting or importing shipments containing wild-caught ornamental fish, invertebrates (including snails and crayfish), and amphibians such as 'water dogs' (tiger salamanders) are required to have permits for these. These shipments require that a completed *Declaration for Importation or Exportation of Fish or Wildlife* (Form 3-177) signed by the exporter or his agent be filed with the US Fish and Wildlife Service law enforcement prior to import or export. In addition, the dealer must provide to the service officer or Customs officer (under 14.54) all shipping documents, all permits, licences or other documents required by the US and required by the foreign country of import or export, and the animals being imported or exported.

Acknowledgements

The author is grateful for the assistance offered by Paul Zajicek and Craig Watson during the preparation of this chapter.

Health and safety

Colin Grist

The average aquarium and the keeping of ornamental fish may appear to be relatively free of hazards but there are several potential dangers to hobbyists and professionals alike. These include faulty equipment, handling hazardous substances, diseased fish and maintaining dangerous species, such as electric eels and venomous lionfish. However, simple precautions are often all that is required to prevent injury and infection.

Faulty equipment

Most standard aquarium equipment is robust and reliable but users should be aware of certain hazards.

Aquarium breakages

Glass is still the most popular material for constructing aquaria, despite being brittle and easily broken. It is a very strong material and when used in aquarium construction is capable of holding a large volume of water. However, it is important to ensure that the correct thickness of glass is used for the volume and, in particular, depth of water since deep water creates greater pressure.

A glass aquarium must always be supported by a strong flat surface, since any unevenness (such as a warped stand or a particle of grit trapped between the base and its support) could cause the base to shatter. A sheet of polystyrene or cork placed beneath the aquarium will reduce these problems. For similar reasons, lifting and carrying an aquarium containing water is not recommended, since the lack of sufficient support could cause the tank to break.

Aquaria constructed from acrylic are becoming more popular, especially for large-scale exhibits. Acrylic is stronger and more robust than glass but sharp edges can be produced if it shatters.

Aquaria built by the major manufacturers undergo rigorous testing and quality control and can be used with confidence.

Electrical faults

Electrical equipment used for fish keeping is generally manufactured to a high standard and is well regulated. Manufacturers' instructions should be followed when installing and using items such as heaters, lights and pumps. In most cases electrical faults will present more problems for the fish within the system than for the personnel maintaining it, since vital heating and filtration may be affected. However, damage to electrical equipment can result in electrocution.

Water is an excellent conductor of electricity and so all equipment should be handled with care, especially if it is submerged or situated near water. Ideally, equipment should be connected to the power supply at a position above the water level and at a sensible distance. Where possible, residual circuit breakers (RCBs) should be used to provide additional protection. In the case of outdoor ponds or public exhibits where power cables are concealed or buried underground, it is important to mark the route and use armour cable trunking in order to prevent future damage by digging or drilling equipment.

Ozone

Many marine aquaria incorporate ozone generators in the filtration system, usually in conjunction with a foam fractionator (protein skimmer). Ozone (O_3) is an unstable form of oxygen produced by passing air over an electrical charge. It is the gas produced during a thunderstorm and has a characteristic pungent odour. It is used as a sterilizing agent but is a very harmful gas and any leakage must be avoided. Large sophisticated systems used in commercial installations have various failsafe mechanisms and automatic shutdown, but smaller domestic units do not. In any event, if odour is detected the ozone generator must be switched off and examined professionally. Ozone very quickly destroys the sense of smell, resulting in an inability to detect the gas, which may then result in brain damage and fatality.

Hazardous substances

Various substances used in fish keeping are hazardous and these include water treatments and disease treatments in particular.

Legislation

This is relevant to employers in the aquarium industry, public aquaria, aquarium shops and commercial aquaculture but also has relevance to veterinarians and owners. The *Control of Substances Hazardous to Health Regulations 1999* (COSHH) as administered by the Health and Safety Executive (HSE) in the UK requires employers to control exposure to hazardous substances in order to prevent ill health amongst workers. In the USA, similar regulations and facilities are administered through the Occupational Safety and Health Administration (OSHA).

The effects of hazardous substances can range from mild eye or skin irritation to chronic lung disease or even death. Asthma can be caused by allergies to substances. Hazardous substances include water and disease treatments, bacteria and other microorganisms, adhesives, paints, cleaning agents, fumes and dust.

To comply with COSHH it is necessary to follow seven steps (Health and Safety Executive, 1999):

1. Assess the risks
2. Decide what precautions are needed
3. Prevent or adequately control exposure
4. Ensure that control methods are used and maintained
5. Monitor exposure
6. Carry out appropriate health surveillance
7. Ensure employees are properly informed, trained and supervised.

COSHH regulates a range of substances regarded as hazardous to health and these are governed by the *Chemicals (Hazard Information and Packaging for Supply) Regulations 1994* (CHIP) whereby such substances are identified by their warning label and for which suppliers must provide safety data sheets. A list of commonly used hazardous substances can be found in the *Approved Supply List* (Health & Safety Executive, 2000).

Practicalities

Certain precautions can be taken when handling substances that are commonly used with aquatic systems.

Salt

Marine aquaria require salt water that can either be natural (e.g. from the sea) or artificially made from pre-prepared dry mixtures. Salt water is abrasive and can cause skin and eye irritations. After being in contact with salt water it is useful to wash with clean fresh water.

Medications

Water treatments and additives and disease medications should all be regarded as potentially hazardous chemicals. They must always be kept hidden and out of reach from children and on commercial premises some may be required by law to be kept in a dedicated lockable cabinet.

Many of these products can be poisonous if taken internally, corrosive, carcinogenic or simply an irritant, depending on the active ingredients. Formaldehyde, malachite green and organophosphates are common medications known to be toxic. Many products incorporate coloured dyes that can stain skin as well as clothing and are often difficult to remove; therefore disposable gloves and other protective garments should be worn. Powdered medications such as antibiotics are harmful if inhaled.

Disinfectants of any kind are, by their very nature, toxic and must not be taken internally. Chlorine-based products are popular sterilizing agents for nets and other aquarium equipment and should only be used in well ventilated areas.

Safety instructions given by manufacturers should be followed and protective clothing used where necessary. Correct disposal procedures must be followed carefully because it may be unlawful to pour certain waste chemicals or water treated with such chemicals down domestic drains.

Adhesives

Certain adhesives are commonly used with aquaria, such as silicone rubber for constructing glass tanks and solvent weld cements for plumbing plastic pipework. These generally produce very strong fumes and must be used in areas where there is good ventilation. Protective clothing must be worn since these products may bond to skin and be difficult to remove.

Zoonoses

There are very few fish diseases that have proved to be zoonotic but research will undoubtedly uncover new cases. Humans become infected by handling diseased fish or contaminated equipment, or by ingesting water from facilities that contain diseased fish. The use of sterilizing equipment, wearing disposable gloves and thorough hand washing should be routine precautions. Public aquaria and commercial aquatic centres must provide dedicated food preparation areas with isolated washbasins.

Several illnesses can be contracted from eating contaminated fish and invertebrates, which may result in food poisoning; signs vary from mild gastroenteritis to death. However, it is not the purpose of this chapter to discuss in detail such zoonotic infections.

Many aquatic microorganisms are potentially zoonotic and these are summarized in Figure 34.1. The most significant bacteria are *Mycobacterium* spp., which cause granulomatous nodules on the hands or fingers (Figure 34.2), i.e. limbs that are in most contact with the aquatic environment. The following precautions can limit the spread of these diseases.

- Use disposable gloves for food preparation, postmortem examinations and handling live fish
- Wear gloves of a suitable length if open wounds are present
- Avoid sharing equipment between systems unless sterilized with bleach at 5000 ppm (10% solution of household bleach) or similar products at the correct concentration and for an appropriate time
- Identify and mark infected systems
- Regard all cadavers as medical or clinical waste and dispose of them carefully
- Immunosuppressed persons should not handle potentially infected materials
- Suitable hand-washing facilities and warning signs should be provided near touch pools in public aquaria (Figure 34.3). However, antiseptic cleansers may provoke allergic reactions in some people.

Bacteria	Importance	Human infection	Treatment
Mycobacteria *Mycobacterium marinum* *M. fortuitum* *M. chelonae*	The most significant zoonotic infection; often called fish tank granuloma, fish fancier's finger or fish handler's disease	Granulomatous nodule, usually on the hands or fingers, which can often heal over several months without treatment. Occasionally a 'sporotrichoid' form is seen, particularly with *M. marinum*, where localized infection is followed by spread to nearby lymph nodes. It may also spread deep into adjacent tissues and produce arthritis, osteomyelitis and tenosynovitis. Immuno-suppressed patients are particularly at risk due to unresponsive T-cells	Current treatment of this disease in humans involves a lengthy course of therapy with co-trimoxazole, tetracycline (in particular minocycline) or rifampicin (often in combination with ethambutol)
Nocardia *Nocardia asteroides* *N. kampachi*	Uncommon and easily confused with mycobacteriosis due to similar clinical signs		
Vibrio *Vibrio* spp.	Occurs in marine and estuarine environments	Human infection through eating infected marine fish, occasionally fatal. Also through contamination of skin wounds	
Aeromonas *Aeromonas hydrophila*	Not common, ubiquitous in aquatic environments	Infections by ingesting contaminated water or direct contact with a wound. Several symptoms can occur but the most common are gastroenteritis and localized wound infection	
Pseudomonas *Pseudomonas fluorescens*	No documented cases, commonly found in freshwater and marine aquarium fish		
Protozoa	No known cases, although *Cryptosporidium* can infect both fish and humans		
Parasites	Nematodes: due to the ingestion of food fish	No risk to people working in aquaria	

Figure 34.1 Zoonotic diseases.

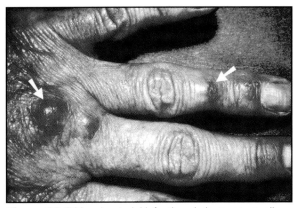

Figure 34.2 Mycobacterial infections in humans usually develop on the hands, as seen on the finger and knuckle in this case. (Courtesy of St John's Institute of Dermatology.)

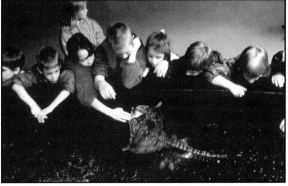

Figure 34.3 Touch pools are popular exhibits in public aquaria containing rays and other placid fish. Appropriate warning signs and hand-washing facilities should be available. (Courtesy of B. Brewster.)

Dangerous species

Many fish and invertebrates are capable of inflicting injury by biting, by using either venomous or non-venomous spines, or by electric shock. With the steady increase in fish keeping and public aquaria, the number of people exposed to these risks is also increasing. Hobbyists are now able to purchase more uncommon and dangerous species through their local retailers.

Bites

Although unusual in aquaria of any size, bites can be inflicted by a variety of fish. In general, this is a result of provocation or when a fish mistakes an aquarist's finger for food. Bite injuries from fish are outlined in Figure 34.4.

Training fish is the best approach to prevent bite injuries. Sharks are generally intelligent fish and can be trained to feed only in a certain place and in a certain way. Similar training of many other fish is also possible. Most bites only require standard treatment for cuts but more

Fish	Nature of injury
Triggerfish	Limited injury but large fish may remove flesh and expose bone
Piranha	Limited injury
Moray eel	Serious bites, often septic due to natural oral bacterial flora
Grouper	Limited injury
Sharks	Nurse shark: powerful crushing jaws, tend to hold on to victim Sand tiger and sandbar shark: not aggressive but powerful jaws and inflict severe lacerations Lemon shark: aggressive Black-tip reef shark: harmless, occasionally nibbles at humans
Barracuda	Severe bites, similar to sharks
Octopus	Very rare; venomous to varying degrees, particularly blue-ringed octopus; parrot-like jaw produces two small puncture holes and localized tingling sensation; profuse bleeding due to anticoagulants in venom
Annelid worms (*Glycera* spp.)	Chitinous jaws capable of penetrating skin; produces painful sensation like a bee sting; numbness and itching for 24–48 hours

Figure 34.4 Dangerous species: bite injuries.

severe injuries from moray eels and sharks will require more attention, since there is potential for loss of limb or, occasionally, death. Bites from octopus and *Glycera* worms should be treated in a similar manner to stings.

Spines and stings

Several species of aquarium fish possess spines, many of which are venomous (Figure 34.5 and 34.6). Some fish (e.g. lionfish) have venomous spines in their dorsal fins, whereas stingrays have venomous spines in the tail. Some catfish have strong spines on their pectoral fins, many of which deliver a powerful venom. Surgeonfish have very sharp, modified scalpel-like scales on their peduncle.

Amongst invertebrates, cone shells have venomous rod-like spines.

Initial treatment involves alleviating pain, produced by a combination of penetration, venom and foreign body reaction from slime and debris. Serious lacerations from rays and catfish should be irrigated with cold sterile saline. Small punctures may require incision prior to irrigation. Suction can be used to remove venom but may prove difficult. Alternatively, the wound should be soaked in hot water for 30–60 minutes, at a temperature as high as the patient can withstand: the heat may help to break down the venom and render it less harmful. Magnesium sulphate added to the water is beneficial or the wound area can be infiltrated with

Fish	Hazard	Injury
Scorpionfish Lionfish Stonefish	Variable dorsal, anal and pelvic spines with venom glands; non-aggressive	Intense pain, impaired local blood supply; lasts several hours. Stone fish: Similar to above but lasts several days; unconsciousness, local skin slough, convulsions, nausea and vomiting, delirium, respiratory distress and death; recovery over months; antivenin is available through Commonwealth Serum Laboratories, Parkville, Australia
Marine stingray	At least one venomous spine on the tail; many can rapidly whip their tail over in a similar manner to a scorpion	Sharp pain, rapid swelling, reduced blood pressure, nausea and vomiting, increased heart rate, muscular paralysis; potentially but rarely fatal
Freshwater stingray	As above	Most dangerous to humans; most severe pain, slow healing lacerations
Catfish (most dangerous are Ariidae, Clariidae and Plotosidae)	Single spine on leading edge of dorsal and pectoral fins; often venomous	Slow-healing lacerations; instant pain with a stinging or scalding sensation (localized or widespread), wound pallor, occasional gangrene; rarely fatal
Surgeonfish	Modified scalpel-like scale on caudal peduncle, some retract into sheath; non-venomous	Injuries very rare in the aquarium as these fish quickly become relatively tame; may cause lacerations
Rabbitfish	Various dorsal, pelvic and anal spines with associated venom glands	Injuries are rare but similar to scorpionfish
Sea urchins Long-spined urchins	Sharp spines in some species; some venomous	Very painful wounds from spines, which often break on penetration and are extremely difficult to remove; venomous species cause muscular paralysis, respiratory distress and occasionally death
Corals Fire coral	Stinging cells (nematocysts)	Instant burning sensation, persists for several hours; other corals cause lacerations that are slow to heal
Jellyfish Anemones	Stinging cells (nematocysts); variable effect depends on venom	Mild irritations, swelling, small skin haemorrhages, nausea and vomiting, salivation, delirium, convulsions, paralysis and respiratory difficulties
Bristleworms	Stinging bristles (setae)	Instant stinging sensation, swelling and numbness for several days
Cone shells	Highly dangerous; venomous 'teeth'	Reduced blood supply, stinging or burning sensations, paralysis, coma and occasionally death

Figure 34.5 Dangerous species: spines and stings.

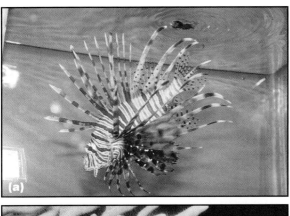
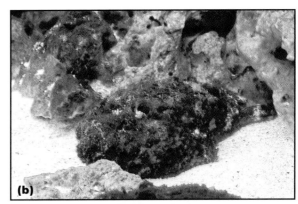
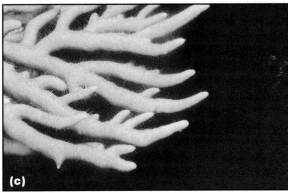
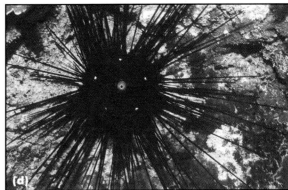

Figure 34.6 (a) The lionfish is a species commonly found in marine aquaria. The highly ornamental fins contain bony rays with venomous stinging cells. (Courtesy of Manor Aquatics; © W.H. Wildgoose.) (b) A stonefish is well camouflaged and has spines that can inject a venom that is rapidly lethal. This species is only occasionally seen outside public aquaria and is the only species for which there is an antivenin available. (Courtesy of London Aquarium; © W.H. Wildgoose.) (c) Fire or stinging coral can inflict very painful wounds that may persist for several weeks. (© W.H. Wildgoose.) (d) Long-spined sea urchins cause deep penetrating injuries. Some species are venomous and the sharp but brittle spines may break off in the wound. (Courtesy of London Aquarium; © W.H. Wildgoose.)

0.5–2% procaine. Wounds should then be covered with an antiseptic sterile dressing. The use of ligatures is not recommended. Antibacterial treatment and inoculation against tetanus may be required. Professional medical help should be sought immediately following stings from dangerous species. Further advice may also be obtained from the Veterinary Poisons Information Service in the UK.

Electric fish

Although incidents of electrocution are very rare, a number of fish species are capable of producing electric charges powerful enough to be of concern to aquarium workers and hobbyists. The most commonly seen in aquaria are the electric eel, electric catfish and several genera of rays. These fish produce electric currents from modified muscle tissues and modified gland cells in the skin. Some species release up to 600 volts for defence and capturing prey while other electric fish produce low voltage currents for orientation.

None of these fish are regarded as being capable of killing a human but care should be taken during handling. Workers should wear arm-length rubber gloves and be accompanied by another person in case of emergency. Electric eels are very tactile and often rub themselves along objects placed in the water, including arms. Accidents involving electric fish species usually result in an uneventful recovery but standard safety procedures following electrocution should be followed.

Water hazards

Pollution

Maintaining water quality in the aquarium is of the utmost importance, for the benefit of not just the fish inhabiting it but also aquarists coming into direct contact. Ingestion of water polluted with chemicals and other substances can be harmful to human health.

Drowning

This is a hazard faced by those who keep ponds, very large aquatic exhibits and open-top pools in public aquaria. In the latter, guard rails should be installed and work should be done whilst accompanied by another person. The following measures help to prevent accidents.

- Effective signage (Figure 34.7) should always be provided to warn people against the dangers of deep water and explain where first aid and safety equipment can be found
- Obstacles (e.g. fences, shrubs, flower-beds) can be positioned so as to make entry into the water difficult, although they are not always practical
- A wide shallow shelf can be created to form a barrier between dry land and deep water. This can also be heavily planted with marsh plants to further deter entry
- Children of all ages must be kept under close supervision

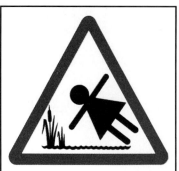

Figure 34.7
Warning signs should be used near garden ponds and other deep-water areas where children in particular are at risk. (© Ornamental Aquatic Trade Association.)

- Safety equipment, such as life-rings, should be available and within easy reach
- If possible, trained personnel should supervise areas around ponds and lakes.

Aquarium diving

Increasingly, public aquaria have tanks so large that divers are required to maintain them. It is very important to have safety protocols in place and this is stipulated in zoo licensing legislation. The situation at different aquaria will vary but it is essential that safety apparatus and diving first aid equipment be readily to hand. All divers, supervisors and first aid staff must be fully trained and conversant with the protocols laid down for their particular establishment. Essentially, there should always be two divers in the water at any one time and a surface supervisor must watch throughout the duration of each dive. The supervisor must be in easy communication (e.g. by radio) with other staff in case of emergency. In some countries, it is required that the supervisor is also in full communication with the divers, both visibly and audibly.

References and further reading

Halstead BW (1959) *Dangerous Marine Animals*. Cornell Maritime Press, Cambridge, Maryland
Health & Safety Executive (1999) *COSHH: A Brief Guide to the Regulations*. HSE Books, Sudbury
Health & Safety Executive (2000) *Approved Supply List*, 6th edn. HSE Books, Sudbury, Suffolk
Nemetz TH and Shotts EB Jr (1993) Zoonotic diseases. In: *Fish Medicine* (ed. MK Stoskopf) pp. 214–220. WB Saunders Co., Philadelphia
Sterba G (1978) *The Aquarist's Encyclopaedia*. Blandford Press, Poole, Dorset

Acknowledgements

The author is grateful to Pete Mohan of Six Flags Aquarium, Ohio, for his personal assistance in the preparation of this chapter.

Appendix 1

Conversion factors

Capacity

1 Imperial gallon	= 4.55 litres
	= 1.20 US gallons
1 US gallon	= 3.78 litres
	= 0.83 Imp gallons
1 litre	= 1000 millilitres (ml)
	= 0.22 Imp gallons
	= 0.26 US gallons
1 millilitre	= 1000 microlitres (μl)
1 cubic metre	= 35.31 cubic feet
	= 1000 litres
	= 220 Imp gallons
	= 265 US gallons
1 cubic foot	= 28.30 litres
	= 6.22 Imp gallons
	= 7.49 US gallons

Mass

1 pound (lb)	= 454 grams (g)
	= 16 ounces (oz)
1 ounce	= 28.35 grams
1 kilogram	= 1000 grams
	= 2.20 lb

Dilutions

1 part per thousand (ppt)	= 1 gram/litre
	= 1 ml/litre
1 part per million (ppm)	= 1 mg/litre
	= 1 ml/1000 litres
	= 1 mg/kg
1 part per billion (ppb)	= 1 microgram/litre
	= 1 microlitre/litre

Temperature

°C	°F
40	104.0
39	102.2
38	100.4
37	98.6
36	96.8
35	95.0
34	93.2
33	91.4
32	89.6
31	87.8
30	86.0
29	84.2
28	82.4
27	80.6
26	78.8
25	77.0
24	75.2
23	73.4
22	71.6
21	69.8
20	68.0
19	66.2
18	64.4
17	62.6
16	60.8
15	59.0
14	57.2
13	55.4
12	53.6
11	51.8
10	50.0
9	48.2
8	46.4
7	44.6
6	42.8
5	41.0
4	39.2
3	37.4
2	35.6
1	33.8
0	32.0

Scientific names of fish and aquatic invertebrates mentioned in the text

Common name	Scientific name
Acara, blue	*Aequidens pulcher*
Angelfish, blue	*Holacanthus bermudensis*
Angelfish, flame	*Centropyge loriculus*
Angelfish, French	*Pomacanthus paru*
Angelfish, freshwater	*Pterophyllum scalare*
Angelfish, passer (king)	*Holacanthus passer*
Angelfish, purple moon	*Arusetta asfur*
Angelfish, queen	*Holacanthus ciliaris*
Angelfish, tropical marine (family)	*Pomacanthidae*
Archerfish	*Toxotes jaculator*
Arowana	*Osteoglossum* spp.
Arowana, Asian	*Scleropages formosus*
Barb, black ruby	*Barbus nigrofasciatus*
Barb, rosy	*Barbus conchonius*
Barb, tiger	*Barbus tetrazona*
Barb, tinfoil	*Barbus schwanefeldi*
Barracuda	*Sphyraena* spp.
Bass, striped	*Morone saxatilis*
Bigeye	*Priacanthus arenatus*
Blenny (family)	*Blennidae*
Blenny, Midas	*Ecsenius midas*
Boney-tongued fish (family)	*Osteoglossidae*
Bream	*Abramis brama*
Bristleworms	*Eurythoe, Hermodice* spp.
Bullhead, brown	*Ictalurus nebulosus*
Butterflyfish (family)	*Chaetodontidae*
Butterflyfish, copper-band	*Chelmon rostratus*
Butterflyfish, four-eyed	*Chaetodon capistratus*
Butterflyfish, Klein's	*Chaetodon kleini*
Butterflyfish, raccoon	*Chaetodon lunula*
Carp (family)	*Cyprinidae*
Carp, black	*Mylopharyngodon piceus*
Carp, common	*Cyprinus carpio*
Carp, Crucian	*Carassius carassius*
Carp, grass	*Ctenopharyngodon idella*
Catfish, Corydoras (armoured)	*Corydoras* spp.
Catfish, channel	*Ictalurus punctatus*
Catfish, electric (family)	*Malapteruridae*
Catfish, red-tailed	*Phractocephalus hemioliopterus*
Catfish, suckermouth	*Plecostomus punctatus*
Catfish, Wels	*Silurus glanis*
Characins (family)	*Characidae*
Cichlids (family)	*Cichlidae*
Cichlid, dwarf	*Apistogramma* spp.
Cichlid, Malawi	*Aulonocara, Nimbochromis, Pseudotropheus* and other spp.
Cichlid, Midas	*Cichlasoma citrinellum*
Cichlid, Pearcii	*Cichlasoma pearcii*
Cichlid, pike	*Crenicichla* spp.
Cichlid, ram	*Papiliochromis ramirez*
Clownfish, common	*Amphiprion ocellaris*
Cone shell (family)	*Conidae*
Coral, fire	*Millepora alcicornis*
Cowfish	*Lactophrys quadricornis*
Crab, anemone	*Neopetrolisthes* spp.
Crab, boxing	*Libia* spp.
Crab, Cameroon	*Cardisoma armatum*
Crab, fiddler	*Uca* spp.
Crab, hermit (family)	*Paguridae*
Crab, red hermit	*Dardanus megistos*
Crab, sponge (family)	*Calappidae*
Crayfish, white-clawed	*Austropotamobius pallipes*
Crayfish, North American signal	*Pacifastacus leniusculus*
Croaker, white	*Genyonemus lineatus*
Damselfish (family)	*Pomacentridae*
Damselfish, yellow-tailed	*Chromis xanthurus*
Danio	*Brachydanio, Danio* spp.
Danio, zebra	*Brachydanio rerio*
Discus	*Symphysodon discus*
Doctorfish	*Labroides dimidatus*
Eel, electric	*Electrophorus electricus*
Eel, European	*Anguilla anguilla*
Eel, green moray	*Gymnothorax funebris*
Eel, moray	*Gymnothorax, Muraena* spp.
Elephantnoses	*Campylomormyrus, Mormyrus* spp.
Fighting fish, Siamese	*Betta splendens*
Flounder (family)	*Bothidae*
Glassfish (family)	*Chandidae*
Goby (family)	*Gobiidae*
Goby, Catalina	*Lythrypnus dalli*
Goby, neon	*Gobiosoma oceanops*
Goldfish	*Carassius auratus*
Gourami	*Colisa, Helostoma, Trichogaster* spp.
Gourami, dwarf	*Colisa lalia*
Gourami, three-spot	*Trichogaster trichopterus*
Grouper (family)	*Serranidae*
Guarti, red-eyed	*Haplochromis* spp.
Gudgeon	*Pseudorasbora parva*
Guppy	*Poecilia reticulata*
Highhat	*Equetus acuminatus*
Ice fish, Antarctic	*Chaenocephalus aceratus*
Jacks	*Caranx* spp.

Common name	Scientific name	Common name	Scientific name
Jellyfish	*Scyphozoans, Cyanae, Dactylometra* spp.	Shark, black-tip reef	*Carcharhinus melanopterus*
		Shark, bonnet-head	*Sphyrna tiburo*
Jelly, moon	*Aurelia aurita*	Shark, lemon	*Negaprion brevirostris*
Jelly, upside-down	*Cassiopeia xamachana*	Shark, nurse	*Ginglymostoma cirratum*
Killifish	*Aphyosemion, Cynolebis, Epiplatys, Nothobranchius* and other spp.	Shark, sandbar	*Carcharhinus plumbeus*
		Shark, sand tiger	*Carcharias taurus*
		Sheepshead, California	*Semicossyphus pulcher*
Koi	*Cyprinus carpio*	Shrimp, anemone	*Periclimenes* spp.
Labyrinthfish (families)	*Anabantidae, Belontiidae, Helostomidae, Osphronemidae*	Shrimp, banded coral	*Stenopus hispidus*
		Shrimp, brine	*Artemia* spp.
Leaf-fish (family)	*Nandidae*	Shrimp, cleaner	*Stemopus, Lysmata* spp.
Lionfish	*Pterois volitans*	Shrimp, peppermint	*Lysmata wurdemanni*
Loaches (family)	*Cobitidae*	Shrimpfish	*Aeoliscus strigatus*
Lobster	*Homarus, Panulirus* spp.	Silver dollars	*Metynnis argenteus*
Lungfish, African	*Protopterus dolloi*	Smelt, rainbow	*Osmerus mordax*
Minnow, common	*Phoxinus phoxinus*	Smoothhound	*Mustelus* spp.
Minnow, White Cloud Mountain	*Tanichthys albonubes*	Snakehead (family)	*Channidae*
Molly (family)	*Poeciliidae*	Squirrelfish	*Holocentrus rufus*
Molly, balloon	*Poecilia molliensis*	Starfish, basket	*Astrophyton muricatum*
Molly, black	*Poecilia sphenops*	Starfish, brittle	*Ophiomastix venosa*
Mormyridae (family)	*Campylomormyrus, Mormyrus* spp.	Starfish, feather	*Himerometra robustipinna*
		Starfish, red knobbed	*Protoreaster lincki*
Mummichog	*Funfulus heteroclitus*	Sterlet	*Acipenser* spp.
Nautilus	*Nautilus* spp.	Stickleback	*Gasterosteus aculeatus*
Octopus, blue ring	*Hapalochlaena maculosa*	Stingray, southern	*Dasyatis americana*
Octopus, common	*Octopus vulgaris*	Stingray, freshwater (family)	*Potamotrygonidae*
Octopus, giant Pacific	*Octopus dofleini*	Stonefish (family)	*Synancejidae*
Orfe	*Leuciscus idus*	Sturgeon	*Acipenser* spp.
Oscar	*Astronotus ocellatus*	Surgeonfish (family)	*Acanthuridae*
Pacu	*Colossoma* spp.	Swordtail (family)	*Xiphiidae*
Paddlefish	*Polyodon, Psephurus* spp.	Tang (family)	*Acanthuridae*
Paradisefish	*Macropodus opercularis*	Tench	*Tinca tinca*
Pearlfish, black-fin	*Cynolebias nigripinnis*	Tetra (subfamily)	*Characidae*
Pencilfish	*Nannostomus, Nannobrycon* spp.	Tetra, cardinal	*Cheirodon axelrodi*
Pencilfish, black-stripe	*Nannostomus harrisoni*	Tetra, neon	*Paracheirodon innesi*
Perch (family)	*Percidae*	Tilapia (family)	*Tilapia*
Pike	*Esox luscius*	Tilapia, Mozambique	*Tilapia mossambica*
Pike-perch	*Stizostedion* spp.	Tilapia, Nile	*Oreochromis niloticus*
Piranha	*Serrasalmus* spp.	Triggerfish (family)	*Balistidae*
Platy	*Xiphophorus* spp.	Trout, brown	*Salmo trutta*
Porcupinefish (family)	*Diodontidae*	Trout, rainbow	*Oncorhynchus mykiss*
Puffer (family)	*Tetraodontidae*	Trumpetfish (family)	*Aulostomidae*
Pumpkinseed	*Lepomis gibbosus*	Tuna	*Thunnus* spp.
Pupfish, desert	*Cyprinodon macularius*	Tuna, bluefin	*Thunnus thynnus*
Rabbitfish (family)	*Siganidae*	Urchin, long-spined	*Diadema, Asthenosoma* spp.
Rainbowfish	*Bedotia, Melanotaenia, Thelmatherina* spp.	Urchin, sea	*Toxopneustes* spp.
		Variatus	*Xiphophorus variatus*
Rasbora	*Rasbora* spp.	Worm, Christmas tree	*Spirobranchus giganteus*
Ray, cownose	*Rhinoptera bonasus*	Worm, feather-duster	*Sabellastarte magnifica*
Ray, southern	*Dasyatis americana*	Wrasse, cleaner	*Labroides dimidiatus*
Roach	*Rutilus rutilus*	Yellowtail	*Seriola quinqueradiata*
Rudd	*Scardinus erythrophthalmus*		
Salmon, coho	*Oncorhynchus kisutch*		
Scallop, flame	*Lima scabra*		
Scats	*Scatophagus* spp.		
Scorpionfish	*Scorpaena* spp.		
Sea apple	*Pseudocolochirus axiologus*		
Sea bass, Mediterranean	*Dicentrarchus labrax*		
Sea bream, gilthead	*Sparus aurata*		
Sea cucumber (family)	*Holothuridea*		
Sea-horse	*Hippocampus* spp.		

Descriptive terms

cyprinid	of the carp family Cyprinidae (e.g. carp, goldfish)
elasmobranch	cartilaginous fish
live-bearers	freshwater fish that give birth to live young (e.g. guppy, molly, platy, i.e. family Poeciliidae)
percoid	perch-like but not in perch family (e.g. pumpkinseed)
salmonid	of the family Salmonidae (e.g. salmon, trout)
teleost	bony fish

Appendix 3

Fish health societies and related organizations

British Veterinary Association
7 Mansfield Street
London W1G 9NQ
UK
Tel: +44 (0) 20 7636 6541
www.bva.co.uk

British Veterinary Zoological Society
c/o Derek Lyons
7 Bridgewater Mews
Gresford Heath
Pandy
Wrexham LL12 8EQ
Clwyd
UK
www.bvzs.org

The Centre for Environment, Fisheries and Aquaculture Science (CEFAS)
Barrack Road
The Nothe
Weymouth
Dorset DT4 8UB
UK
Tel: +44 (0) 1305 206600
www.cefas.co.uk

European Association of Fish Pathologists
c/o David Bruno (Secretary)
FRS Marine Laboratory
Victoria Road
Aberdeen AB11 9DB
UK
Tel: +44 (0) 1224 295615
www.ifremer.fr/eafp

Fisheries Research Services
FRS Marine Laboratory
Victoria Road
Aberdeen AB11 9DB
UK
Tel: +44 (0) 1224 876544
www.marlab.ac.uk

Fish Veterinary Society
c/o Edward Branson (President)
Red House Farm
Llanvihangel
Monmouth
Gwent NP5 4HL
UK
www.fishvetsociety.org.uk

Institute of Aquaculture
University of Stirling
Stirling FK9 4LA
UK
Tel: +44 (0) 1786 467878
www.stir.ac.uk/Departments/NaturalSciences/Aquaculture

International Association for Aquatic Animal Medicine
c/o Frances Gulland (President)
The Marine Mammal Center
Marin Headlands
Golden Gate National Recreation Area
Sausalito
CA 94965
USA
+1 415 289 7325
iaaam.org

Ornamental Aquatic Trade Association
Unit 5
Narrow Wine Street
Trowbridge
Wiltshire BA14 8YY
UK
Tel: +44 (0) 1225 777177
www.ornamentalfish.org

Registry of Tumors in Lower Animals
Department of Pathology
George Washington University Medical Center
2300 I Street N.W.
Washington DC 20037
USA
fact.gwumc.edu/tumour

Royal College of Veterinary Surgeons
Belgravia House
62–64 Horseferry Road
London SW1P 2AF
UK
Tel: +44 (0) 20 7222 2001
www.rcvs.org.uk

A more detailed list of American and worldwide fish diagnostic laboratories can be found in Stoskopf (1993) *Fish Medicine*, pp. 823–828 (W.B. Saunders Co., Philadelphia)

Index

Abandonment of Animals Act 1960, 276–7
Abdomen, examination of, 88
Abdominal enlargement, 130–2
  ascites, 131–2
  blood, 132
  gastric foreign body, 131
  intestinal obstruction, 132
  neoplasia, 130
  obesity, 131
  ovarian disorders, 132
  parasites, 132
  polycystic kidneys, 131
  swim-bladder disorders, 130–1
Abnormal pitch, 159
Abscesses, 128
Acanthamoeba spp., 167
Acanthamoeba polyphaga, 171
Acanthocephalans, 175, 180
Accidents, 165–6
  asphyxia, 166
  electrocution, 166
  escape, 165
  water loss, 166
Acetazolamide, 246
Acetic acid, glacial, 243
Achlya spp., 195, 200
Acid–base balance, 137
Acriflavine, 244, 247
Activated carbon, 54, 246
Additive genetic variance, 233
Additive traits, 233
Adhesives, toxicity of, 286
Adverse drug reactions, 257
Aeration of aquaria, 38
  see also Filtration systems; Oxygen
Aerococcus viridans, 273
Aeromonas spp., 153
Aeromonas caviae, 186, 187
Aeromonas hydrophila, 58, 129, 130, 185, 186, 187–8, 189, 287
Aeromonas salmonicida, 118, 185, 187
  subsp. *achromogenes*, 188–9
Aeromonas sobria, 186, 187
Aggression, 161, 211
Air pumps, 30
Albinism, 113
Alcohol disinfectants, 255
Algae, 165, 200
Algal bloom, 35, 206, 210
Algicides, 217
Alkalinity, 3–4, 210
  and metal toxicity, 215
  see also pH
Alleles, 233
Alphaxolone–alphadalone, 82
Aluminium, 214
Amikacin, 244
Amino acid deficiency, 228

2-Amino-4-phenylthiazole, 78
Ammonia, 7, 55, 206–7
  and anorexia, 156
  measurement, 7
  and pH, 2
  toxicity, 7, 140, 157
Ammonium chloride, 246
Amoebae, 167, 171
Amoxycillin, 244, 247
Amyloodinium spp., 116, 167
Amyloodinium ocellatum, 141, 143, 167–8
Ana-aki-byo, 204
Anabaena spp., 200
Anaemia, 141, 158
  nutritional causes, 228
Anaesthesia, 76–7, 259
  consent forms, 77
  health and safety, 77
  induction, 77
  inhalation, 77–81
    anaesthetic agents, 77–9
    artificial ventilation systems, 80–1
    direct application, 79
    emergency resuscitation, 81
    maintenance of water quality, 79
    procedure, 79
    recovery, 81
  invertebrates, 268
  legislation, 77
  maintenance, 77
  monitoring, 77
  non-chemical, 82
  parenteral, 81–2
  preparation, 76–7
  recovery, 77
Analgesia, 76, 246, 261
Anatomy, 123–5, 259
  body cavity, 124
  cardiovascular system, 125
  digestive system, 124–5
    liver, 124–5
    oral cavity, 124
    stomach and intestinal tract, 124
    swim-bladder, 125
  endocrine system, 125
  eye, 147–9
    choroid, 147
    cornea, 147
    globe, 147
    iris, 149
    lens, 149
    light response, 149
    retina, 147–8, 149
    sclera, 147
  musculoskeletal system, 123–4
  reproductive system, 125
  respiratory tract, 135–6

  skin, 110–11
  urinary system, 125
Anchor worm *see Lernaea*
Anemones, 270
  colonial, 270–1
  disc, 270
  diseases of, 270, 271
  feeding, 270, 271
  new stock, 270
  stings, 288
  water quality, 270, 271
Angelfish, black, 235
Anguillicola spp., 179
Animal Transport Regulations, 12
Animal Welfare Act, 283
Animals (Scientific Procedures) Act 1986 as amended, 277
Anisakis spp., 175
Annelid worms, 175, 180, 288
Anodonta spp., 181
Anorexia, 156, 238
  causes
    ammonia, 156
    bacteria, 156
    dehydration, 156
    parasites, 156
    pH, 156
    predation, 156
  in sharks, 56
Antibacterial agents, 244–5
Antibiotics, 242
  in-water medication, 239
  sensitivity testing, 98–9, 186–7
Antifungal agents, 246
Antiparasitic agents, 243–4
Aphanizomenon spp., 200
Aphanomyces spp., 195, 200
Aphanomyces astaci, 273
Apicomplexa, 167
Apiosoma spp., 167, 170
Apiosoma piscicolum, 170
Aquaria
  breakages, 285
  cleaning and disinfection, 74
  examination of, 71
  filtration systems, 19–20
  freshwater *see* Freshwater aquaria
  marine *see* Marine aquaria
  public *see* Public aquaria
Aquarium diving, 290
Aquatic environment, 1–8, 63, 69–74
  alkalinity, 3–4
  chloramine, 8
  chlorine, 8
  density, 2
  dissolved gases, 4–5, 208–10
    see also Carbon dioxide; Chlorine; Nitrogen; Oxygen
  domestic hazards, 8

hardness, 3
metals, 8
nitrogenous compounds, 6–8
    see also Ammonia; Nitrate;
    Nitrite
pesticides, 8, 216
pH see pH
physical properties, light, 2
ponds see Ponds
salinity see Salinity
sound, 2
surface tension, 2
temperature see Temperature
see also Environmental disorders
Aquatic invertebrates see Invertebrates
Aquatic traders see Dealers
Argulus spp., 113, 114, 150, 153, 175, 182
Argulus foliaceus, 182
Artemia spp., 271, 272
Artemia salina, 272
Artificial ventilation systems, 80–1
    non-recirculating, 80
    recirculating, 80–1
Ascites, 120, 131–2
Asellus, 8
Asphyxia, 166
Atractolytocestus spp., 175
Atropine, 246
Aurantiactinomyxon ictaluri, 158
Aureobasidium spp., 200
Autosomal chromosomes, 233
Azamethiphos, 247
Aztreonam, 244

Bacterial disease, 113, 185–93
    abnormal swimming behaviour, 157
    anorexia, 156
    bruising, 114
    causal factors, 185
        bacterial virulence, 185
        stress, 185
    clinical signs, 186
    diagnosis, 186–7
        antibiotic susceptibility tests, 186–7
        clinical outcome, 187
        identification, 186
        interpretation, 186
        sampling, 186
    gill disease, 158
    gill necrosis, 142–3
    mouth ulcers, 126
    prevention, 185
    skin texture changes, 120
    swellings, 116
    see also Bacterial pathogens
Bacterial filters, 238
Bacterial gill disease, 191
Bacterial pathogens, 187–93
    Aeromonas salmonicida subsp.
        achromogenes, 188–9
    Chlamydia, 192–3
    Cytophaga–Flavobacterium–
        Flexibacter group, 190–1
    Edwardsiellae, 191–2
    motile aeromonads, 187–8
    mycobacteria, 190
    Nocardiae, 192
    Photobacterium damsela subsp.
        piscicida, 192
    pseudomonads, 188
    streptococci, 191
    vibrios, 189–90
Bacteriology, 96–9
    antibiotic sensitivity testing, 98–9

bacteriological identification, 98
inoculation of culture plates, 97–8
respiratory disease, 140
sampling, 97
sampling equipment, 97
serology, 98
skin, 112
stained tissue smears, 99
Ballottement, 125
Barley straw, 70, 200, 216
Barracuda, 288
Batch screening, 254
Behaviour, 73
    see also Behavioural changes;
    Compatibility of captive species
Behavioural changes, 155–61
    aggression, 161
    colour change, 161
    feeding behaviour, 156–7
        anorexia, 156
        dysphagia, 156
        pica, 156–7
    reproductive behaviour, 160–1
        lip-lock, 160
        spawning, 160–1
    swimming behaviour, 157–60
        abnormal buoyancy, 158–60
        abnormal schooling, 157
        clamped fins, 160
        coughing, 160
        flashing, 160
        hanging or drifting, 160
        jumping, 160
        piping, 157–8
        spinning, surfing and
            disorientation, 157
    toxins, 213
Benedenia spp., 120, 175, 176
Benzocaine, 78
Binding agents, 252
Biocides, 216–17
Biological filtration, 54
Biological oxygen demand, 4
Biopsy, 265
Birnaviruses, 204
Bites, 287–8
Black spot, 116, 177, 178
Bleeding
    into body cavity, 132
    into opercular cavity, 145
Blood sampling, 96
Bodonidae, 167, 168–9
Body cavity, 124
    bleeding into, 132
    see also Internal disorders
Body shape, abnormal, 128–32
    abdominal enlargement, 130–2
    body wall lesions, 128
    spinal lesions, 129–30
Boreholes, 214
Bothriocephalus spp., 132, 175
Bothriocephalus acheilognathi, 178
Branchioblastoma, 145
Branchiomyces spp., 143, 197–8
Branchiomyces demigrans, 197–8
Branchiomyces sanguinis, 197–8
Branchiurans, 175, 182
Breeding, 231–2
    aquarium fish
        freshwater, 42
        marine, 49
    broodstock, 14
    bubble-nest builders, 232
    cichlids, 232
    egg incubation, 15
    egg scatterers, 232

larval husbandry, 15–16
live-bearers, 231–2
manipulation of, 14–15
pond fish, 34
Bristleworms, 288
Bronopol, 246, 247
Broodstock, 14
    conditioning, 231
    disorders of, 231
Brooklynella spp., 120, 167
Brooklynella hostilis, 141, 170
Bruising, 114
Bubble-bead filters, 28
Bubble-nest builders, 232
Bucephalus spp., 175
Buffering capacity of water, 2, 3–4
Buoyancy, abnormal, 158–60
    abnormal pitch, 159
    excess negative buoyancy, 159
    excess positive buoyancy, 158–9
    listing, 159
Butorphanol, 246, 261

Cadmium, 214
Caligus spp., 175
Caligus elongatus, 181
Camallanus spp., 115, 133, 175, 179
Camouflage, 161
Campylobacter spp., 58
Capillaria spp., 133, 175, 179, 226
Capillostrongyloides spp., 179
Capriniana spp., 167, 170
Capriniana piscium, 170
Carbohydrates, dietary, 225
Carbon dioxide, 5, 209
    anaesthesia, 78
    and pH, 2
Cardinal tetra, 41
Cardiovascular system, 125
Carp, 31
Carp pituitary extract, 246
Carp pox, 117, 202
Cataracts, 151–2
Catfish, 288
Ceratomyxa spp., 173
Cestodes, 175, 178–9
Chasing, 161
Chemical filtration, 54
Chilodonella spp., 23, 120, 141, 167, 170
Chilodonella hexasticha, 170
Chilodonella piscicola, 170
Chitin inhibitors, 182
Chlamydia spp., 187, 192–3
Chloramine-T, 8, 210, 243, 244, 255, 257
Chlorhexidine, 255
Chlorine, 8, 210, 217
    and pH, 2
    toxicity, 140, 214
Chlorinity, 6
Chloromyxum spp., 173, 174
Chloroquine diphosphate, 243
Choroid, 147
Christmas-tree worms, 272
Chromatoblastomas, 220
Chromosomes, 233
Cichlid bloat, 132
Cichlids, 232
Ciliates, 167, 169–71
Clamped fins, 160
Cleaner fish, 253
Cleaning
    aquaria, 43, 74
    ponds, 34

Client records, 65–7
Clinic visits, 63, 64
Clinical examination, 85–9, 93
    abdomen, 88
    eyes, 87–8
    general appearance, 86
    gills, 88
    heart, 88
    for internal disorders, 125
    mouth, 87
    olfactory openings, 87
    opercular cavity, 88
    preliminary, 85
    skeleton, 89
    skin, 86–7
    sudden death, 163
    vent, 88–9
Clinostomum spp., 116, 128, 175, 177
Clove oil, 78
Coccidians, 171–2
Coldwater disease, 191
Coldwater systems
    stocking levels, 22
    water quality, 21
Colour change, 87, 112–14, 161
    bruising, 114
    camouflage, 161
    courtship, 161
    and diet, 226
    disease, 161
    generalized inflammation
        septicaemia, 112, 113
        spring viraemia of carp, 112–13
    localized inflammation
        bacteria, 113
        parasites, 113
        sunburn, 113
    loss of colour
        albinism, 113
        epidermal hyperplasia, 114
        excess mucus, 114
        management problems, 113
        mycobacteriosis, 113
        neon tetra disease, 114
Compatibility of captive species, 41, 48,
    73
Computed tomography, 107
    internal disorders, 126
Cone shells, 288
Connective tissue neoplasia, 221
Consent forms, 77, 258, 260
Control of Substances Hazardous to
    Health Regulations 1999, 279
Convention on International Trade in
    Endangered Species (CITES), 278
Copepods, 144, 175, 181–2
Copper, 8, 214
Copper sulphate, 243
Coral fish disease, 143
Corals, 268–70
    diseases of, 269–70
    feeding, 269
    light, 269
    new stock, 269
    stinging, 288
    water quality, 269
Cornea, 147
Corneal ulceration, 150–1
Coronavirus, 204
Cotton-wool disease *see Saprolegnia*
Cough reflex, 138, 160
Courtship, colour changes associated
    with, 161
Crabs, 272–3
Crustaceans, 175, 181–3
    branchiurans, 182

copepods, 144, 181–2
    feeding, 272, 273
    freshwater, 273
    isopods, 144, 182–3
    marine, 272–3
    water quality, 272
Cryptobia spp., 132, 141, 167, 168–9
Cryptobia agitans, 169
Cryptocaryon spp., 120, 150, 167
Cryptocaryon irritans, 115–16, 141, 143,
    171
Cuticle, 111
Cypermethrin, 247
Cytophaga spp., 118, 142, 158, 190–1
Cytophaga psychrophila, 191

Dactylogyrus spp., 141, 175, 176
Dangerous species, 287–9
    bites, 287–8
    electric fish, 289
    stings, 288–9
    see also Sharks
Daphnia, 16, 233
Dealers, 17, 19–24
    disease control, 23
    filtration systems, 19–20
        aquaria, 19–20
        pond systems, 20
    health problems, 23
    recommendation, 67
    stock management, 22–3
    stocking levels, 21–2
        coldwater, 22
        marine, 22
        tropical freshwater, 21–2
    veterinary approach, 23–4
    water quality management, 20–1
        and effect of transportation, 21
Dehydration, and anorexia, 156
Density of water, 2
Dental overgrowth, 127
Dermis, 111
Dermocystidium spp., 199–200
Dermocystidium koi, 115, 118, 199–200
Dermocystidium salmonis, 199–200
Dermophthirius spp., 175, 176
Detergents, 120
Developmental anomalies, 223–4
Dexamethasone, 246
Dichlorvos, 214
Diet,
    and colour, 226
    and health, 256
    inappropriate, 227
Dietary deficiencies, 56
    see also Malnutrition; Nutritional
        disorders
Diflubenzuron, 182, 243
Digeneans, 175, 177–8
Digestive system, 124–5
    liver, 124–5
    neoplasia, 222
    oral cavity, 124
    stomach and intestinal tract, 124
    swim-bladder, 125
Dinoflagellates, 143
Diphyllobothrium spp., 175
Diplostomum spp., 151, 175, 177, 178
Discocotyle sagitta, 176
Discus, 40, 41
Disease control, 23
    marine aquaria, 50
    ponds, 33
Disease control legislation, UK, 277
Diseases of Fish Act 1937, 277

Diseases of Fish Act 1983, 277
Disinfectants, 23, 74, 255–6
Disorientation, 157
Dissolved gases, 4–5, 208–10
    see also Carbon dioxide; Chlorine;
        Nitrogen; Oxygen
Diuron, 283
Domestic hazards, 8, 216
Domestic water supply, 214
Dominant genetic variance, 233
Dominant traits, 233
Doppler pulse ultrasound, 77, 88
Doxapram, 246
Drifting, 160
Dropsy, 120, 170
Drowning, 289–90
Drug resistance, 238
Dysphagia, 156
Dyspnoea, 137
Dystocia, 132

E-test, 99
EC Zoos Directive, 278
Echinoderms, 273–4
Echinorhynchus spp., 175
Echinorynchus truttae, 180
Ectoparasites, 141–2
    examination for, 94–6
        gill preparations, 95–6
        skin preparations, 94–5
    gills, 143–4
Edwardsiella spp., 187, 191–2
Edwardsiella ictaluri, 119, 157, 191–2
Edwardsiella tarda, 58, 158, 159, 191–2
Egg binding, 132, 232
Egg hatching, 231
Egg incubation, 15
Egg layers, 232
Eimeria spp., 167
Eimeria anguillae, 172
Eimeria rutili, 172
Electric conductivity, 5–6
Electric fish, 289
Electrical faults, 285
Electrical shock, 210–11
Electro-anaesthesia, 82
Electrocardiography, 126
Electrocution, 166
Emaciation, 133–4
Emamectin, 247
Endocrine system, 125
Endoscopy, 108, 266
    internal disorders, 126
Enrofloxacin, 245
Enterococcus spp., 191
Enucleation, 264
Environment *see* Aquatic environment
Environmental disorders, 205–12
    algal overgrowth, 210
    chlorine and chloramine, 210
    dissolved gases, 208–10
    electrical shock, 210–11
    flooding and runoff, 211
    hardness and alkalinity, 210
    nitrogenous compounds, 206–7
    physical damage, 211
    salinity, 207–8
    sunburn, 211
    water quality, 205–6
Environmental improvement, 237–8, 253
Environmental Protection Act 1990, 279
Epidermal hyperplasia, 114, 127
Epidermis, 111
Epistasis, 233
Epistatic genetic variance, 234

Epistylis spp., 167, 170, 226
Epistylis iwoffi, 170
Epitheliocystis, 116, 144
Equipment
    bacterial sampling, 97
    faulty, 285
    ponds, 30
    radiography, 103
    ultrasonography, 105
Ergasilus spp., 141, 175, 181
Eroded mouth syndrome, 190
Erpocotyle laevis, 176
Erysipelothrix spp., 58
Erythromycin, 245, 257
Erythrophores, 111
Erythrophoroma, 221
Escape, 165, 211
Escherichia coli, 58
Etomidate, 78
Eustrongylides spp., 175, 226
Euthanasia, 61, 82–3
    by owners, 83
    invertebrates, 268
Exophiala spp., 200
Exophthalmos, 152
Eyes, examination of, 87–8
    see also Ocular disorders

Faeces, abnormal, 132–3
Failure to respond to treatment, 257
Feather duster worms, 272
Federal Environment Pesticide Control
    Act, 282–3
Federal Food, Drug, and Cosmetic Act,
    281–2
Feeding, 74
    see also Diet; Nutrition
Feeding behaviour, 156–7
    anorexia, 156
    dysphagia, 156
    pica, 156–7
Feeding regimen, 226–7
Fenbendazole, 243
Fenthion, 283
Fibroma, 118
Fighting, 211
Filtration media
    ponds, 28–30
    flow rates, 29
    retention time, 29–30
Filtration systems, 19–20, 71–2
    freshwater aquaria, 19–20, 38–41
        foam filters, 38–9
        hang-on filters, 40
        power filters, 39–40
        trickle filters, 40–1
        undergravel filters, 39
    for invertebrates, 267
    marine aquaria, 46–8
        power filters, 46
        sand filters, 47
        trickle filters, 46, 47
        undergravel filters, 46
    ponds, 20, 26–8, 71–2
        bubble-bead filters, 28
        fluidized filters, 28
        gravity-fed filters, 26–7
        pump-fed external filters, 26
        trickle tower filters, 28
        undergravel filters, 27–8
        vegetable filters, 28
    public aquaria, 53–5
        biological filtration, 54
        chemical filtration, 54
        mechanical filtration, 53–4

Fin nipping, 121, 161
Fin rot, 120, 121, 191
Fins, 87
    clamped, 160
Fire coral, 288
First aid, 238
    non-medical, 64
Fish Diseases Act 1937, 12
Fish Health Regulations 1997, 12
Fish health societies, 294
Flagellates, 167
    bodonids, 168–9
    hexamitids, 169
    oodinids, 167–8
    trypanosomes, 168
Flashing, 138, 160
Flavobacterium spp., 118, 142, 153, 158,
    190–1
Flavobacterium branchiophilum, 142,
    191
Flavobacterium columnare, 115, 119,
    120, 121, 126, 190, 191
Flexibacter spp., 118, 142, 158, 190–1
Flexibacter maritimus, 190, 191
Flooding, 211
Florfenicol, 245, 247
Fluidized filters, 28
Flukes, 23
Foam filters, 38–9
Foam fractionation, 30, 54
Foreign bodies, 127, 131, 145
    and anorexia, 156
Formalin, 243, 246, 247, 257
    neutral buffered, 100
Freshwater aquaria, 37–44
    aeration, 38
    decor, 38
    filtration, 38–41
        foam filter, 38–9
        hang-on filters, 40
        power filter, 39–40
        trickle filters, 40–1
        undergravel filter, 39
    health problems, 44
    heating, 37–8
    holidays, 44
    lighting, 38
    maintenance, 43–4
        cleaning, 43
        partial water changes, 43
        plants, 43–4
        procedures, 43
        water quality, 43
    plants, 41
    positioning, 37
    selection, 37
    see also Marine aquaria
Fry, 231, 233
Fumagillin, 243
Fungal disease, 115, 195–200
    gill necrosis, 143
    ocular disorders, 154
    swellings, 116
    see also specific fungi
Furazolidone, 245

Gaffkaemia, 273
Gas accumulation, 152–3
Gas bubble disease, 117, 152–3, 165, 209
Gas exchange, restricted, 164
Gases, toxic, 217
    see also Chlorine; Hydrogen
    sulphide
Gastric emptying time, 252
Gastrointestinal disease, 158

Gavage, 241
Genes, 233
Genetic characteristics, 233–4
Genetics, 233–6
    and disease, 234–6
    fancy goldfish, 234–5
Genotype, 233
Gentamicin, 245
    toxicity, 217
Gill disease, 158
Gill flukes, 143
Gill rot, 143, 197–8
Gills
    biopsy, 139
    brown coloration, 143
    chrondroma, 145
    clubbed, 228
    colour change, 140–3
    examination, 88
        for ectoparasites, 95–6
    hyperplasia, 142, 144
    hypertrophy, 142, 144
    metal toxicity, 215
    necrosis, 142–3
    neoplasia, 145
    normal gross appearance, 140
    sample examination, 112, 139
    swellings, 144–5
    visible ectoparasites, 143–4
    see also Respiratory disease
Globe, 147
Glugea spp., 144, 150, 167, 173
Glycera spp., 288
Glyphosate, 214
Gnathia spp., 182–3
Goitre, 128, 145
Gold dust disease, 116
Goldfish, 41
    genetic disorders, 234–5
    varieties, 31
Gonadectomy, 265
Goussia spp., 167
Goussia aurata, 172
Goussia carpelli, 172
Goussia metchnikovi, 172
Goussia sinensis, 172
Goussia subepithelialis, 172
Granulomas, 128
Gravel cleaners, 39
Gravity-fed filters, 26–7
Grouper, 288
Guppy, 41
Guppy killer, 120
Gyrodactylus spp., 120, 141, 171, 175

Haematoma, 128
Haemolytic anaemia, 141
Haemorrhage *see* Bleeding
Haemorrhagic anaemia, 141
Halothane, 78
Hang-on filters, 40
Hanging, 160
Hardness of water, 3, 210
    abnormality, 3
    measurement, 3
    and metal toxicity, 215
    requirement, 3
Hartmanella spp., 167
Hatch rates, 232–3
Hazardous substances
    adhesives, 286
    legislation, 285–6
    medications, 286
    salt, 286
    zoonoses, 286–7

Head and lateral line erosion syndrome, 119, 204
Head standing, 159
Head-down, 159
Health controls for fish farming, 13–14
Health problems
  dealers, 23
  freshwater aquaria, 44
  marine aquaria, 51
  ponds, 35–6
Health and safety, 285–90
  dangerous species, 287–9
  faulty equipment, 285
  hazardous substances, 285–7
  water hazards, 289–90
Heart, examination of, 88
Heating
  freshwater aquaria, 37–8
  invertebrate needs, 267
  marine aquaria, 45
Hemiclepsis marginata, 168
Henneguya spp., 116, 128, 144, 150, 173
Herbal remedies, 254
Herbicides, 217
Heritability, 234
Herpesvirus diseases, 202–3
Heterosporis spp., 167, 173
Heterosporis finki, 173
Heterosporis schuberti, 173
Hexacapsula spp., 173
Hexamita, 133, 169
Hexamitidae, 167, 169
Histopathology, 100–1
  skin, 112
History taking, 63–4
Hoferellus carassii, 174
Hole-in-the-head, 119, 191
Home visits, 63
Household chemicals, 216
Hovering, 137
Hydrogen peroxide, 243, 246, 247
Hydrogen sulphide, 209–10, 214, 217
Hyperaemia, 121
Hyperthermia, 165, 205
Hypodermis, 111
Hypoplastic anaemia, 141
Hypothermia, 205
  anaesthesia, 82
Hypoxaemia, 208
Hypoxia, 157
  sudden death, 164
Hysterothylacium spp., 175

IATA regulations, 10
Ich *see Ichthyophthirius multifiliis*
Ichthyobodo spp., 23, 120, 167, 168–9
Ichthyobodo necator, 141, 169
Ichthyophonus spp., 133, 198–9
Ichthyophonus hoferi, 116, 128, 129, 198–9
Ichthyophthirius spp., 120, 150, 167, 226
Ichthyophthirius multifiliis, 33, 115, 141, 143, 158, 170–1
Imaging techniques, 103–8
Immuno-stimulants, 254
Import of Live Fish (England and Wales) Act 1980, 12, 277
In-feed medication, 240–1
  bodyweight, 240
  dose rate, 240
  feeding rate, 240
  interval, 240–1
  methods, 241
    gelatin-treated food, 241

ice-cube method, 241
    medicated food items, 241
    pre-medicated feed, 241
    soaking pellet food, 241
    surface-coating of pellet food, 241
In-water medication, 239–40
  absorption, timing and weather, 239
  antibacterial drugs, 239
  distribution, 239–40
  permanent baths, 239
  short dips, 239
Inbreeding, 236
Infection
  sudden death, 165
  see also Parasites
Inhalation anaesthesia *see* Anaesthesia
Injection, 241–2
Instruments, surgical, 259
Internal disorders, 123–34
  abnormal body shape, 128–32
    abdominal enlargement, 130–2
    body wall lesions, 128
    spinal lesions, 129–30
  anatomy, 123–5
    body cavity, 124
    cardiovascular system, 125
    digestive system, 124–5
    endocrine system, 125
    musculoskeletal system, 123–4
    reproductive system, 125
    urinary system, 125
  emaciation, 133–4
    chronic disease, 133–4
    starvation, 133
  investigations, 125–6
    clinical examination, 125
    electrocardiography, 126
    endoscopy and laparotomy, 126
    laboratory samples, 126
    radiography, 126
    ultrasonography, 126
  oral lesions, 126–8
  vent, 132–3
    abnormal faeces, 132–3
    inflammation, 133
    protrusion, 133
    visible parasites, 133
Intestinal obstruction, 132
Intestinal tract, 124
Invertebrates, 267–74
  anaesthesia, 268
  anemones, 270
    colonial, 270–1
    disc, 270
  corals, 268–70
  crustaceans
    freshwater, 273
    marine, 272–3
  disease of, 256, 268
  echinoderms, 273–4
  environment
    filtration, 267
    heating, 267
    lighting, 267
    'living rock', 267
    maintenance, 267
    salinity, 267
    water movement, 267
  euthanasia, 268
  jellyfish, 271
  molluscs, 271
  in ponds, 33
  worms, 272
Iodine, 245
Iodophores, 255

Iridophores, 111
Iridoviruses, 204
Iris, 149
Iron, 8, 214
Isoflurane, 78
Isolation facilities, 254
Isopods, 144, 175, 182–3
Itraconazole, 154, 246
Ivermectin, 243

Jaubert system, 46, 47
Jellyfish, 271
  stings, 288
Jumping, 160, 211

Kanamycin, 245
Keratitis, 150
Ketamine hydrochloride, 82
Khawia spp., 175
Khawia sinesis, 178
Kidney
  biopsy, 265
  metal toxicity, 215
Kidney enlargement disease, 174
Koi, 31, 32
  radiography, 103
  scale pattern in, 235
Koi herpesvirus, 202
Koi shows, 36
Kudoa spp., 173

Laboratory investigations, 91–101, 111–12
  bacteriology, 96–9
    antibiotic sensitivity testing, 98–9
    bacteriological identification, 98
    inoculation of culture plates, 97–8
    sampling, 97
    sampling equipment, 97
    serology, 98
    stained tissue smears, 99
  blood sampling, 96
  clinical examination, 93
  ectoparasite examination, 94–6
    gill preparations, 95–6
    skin preparations, 94–5
  gill sample examination, 112
  histopathology, 100–1
  internal disorders, 126
  mycology, 101
  ocular disorders, 149–50
  parasitology, 99–100
  postmortem examination, 93–4
  respiratory disease, 139
  skin scrape examination, 111
  virology, 101
  water quality, 91–3
    basic parameters, 92–3
    sampling technique, 92
Lactococcus spp., 191
Lampsilis spp., 181
Laparotomy, 126
Larvae, 231, 233
Lead, 8, 214
Leech traps, 253
Leeches, 114, 144, 180
Legionella pneumophila, 58
Legislation
  hazardous substances, 285–6
  UK, 275–9
    disease control, 277
    medicines, 275–6
    veterinary, 275

welfare, 276–7
wildlife-related, 278
zoos, 277–8
US, 281–3
medicines, 281–3
veterinary, 281
welfare, 283
wildlife-related, 283
Lemaeenicus spp., 175
Lens, 149
Lenticulopathy, 152
Lepeophtheirus spp., 175, 181
Lernaea spp., 113, 114, 150, 153, 175
Lernaea cyprinacea, 181
Leteux-Meyer mixture, 243
Leucophores, 111
Levamisole, 243
Lice *see Argulus*
Life support systems, 53–5
closed, 53, 54
open, 53
see also Filtration systems; Water
quality
Lifespan
aquarium fish
freshwater, 42
marine, 48
pond fish, 33
Light, 2
Light response, 149
Lighting
for corals, 269
freshwater aquaria, 38
for invertebrates, 267
marine aquaria, 46
Lignocaine, 78
Ligula spp., 132, 175
Lime, 256
Lindane, 214
Lionfish, 287
Lip-lock, 160
Lipids, dietary, 225
Listing, 159
Live foods, 42, 226
Live sand filtration, 46, 47
Live-bearers, 231–2
Liver, 124–5
biopsy, 265
metal toxicity, 215
'Living rock', 267
Lobsters, 272–3
Lufenuron, 243
Lymphocystis, 117, 144, 154, 203–4

Magnetic resonance imaging, 107–8
internal disorders, 126
Malachite green, 246, 257
ocular disorders, 154
toxicity, 140, 217
Malawi bloat, 132
Malicious poisoning, 218
Malnutrition, 129
and ocular disorders, 154
see also Nutritional disorders
Marine aquaria, 45–51
captive species, 48–50
breeding, 49
compatibility, 48
disease prevention, 50
lifespan, 48
nutrition, 49
stocking levels, 48–9
construction, 45
heating, 45
lighting, 46

maintenance, 50–1
common health problems, 51
medication, 51
need for experience, 51
procedures, 50–1
stocking levels, 22
tanks, 45–6
water changes, 74
water management, 46–8
filtration systems, 46–8
salinity, 46
water quality, 46
water quality, 21
see also Freshwater aquaria
Martigifera spp., 181
Mebendazole, 244
Mechanical filtration, 53
Medication, 23, 74
marine aquarium fish, 51
pond fish, 36
public aquarium fish, 57–8
Medicines Act 1968, 275–6
Medicines legislation
UK, 275–6
US, 281–3
Medicines (Restrictions on the
Administration of Veterinary
Medicinal Products) Regulations
1994 (SI 1994/2987)
as amended by SI 1997/2884
(Amelia 8), 276
Melanoma, 221
Melanophores, 111
Metal toxicity, 8, 130, 214–15
clinical signs and pathological
effects, 215
factors affecting, 214–15
see also individual metals
Metazoan parasites, 175–83
acanthocephalans, 180
annelids, 180
cestodes, 178–9
crustaceans, 181–3
digeneans, 177–8
molluscs, 181
monogeneans, 175–7
nematodes, 179–80
Methaemoglobinaemia, 143
Methylene blue, 245,
Metomidate, 78
Metronidazole, 244
Microchip implants, 266
Microcotyle spp., 141, 175
Microcystis spp., 200
Micronutrient deficiency/excess, 227–8
Microsporeans, 167, 172–3
Microworms, 233
Mineral deficiency, 56, 228
Minerals, dietary, 226
Minimum inhibitory concentration (MIC),
99
Molluscicides, 217
Molluscs, 175, 181, 271
diseases of, 271
feeding, 271
water quality, 271
Monogeneans, 175–7
Moray eel, 288
Motile aeromonads, 187–8
Mouth, 124
examination of, 87
lesions of, 126–8
deformity, 127–8
obstruction, 127
ulceration, 126–7
Mouth fungus, 115, 119, 120, 126

Mouth rot, 126, 127
Mouth-brooding, 127
MS222, 78, 247
Mucus
excess, 114, 120, 141
lack of, 120
Musculoskeletal system, 123–4
Mycobacteriosis, 113
Mycobacterium spp., 153, 187, 227
Mycobacterium chelonae, 287
Mycobacterium fortuitum, 58, 190, 287
Mycobacterium marinum, 58, 190, 287
Mycology, 101
Myxidium spp., 173
Myxobacterium spp., 190–1
Myxobolus spp., 116, 128, 173
Myxobolus cerebralis, 157, 175
Myxobolus cyprini, 173
Myxobolus ellipsoides, 129
Myxobolus heterospora, 150
Myxobolus hoffmani, 150
Myxobolus koi, 173
Myxobolus scleroperca, 150
Myxococcus spp., 190–1
Myxosoma spp. *see Myxobolus* spp.
Myxosporeans, 173–5
Myzobdella spp., 175, 180

Neascus spp., 116, 175
Nematodes, 175, 179–80
Neobenedenia spp., 120, 150, 175, 176
Neomycin, 245, 257
Neon tetra disease, 114, 128
Neoplasia, 127, 130, 219–23
and anorexia, 156
body wall, 128
connective tissue, 221
digestive system, 222
gills, 145
nervous system, 221–2
ocular, 154
reproductive system, 222–3
skin, 117–18, 219–21
papilloma, 219–20
pigment cells, 220–1
surgery, 262–3
urinary system, 222
vascular system, 221
Nervous system, neoplasia, 221–2
Nets, 30
New tank/pond syndrome, 7, 35, 157
Niclosamide, 283
Nifurpirinol, 245, 257
Nitrate, 8, 55, 207
measurement, 8
toxicity, 8
Nitrite, 7–8, 55, 207
measurement, 8
toxicity, 8, 158
Nitrobacter, 6, 8
Nitrofurazone, 245
Nitrogen, 4–5
measurement, 4
supersaturation, 5
Nitrogenous compounds, 6–7, 206–7
see also Ammonia; Nitrate; Nitrite
Nitrogenous waste, excretion of, 137
Nitrosomonas, 7
Nocardia spp., 153, 187
Nocardia asteroides, 192, 287
Nocardia kampachi, 192, 287
Nuptial tubercles, 115, 121
Nutrition
anemones, 270, 271
corals, 269

crustaceans, 272, 273
deficiencies in *see* Malnutrition
echinoderms, 274
feeding regimen, 226–7
freshwater aquaria, 42
jellyfish, 271
live foods, 42, 226
marine aquaria, 49
molluscs, 271
ponds, 33–4
public aquaria, 55–6
dietary deficiencies, 56
energy requirements, 55–6
feeding regime, 55
worms, 272
Nutritional disorders, 227–9
excessive or inadequate feeding
rates, 227
inappropriate diet, 227
investigation of, 228–9
poor quality/contaminated food, 227
specific micronutrient deficiency/
excess, 227–8
see also Malnutrition
Nutritional requirements, 225–6
carbohydrates, 225
lipids, 225
minerals, 226
proteins, 225
vitamins, 226
Nutritional supplements, 255
Nystatin, 257

Obesity, 131
Octopus, 288
Ocular disorders, 147–54
anatomy, 147–9
choroid, 147
cornea, 147
globe, 147
iris, 149
lens, 149
light response, 149
retina, 147–8, 149
sclera, 147
cataracts, 151–2
causative agents, 153–4
bacteria, 153–4
fungi, 154
malnutrition, 154
neoplasia, 154
parasites, 153
trauma, 154
viruses, 154
corneal ulceration, 150–1
exophthalmos, 152
gas accumulation, 152–3
investigations, 149–50
keratitis, 150
lenticulopathy, 152
nutritional causes, 228
retinopathy, 152
scleral infections, 150
uveitis, 152
Olfactory openings, examination of, 87
Oodinidae, 167, 167–8
Opercula
deformity of, 145–6
nutritional causes, 228
examination of, 88
flaring of, 137
Oral *see* Mouth
Orfe, 31
Organic compounds, 215–16
Organochlorines, 129, 214

Organophosphates, 129, 214
Ormetoprim, 245, 247
Ornamental fish, 9–12
categorization and origin, 9
global exports, 10
global imports, 10
global industry, 9–10
IATA regulations, 10
United Kingdom, 10–11
aquatic hobby, 11
legislative controls, 11–12
Ornamental fish farming, 13–18
distribution, 17–18
costs of, 18
dealer selection and sales, 17
packing and transportation, 17–18
within UK, 18
health controls, 13–14
problems, 14
production, 14–17
egg incubation, 15
growing-on, 16
health checks and water quality
monitoring, 17
larval husbandry, 15–16
manipulation of breeding, 14–15
pond management, 16–17
selection for breeding, 14
Ortholinea spp., 173
Oscar, renal tumour, 130, 222
Oscillatoria spp., 200
Osmotic control, 137
Osmotic imbalance, 213
Ovarian disorders, 132
Ovarian prolapse, 265
Oxidation–reduction potential, 54
Oxolinic acid, 245, 247
Oxygen, 4, 208–9
abnormality, 4
biological oxygen demand, 4
dissolved, 55
measurement, 4
requirement, 4
supersaturation, 4
Oxygen saturation, reduced, 164
Oxytetracycline, 245, 247, 257
toxicity, 217
Ozone, 47, 48, 54
as disinfectant, 256
toxicity, 140, 285

Packing of live fish, 17–18
Papilloma, 117, 145, 219–20
Papillosum cyprini, 202
Paramoeba spp., 167, 273
Paramoeba pemaquidensis, 171
Parasites, 113, 114–15, 120, 167–83
abdominal enlargement, 132
abnormal swimming behaviour, 157
anorexia, 156
gill disease, 158
gill necrosis, 143
gill swellings, 144
manual removal of, 254
metazoan, 175–83
acanthocephalans, 180
annelids, 180
cestodes, 178–9
crustaceans, 181–3
digeneans, 177–8
molluscs, 181
monogeneans, 175–7
nematodes, 179–80
myxozoan, 173–5
ocular disorders, 153

oral obstruction, 127
protistan, 167–73
amoebae, 171
ciliates, 169–71
coccidians, 171–2
flagellates, 167–9
microsporeans, 172–3
skin swellings, 116
Parasitic cysts of body wall, 128
Parasitology, 99–100
Parvicapsula spp., 173
*Pasteurella piscicida see Photobacterium
damselae* subsp. *piscicida*
Peat, 246
Peduncle disease, 191
Periorbital gas *see* Gas bubble disease
Peroxygen compounds, 256
Pesticides, 8, 216
Pet Animals Act 1951, 12, 276
Pet Animals Act 1951 (Amendment) Act
1982, 276
pH, 2, 206
and anorexia, 156
fluctuating, 2
high, 2, 206
low, 2, 206
measurement, 2
and metal toxicity, 215
public aquaria, 54
requirements, 2
Pharmacokinetics, 252–3
Phenotype, 233
2-Phenoxyethanol, 78
Philometra spp., 175, 179
Phoma spp., 200
Photobacterium damselae subsp.
piscicida, 187, 192
Photosynthesis, reduced, 164–5
Physical injury *see* Trauma
Pica, 156–7
Pigment cell tumours, 117–18, 220–1
Pine-cone disease, 120
Piperazine, 244
Piping, 137, 157–8
Piranha, 288
Piscicola spp., 114, 175, 180
Piscicola geometra, 168
Piscinoodinium spp., 116, 141, 143, 167
Piscinoodinium pillulare, 167–8
Pithing, 83
Plants
aquaria, 41
maintenance, 43–4
ponds, 33, 35
Plecostomus, 159
Pleistophora spp., 167, 172
Pleistophora hyphessobryconis, 114,
128, 173
Pollution, 289
Polycystic kidneys, 131
Pomphorhynchus spp., 175, 180
Pond heaters, 30
Pond vacuums, 30
Ponds, 25–36, 69–70
breeding, 34
construction, 25, 70
design, 69–70
equipment, 30
filtration media, 28–9
flow rates, 29
retention time, 29–30
filtration systems, 20, 26–8, 71–2
bubble-bead filters, 27
fluidized filters, 27
gravity-fed filters, 26–7
pump-fed external filters, 26

trickle tower filters, 27
undergravel filters, 27–8
vegetable filters, 27
maintenance, 34–5
cleaning, 34
seasonal aspects, 35
water testing, 34
winter maintenance, 34–5
nutrition, 33–4
ornamental fish farming, 16–17
position, 25, 69
size, 25–6, 238
stocking levels, 30–3
disease prevention, 33
invertebrates and amphibians, 33
lifespan, 33
planting, 33
water changes, 74
Pop eye, 152
Posthodiplostomum spp., 175, 177
Postmortem examination, 93–4
respiratory disease, 139–40
skin disease, 112
sudden death, 164
Potassium permanganate, 244, 245,
246
Povidone–iodine, 245
Power filters, 39–40, 46
Praziquantel, 244
Predation
anorexia, 156
sudden death, 166
Prophylaxis, 23, 57, 255–6
Proprietary medications, 242, 247–51
Protection of Animals Act 1911 (1912
Scotland), 276
Protection of Animals (Anaesthetics)
Acts 1954 and 1964, 276
Protein skimmers, 30, 47, 48
Proteins, dietary, 225
Protistan parasites, 167–73
amoebae, 171
ciliates, 169–71
coccidians, 171–2
flagellates
bodonids, 168–9
hexamitids, 169
oodinids, 167–8
trypanosomes, 168
microsporeans, 172–3
Prymnesium parvum, 200
Pseudanthocotyloides, 176
Pseudobranchectomy, 264
Pseudocaligus brevipedis, 181
Pseudomonads, 188
Pseudomonas spp., 58, 153, 187
Pseudomonas anguilliseptica, 188
Pseudomonas chloraphis, 188
Pseudomonas fluorescens, 186, 188,
189, 287
Pseudomonas pseudoalcaligenes, 188
Public aquaria, 53–62
dangerous species, 59–61
disease treatments, 57–8
fish removal, 61
life support systems, 53–5
closed, 53
filtration methods, 53–4
lighting and noise, 55
open, 53
water quality, 54–5
nutrition, 55–6
dietary deficiencies, 56
energy requirements, 55–6
feeding regime, 55
quarantine, 56–7

new arrivals, 56–7
prophylactic medication, 57
records, 57
record keeping, 58–9
zoonoses, 58
Pump-fed external filters, 26
Pumps, 30
Pyrethrum, 214

Quadrula spp., 181
Qualitative inheritance, 233
Quantitative inheritance, 233–4
Quarantine, 74, 255
new arrivals, 42, 56–7
prophylactic medication, 57
public aquaria, 56–7
records, 57
Quaternary amines, 255
Quinaldine, 78

Rabbitfish, 288
Radiography, 103–5
contrast studies, 103–4
equipment, 103
internal disorders, 126
interpretation, 104
safety, 104–5
technique, 103
Rainwater, 213
Ramirez's dwarf cichlid virus, 204
Rapid tissue necrosis of corals, 269
Recessive traits, 233
Record keeping, 58–9
Red worm, 179
Red-tail disease, 273
Red-tailed catfish, foreign body, 131
Redox value, 47
Refractive index, 5
Reovirus, 204
Reproductive behaviour, 160–1
lip-lock, 160
spawning, 160–1
see also Breeding
Reproductive problems, 232–3
egg binding, 232
hatchability, 232–3
larvae and fry, 233
spawning failure, 232
Reproductive system, 125
neoplasia, 222–3
Respiration, 136–7
unilateral, 138
Respiratory disease, 135–46
anaemia, 141
anatomy, 135–6
clinical signs, 137–8
environmental hypoxia, 140
investigations, 138–40
clinical history, 138
laboratory tests, 138–40
observation, 138
physical examination, 138–9
physiology, 136–7
acid–base balance, 137
nitrogenous waste excretion, 137
osmotic control, 137
respiration, 136–7
toxins, 140
viral, 140
see also Gills
Respiratory distress, 213
Restraint, 75
Resuscitation, 81
Retina, 147–8, 149

Retinopathy, 152
Reverse osmosis, 21
Rhabdovirus carpio, 112–13, 201–2
Rhizopus spp., 200
Rivers, 214
Rotenone, 214
Rotifers, 16
Rudd, 31
Runoff, 211
Rust disease, 116

Sabellid fan worms, 272
Saddleback syndrome of tilapia, 235–6
Salinity, 5–6, 207–8
invertebrate needs, 267
marine aquaria, 46
measurement, 5–6
medicinal use, 6
public aquaria, 55
requirement, 6
Salmincola spp., 141, 175
Salmonella spp., 58
Salt, hazards of, 286
see also sodium chloride
Sand pressure filters, 30, 47
Sanguinicola spp., 143, 175, 177, 178
Saprolegnia, 115, 126, 143, 154
Saprolegnia parasitica, 196
Saprolegniasis, 195–7
characteristics, 195–6
clinical signs, 196
control, 197
diagnosis, 197
pathology, 196
treatment, 197
Sarafloxacin, 245, 247
Scales, 87
raised, 120
Schooling, abnormal, 157
Scientific names, 292–3
Scintigraphy, 107
Sclera, 147
Scleral infections, 150
Scorpionfish, 287
Sea urchins, 288
Sea water, 214
Sedation, 82
Self-trauma, 211
Septicaemia, 112, 113
Serpulid worms, 272
Sex-linked genes, 233
Sharks, 59–60
anorexia in, 56
bites, 288
blood sampling, 60
energy requirements, 55–6
Shrimps, 272–3
Skeleton, examination of, 89
Skin
anatomy, 110–11
cuticle, 111
dermis, 111
epidermis, 111
examination of, 86–7
external features, 110
histological structure, 110–11
hypodermis, 111
laboratory tests, 111–12
Skin disease, 109–22
colour change, 112–14
bruising, 114
generalized inflammation, 112–13
localized inflammation, 113
loss of colour, 113–14
fin lesions, 121–2

spots, 115–16
　　black spot, 116
　　epitheliocystis, 116
　　nuptial tubercles, 115
　　velvet, 116
　　white spot, 115–16
swellings, 116–18
　　neoplasia, 117–18, 219–21
　　nodular lesions, 116–17
texture changes, 120
visible pathogens, 114–15
　　fungi, 115
　　parasites, 114–15
Skin scrape examination, 111
Skin ulcers, 118–19
　　surgery, 261–2
Slime disease, 114, 120, 170
Sock nets, 75
Sodium bicarbonate, 246
Sodium chloride, 244, 246
Sodium hydroxide, 256
Sodium hypochlorite, 256
Sodium ion-selective meter, 6
Sodium thiosulphate, 246
Sound, travel in water, 2
Spawning, 160–1, 231
　　failure of, 232
Specific gravity, 5
Sphaerospora spp., 144, 173
Sphaerospora molnari, 174
Sphaerospora renicola, 174, 175, 201
Spinal lesions, 129–30
　　acquired, 129–30
　　congenital, 129
　　nutritional causes, 228
Spinning, 157
Spironucleus spp., 119, 133, 158, 167, 169
Spironucleus vortens, 169
Spirulina spp., 226
Sporocytophaga spp., 190–1
Spots, 115–16
Spring viraemia of carp, 112–13, 201–2
Springs, 214
Staphylococcus spp., 153
Starfish, 273–4
Starvation, 133
Stingrays, 60–1, 287
Stings, 288–9
Stock management, 22–3
Stock selection, 255
Stocking levels, 21–2, 72–3
　　aquaria
　　　　freshwater, 42
　　　　marine, 48–9
　　ponds, 30–3
Stomach, 124
Stonefish, 287
Streams, 214
Streptococcus spp., 153, 187, 191
Streptococcus iniae, 157
Stress, 23
　　and bacterial disease, 185
Structural genes, 233
Styrene, 216
Subcutaneous fluid-filled cavity, 128
Sudden death, 163–6
　　accident, 165–6
　　　　asphyxia, 166
　　　　electrocution, 166
　　　　escape, 165
　　　　water loss, 166
　　environmental effects, 164–5
　　　　gas bubble disease, 165
　　　　hyperthermia, 165
　　　　hypoxia, 164–5
　　　　noxious algae, 165

　　　　toxins, 165, 213
　　infection, 165
　　investigations, 163–4
　　　　clinical examination, 163
　　　　clinical history, 163
　　　　postmortem examination, 164
　　　　water samples, 164
　　predation, 166
Sulphadiazine/trimethoprim, 245
Sulphadimethoxine/ormetoprim, 245,
Sulphadoxine/trimethoprim, 245, 247
Sulphamerazine, 247
Sulphonamide toxicity, 217
Sunburn, 113, 211
Surface tension, 2
Surfing, 157
Surgeonfish, 288
Surgery, 259–66
　　anaesthesia *see* Anaesthesia
　　anatomy, 259
　　consent forms, 260
　　instrumentation, 259
　　postoperative care, 261
　　preoperative preparation, 260
　　presurgical investigation, 259
　　procedures
　　　　diagnostic biopsy, 265
　　　　endoscopy, 266
　　　　enucleation, 264
　　　　gonadectomy, 265
　　　　lacerations and skin injury, 264–5
　　　　masses, 262–3
　　　　ovarian prolapse, 265
　　　　skin ulcers, 261–2
　　　　swim-bladder disorders, 265
　　　　telemetry implants, 266
　　techniques, 260
　　wound closure, 260
Surgical staples, 260
Sutures, 260
Swellings, 116–18
　　Dermocystidium infection, 118
　　gills, 144–5
　　mouth, 127
　　neoplasia, 117–18
　　　　carp pox, 117
　　　　fibroma, 118
　　　　papilloma, 117
　　　　pigment cell tumours, 117–18
　　nodular lesions
　　　　bacteria, 116
　　　　fungi, 116
　　　　gas bubble disease, 117
　　　　lymphocystis, 117
　　　　parasites, 116
　　　　vesicles, 116
　　subcutaneous fluid-filled cavity, 118
　　surgery, 262–3
　　see also Neoplasia
Swim-bladder disease, 125, 130, 158
　　surgery, 265
Swimming behaviour, 157–60
　　abnormal buoyancy, 158–60
　　abnormal schooling, 157
　　clamped fins, 160
　　coughing, 160
　　flashing, 160
　　hanging or drifting, 160
　　jumping, 160
　　piping, 157–8
　　spinning, surfing and disorientation,
　　　　157

Tachypnoea, 137
Tail waving, 159
Tail-up, 159

Tanks *see* Aquaria
Tapeworms, 178–9
Teflubenzuron, 247
Telangiectasis, 145
Telemetry implants, 266
Temperature, 205
　　abnormality, 1
　　and metal toxicity, 215
　　manipulation for parasite control, 253
　　ponds, 35
　　public aquaria, 54
　　requirements, 1
Tench, 31
Territorial behaviour, 161
Tet disease, 120, 170
Tetracapsula spp., 173
Tetracapsula bryosalmonae, 173, 174,
　　175
Tetracapsula bryozoides, 174
Tetrahymena spp., 141, 150, 167
Tetrahymena corlissi, 120, 170
Texture changes, 120
Thecamoeba spp., 167
Thecamoeba hoffmani, 171
Thelohania spp., 273
Therapeutics, 237–57
　　adverse reactions, 256–7
　　aquatic invertebrates, 256
　　choice of drug, 242
　　consent forms, 258
　　environmental improvement, 237–8
　　failure to respond, 257
　　first aid, 238
　　health and safety, 257–8
　　legislation, 258
　　routes of administration, 238–42
　　　　gavage, 241–2
　　　　in-feed medication, 240–1
　　　　in-water medication, 239–40
　　　　injection, 241
　　　　topical preparations, 242
　　specific medication, 238
　　supportive treatment, 254–5
Thyroid hyperplasia, 56
Tilapia, saddleback, 235–6
Tissue adhesive, 260
Tissue samples, 218
Toltrazuril, 244
Topical preparations, 242
Toxaphene, 214
Toxins, 213–18
　　abnormal swimming behaviour, 157
　　biocides, 216–17
　　clinical signs, 213
　　gases, 217
　　investigation of, 217–18
　　metals, 214–15
　　organic compounds, 215–16
　　sudden death, 165
　　therapeutic agents, 217
　　water sources, 213–14
Traders *see* Dealers
Transportation of live fish, 17–18, 41–2
　　effect on water quality, 21
　　sedation for, 82
Trauma, 23, 114, 119
　　mouth ulcers, 126
　　ocular disorders, 154
　　spinal lesions, 129
　　surgery, 264–5
Triaenophorus spp., 175
Tricaine methane sulphonate, 78, 247
Trichlorfon, 214, 244
Trichodina spp., 23, 120, 167, 170
Trichodina truttae, 170
Trichodinella spp., 120, 167, 170

Trichodinella epizootica, 170
Trichodinids, 170
Trichophrya spp., 141
Trickle filters, 28, 30–1, 46, 47
Trifluralin toxicity, 130
Triggerfish, 288
Tropical freshwater systems
    stocking levels, 21–2
    water quality, 21
    see also Freshwater systems
Trypanoplasma spp., 167, 168–9
Trypanoplasma salmositica, 169
Trypanosoma spp., 167
Trypanosoma carassii, 168
Trypanosomatidae, 167, 168
Tuberculosis, 113
Tubifex, 157, 226

Ulcerative keratitis, 150–1
Ulcers
    mouth, 126–7
    skin, 118–19
Ultrasonography, 105–7
    equipment, 105
    internal disorders, 126
    interpretation, 106
    safety, 106–7
    technique, 105–6
Ultraviolet lamps, 30, 47
Ultraviolet radiation, 211
Ultraviolet sterilization, 54, 253, 255, 256
Undergravel filters, 27–8, 39, 46
Unicapsula spp., 173
Unilateral respiration, 138
Unio spp., 181
Unioida spp., 175
United Kingdom
    aquatic hobby, 11
    aquatic industry, 10–11
        pet shops, 11
        supply chain, 10–11
        water quality standards, 11
    fish distribution in, 18
    legislative controls, 11–12, 275–9
United States, 281–3
Urinary system, 125
    neoplasia, 222
Uronema spp., 120, 141, 167
Uronema marinum, 170
Uveitis, 152

Vaccines, 256
Vagococcus spp., 191

Vahikampfia spp., 167
Vascular tumours, 221
Vegetable filters, 28
Velvet disease, 116, 143
Venomous fish, 61
Vent
    disorders of, 132–3
        abnormal faeces, 132–3
    examination of, 88–9
Venturis, 30
Verticillium spp., 200
Vesicles, 116
Veterinary Checks Directive, 12
Veterinary legislation
    UK, 275
    US, 281
Veterinary Surgeons Act 1966, 275
Veterinary Surgeons Act 1966 (Schedule
    3 Amendment) Order 1988, 275
Vexillifera spp., 167
Vexillifera bacillipedes, 171
Vibrio spp., 153, 187, 287
Vibrio alginolyticus, 189
Vibrio anguillarum, 189
Vibrio damsela, 189
Vibrio fluvialis, 58
Vibrio ordalii, 189
Vibrio parahaemolyticus, 58, 189
Vibrio salmonicida, 189
Vibrio vulnificus, 58, 189
Viral diseases, 201–4
    abnormal swimming behaviour, 157
    herpesvirus disease, 202–3
    lymphocystis, 203–4
    ocular disorders, 154
    spring viraemia of carp, 201–2
Viral erythrocytic necrosis virus, 204
Virology, 101
Vitamin deficiency, 56, 228
Vitamins, dietary, 226

Water changes, 74
    partial, 43
Water hazards, 289–90
Water loss, 166
Water movement, 267
Water purifiers, 30
Water quality, 254
    for anemones, 270, 271
    coldwater, 21
    for corals, 269
    for crustaceans, 273
    dealers, 20–1
    disorders of, 205–6

    hyperthermia, 205
    hypothermia, 205
    pH, 206
    temperature, 205
    during anaesthesia, 79
    for echinoderms, 274
    and effect of transportation, 21
    freshwater aquaria, 43
    for invertebrates, 267
    for jellyfish, 271
    marine aquaria, 21, 46
    for molluscs, 271
    ornamental fish farming, 17
    ponds, 34
    public aquaria, 54–5
    and skin disease, 120
    testing, 73, 91–3, 111
    tropical freshwater, 21
    UK standards, 11
    for worms, 272
Water samples, 164, 218
Water sources, 213–14
Water test kits, 30
Welfare legislation
    UK, 286–7
    US, 283
White grub, 178
White spot, 115–16, 141, 143
Wildlife and Countryside Act 1981, 12, 278
Wildlife-related legislation
    UK, 278–9
    US, 283
Winter maintenance of ponds, 34–5
Wood preservatives, 216
Worms, 272
Wound closure, 260

Xanthophores, 111

Yellow grub, 128, 178
Yersinia enterocolitica, 58

Zeolite, 246
Zinc, 214
Zoo legislation, 277–8
Zoo Licensing Act 1981, 277–8
Zoonoses, 58, 286–7
Zooplankton, 16
Zuger jars, 15